AF866379

The Magical and Sacred Medical World

The Magical and Sacred Medical World

Edited by

Éva Pócs

Cambridge Scholars Publishing

The Magical and Sacred Medical World

Edited by Éva Pócs

This book first published 2019

Cambridge Scholars Publishing

Lady Stephenson Library, Newcastle upon Tyne, NE6 2PA, UK

British Library Cataloguing in Publication Data
A catalogue record for this book is available from the British Library

Copyright © 2019 by Éva Pócs and contributors

All rights for this book reserved. No part of this book may be reproduced, stored in a retrieval system, or transmitted, in any form or by any means, electronic, mechanical, photocopying, recording or otherwise, without the prior permission of the copyright owner.

ISBN (10): 1-5275-2252-0
ISBN (13): 978-1-5275-2252-7

Style edited by Andrew Rouse
Index prepared by Ágnes Maléth
Editorial assistant: Andrea Zombory

The publication of this volume has received funding from the European Research Council under the European Union's Seventh Framework Programme (FP7/2007-2013) / ERC grant agreement № 324214.

TABLE OF CONTENTS

LIST OF ILLUSTRATIONS

PREFACE

ÉVA PÓCS

The conference which lends its title to the present volume was held in the city of Pécs and was organised by the Department of Ethnography and Cultural Anthropology of Pécs University in September 2009. This collection of papers presents, in line with the purpose of the conference, the sacred and magical aspects of ethnomedicine. The subject area itself was identified by the common points between religious anthropology, ethnomedicine and medical anthropology, focusing on topics like magical and religious concepts of health and disease, causes of disease, various illnesses, religious and magical averting and healing rites, healing gods, saints and holy places and, last but not least, the part that these play in the society, religion, mentality and everyday life of a community, as well as their various representations in folklore, literature or art.

We know of a wide range of different phenomena within the religious and magical aspects of European ethnomedicine; nevertheless, there are not many works of a high theoretical standard that place these in a broader religious, anthropological, folkloristic, social or historical context. Considerable advances have been made over recent decades (e.g. in studying the relevant aspects of shrines, possession, shamanism or witchcraft, or the study of bewitchment and charms, or in processing the historical records of a narrower area such as medicine in the region of Naples and summarising its medical "holy system"). Nevertheless, there has been a scarcity of interdisciplinary works that could equally well take into account considerations of medicine, folklore studies or religious studies. Apart from a few well-known Italian and Greek examples, there have been hardly any investigations into contemporary healing practices using modern anthropological methodology and extended fieldwork (and where there have been such efforts, e.g. in Karelia, they have still gone unpublished), in spite of the fact that Europe offers no fewer opportunities for such research than the non-European traditional societies. Thus, it is natural that we welcomed accounts of such research endeavours at the conference, as well as in the present volume. These papers present the local systems and connections of various phenomena and describe the part they play in their local societies, or they analyse broader connections of medical phenomena in terms of religious ethnology, medical history, medical anthropology and folklore. The volume includes, without restrictions of a methodological, temporal or geographical nature, works from the fields of folklore studies, anthropology, cultural history, comparative historical and textual philology, as well as research findings which use the latest methods of analysis in textual folklore or are based on archival research or fieldwork in or outside of Europe. Besides anthropologists and folklore researchers, representatives of psychiatry, literary scholarship and linguistics were also welcome to contribute. Our goal was that each of the four chapters of the book should present one subject matter from a multiplicity of angles and within broad time frames, preferably featuring several regions of Europe.

Part 1 of the book is devoted to concepts of disease, within which demonic causes of disease have played a special role throughout the recorded past of Europe and the ancient Orient right up until the present day. The most varied forms of assaults from demons against the human world have been known, both in the pre-Christian religions and the accompanying folk beliefs, and in Christianity—the chapter also offers samples of these. *Janine Rivière* has examined notions of the night-time demon known by names such as *Mahr/mare/mara* and *nightmare*, as well as the pressure exerted by these demons and experienced by humans. She looks at the way in which the demon, known to assault its victims sexually, appears in the medical theories and popular experience of early modern England, and how these parallel sets of ideas mutually influence each other. *Svetlana Tsonkova* explores a disease demon called the *nezhit*, which often appears in late Medieval and early modern Bulgarian charm texts. She identifies the kind of divine healing and averting procedures in whose context these demons, already known from magical texts of the ancient Orient, tend to appear, and she describes the kinds of remedies offered against them by the healing texts and by contemporary practice. *Laura Iancu* summarises the results of her extended fieldwork in Moldova when analysing the disease concepts of the Roman Catholic population of Magyarfalu (Arini) as part of the world view of that community and within the broader social system of magical and religious healing. She offers a detailed analysis of the role of a specific demonic cause of disease also mingled with the figure of the Christian devil referred to as *rossz* or *nem tiszta* [literally "evil" or "not pure"] and the diseases and healing methods associated with this demon.

The dualistic figure of the Eastern European witch, a simultaneously human and demonic figure, represents at once the category of demonic perpetrators of disease and the class of harmful humans. In her paper, *Katerina Dysa* presents early modern examples of witchcraft from the Ukraine and Poland. She analyses the chain of events of the witch performing maleficium and then the healing of this condition through the prism of the everyday tensions and conflicts of past religious communities. Referring to cases of magical healing, she draws attention to the way in which natural and magical causes of disease were conflated and treated in the same way in past societies. *József Gagyi* analyses contemporary witchcraft in villages of the Székler Land region and points out certain alternative causes of disease living alongside each other through the exploration of a case in which the community gave preference to a breach of taboo rather than an explanation of disease based on bewitchment.

Another dualistic figure, half demon, half human, that has played a significant part in popular belief in Eastern Europe is the vampire. A paper by *Ádám Mézes* treats a phenomenon which provoked panic in the Carpathian Basin in the eighteenth century—fear of assault by vampires. The author analyses the investigations into vampire belief that were commissioned during the reigns of emperors Charles VI and Maria Theresa. He also reviews a work called *Visum repertum* written by a surgeon called Georg Tallar as part of the state control mechanism. This forms part of an effort to reconstruct the activity and participants of the medical committee which was examining the vampire phenomenon, and to interpret cases of latter-day vampirism in the context of the processes of the enlightenment, the expansion of state control, medicalisation and secularisation.

Part 2 describes some of the human agents and rituals, in and outside Europe. It discusses methods of magic and healing and the overall activity of rural healers and clerical and lay representatives of elite culture, as well as their related views and doctrines. All of these have existed and functioned in close interaction and with mutual influence since antiquity, from the Middle Ages right up until early modern times. *Christa Agnes Tuczay* examines a whole sequence of mostly ancient Greek and medieval German literary and linguistic records from the point of view of the activity of specialists of sacred communication and mediumism. She presents methods of this special kind of perception and related healing techniques in a classification which follows the categories of divination by offering a number of interesting examples of divining mediums possessed by spirits. *Ane Ohrvik* describes a few noted instances from eighteenth-

and nineteenth-century Norwegian MS recipe books, by analysing the roles of the different types of healers and the plurality of contemporary healing practice.

Madis Arukask's paper on the Vepsian "cunning man" (*tedai*) brings us back to the present age and describes the dialogue between the collecting ethnographer in search of archaic textual relics and contemporary society which is concerned with the survival or extinction of certain elements of traditional healing. The universal character of witchcraft and magic, and the similarities which overarch great expanses of space and time have been a constant source of wonderment for researchers—the papers in this section may have a similar effect. *Gábor Vargyas* offers a piece in which he analyses the social role of the shamans of the *Bru* tribe in Vietnam from the point of view of the inherent ambivalence of their activity. In this way, he draws attention to the dual role of bewitchment and healing carried out by magicians and shamans, which is also a universal trait well known in the systems of European witchcraft. *Krisztina Kehl-Bodrogi* reports on her fieldwork in Uzbekistan and analyses the recovery of religious healing in the period after the dissolution of the Soviet Union and the country's independence. Her case study sheds light on the way in which, besides the increase in religious beliefs, various phenomena of New Age spiritualism are also gaining ground.

Two papers are concerned with exorcisms performed by priests according to a routine fixed in the liturgy. By practising exorcism, the church was carrying out an anti-demon activity which used and integrated both the textual legacy of the anti-demon practice of oriental antiquity together with the Hellenistic belief in demons, and the formulas of popular magic used to expel illness demons and send them out of the body. This ecclesiastical practice played a role identical to that of lay, popular healing methods and both were performed in the same spheres of private and public lives: to render assistance in the crisis situations of human life. The paper of *Dániel Bárth* sheds light on the contours of these practices by presenting an extremely significant, though so far unprocessed, Hungarian source: part of a Benedictine manuscript collection, written in eighteenth-century Hungary, held at the Benedictine Pannonhalma Archabbey. The healing and exorcising priest became practically extinct in the area of western Christianity by the twentieth century, contrary to the practice of the Eastern Church. *Tünde Komáromi*'s paper makes a Christian perpetrator of disease its focus and she writes about Satan as he comes to possess humans. Reporting on her fieldwork which she had carried out in Russia, she describes rituals of exorcism practised in the monastery of the Holy Trinity and offers a portrait of an exorcising priest of nationwide renown. Her analysis places all of this in the context of the symptomatology of contemporary Russian society.

Part 3 is about the healing effect of deities and saints. The rural cultures of Europe are known to have featured a whole range of non-Christian demonic beings with goddess traits, such as the fairies of the Balkans, the figure of *Luca (Lucy)* known among the Hungarians, the German-Austrian *Perchta* or the Russian *Friday women* who assault and sicken people as a punishment for breaches of taboo. *Mirjam Mencej* offers us a broad-ranging description of these "divine" concepts of disease. The author places the main focus on Slovenian belief figures who punish people for breaking known taboos, while she also draws conclusions regarding the symbolic significance of thread and spinning.

The healing effect of deities and saints, most potent in the vicinity of sacred spots such as their graves, relics, images and statues, prevalent since antiquity and all the way to the most contemporary shrines, constitutes one of the key chapters in the history of magical healing. *Emanuela Timotin* peruses Romanian charm texts from MS records from the seventeenth to the nineteenth centuries and analyses the role of healing saints that feature in these texts (Saint Cosmas and Damian, Simeon, Cyprianus etc.). She explores the roots of this tradition in the hagiography of the saints in question and involves textual parallels from the orally transmitted textual legacy of the most recent period.

Éva Pócs's paper on dream healing offers a review of healing by incubation in Europe and discusses the non-Christian variants of the phenomenon and cases of dream healing not related to sacred spots, offering a pan-European review overarching several epochs. She then goes on to analyse cases of dream battles between the healing and harmful spirits which emerge from the documentation of witchcraft trials of the early modern period. *Albena Georgieva* explores cases of healing reported to have taken place at Bulgarian shrines from the point of view of the emanating effect of the saint. She also analyses the significance of narratives that emerge in the wake of such instances of healing by incubation and other influences in sustaining knowledge of the history of the shrine and initiating newcomers into its community.

The papers in *Part 4* present vital aspects of European antiquity and the ancient Orient which constitute the very roots, indeed the archaic foundations, of European ethnomedicine and which in certain respects are in fact alive to this very day. *Nora Zergi* contributes to an ongoing debate about the identification of a plant, the *moly*, which appears in the works of

Homer, by making an interesting proposal. *Anna Tóth* asks an exciting question in the context of Greek and Roman statues of deities—how and why did people start to attribute healing power to these in late antiquity? *Ildikó Csepregi* explores more general issues of religious taboo and religious scepticism in the course of her examination of cases of incubation, and sleeping at a holy place and experiencing recovery, reconstructed from late antique and medieval material. Incubation dreams often include pork, a taboo in several religions, used as a medication in spite of that injunction.

The last two papers bring us back to the present time. *Judit Kis-Halas* offers a case study about a new method of healing, "spirit surgery" or *psychotronics* from Baranya County, Hungary, using a great deal of illustrative material. This method bears some shamanistic traits ("soul journeys" to the heavenly Jerusalem and carrying out operations there) and is highly popular—so much so that a number of traditional healers have integrated it into their toolkit and use it in combination with their previous range of methods. Two of our authors—*József Vas* and *Noémi Császár*—are psychiatrists and rely on the day-to-day experience of the working therapist when they describe a successful psychiatric method for treating grave psychological conditions which utilises certain archaic elements of spirituality for, as it were, medical purposes.

Naturally, neither the conference nor the resulting volume could exhaust every possible aspect of such an extensive central theme—we must make do with the "taster" that we have been offered through the above examples. However heterogeneous and colourful the material, we hope that the present collection is helpful, not by transmitting the entire system of sacred and magical healing, but by bringing the reader closer to the crucial questions of contemporary European research and by further broadening the still rich and colourful horizon of "magical and sacred medicine" in Europe.

1. MAGICAL AND SUPERNATURAL CAUSES OF ILLNESSES

"HAG-RIDING": DEMONS OF DESIRE OR SYMPTOMS OF DISEASE? MEDICAL THEORIES AND POPULAR EXPERIENCES OF THE NIGHTMARE IN PREMODERN ENGLAND

JANINE RIVIÈRE

> In thoughts from the Visions of the night, when deep sleep falleth upon Men, Fear came upon me, and Trembling, which made all my Bones to shake. Then a Spirit passed before my face; the hair of my flesh stood up. (Job. 4:13–15).

> In this disease, the patient, in time of sleep, imagines he feels an uncommon oppression or weight about his breast or stomach, which he can by no means shake off. He groans, and sometimes cries out, though oftener he attempts to speak in vain. Sometimes he imagines himself engaged with an enemy, and, in danger of being killed, attempts to run away, but finds he cannot. (William Buchan. *Domestic medicine....* London, 1772; Oldridge 2002).

Terrifying dreams frequently wakened premodern English men and women from their sleep. On Friday the 16th of July 1658, Thomas Vaughan, the rector of St Bridget's Church, Oxford, had the following nightmare, "I was pursued by a stone horse, as my deare wife dreamed, before shee sickened, and I was griviously troubled all night with a suffocation att the Heart, which continued all next day most violently, and still it remaines, but with some little remission" (Vaughan 1941, f.107; Marilla 1944). Vaughan is describing a kind of dream that premodern English people knew as the nightmare, a specific form of bad dream. Today, this form of the nightmare is understood as a form of sleep disorder that modern scientists define as sleep paralysis. This is an experience that typically occurs in hypnagogic (before falling asleep) states or hypnopompic (before waking up) states and results in feelings of intense terror, physical paralysis and the sense of being suffocated.[1] As historians Owen Davies and Willem de Blécourt have suggested, premodern accounts of the nightmare, often associated with witchcraft, can be attributed to incidents of sleep paralysis (Davies 2003; de Blécourt 2003).

But what exactly is sleep paralysis? The most respected expert in this field is the psychologist Dr Allan Cheyne, who has collated thousands of records of sleep paralysis and associated experiences. Cheyne defines sleep paralysis as "a period of paralysis upon waking or falling asleep and is often accompanied by terrifying hallucinations" (Cheyne 2002). The links between sleep paralysis and premodern and modern experiences of the nightmare, *incubus* or "hag-riding" were only made by the folklorist David Hufford in the 1970s when he studied beliefs in the "Old Hag" in Newfoundland (Hufford 1982). Since then, neurologists, psychologists, sociologists and anthropologists have studied this phenomenon in a variety of cultures. It has been found that across cultures, sleep paralysis incorporates a strikingly consistent series of symptoms, including intense terror, a sensed or seen malevolent presence, physical and/or verbal paralysis, and physical or sexual assault by an unknown being (Cheyne 2001; Cheyne, Newby-Clark and Rueffer 1999; Cheyne 2005). Like premodern experiences of the nightmare, modern sufferers of sleep paralysis are often confused as to whether they are dreaming or waking.

This essay will chart medical understandings of the nightmare from the mid-sixteenth to the mid-eighteenth century in order to show that the discourse on the nightmare reflects important cultural shifts and tensions in contemporary attitudes, particularly in medical circles, to dreams and the discernment of dreams. At the beginning of the seventeenth century, intellectual discussions regarding the nightmare within the discourses on dreams, witchcraft and medical literature reveal cultural tensions between a supernatural and natural aetiology of dreams. However, by the mid-eighteenth century, the supernatural causes of the nightmare had been largely undermined by a purely medical and physiological explanation in learned discourse. What this indicates is that the traditional belief in the supernatural nature of the nightmare was increasingly less acceptable in learned discourse due to the rise of materialist, medical theories of the body and mind.

Similarly, there is an inherent tension in the idea that dreams and the nightmare are caused by either exterior or interior forces that act upon the mind/soul in sleep. In line with the intellectual reaction against the popular

---

[1] For modern studies of sleep paralysis see: Cheyne 2005; Cheyne, Newby-Clark and Rueffer 1999; Cheyne 2002; Yeung, Xu and Chang 2005; Szklo-Coxe, Young, Finn and Mignot 2007; Semiz, Basoglu, Ebrinc and Cetin 2008).

belief in prognostic dreams, the discourse on the nightmare followed a similar trend of demoting the supernatural to the level of superstition. (This is a pattern that Lucia Dacombe noted in her study of dreams in eighteenth-century medical discourse. Dacombe 2004). However, as is apparent in modern cultures today, both the natural and supernatural theory of the nightmare coexisted and, rather than decline, actually continued from the sixteenth well into the eighteenth centuries in spite of important developments in natural philosophy and medicine. Premodern folk continued to believe in the existence of nocturnal demons who assaulted sleeping humans in the vulnerable state of sleep.

The issue of dream discernment in the eighteenth century subtly shifted from being centred on discriminating between divine and demonic dreams, to distinguishing natural from supernatural dreams. Premodern people tried to understand the cause and meaning of the nightmare. Was the nightmare the result of natural imbalances in the body or was it indeed the terrifying assaults of real malevolent beings? Discernment was thus also a problematic and ambiguous issue for victims of the nightmare as a manifestation of the demonic in daily life. Questions about the cause of the nightmare also oscillated between the discernment of supernatural, preternatural and natural agents, which centred on the inherent problem of distinguishing reality from fantasy and the imagination. Was it a real experience, proof of the demonic or the supernatural, occurring in waking life or was it merely a projected fantasy of the sleeper manifesting in terrifying dreams? As this essay seeks to show, accounts and theories of the nightmare can also reveal important insights into premodern men and women's fantasies about sex and sexuality. As contemporary writers themselves acknowledged, victims of the "Mare" often reported being sexually assaulted. In the history of dreams, the nightmare is the dark other of the divine dream, offering us glimpses into the terrifying fears and anxieties of past people.

In seventeenth- and eighteenth-century England there was a close correlation between witchcraft beliefs and beliefs about the "Mare". The older associations between witchcraft and the supernatural assaults of night demons or spirits are still apparent in several modern cultures. For example, David Hufford found that modern Newfoundlanders still believe that the "Old Hag" is sometimes sent by an individual with a grudge against the victim. They also believe that by saying the "Lord's prayer backwards in the name of the devil" it was possible to "hag" someone (Hufford 1982, 4). A recent transcultural study of sleep paralysis among African Americans also shows that many people still refer to the encounter as "being ridden by the witch". They counteract the threat by placing a broom at the bedroom door so that the witch will "be kept busy counting straws" rather than attacking the sleeper (Paradis and Friedman 2005).

Victims recall the sense of terror associated with the nightmare or sleep paralysis as being acute and debilitating. John Bond, an eighteenth-century Scottish physician and chronic sufferer of the nightmare, recalled suffering "strong palpitations, great Anxiety, Languor, and Uneasiness" during and after the experience (Bond 1753, 2). In fact, the terror associated with sleep paralysis has become recognised as one of its defining features, being reported by 66–88 per cent of subjects studied (Parker and Blackmore 2002). Cross-cultural studies in psychiatry have revealed both differences and significant similarities in cultural beliefs and explanations of sleep paralysis (Hufford 2005; Law and Kirmayer 2005; De Jong 2005; McNally and Clancy 2005: 113–22; Hinton, Pich, Chhean and Pollack 2005; Paradis and Friedman 2005; Yeung, Xu and Chang 2005). For example, whilst Newfoundlanders believe that sleep paralysis, known by them as the "Old Hag", involves a supernatural assault by a spirit of a witch, traditional Japanese culture refers to the *kanashibari,* in which the sleeper is attacked by the spirits of the dead (Hufford 1982; Schegoleva 2001). Common to all cultures is the persistence of the belief that sleep paralysis, despite modern scientific research, is in fact a supernatural assault by a malevolent being.

Whilst some scientists assert that sleep paralysis is merely the result of physiological malfunctions of the brain—specifically the limbic system or visual cortex—it remains that science has still not fully solved the mystery of how perfectly healthy individuals can have experiences involving full-blown "hallucinations" of demonic beings assaulting them (Cheyne 2001). David Hufford has suggested that culture, rather than forming or shaping experience according to prescribed cultural models, is shaped by the experiences themselves. That is to say that experiences of sleep paralysis give rise to cultural beliefs and not vice versa (Hufford 2005). Cheyne suggested as much in his article on the "ominous numinous" (Cheyne 2001). Read in this light then, cultural beliefs and individual experiences of the "Mare" or *incubus* in the premodern period can serve as a vital way for historians to understand how experiences shape culture and vice versa. Owen Davies believes that early modern accounts of the nightmare and witchcraft beliefs were inherently shaped by experiences of sleep paralysis (Davies 2003).

Certainly, there is a striking resemblance between modern descriptions of sleep paralysis across cultures and early modern accounts of witchcraft and the "Mare". Reginald Scot in his *Discoverie of Witchcraft* (1584) included the account of a priest who recalled, "There cometh unto mee, almost everie night, a certeine woman, unknowne to me, and lieth so heavie upon my brest, that I cannot fetch my breth, neither have anie power to crie, neither doo my hands serve me to shoove hir awaie, nor my feete to go from hir" (Scot 1584, 66). Modern sleep research has compiled hundreds of remarkably similar narratives of sleep paralysis. The following account is from a 35-year-old Moroccan male from a study on sleep paralysis in 2005.

> Once a week an old lady comes to him without him knowing whether he is awake or asleep. Sometimes it is a being that he cannot describe. It goes on top of him, holds him and tries to strangle him. ... Mohammed described his attack as follows: "When I lie on my back I either hear ringing in my ears or I hear the doorbell ringing. ... My heart is pounding and my body feels agitated and trembles as if I am getting shocks, or as if I am being put under narcosis. From time to time, it seems as if someone is pressing on my body. Sometimes I see a scary old witch with a skinny head, long dirty hair, dirty teeth and old black clothes coming towards me. She spreads out her hands towards me to strangle me and she is so strong that I cannot push her away from me" (De Jong 2005: 83).

Whilst our modern understanding of nightmares refers to any kind of terrifying dream, up until the last century, the nightmare was believed to be either a specific kind of supernatural nocturnal assault, or an illness in which the person "affected with this disease does dreame, that they are set upon or Tortured with some great weight lying upon them" (Anon., Sloane 1821, f. 91). In addition to the nightmare as a specific kind of dream encounter, premodern writers also spoke of "fearful dreams" and "demonic dreams". "Fearful dreams" referred to terrifying dreams which were not necessarily ascribed to the Devil. "Demonic dreams" on the other hand were dreams sent by the Devil that were not always terrifying, since the Devil might send a dream in the disguise of an Angel of Light.

Many premodern English accounts of the nightmare come from witchcraft trials. In these accounts, a common alternate term for the nightmare is being "witch-ridden". In an English witchcraft trial in York in 1595, Dorothy Jackson accused her neighbour of witchcraft, claiming that she was "ridden with a witch three times of one night, being thereby greatly astonished and upon her astonishment awakened her husband". Nicolas Raynes in a Northumberland trial accused Elizabeth Fenwick of "hag-riding" his wife who, "after being threatened, has been continually tormented by Elizabeth, a reputed witch, who rides on her, and attempts to pull her on to the floor" (Davies 2003, 186). Similarly, in March 1649/50, the child of Sara Rodes of Bolling, Yorkshire, suffered from a serious nocturnal assault, which she believed was an attack of witchcraft. Sleeping in the same bed, Rodes woke one evening to find her child trembling and terrified saying, "Mother, Sikes wife came in att a hole att the bedd feete, and upon the bedd, and tooke me by the throate, and wold have put her fingers in my mowth, and wold needs choake me" (Davies 2007, 146).

Reports of witches "riding" or assaulting their victims in sleep also occur in early modern French, Dutch and German accounts. Lyndal Roper informs us of several German cases from Augsburg, where pregnant women complained of witches tormenting them at night by pressing down on their chests after they had recently given birth (Roper 1994, 209). Robin Briggs also notes the cases of several witch trials in Lorraine, whereby victims claimed to be assaulted by supernatural beings, including animals and witches. For example, in 1601 Jacotte Simon claimed that whilst lying in bed after her husband had left, she "felt something press down on her". When she made the sign of the cross with her tongue, since she could not move her body, her assailants relented somewhat, yet continued to press her into the bed until her husband entered the room (Briggs' account, quoted in Davies 2003, 185).

One of the most intriguing and full accounts of an early modern sleep paralysis case came to the attention of English readers in 1689, when William Salmon translated the case notes of the esteemed Dutch physician Isbrand van Diemerbroeck (1609–1674) (Kompanje 2008; Salmon 1694). Within this text is Diemerbroeck's case notes of a 50-year-old woman who suffered from the nightmare.

> A woman of fifty years of age, in good plight, fleshy, strong and plethoric, sometimes troubled with a headache, and cattarrhs falling upon her breast in the winter, molested with no catarrhs, but very sore in the daytime, but in the night-time, when she was composing her self to sleep, sometimes she believed the devil lay upon her and held her down, sometimes that she was choaked by a great dog or thief lying upon her breast, so that she could hardly speak or breath, and when she endeavoured to throw off the burthen, she was not able to stir her members. And while she was in that strife, sometimes with great difficulty she awoke of her self, sometimes her husband hearing her make a doleful inarticular voice, waked her himself; at what time she was forced to sit up in bed to fetch her breath; sometimes the same fit returned twice in the night upon her going again to rest (Salmon 1694, 183–5).

Whilst the woman understood herself to be "overlay'd by some Demon, thief or other ponderous Body", Diemerbroeck believed her to be suffering from the medical disease of the *incubus,* which was caused by "the collected vapours being condensed in the head" (Salmon 1694, 183–5). Although the terms "Mare", nightmare or "witch-riding" were used in popular accounts, in medical works, physicians referred to the same experience as a disease known as the *incubus*. The notable discrepancies between the medical prognosis of Dimerbroeck and the beliefs of his patient reflect the ongoing tensions between the supernatural and medical theory of the nightmare.

The belief that experiences of the nightmare were supernatural assaults versus the medical theory that it was a disease coexisted in the premodern period and survive to this day. In many ways, the tension between modern scientific theories of sleep paralysis and the continuing cultural beliefs in the supernatural nature of the nightmare is a continuation of premodern debates. What this essay aims to show is how these two parallel views of the nightmare coexisted in premodern English culture.

According to modern sleep research, 25 to 40 per cent of persons experience one or more incidents of sleep paralysis in their lives (Cheyne, Newby-Clark and Rueffer 1999). If we accept that our fundamental psychological make-up is not all that different at the basic phenomenological level from premodern people, then it stands to reason that numerous premodern men and women also experienced sleep paralysis. Early modern narratives of dreams, nightmares, and more specifically the nightmare, indicate that our basic psychic structure and preoccupations have not changed, even if our cultural understandings of mental aspects of life have definitely evolved. This is not to assert by any means that there are no differences between past and present people; rather I am suggesting that historians have neglected to fully explore or acknowledge our common human and psychic infrastructure (Roper 1994).

The surviving premodern English accounts of the nightmare report remarkably similar symptoms to modern accounts of sleep paralysis: intense fear, paralysis, a sense of oppressive weight and frequently a feeling of something creeping up on them. Unfortunately, few detailed accounts of premodern nightmare experiences are recorded. Most accounts are fragmentary and appear in witchcraft accounts and trial records or in the clinical notes of physicians like Richard Napier, who meticulously recorded the prognosis and symptoms of his diverse clientele. However, as Carolyn Walker Bynum astutely noted in her important work on medieval female mystics, history is in truth, always fragmentary (Bynum 1992).

In early modern England, the nightmare or "*incubus*" was a term used to refer to a specific experience whereby the victim suffered a "fearful dream" or sometimes a lucid encounter in which they were temporarily paralysed and assaulted by a male (*incubus*) or female (*succubus*) night demon, witch or the Devil. As this chapter will illustrate, this definition lost currency in some medical and learned circles in the course of the seventeenth century. By the mid-eighteenth century, the idea that the nightmare was a disease rather than a real encounter had become dominant in medical discourse. However, whilst there was a definite shift towards a somatic theory of the nightmare, the idea that it was merely a bad dream or hallucination, and not a real encounter as a result of a physiological disease, had been around since at least the fifteenth century.

As Ernest Jones, the early psychoanalyst, argued in his important, though controversial work, the nightmare was historically and culturally inextricably linked to beliefs and experiences of *incubi* or *succubi* (Jones 1951, 77. Note: it is important to recognise that Jones' predominant agenda was to establish psychoanalysis as a credible science in this work). Early modern English and Continental definitions of the nightmare also show these patterns and support Jones' conclusions about the common etymology of the nightmare being linked to the Anglo-Saxon word "Mara" meaning "crusher" (Jones quoted in Hufford 1982, 53). Thomas Blount's dictionary from 1661, the *Glossographia,* defined the nightmare as "a kind of disease commonly called the Elfe, or Night-Mare with which whoever is affected, he supposes himself to be invaded by some spirit, which leaning hard upon him, stops the passage of the breath" (Blount 1661). Similarly, showing the twofold medical and supernatural theory of the nightmare, Elisha Coles' English dictionary of 1677 defined the word "*incubus*" as "the Devil (in Mans shape) lying with women, as Succubus with men, also the Night-mare, or raw humours from the stomach troubling the brain and animal spirits, that the body cannot move" (Coles 1677). The premodern English understanding of a nightmare was thus a shifting cultural category for a specific kind of dream experience. As this chapter will demonstrate, physicians increasingly asserted that the nightmare was a symptom of a specific disease, rather than a supernatural assault by night demons as was popularly believed.

Terror and fantasy: "hag-riding" and experiences of the nightmare

The nightmare as a male (*incubus*) or female (*succubus*) demon was a terrifying figure that haunted the dreams and sleep of early modern people. Drawing on the writings of the ancient Greeks, the nightmare survived in learned medical and folk beliefs through the medieval into the early modern period. In late medieval and early modern medical writings, the nightmare was understood as a "disease bredde and engendered by overmuch excess of drinking, and by a continuall and long cruditie or rawness of the stomacke" (le Loyer 1605, 102). This theory drew on the ideas of Galenic medicine and was accepted by numerous writers.

Galen had expounded a medical theory of the four humours (blood, phlegm, choler, melancholy) that explained all diseases and prescribed cures based on this system. The humoural system was founded on the idea of the symbiotic relationship between the macrocosm and the microcosm. All things existed in a delicate balance of cause and effect and the movements of the planets and stars affected human beings and their inner physiologies as a result. Personality as well as behaviour were explained according to this schema and mental illness as well as biological disease were the consequences of imbalances in the four humours. Early modern people thus had a distinctly different idea of the relationship between the body, self and exterior world than we do today. Their idea of the self and the complex relationship between body, mind and soul was distinctly more of a fluid, symbiotic relationship.

The exterior world mysteriously impacted on the body and mind of the individual. The movements of the planets, the quality of the air and varying temperatures caused direct shifts in individual behaviour and health. The body itself was understood to be in a state of delicate balance, sensitive to the moon, sun and planets as well as subtle alterations in temperatures and the five elements. Personality and behaviour were equally more volatile and subject to dramatic changes as a result of imbalances in the body's humours and temperature. The self as we know it as a supposed unified, self-contained and intangible entity was understood quite differently and subject to a more complex range of external stimuli. Before Freud and modern dream theory, dreams were understood as expressions, not of the internal struggles of the psyche between unconscious and conscious forces, but rather produced and affected by a complex range of exterior and interior forces. Yet, whilst understandings of dreams subtly and slowly changed, experiences themselves remained remarkably similar in narrative accounts.

Typically, the victim of the nightmare felt great pressure on the chest, had trouble breathing, could not move nor cry out of fear and saw a terrifying demonic being coming towards them. In 1583 Phillip Barrough wrote in his medical work, *The methode of physicke*, "Ephialtes in Greeke, in Latin Incubus and Incubo. It is a disease, where as one thinketh him selfe in the night to be oppressed with a great waight, and beleeveth that some thing commeth upon him, and the pacient thinketh himselfe strangled in this disease. It is called in English the Mare" (Barrough 1583, 34). The feeling of terror and an oppressive weight upon the chest recurs in physicians and victims' descriptions of the nightmare. Similarly, the person who suffered such attacks also struggled against temporary paralysis of the body and an inability to speak or cry out. In addition to English prescriptive treatises, Continental medical works were popular in England and frequently translated into English. These tracts typically included discussions of the causes, symptoms and "physick" of common diseases. According to the late sixteenth-century medical work by Hieronymus Brunschwig, "the disease called Incubus/that is the Mare/ whych is a sycknesse or fantasye oppressinge a man in his slepe/ that him semeth a great weyght lye upon his body/ wherefore he groneth and sigheth/but can not speake" (Brunschwig 1561, 10). Here we can see the complex blending of popular and medical knowledge.

The history of emotions is receiving increasing interest by historians (Rosenwein 2003; Reddy 2001; Ray 2001; Oatley 2004; Gross and Gross 2006; Gouk and Hills 2005; Stearnes 1986; Stearnes and Stearnes 1988). A cultural history of the nightmare can help us to understand how early modern people experienced terror, fear, anxiety and dread as a debilitating emotion. Feelings of helplessness and of complete paralysis, in addition to the sight of a terrible being coming to assault the victim, are descriptions which physicians consistently include in their symptoms of the nightmare. These symptoms are curiously analogous and indicate the primacy of the emotion of terror in nightmare experiences. Furthermore, the symptoms associated with the nightmare are also clearly indicative of the body's primal physiological response to intense fear and terror. Those afflicted with the "Mare" were reported to sweat profusely, lose the power of speech, become immobile, breathless and feel suffocated (see for example: Bayfield 1663, 65; Bruele 1632, 51; Gardiner 1611, 55).

As mentioned earlier, individual accounts of the nightmare are unfortunately rare from this period. However, the notes of the physician Richard Napier show that men, women and children of all ages, from all kinds of backgrounds, consistently complained of "fearfull dreams" and being afraid at night in the dark, lest some "divel" attack them. Napier's notebooks include one incident whereby a woman suffered from the nightmare proper. Elizabeth Banebery, aged 22 of Fenny, Stratford, saw Napier in 1618 about several symptoms following a difficult pregnancy and Napier concluded that the indications were symptomatic of a mental disorder rather than a physical disease, noting she was "mightily afflicted in mind, not sick in Body" (Crawford and Gowing 1999, 275). She complained of dreams that made her "mopish" and that she would suffer violent mood swings. On one occasion she was "tempted to kill herself and had a knife in her hand". On March 13th Banebary confided in Napier, "after her child birth fell with a dream and was frighted as if something lay upon her and since has been troubled with worldly matters” (Crawford and Gowing 1999, 276). This was clearly by seventeenth-century terms a serious bout of the nightmare or *incubus*.

Authors of medical works complained that the “vulgar” sort still held to the belief that the nightmare was in fact a supernatural, real assault of a male or female demon. These comments indicate the continuity of the popular belief in the reality of the nightmare as a supernatural physical, psychic and sexual assault. In 1630 Richard Bernard wrote a tract giving advice to English magistrates on how to deal with witchcraft trials. On the subject of bewitchment, Bernard wrote that,

> Because of the strong imagination of such as suspect themselves to be beewitched, which will make them think verily that they see strange apparitions: and for feare will dreame of the suspected, and so may cry out, and talke of him or her in their fearefull dreames, the fantasie being oppressed. And if the disease called the Mare, happen to such an one, then their sweating, their moving and struggling, with an imagination of one creeping upon them, from the feete to their brest, (they a waking in feare and trembling) wil make them say & sweare too that they are bewitched (Bernard 1630, 195–196).

Pierre le Loyer, a French expert on ghosts, and much admired in England, wrote that victims of the nightmare “imagin some man or woman of an exceeding great and wonderful stature dooth stop their mouth for feare they should cry. They move their armes and their legges to and fro in their bedde, thinking so to chase and heare them speake unto them” (le Loyer 1605, 102). The accompanying terror associated with the experience of the nightmare is understandable in light of these accounts showing that persons afflicted frequently believed themselves helplessly the prey of terrifying night demons. As late as 1689, Thomas Tryon commented that the vulgar still believed the nightmare was a supernatural assault of demons (Tryon 1689, 24–25).

As mentioned earlier, experiences of the nightmare or *incubus* were also linked in popular beliefs and learned lore to incidents of witchcraft (see for example: Davies 2003; de Blécourt 2003). In the north-east of England in 1660, Elisabeth Simpson was accused of “hag-riding” Frances Mason who complained that whilst in bed “where she lay miserably tormented, crying out that the said Elisabeth did pinch her heart and pull her in pieces”. Similarly, using almost identical descriptors, Jane Milburne testified in 1663 that Dorothy Stranger bewitched her “soe intollerably that she could not rest all the night and was like to teare her very heart in peeces and this morning left her” (Oates 2003, 220). As in modern accounts of sleep paralysis, premodern experiences of the “Mare” also included tales of being assaulted by demonic animals. Edward Wayman, a Fifth Monarchist, reported an experience of the nightmare, which he believed to have been his "first call".

> My first call was upon a dream, which I had of a great black terrible dog, which seized upon me, and took hold of my ear fast, which I thought was the Devil; at which, I waked with screeks and cries, and such frights, as for three weeks I thought that I should have gone distracted; for I found this was sent to raise me out of my sins, which were after set so before me, so that I was a long time afflicted (Rogers 1653, 409).

Those who experienced terrifying dreams also frequently spoke of fearing supernatural assaults of the Devil or thought of themselves as bewitched. Ellen Greene, aged 34, of Fentraiton [sic] in Cambridge told Napier she was "haunted by an ill spirit, whom she saith he speaketh to her" on August 8th 1634. Another patient of Napier's, Mr Thomas Amstron of Catnoll, aged 30, was "distracted this 14 nights, fearfull of every thing specially by night, dispairing better with company, cannot sleep well" (Napier, *Ashmole* 412). These accounts support Owen Davies' and Willem de Blécourt's arguments about the way that premodern experiences of "sleep paralysis" gave rise to witchcraft beliefs.

English men and women frequently seemed to be suffering from nightmares and had difficulty sleeping, being "troubled in mind" by terrifying images seen in sleep which resulted in chronic fear, insomnia and anxiety. Children were also prey to "night terrors" (Nash 1594). One of Napier's clients was Joseph Sparo, an 11-year-old boy whose parents sent him to Napier in 1602 since he was "fryghtfull in the night" (Napier, *Ashmole*, 221, f. 223). However, it was not only the young who suffered bad sleep and petrifying dreams: Napier also reports that Old Goody Child of Aspley, aged 79, was "troubled in mynd" and "fearfull of some devill, cannot sleep" (Napier, *Ashmole* 217, f. 30). While these accounts provide clues to premodern English mental life, these experiences are more likely incidents of ordinary bad dreams rather than the nightmare proper. Interestingly, insomnia was clearly a common complaint among seventeenth-century people.

John Bond's important medical tract, *On the Incubus or Nightmare* (1753) reflects the mid-eighteenth century medical consensus that the nightmare was solely the result of complex imbalances in the body, a disease that resulted in temporary paralysis and intense feelings of dread. Little is known about John Bond, other than that he was a Scottish physician who submitted a Latin version of his work on the Incubus for his Doctorate at the University of Edinburgh. As mentioned earlier, Bond was also himself a chronic sufferer of the nightmare (Dacombe 2004, 408). In his preface, he confessed the reason for writing his work, "Being much afflicted with the Night-mare, self-preservation made me particularly inquisitive about it. In consulting the ancient Physicians, I found little information concerning it, except dreadful prognostics; nor could a rational account of it be expected from them, as they were unacquainted with the circulation of the blood" (Bond 1753: preface).

Bond believed that the paucity of medical knowledge about the nightmare was the result of the lack of empirical studies of the disease and was also due to the fact that previous authors had not experienced the phenomenon themselves. He used contemporary advancements in knowledge about the circulation of the blood to suggest, contrary to previous medical theories, that "the Night-Mare is commonly, and, I believe, justly, attributed to a stagnation of the Blood; but how this stagnation is produc'd has not been explain'd, so far as I know, in a satisfactory manner" (Bond 1753).

Within his important text, Bond included multiple accounts of individuals who suffered the nightmare, believing them to be assaults of the Devil or night demons. This indicates the continuity of popular belief in the supernatural cause of the nightmare even until the mid-eighteenth century. Interestingly, Bond included testimonies of the nightmare reported by numerous women, presumably his patients or those of his colleagues, which he believed occurred "before the eruption of the Menses".

> A young Lady, of a tender, lax habit, about fifteen, before the Menses appear'd, was seiz'd with a fit of this Disease, and groan'd so miserably that she awoke her Father, who was sleeping in the next room. He arose, ran into her chamber, and found her lying on her Back, and the Blood gushing plentifully out of her Mouth and Nose. When he shook her, she recover'd, and told him she thought some great heavy Man came to her bedside, and, without farther ceremony, stretched himself upon her. She had been heard moaning in sleep several nights before (Bond 1753).

Bond believed that this woman suffered the nightmare due to an excess of menses or blood that was subsequently cured when "she had a copious eruption of the Menses, which, for that time, remov'd all her complaints" (Bond 1753). The build-up of blood in the body, according to Bond's theory, oppressed the brain resulting in hallucinations of the nightmare. Once the proper balance of blood in the body was restored, the nightmare ceased.

The sexual nature of the nightmare is implicit here in the descriptions of "heavy" male beings lying on the sleeper. Similarly, in this excerpt, the nightmare is conceived of as a symptom of a particularly feminine ailment. Bond includes several other accounts of women who also experienced fits of the nightmare before menstruation, supporting his theory that the disease was caused by excessive blood in the body. According to Bond then, the *incubus* was a purely physiological disease that was caused by excessive blood in the body. The sense of suffocation and physiological paralysis was caused by blood oppressing the heart and lungs, resulting in a sense of oppressive weight on the chest of the afflicted.

Demons of desire: succubi and incubi

While physicians continued to subscribe to a medical theory of the nightmare, other writers such as Thomas Heywood (1573–1641), the English playwright and poet, used stories of *incubi* or *succubi* to support belief in the world of spirits against the threat of atheism (Kathman 2004). Heywood defended the belief in the reality of *incubi*, *succubi*, witches, and angels in his work, *The hierarchie of the blessed Angells,* published in 1635. According to Heywood, "that there are such Spirits as we call Incubi and Succuba, there are histories both many and miraculous" (Heywood 1635, 539). Heywood compiled his accounts of *incubi* from the *Malleus Maleficarum*, the lives of the Church Fathers, Boethius, and contemporary accounts. He drew from key demonological works to prove that men and women were actually visited by male and female night demons. For example, one account Heywood takes from Boethius informs us of "a Maid of a noble family" in Scotland who was "found with child" and afterwards confessed to being visited nightly by a "beautiful young man" who turned out to be a nefarious incubus (Heywood 1635: 541). Heywood's support for the belief in *incubi/succubi* indicates that some members of the educated and upper classes also subscribed to the belief in the reality of night demons.

Women were not the only ones to become the sexual prey of "lewd demons". Heywood also includes the tale of a French nobleman "given over to voluptuousnesse" who encountered a succubus one evening on a walk in Paris and he took her home and had sex with her. On waking, the man found that his new lover was in fact dead. The woman he had slept with turned out to be the corpse of a recently executed witch (Heywood, 1635, 542–3). These tales of the nightmare illustrate traditional beliefs about the reality of *incubi/succubi* and their common links to sex and witchcraft. It is significant that popular accounts of the nightmare and early definitions include sexualised descriptions of "hag-riding", "venery" and "seminal emissions". The sexualised aspects of the nightmare experience remained implicit but faded from view in medical accounts as somatic theories began to supplant supernatural aetiologies in the later seventeenth century.

Ernest Jones has traced the etymology and history of the nightmare showing how in the early modern and medieval periods, the sexual nature of the nightmare was explicit, whilst in later works, this facet became obscured and disappeared in favour of a purely physiological explanation (Jones 1951, 88). This is certainly supported by the evidence of English writings. In 1582 Stephen Bateman commented in his reworking of the thirteenth-century medical treatise ascribed to Bartholomew the Englishman that the nightmare involved individuals being "molested with Incubi & Succubi" who "do defile the body in ye night" (Bartholomaeus 1582, 84). The sexual component of the nightmare was clearly explicit in some works yet implicit in others. In the *Anatomy of Melancholy,* Robert Burton noted that "such are as troubled with Incubus, or witch-ridden, as we call it, if they lie on their backs, they suppose an old woman rides them" (Burton 1621, 122–3).

One way of understanding the nightmare experience is to apply psychological interpretations that were not unknown to early modern people. That means by considering the experience of the nightmare as reflections of early modern men and women's sexual fantasies and anxieties. Early modern writers show a clear awareness of the erotic features of the *incubus* experience. Writers like Thomas Heywood and the authors of the infamous *Malleus Maleficarum,* Jacob Sprenger and Heinrich Kramer, referred to the numerous histories where entire convents of nuns were plagued by the sexual assaults of *incubi*. Heywood also includes several accounts of men being sexually assaulted or consenting to carnal relations with *succubi*, most often priests or gentlemen (Heywood 1635, 539–43). Additionally, the older English definitions of the "Mare" also include references to "Hag-Riding" and being "witch-ridden", which do little to hide the sexual components of this encounter. For these authors, the nightmare was a real experience rather than an imagined one in which victims were viciously assaulted by "lewd" and malevolent night demons.

The erotic nature of traditional beliefs in the nightmare is also evident in contemporary discussions about male nocturnal "emissions" that were the result of sexual dreams frequently ascribed to the visitations of *succubi*. Thomas Walkington referred explicitly to the erotic facets of the nightmare advising that abstinence from excessive "seminal emissions" was the best cure: "There is an other diet for Venus: we must not spend our selves upon common curtizans: wee must not be like Sparrowes, which ... goe to it eight times in an hower, nor like Pigeons, which twain are fained of the Poets to draw the chariot of Cytheraea" (Walkington 1607, 30). Moreover, as James Ferrand commented in his *Epotomania, or, a Treatise discoursing of the essence, causes, symptomes, prognosticks, and cure of Love or Erotique Melancholy* (1640), "This Disease takes them commonly in their first sleepe, when as the thick grosse vapors which are carried up to the Braine, stop the Nerves that serve for speech and Respiration: by which meanes the parties thus troubled, think they have a heavy burthen lying upon them, or else some Divell, or Witch, that would attempt a breach upon their Chastity" (Ferrand 1640, 211). The erotic nature of the nightmare for most people was self-evident and perhaps the most terrifying aspect of the experience.

King James I wrote at length of *incubi* and *succubi* as "spirits" that "haunt(s) most of the Northerne and barbarous parts of the world". Redolent of the tendency of early modern people to externalise the darker aspects of sexuality in supernatural others such as the witch, the Devil and demons, James presents *incubi* and *succubi* as "lewd" demons who stole the semen of men in order to procreate with witches in sadistic sexual encounters that are such a classic facet of early modern demonology (James I 1603, 65–8). According to James, in some instances, the Devil steals the "sperme" from dead or living men and uses it to impregnate women. However, reflecting the demonic inversion of normal procreation, sex with the Devil was frequently "intollerably colde" and lacking the passionate warmth of human copulation (James I 1603, 66). Thus, sex with demons for women as well as men was often described as terrifying, cold, inhuman and most often infertile. Should a woman become pregnant with the child of an *incubus*, the baby was often a monster or, in the case of legends, a magician or sorcerer like Merlin.

The late medieval *Malleus Maleficarum* (1486) devotes considerable length to the question of whether *incubi* or *succubi* can inhabit bodies or conceive children by "filthy acts" with witches by stealing the semen from human men. The two inquisitors conclude that this was possible in certain circumstances. However, more importantly, they saw the sexual relations between demons (*incubi/succubi*) and human women as a key feature and sin of witches. According to the *Malleus'* authors, *incubi* had "carnal relations" with men and women "not for the sake of pleasure but for the sake of corrupting". Unlike later demonological works, Sprenger and Kramer believed that sex with demons was a source of some pleasure for witches (Mackay 2009: 307–11). As demons of desire, the nightmare in male or female form could be interpreted as an externalised projection of male and female sexual desires and anxieties that became more internalised in the eighteenth century.

Another way of reading early modern ideas and experiences of the nightmare is as expressions of collective anxieties about sexuality. The sense of helplessness, oppression, and terror in the face of being "hag-" or "witch-ridden" by an ugly old woman or demonic male can be read as the projected individual and cultural fears of men and women about the other sex's darker desires. (Charles Zika has argued that the sexualised representations of witches' bodies in art are also redolent of early modern fantasies and fears about old women's bodies. Zika 2002). Whilst I would not go so far as to interpret this experience as repressed oedipal desires, I will suggest that we can note the discernable gendering and manifestation of sexual desire and anxiety in supernatural interpretations of the nightmare. In the throes of the nightmare, the male victim was in a terrifying state of physical paralysis in which the figure of a "hag" or female demon "rode them". In women's narratives of the nightmare, they were assaulted by a preternatural demonic male figure in what was ostensibly a rape-like scenario. Unable to move, the female victim was paralysed as the demonic male being crept into their chambers and did as they pleased, often strangling or sexually assaulting them.

Ernest Jones has interpreted this as the classic projection of male fantasies and anxieties about sex that certainly makes sense when one reads accounts of the "Mare" as written by physicians regarding their clients' experiences. Sex with the "Mare" was infertile and frightening, so that the victim "can scarce draw his breath" and he "doth imagine that he is assaulted & opprest by some thing for hee thinks that somewhat doth sit upon his brest". The sufferer also "cannot speak a word although he endeavor to his utmost power ... sometimes he groanes, as they doe that weep" (Bruele 1632, 51). The curiously consistent theme of being assaulted by a woman, usually supernaturally beautiful or old and ugly does suggest darker elements of masculine desire in addition to masculine sexual anxieties about the "woman on top" (Breitenberg 1996). However, this paradigm could also be applied to women's experiences of the "nightmare", since both sexes experienced the nightmare as an assault by a demonic being of the opposite sex. Whilst most encounters involved heterosexual sexual assaults, often female victims were attacked by female witches. This is perhaps due to the fact that the stereotypical figure of the witch was closely associated with females. If we apply the theory that experiences of the nightmare express projected individual and collective anxieties about sexuality, these encounters could be read as featuring cultural stereotypes of the sexual perversion and sexuality of the witch.

An example of a premodern account of a male's terrifying encounter with a supernatural sexual assault of female spirits can be found in Richard Bovet's tract, *Pandaemonium, or the Devil's Cloyster* (1684). According to the tract, which was a collation of supernatural tales, there was an incident in a Nobleman's house in the west of England. One evening, one of the ladies' footmen complained of a headache and retired to bed. The Lady later passed her servant's room to find the door open and:

> saw the poor young Man lying speechless on the Bed, his Eyes were staring very wide, and fixed on one side of the Room, his Hands were clutched, his Hair erected, and his whole body in so violent a sweat ...; all the Clothes of the Bed were flung ... his very shirt was drawn off his Body ... and it was near half an hour before he could recollect himself ... He told us that he lay about half an hour, endeavouring to compose himself to sleep, but could not ... that about that time there came into the Room to him two in appearance of very beautiful young Women, whose presence enlightened the place, as if it had been day ... That they had endeavoured to come into the Bed to him ... which he resisted with all the power he could, striking at them several times with his Fists ... yet they were so strong, that they drew all the Bed-clothes off him, though he endeavoured with all his force to hold them, that after that they had stripped him of his shirt; and he had contested so long with them, that he concluded within himself he should die under their violences, during all that time he had no power to speak, or call for aid (Bovet 1684, 223–34).

Although an encounter with two beautiful women in the private realms of the bedroom might seem tantalizingly erotic, in this case, the young man was terrified and had struggled in vain against their preternatural advances. In this way, his masculine physical strength was overcome by the unnatural physical powers of the two women who were showing a striking, and hence supernatural, gender inversion of the woman on top or female in the role of sexual aggressor. The anxiety generated by women in men in situations of sexual aggression and power has been astutely studied by Katherine Hodgkin, among others, and is part of the historiographical debate about the "crisis in gender" in the early modern period. Whilst I would not suggest experiences of the nightmare illustrate a crisis in gender relations, they do reveal deep-rooted anxieties in *both* men and women about the darker aspects of sexuality.

The involvement of fantasy and the "imagination" in the production of the nightmare was a theory which early modern physicians and other writers also supported. This was linked to the natural theory of dreams. According to Robert Burton, who advocated the predominant view,

> This we see verified in sleepers, which by reason of abundance of humors and concurse of vapours troubling the Phantasie, imagine many times absurd and prodigious things, and in such are troubled with Incubus, or witch-ridden, as we call it, if they lie on their backs, they suppose an old woman rides them, and sits so hard upon them, that thy are almost stifled for want of breath; when there is nothing but a concourse of bad humours which trouble the Phantasie (Burton 1621, 35).

The faculty of "phantasie" as a subordinate facet of the imagination was one which other writers also believed produced visual hallucinations like the nightmare. Richard Bernhard noted that "a strong imagination" led the fearful to dream of the suspected witch due to "the fantasie being oppressed". On the subject of the "Mare" he also supports the increasingly popular view that this too was the result of the imagination and faculty of "Phancy" (Bernard 1630, 205).

Hallucinations produced by the overactive imagination or "fantasie" were also believed to lie behind common encounters with ghosts, witches, spirits, and apparitions. As a popular 1605 English translation of Pierre le Loyer's *De Spectris* put it, "It resteth now that we speake of the Fantasie, which is no other thing, but an Imagination or impression of the Soule, of such formes and shapes as are knowne: or of such shall be imagined, without any sight had of them" (le Loyer 1605, 3). According to le Loyer, the nightmare was a hallucination caused by the combined forces of indigestion and a "corrupted" imagination or "fantasie" in which the person afflicted imagined "that they are enticed and solicited by them [*incubi/succubi*] to actes of venery" (le Loyer 1605, 102). Read in this context, the idea that experiences of nightmares reflected male or female fantasies about sexual desire is neither anachronistic nor untenable.

The somatisation of dreams: physic and medicine

Increasingly throughout the seventeenth, and becoming more dominant in the early eighteenth century, medical theories of the nightmare were eclipsing popular supernatural aetiologies, at least in learned discourses. Natural or medical theories of the nightmare are usually a combination of the new theories of the mind and the Galenic humoural system. As Richard Kagan showed, medical theories of dreams had only gained currency in the twelfth century with the rediscovery of ancient classical texts by medieval scholars (Brown 1999, 55). In the early modern period, this schema of dreams had become increasingly popular among educated writers.

"Fearful dreams" and the nightmare were often associated with bouts of melancholy, as Robert Burton's *Anatomy of Melancholy* and numerous other premodern medical treatises assert. According to Burton in his discussion of the imagination, "in Melancholy men this faculty is most powerfull and strong, and often hurt, producing many monstrous and prodigious things, especially if it be stirred up by some terrible object" (Burton 1621, 36). Additionally, Burton also argued that indigestion also caused fearful dreams and bouts of the incubus: "Hare, a black meat, melancholy & hard digestion, it breeds Incubus often eatem & causeth feafull Dreames, & so doth all Venison, & is condemned by a Jury of Physicians" (Burton 1621, 88). Other foods believed to cause terrible dreams included beans, peas, and fruits since "they fill the braine ... with gross fumes, breed black thick blood, and cause troublesome dreames" (Burton 1621, 92). In line with the natural theory of dreams, which asserted that dreams were frequently merely the by-products of indigestion, Burton advised sufferers of melancholy to avoid sleeping too much on a full stomach: "if it be used in the day time, or upon a full stomacke, the body ill composed to rest, or after hard meates, it increaseth fearfull dreames, Incubus, night walking, crying out, and much unquietness" (Burton 1621, 118).

The Cambridge-trained physician, Timothy Bright, who wrote *A treatise of melancholy* (1586) had also recognised "fearful dreams" and the nightmare as symptoms of melancholy and indigestion (Bright 1613, 238). Bright attributed more significance to the power of the mind over the body than vice versa, arguing that terrible dreams were one of the many "Whelpes of that Melancholicke litter".

> So easily is the bodie subject to alteration of the mind, and soone looseth with anguish and distraction thereof, all the support of his excellencie. Besides this in you, vaine feares, and false conceits of apparitions, imagination of a voice sounding in your eares, frightfull dreames, distrust of the consumption, and putrifying of one part of another of your bodie, and the rest of this crue are of molestation, which are Whelpes of that Melancholicke litter, and are bred of the corrupted state of the bodie altered in Spirit in Bloud, in substance and complexion, by the abundance of this setling of the Bloud we call Melancholy. This increaseth the terrour of the afflicted minde, doubling the feare and discouragement (Bright 1613, 238).

Therefore, for Bright, experiences of fearful dreams like those seen in the nightmare were merely the result of corrupted faculties of the mind and imbalances in the body.

Black thoughts, sadness, madness and terrible visions of the devil, demons and witches were common symptoms of the melancholic person who was under siege by an "abundance" of black humour. The mind was labouring in the prison of the body while the senses were deceived.

> This meanes, (I mean the outward meanes of consolation and cure) must needs passe by our senses to enter the minde, whose instrument being altered with by the humour, and their sincerity stained with the obscure and darke spots of Melancholy, receive not indifferently the medicine of consolation. So it both mistaketh that which it apprehendeth, and delivereth it imperfectly to the mindes consideration. As their Braines are thus evill disposed, so their hearts in no better case, and acquainted with terrour, and overthrowne with that fearful passion, hardly set free the cheerful Spirits, feebled with the corporeal prison on the bodie, and hardly yeelde to perswasion of comfort, whatsoever it bringeth of assurance (Bright 1613, 239).

The terror that the melancholic person felt was the complex result of the body's effects on the mind. A false perception of reality was the result of the body's noxious fluids rising from the stomach to suffuse the brain with deceptive images.

Medical theories based on Galenic medicine that privileged the humours as the site of all health and disease argued that the nightmare was merely the result of vapours rising from the stomach to the brain, heart and lungs. Understood in this way, the nightmare was ultimately a disease rather than a supernatural assault. According to Edmund Gardiner in his work *Phisicall and approved medicines* (1611), "this disease of the night-Mare ... it commeth by meanes of certaine grosse and thicke vapours, which doe partly intercept, and hinder the free passage of the spirits animall" (Gardiner 1611, 55). Thomas Walkington also subscribed to humoural imbalances, asserting that the nightmare "is nothing else but a disease proceeding of grosse phleume in the orifice of the stomach, by long surfet, which sends up could vapors to hinder the passage of the spirits decending" (Walkington 1607, 29–30).

Dr Willis was another physician who used his knowledge of medicine and "physick" to sell handy medical reference books to the public (Willis 1684). John Bond had read Willis carefully in order to more fully understand his own affliction (Bond 1753). According to Willis's *Practice of Physick* (1684), the nightmare was in fact a "distemper" of the brain.

> In truth, the Symptoms which are wont to be raised up in the distemper called the Incubus or Night-mare, viz. loss of speech, and a mighty weight or load that seems to lye upon the breast, proceed altogether from the

> morbisick matter fixed in the confines of the Cerebel, and obstructing the passages of the Spirits destinated for the Pracordia (Bond 1753, 92).

Physicians offer variations on these themes, some according more influence to the brain, others the stomach. Jeremy Collier wrote in his *Miscellanies upon moral subjects* (1695) that "the fumes of Indigestion, insensible Abatements of Health, sudden Changes of Weather, affect the Brain, though they make no sensible Impression elsewhere" (Collier 1695, 35).

Not all medical works in this period were written by "eminent phisitians"; Burton himself was a scholar and Dean of Oxford and was a cleric rather than a physician (Burton 1621). For the less educated, works such as *The Problems of Aristotle* were perennially popular titles on the book market. This work ascribed to Aristotle was first published in 1595 and went through no less than eleven editions by 1684 (Anonymous 1595). Indicative of the way that early modern writers split the body into parts, in the sections "Of the Head" and "Of Backs" are discussions of the *incubus*. (For an excellent history of the body in parts see: Hillman and Mazzio 1997). The author of this work combines the twofold medical theory of the "nightmare", ascribing it to both the result of humoural imbalances of the body and the corruption of "the fantasie" or imagination. The format of the book is dialectical.

> Q. Why hath a man which lieth on his backe horrible Visions?
> A. Because then the passage or sinewe of the fantasie is open, which is in the forepart of the braine, and so the fantasie is destroyed, and then those visions followe. Another reason is, because that when a man dooth lye on his backe, the humours are disturbed and moved upward where the fantasie is, which is so by that meanes is disturbed.
> Q. Why is it naught to lie on the backe?
> A. Because, as the Phisitions do say, that doth dispose a man to leprosie, madnes, and to an *Incubus*. Where you may note, that *Mania*, or madnes is the hurt or disturbance of the forepart of the braine, with a taking away or deprivation of the imagination: but *Incubus*, that is, the nightmare, is a passion of the heart, when a man dooth thinke himselfe to bee strangled in his sleepe, and somewhat lie heavie upon his stomacke, which he would put off (Anonymous 1597).

In this way, we can see that in the later period of the seventeenth century, most medical writers argued that the nightmare was not supernatural in origin but merely a disease that was the result of either the body's natural processes, like indigestion, and/or the hallucination of a "corrupted" imagination.

During the first half of the eighteenth century, this trend continued and more complex medical theories replaced older notions of the nightmare. In an anonymous work "by a physician" *A Treatise of Diseases of the Head, Brain & Nerves* (1714), the nightmare was seen to be the forerunner of an "apoplexy" in which "persons [are] subject to Lethargies or Vertigoes". Chapter XI offered an entire section devoted to the "*Incubus* or Night-mare" that described the symptoms, cause and cure of this disease. "The Night-mare, or as some call it, the Hag, is a Nocturnal Disease arising from thick Vapours which chiefly obstruct the hinder part of the Brain, by which the Flux of Animal Spirits being stop'd Breathing is hinder'd" (Anonymous 1714, 73). In 1707 Andrew Bell published a new edition of Thomas Tryon's earlier *Treatise on Dreams* (1689) retitled as *Nocturnal Revels: or, a General History of Dreams.* Appended to the original treatise was an extensive section of oneiromancy. This work completely denigrated the supernatural aetiology of nightmares.

> As for those that in their Sleep are troubled with the Incubus or Nightmare, they seem to be of a Temper quite contrary to the former, and are Melancholy, of few and gross Spirits, and abounding with Phlegm; ... This Disease being an Obstruction of Motion, or an interception, especially of Breathing and Speech, with a false Apprehention of some heavy thing lying upon their Breasts, ... occasioned by reason that the free penetration of the Spirits to the Nerves, is hindred, the Passage being stopt by a surcharge of the aforesaid Humours (Anonymous 1707, 13–4).

Here we see the common commingling of medical theories of the nightmare that incorporated humoural medicine with contemporary notions of melancholy.

The dangers of excess: cures and prophylactics

Redolent of popular medical views of health and disease, the dangers of excess were also used to explain the moral and physiological causes of the nightmare. This had been a popular theory in seventeenth-century medical and prescriptive works. In 1651 Thomas Hobbes had drily written off belief in the nightmare as supernatural as mere superstition. To Hobbes, the real causes were that this disease "springing from Gluttony, it makes men believe they are invaded, opprest, and stifled with a great weight" (Hobbes 1651, 184). The dangers of excess included the sins of excessive drinking, eating, sex and even sleep. This is reflective of the way that diseases in this period were part of the moral cosmology and idea of God's retribution for excess and sin. The body was a moral prison or potential vehicle of punishment for those indulging in excessive appetites.

Within this culture, the nightmare was viewed as a just retribution for morally and physiologically dangerous excesses. Sexual excess was, according to Thomas Walkington, something to be seriously tempered and abstained from lest the body give rise to nightmares (Walkington 1607, 30). Phillip Barrough also urged against the dangers of excess since "this vice [the nightmare] is caused of excesse of drinking, and continuall rawnes of the stomacke" (Barrough 1583, 34). Thus, according to Barrough, drunks, fat men and children were the chief victims of this "vice". Mention of the perceived contemporary attitudes towards sexual excess in the particular form of masturbation is not remiss here, since the nightmare was a long held kind of private sexual fantasy resulting frequently in "nocturnal emissions" and suggestive of involuntary masturbation. Thomas Laqueur has argued that cultural anxieties about the dangers of sexual excess were prevalent in seventeenth- and particularly eighteenth-century England resulting in a discreet campaign in print to curb this taboo vice (Laqueur 2004). Theories and experiences of the nightmare as the reflection of sexual fantasies and anxieties of premodern people can offer us important insight into seventeenth- and eighteenth-century ideas of the body, mind and sexuality.

Sex as an appetite of the body is inherently linked to the body's desire for food and drink. John Bond included the following account of an eighteenth-century "corpulent clergyman" who, due to his excessive love of food and drink, suffered intense bouts of the nightmare.

> A corpulent Clergyman, about fifty years old, who is very fond of strong beer and flesh suppers, but so subject to the Night-mare, that he is obliged to stint himself to a certain quantity every night; whenever he happens to take an over-dose, he groans so loudly that he often wakens all the People in the house. He has assured me, that, in these fits, he imagin'd the Devil came to his bedside, seiz'd him by the Throat, and endeavoured to choack him. Next day he observ'd the black impressions on his hard Fingers on his Neck (Bond 1753, 55).

Excessive indulgence also led to dangerous overabundances of the body's natural fluids. William Salmon argued that the nightmare caused "an over-redundancy of Blood in the whole Body" (Salmon 1694, 184). Thomas Tryon also noted that the *incubus* caused an abundance of "Phlegm" in the body in addition to "a surcharge of Humors" that impeded the animal spirits resulting in a temporary paralysis of the body's natural workings (Tryon 1689, 24–5). The physician, Helkiah Crooke, also believed that the nightmare was caused by “a great quantity and notable thickness” of humours that “strangled” the “animal spirits” residing in the “ventricles” of the brain. The dangers of excess therefore led to the deadly commingling of humoural fluids in the stomach that rose to the brain causing the hallucination of the nightmare and the sense of physical oppression and temporary paralysis in sleep.

Moderation was seen to be the key to good health in premodern English physic. When all else failed, moderating the body’s excessive appetites was viewed as essential for the well-being of the overall person. Robert Bayfield, an English physician, suggested that the best prophylactic was “a slender diet” in addition to avoiding the supine position (Bayfield 1663, 65). *The Problems of Aristotle* also advised “the best Physick is, to use temperance in eating and drinking” (Anonymous 1595). In his important work on “nocturnal revels”, Andrew Bell advised,

> The cure is to be effected by a Regular Diet, and such as may generate good Spirits; and prevent the Encrease of Melancholy and Phlegm; avoid full suppers, and Excess in Liquors, which oft occasion this disease: Use convenient Purging, and sometimes breathing a Vein may be convenient; especially in Women, in certain Obstructions peculiar to that Sex. The Black Seeds of the Male Piony are much commended in this Distemper (Anonymous 1707, 14).

Francis Bacon also recommended a powder of the “peony” seed be used as a cure for the nightmare, as did Nicholas Culpepper in his work *The English Physician* (1652) (Bacon 1627, 259; Culpepper 1652, 193).

The general consensus of physicians for a prophylactic against the *incubus* was therefore to counsel moderation or a “slender diet” especially for supper. Drinking liquors or excessive alcohol in any form was to be avoided, as was “gluttony”. The dangers of excess were believed to result in serious bouts of the nightmare that could become chronic and lead to more serious illnesses such as “epilepsie”, “palsy” or “apoplexy”. Phillip Barrough urged “it is good to remedie this evill at the first: for if it continewe, it induceth and sheweth before some grevous disease, as the Apoplexie, the falling sickness, or madnesse” (Barrough 1583, 34). Authors also advised sleeping on one’s side and to at all costs avoid the “supine” position since this could often lead to the nightmare. Thomas Coohan advised moderation in sleep. A healthy human should sleep no more than “7.8 or 9 hours” a night, should always sleep at night and not indulge in daytime naps. Similarly, the anonymous author of the tract, *Directions and Observations relative to Food, Exercise and Sleep* (1772), recommended no “less than six nor more than nine Hours a Day” of sleep.

The popular work of the M.D. William Buchan, *Domestic Medicine* (1769), urged moderation in sleep, promoting what historian Lucia Dacombe defined as a form of "bodily domestication" (Buchan 1772, 108; Dacombe 2004). Buchan advised his readers, "sleep, as well as diet, ought to be duly regulated. Too little sleep weakens the nerves, exhausts the spirits, and occasions diseases; and too much renders the mind dull, the body gross, and disposes it to apoplexies, lethargies, and such like" (Buchan 1772, 108). The custom of some "indolent and slothful" people who indulged in "lolling a-bed" for eight or nine hours was therefore conducive to a weak and disease-prone constitution (Buchan 1772, 108). The ideal sleep, according to eighteenth-century physicians and philosophers like John Locke, was a dreamless one (Dacombe 2004). Coohan also advised sufferers of the nightmare or "terrible dreams" to avoid eating leeks, onions and beans since they raised up "ill dreams" (Coohan 1636, 31, 63–5 and 275). The dangers of excess could therefore be tempered and the nightmare cured, according to English physicians, by moderation of all the body's appetites.

Conclusion

Although in religious discourse the supernatural origins of dreams were difficult to discredit, the medical discourse on dreams tells a different story. Medical tracts dreams, and the nightmare in particular, were more confidently relegated to the realms of the body and the physiological. This was a pattern that increased throughout the period of the seventeenth century. In learned discourse, the medical model of dreams, first appearing in the twelfth century, increasingly supplanted the supernatural and oneirocritic interpretation of dreams. The shift from supernatural to natural theories of the nightmare and dreams is also indicative of the development of empirical science, or natural philosophy, among groups of physicians and other intellectuals. What is notable is that in medical works, the nightmare, rather than being understood as an attack by demons or the devil, was increasingly argued to be merely the result of natural, and therefore rational and scientifically explicable by-products of the body or mind/soul. Whilst in the seventeenth century the supernatural causes of the nightmare were acknowledged according to early modern demonological lore, by the mid-eighteenth century, this discussion was diminished in learned works to being merely part of the etymology of the medical term *incubus*.

However, beliefs in the nightmare as the supernatural assaults of demons continued among the broader populace and reflect the complex commingling of various discourses and dream cultures. Before the eighteenth century, the nightmare was typically understood as an incident, whereby an old, ugly woman or “hag” attacked the male sleeper in a terrifying dream in which they “rode” the victim, assaulting them by sitting on their chest. The victim of the nightmare was “oppressed” by this being so that they were paralysed with fear and the weight of the “Hag” so that any physical movement or defence was impossible. Typical symptoms of the nightmare encounter included a profound sense of dread, physical paralysis, terror and breathlessness.

However, aside from illustrating these subtle cultural shifts in thinking about dreams and the somatisation of dreaming, the medical discourse on dreams also reflects a distinctly gendered paradigm. By being delegated to “superstition” and “vulgar” belief, the older supernatural ideas and experience of the nightmare show the imposition of the masculine and rational discourse of science or natural philosophy over a feminised discourse. Similarly, and more poignantly, the experience of the nightmare as “hag-riding” reflects the deeply rooted cultural anxieties about male and female sexuality. By seeking to override this belief or understanding of the nightmare as merely the adverse result of indigestion or “lying on one’s back”, medical understandings of dreams sought to eradicate male anxieties about female sexuality through the decidedly masculine discourse of natural philosophy and the “new science”. Men like John Bond, who suffered chronic bouts of the nightmare, fought their male anxieties and feminised the discourse of the supernatural by advocating a medical view of the “Mare” thus engendering it as neither terrifying nor supernatural. In this way, writers like Bond nullified the deep psychological terror that this terrifying experience raised in sufferers as well as inadvertently contributing to the cultural hegemony of the masculine, medical discourse. For women, a somatic theory of the nightmare also helped to alleviate their anxieties about aggressive sexuality, projected onto the form of the demonic male being who assaulted them physically and sexually in their sleep.

The surviving fragmentary accounts of the nightmare show that people predominantly understood experiences of the nightmare as real malevolent assaults. This is particularly apparent in the demonological lore and witchcraft trials. The early modern cosmology was one in which the Devil and his minions were actively at work to terrify, torment and subvert good Christians into sin, heresy and dissent. Medieval and early modern peoples, when experiencing the nightmare, believed they were really attacked in their sleep by female or male demons who sat on their chests in what was implicitly a case of supernatural sexual assault. In classical culture, cases of demonic assault by *succubi/incubi* were understood primarily as supernatural assaults of demons. This tradition was embedded into the early modern core of demonological beliefs by intellectuals, and it may be assumed, was also incorporated into the popular lore of witchcraft.

During the sixteenth and seventeenth centuries, instances of the nightmare occur in accounts of witchcraft, seeing the being of the witch supplanting or blurring with the idea of the female demon. The bewitched were, in this sense, attacked by a female witch in their sleep resulting in deep terror and the sense of helplessness that such attacks invariably raised. Unlike in cases where the victim believed themselves assaulted by an unknown demon, witchcraft nightmares allowed the victim the possibility of defence through either counter-magic or a witch trial. In either case, whether the person afflicted with nightmares believed they had been assaulted by witches or *succubi/incubi*, they still typically believed the experience had been real, rather than dreamed.

By questioning and undermining the reality of the nightmare experience, as not just a supernatural encounter but as a "real" experience, medical theories of dreams served to console sufferers of the nightmare that their experience was merely a natural by-product of the workings of the body and thus "just a dream". The most alarming possibility that this medical view of the nightmare could raise was that a natural disease was imminent. In this way, the medical view of the nightmare served to console the sufferer, giving the possibility of a cure and incorporating the nightmare into the realms of physic. Medical writers were therefore subsuming "fearful dreams" and the nightmare in the realms of natural philosophy and medicine and thus taking them away from the worlds of religion, demonology and popular belief. In this way, the nightmare shifted in contemporary belief, at least in medical circles, as being the treatable symptoms of disease and was thus firmly placed in the realms of the body.

This medical view of the nightmare was part of the masculine scientific discourse that came to dominate seventeenth- and eighteenth-century intellectual thought. The literature on the nightmare also reveals another interesting insight into early modern cultural shifts in intellectual thinking. Works on the body, mind and health, as well as dreams, reveal a tendency towards the feminisation or "vulgarisation" of the irrational, superstitious and supernatural. The rise of Baconian empirical thought and material science long heralded as the bastion of the "Enlightenment" served to uphold reason as the most worthy faculty that man possessed. Reason was upheld as the masculine faculty *par excellence*, which women had less access to being held captive by their emotions and imaginative faculties. The faculty of the imagination, linked to the faculty of fancy ("phancy"), was demoted as being a lesser, irrational facet of the mind that undermined the higher workings of "reason". In this way, human experiences such as dreams and the nightmare, traditionally linked to these lesser faculties, were demoted as irrational and feminised. Thus, the nightmare was viewed as a feminine, irrational symptom not only of the body but also of the mind. Men who suffered bouts of the *incubus* were thrashing in the throes of the imbalances and imperfections of their bodies and minds, held captive by their feminine imaginative faculty. Thus, even if the nightmare was no longer viewed as a real attack of a female demon, in medical works, this demon had become interiorised and absorbed into the rational model of the mind and body.

By the mid-eighteenth century, the wholesale belief in the reality of witchcraft, witches, and the Devil and their active role in terrorising early modern people began to slowly decline, at least in some intellectual circles. Whilst I would not suggest that the rise of so-called "rational science" led to the decline of magical world views, I would suggest that the period of "Enlightenment" did result in intellectual shifts in attitudes towards the supernatural, above all in their understanding of dreams. This is particularly apparent in medical circles and medical treatises on anatomy, the body and the mind. Although research by Owen Davies and Willem de Blécourt has shown that beliefs in witchcraft had not in fact declined by the mid-eighteenth century, certainly there were shifts towards an increasing criticism and scepticism of magical beliefs among intellectuals (de Blécourt and Davies 2004).

Belief in the supernatural did not wane in this period but rather was evolving into the kinds of new forms that Alex Owen discusses in his study of the occult in nineteenth-century England (Owen 2004). The medical and natural theory of dreams going back to Aristotle, Galen and Hippocrates was raised up above the parallel tradition of the supernatural. Thus, magical world views did not decline but rather were lowered from being acceptable intellectual systems of thought and were supplanted with newer empirical and medical models. What the discourse and debates about the meaning of dreams indicates is this complex interplay of parallel traditional theories of dreams—the natural and the supernatural. As Alexandra Walsham has shown, ideologies and beliefs at ground level operate in more complex ways than allowed for by models of "rise" or "decline" (Walsham 1999). Such models are oversimplistic and miss much of the complex interplay of negotiation that operates in historical cultures. A history of dream cultures, or cultural thought about dreams, reveals this complex negotiation.

References

Anonymous. 1595. *The Problems of Aristotle with other Philosophers and Phisitions*. Edinburgh: Printed by Roger Waldgrave.

Anonymous. 1597. *The Problems of Aristotle with other Philosophers and Phisitions.* London: Printed for Arnold Hatfield.

Anonymous. 1707. *Nocturnal Revels: or, a General History of Dreams in two parts.* London: Printed for Andrew Bell.

Anonymous. 1714. *A treatise of diseases of the Head, Brain & Nerves.* London: Printed and sold, by the Author's Appointment, at the Hatch with blue Spikes, near the Square in Haydon-yard in the Minories.

Anonymous. 1821. "Of the Cramps and of the Nightmare." British Library Manuscript, Sloane.

Bacon, Francis. 1627. *Sylva sylvarum: or A naturall historie in ten centuries.* London: Printed by John Haviland and Augustine Mathewes for William Lee.

Barrough, Philip. 1583. *The methode of phisicke conteyning the causes, signes, and cures of inward diseases in mans body from the head to the foote.* London: By Thomas Vautroulliere.

Bartholomaeus, Anglicus. 1582. *Batman uppon Bartholome his booke De proprietatibus rerum, newly corrected, enlarged and amended.* London: Imprinted by Thomas East.

Bayfield, Robert. 1663. *Tes iatrikes kartos, or, A treatise de morborum capitis essentiis & pronosticis adorned with above three hundred choice and rare observations*. London: Printed by D. Maxwel and are to be sold by Richard Tomlins.

Bernard, Richard. 1630. *A guide to grand-jury men divided into two books: in the first, is the authors best aduice to them what to doe.* London: Printed by Felix Kyngston for Edw. Blackmore.

Blécourt, Willem de. 2003. "Bedding the Nightmare: somatic experience and narrative meaning in Dutch and Flemish legend texts." *Folklore* 114: 227–45.

Blécourt, Willem de, and Owen Davies. 2004. *Witchcraft continued: popular magic in modern Europe*. Manchester, and New York: Manchester University Press.

Blount, Thomas. 1661. *Glossographia, or, A dictionary interpreting all such hard words of whatsoever language now used in our refined English tongue with etymologies, definitions and historical observations on the same.* London: Printed by Tho. Newcombe for George Sawbridge.

Bond, John. 1753. *An essay on the incubus, or night-mare*. London: D. Wilson and T. Durham.

Bovet, Richard. 1684. *Pandaemonium, or, The devil's cloyster being a further blow to modern sadduceism, proving the existence of witches and spirits.* London: Printed for J. Walthoe.

Breitenberg, Mark. 1996. *Anxious masculinity in early modern England.* Cambridge: Cambridge University Press.

Bright, Timothie. 1613. *A treatise of melancholy Containing the causes thereof, and reasons of the strange effects it worketh in our minds and bodies: with the physicke cure, and spirituall consolation for such as have thereto adjoyned afflicted conscience.* London: Printed by William Stansby.

Brown, Peter. 1999. *Reading dreams: the interpretation of dreams from Chaucer to Shakespeare.* Oxford: Oxford University Press.

Bruele, Gualtherus. 1632. *Praxis medicinae, or, the physicians practice wherein are contained inward diseases from the head to the foote: explayning the nature of each disease, with the part affected; and also the signes, causes, and prognostiques*. London: Printed by John Norton, for William Sheares.

Brunschwig, Hieronymus. 1561. *A most excellent and perfecte homish apothecarye or homely physik booke, for all the grefes and diseases of the bodye. Translated out the Almaine speche into English by Jhon Hollybush.* Edited by John Hollybush, imprinted at Collen: By [the heirs of] Arnold Birckman.

Buchan, William. 1772. *Domestic Medicine: or, a treatise on the prevention and cure of diseases by regimen and simple medicines*. London: Printed for W. Stahan; T. Cadell.

Burton, Robert. 1621. *The anatomy of melancholy what it is. With all the kindes, causes, symptomes, prognostickes, and severall cures of it.* Oxford: Printed by John Lichfield and James Short, for Henry Cripps.

Bynum, Carolyn Walker. 1992. *Fragmentation and Redemption: essays on gender and the human body in medieval religion.* New York: Zone Books.

Cheyne, J. A. 2001. "The ominous numinous: sensed presence and 'other' hallucinations." *Journal of Conscious Studies* 8 (5): 1–18.

—. 2002. "Situational factors affecting sleep paralysis and associated hallucinations: position and timing effects." *Journal of Sleep Research* 11: 169–77.

—. 2005. "Sleep paralysis episode frequency and number, types, and structure of associated hallucinations." *Journal of Sleep Research* 14: 319–24.

Cheyne, J. A., Ian R. Newby-Clark, and Steve D. Rueffer. 1999. "Relations among hypnagogic and hypnopompic experiences associated with sleep paralysis." *Journal of Sleep Research* 8: 313–7.

Coles, Elisha. 1677. *An English dictionary explaining the difficult terms that are used in divinity, husbandry, physick, phylosophy, law, navigation, mathematicks, and other arts and sciences*. London: Printed for Peter Parker.

Coohan, Thomas. 1636. *The Haven of Health*. London: Printed by Anne Griffin for Roger Ball.

Collier, Jeremy. 1695. *Mischellanies upon Moral Subjects* [sic.]. London: Printed for Sam Keeble.

Crawford, Patricia, and Laura, Gowing, eds. 1999. *Women's worlds in seventeenth-century England*. London and New York: Routledge.

Culpepper, Nicholas. 1652. *The English Physitian, or, an Astrologo-Physical Discourse of the Vulgar Herbs of this Nation.* London: Printed by Peter Cole.

Dacombe, Lucia. 2004. "'To what purpose does it think': dreams, sick bodies and confused minds in the Age of Reason." *History of Psychiatry* 15 (4): 395–416.

Davies, Owen. 2003. "The nightmare experience, sleep paralysis, and witchcraft accusations." *Folklore* 114: 181–203.

—. 2007. *The Haunted: a social history of ghosts*. Houndsmills, and New York: Palgrave Macmillan.

De Jong, Joop T. V. M. 2005. "Cultural variation in the clinical presentation of sleep paralysis." *Transcultural Psychiatry* 42 (1): 78–92.

Ferrand, James. 1640. *Epotomania: or a Treatise Discoursing of the Essence, Causes, Symptomes, Prognosticks, and Cure of Love or Erotique Melancholy.* Oxford: Printed by L. Luchfield and are to be sold by Edward Forrest.

Gardiner, Edmund. 1611. *Phisical and approved medicines, as well in meere simples, as compound observations.* London: Printed [by E. Allde] for Methew Lownes.

Gross, Daniel, and M. Gross. 2006. *The secret history of emotion: from Aristotle's Rhetoric to modern brain science.* Chicago: University of Chicago Press.

Heywood, Thomas. 1635. *The hierarchie of the blessed angells*. London: Printed by Adam Islip.

Hillman, David, and Carla Mazzio. 1997. *The body in parts: fantasies of corporeality in early modern Europe.* London: Routledge.

Hinton, Devon E., Vuth Pich, Dara Chhean, and Mark H. Pollack, 2005. "'The ghost pushes you down': sleep paralysis-type panic attacks in a Khmer refugee population." *Transcultural Psychiathry* 42 (1): 46–77.

Hobbes, Thomas. 1651. *Philosophicall rudiments concerning government and society*. London: Printed by J.G. for R. Royston.

Hufford, David J. 1982. *The terror that comes in the night: an experience-centred study of supernatural assault traditions.* Philadelphia: University of Pennsylvania Press.

—. 2005. "Sleep paralysis and spiritual experience." *Transcultural Psychiatry* 42 (1): 11–45.

James I. 1603. *Daemonologie in forme of a dialogue, divided into three book.* London: Printed by Arnold Hatfield for Robert Waldgrave.

Jones, Ernest. 1951. *On the nightmare.* New York: Liveright.

Kathman, David. 2004. "Heywood, Thomas (*c.*1573–1641)." In *Oxford Dictionary of National Biography*, edited by H. C. G. Matthew, and Brian, oldalszám. Harrison, Oxford: OUP. http://www.oxforddnb.com.myaccess.library.utoronto.ca/view/article/13190, accessed January 27, 2010.

Kompanje, E. J. O. 2008. "'The devil lay upon her and held her down': Hypnagogic hallucinations and sleep paralysis described by the Dutch physician Isbrand van Diemerbroeck (1609–1674) in 1664." *Journal of Sleep Research* 17: 464–7.

Laqueur, Thomas. 2004. *Solitary Sex: a cultural history of masturbation.* New York: Zone Books.

Law, Susan, and Laurence J.Kirmayer. 2005. "Inuit interpretations of sleep paralysis." *Transcultural Psychiatry* 42 (1): 93–112.

Loyer, Pierre le. 1605. *A treatise of specters or straunge sights, visions and apparitions appearing sensibly unto men.* London: Printed by Val. S[immes] for Mathew Lownes.

Mackay, Christopher, trans. 2009. *The Hammer of Witches: a complete translation of the Malleus Maleficarum*. Oxford: Oxford University Press.

Marilla, E. L. 1944. "Henry and Thomas Vaughan." *The Modern Language Review* 39 (2): 180–3.

McNally, R. J., and Clancy, S. A. 2005. "Sleep Paralysis, Sexual Abuse and Space Alien Abduction." Transcultural Psychiatry 2005 (1): 113–22.

Napier, Richard. [16??]. "Medical Notes." Bodleian Library, *Ashmole* 412.

—. [16??]. "Medical Notes." Bodleian Library, *Ashmole* 221.

—. [16??]. "Medical Notes." Bodleian Library, *Ashmole* 217.

Nash, Thomas. 1594. *The terrors of the night or, A discourse of apparitions.* London: Printed by John Danter for William Jones.

Oates, Caroline. 2003. "Cheese gives you Nightmares: Old Hags and Heartburn." *Folklore* 114: 205–25.

Oatley, Keith. 2004. *Emotions: a brief history.* Oxford: Blackwell.

Oldridge, Darren. 2002. "Protestant conceptions of the Devil in Early Stuart England." *History* 85: 32–46.

Owen, Alex. 2004. *The place of enchantment: British Occultism and the Culture of the Modern.* Chicago: Chicago University Press.

Parker, Jennifer D., and Susan J. Blackmore. 2002. "Comparing the content of sleep paralysis and dream reports." *Dreaming* 12 (1): 45–59.

Paradis, Cheryl M., and Steven Friedman. 2005. "Sleep paralysis in African Americans with panic disorder." *Transcultural Psychiatry* 42 (1): 123–34.

Ray, Rajat Kant. 2001. *Exploring emotional history: gender, mentality and literature in the Indian awakening.* New Delhi, New York: Oxford University Press.

Reddy, William M. 2001. *The navigation of feeling: a framework for the history of emotions*. Cambridge: Cambridge University Press.

Rogers, John. 1653. *Ohel or Beth-shemesh A tabernacle for the sun, or, Irenicum evangelicum.* London: Printed for R.I. and G. and H. Eversden.

Roper, Lyndal. 1994. *Oedipus and the Devil: witchcraft, sexuality and religion in early modern Europe*. London: Routledge.

Rosenwein, Barbara H. 2003. *Emotional communities in the early middle ages.* London: Cornell University Press.

Salmon, William. 1694. *The Anatomy of Human Bodies; comprehending the most Modern Discoveries and Curiosities in that Art*. London: Printed for W. Whitwood at the Angel and Bible in Little Britain.

Schegoleva, Anna. 2001. *Sleepless in Japan: the kanashibari phenomenon*. Oxford: Oxford Brookes University.

Scot, Reginald. 1584. *The discoverie of witchcraft.* London: by [Henry Denham for] William Brome.

Semiz, Umit B., Cengiz Basoglu, Servet Ebrinc, and Mesut Cetin. 2008. "Nightmare disorder, dream anxiety, and subjective sleep quality in patients with borderline personality disorder." *Psychiatry and Clinical Neurosciences* 62: 48–55.

Stearnes, C. Z., and P. Stearnes. 1988. *Emotion and social change: toward a new psychohistory*. New York: Holmes & Meier.

Stearnes, Peter. 1986. *Anger: the struggle for emotional control in America's history*. Chicago: University of Chicago Press.

—. 1989. *Jealousy: the evolution of an emotion in American history*. New York: New York University Press.

—. 1998. *An emotional history of the United States*. New York: New York University Press.

—. 1999. *Battleground of desire: the struggle for self-control in modern America*. New York: New York University Press.

Szklo-Coxe, Mariana, Terry Young, Laura Finn, and Emmanuel Mignot. 2007. "Depression: relationships to sleep paralysis and other sleep disturbances in a community sample." *Journal of Sleep Research* 16: 297–312.

Tryon, Thomas. 1689. *A treatise of dreams & visions wherein the causes, natures, and uses, of nocturnal representations, and the communications both of good and evil angels, as also departed souls, to mankind. Are theosophically unfolded.* London: s.n.

Vaughan, Thomas. 1741. *Alchemical notes.* British Library, Sloane f.107.

Walkington, Thomas. 1607. *The optick glasse of humors. Or The touchstone of a golden temperature.* London: Imprinted by John Windet for Martin Clerke.

Walsham, Alexandra. 1999. *Providence in early modern England.* Oxford: Oxford University Press.

Willis, Thomas. 1684. *Dr Willis's Practice of Physick, Being the whole Works of that Renowned and Famous Physician.* London: T. Dring, C. Harper, and J. Leigh.

Yeung, Albert, Yong Xu, and Doris F. Chang. 2005. "Prevalence and illness beliefs of sleep paralysis among Chinese psychiatric patients in China and the United States." *Transcultural Psychiatry* 42 (1): 135–45.

Zika, Charles. 2002. *Exorcising our demons: magic, witchcraft and visual culture in early modern Europe.* Leiden: Brill.

BURNT WITHOUT FIRE: THE ILLNESS DEMON IN BULGARIAN LATE MEDIEVAL MAGICAL TEXTS

SVETLANA TSONKOVA

Introduction

Supernatural perpetrators of illnesses have appeared in many traditions throughout human history. They are called by different names and may cause a variety of diseases or damage to the health of both humans and animals. Being extremely harmful and dangerous, and threatening a crucial aspect of human existence, these malevolent agents occupy a key position among supernatural beings. In connection with this, the counteraction to these perpetrators constitutes an important part of magical practice (Barb 1966; Spier 1993).

The object of this article is one such malevolent supernatural agent—the *нежит* (henceforth the *nezhit)*, an illness demon, as it appears in a group of late medieval Bulgarian magical texts. Here I shall focus on two issues. Firstly, to present the specific characteristic features of the *nezhit*, as preserved in the Bulgarian textual source materials. It is an interesting and powerful figure with a complex image and behaviour. It also interacts with supernatural agents, humans and animals on several levels. On account of these reasons, the *nezhit* is definitely worth being included in the long list of supernatural perpetrators of illness.

Secondly, my article deals with the various means of protection against the *nezhit* through the use of texts and objects. I am also especially interested in one particular aspect: how the textual source material refers to the use of magical objects as protective amulets. This issue relates to my interest in aspects of the practical daily life of magic and magical texts. To my mind, the texts about the *nezhit* provide good examples of positive practical magic.

The source materials

The source materials for this article are twelve texts dealing with the *nezhit*. They are preserved in *Trebnik* (Euchologion) № 622, a seventeenth-century manuscript kept in the St. St. Cyril and Methodius National Library in Sofia. The manuscript is described and partially published by B. Tsonev in the second volume of his *List and Description of the Slavic manuscripts in the National Library in Sofia* (Tsonev 1923, 132–8. This publication includes all twelve texts about the *nezhit* available in the manuscript). On the basis of some parts of the content and of some philological peculiarities, Tsonev regards the manuscript to have been written and used in Macedonia (Tsonev 1923, 138). So far, there is no more detailed research on the place of origin and the dating of this particular prayer book, and these questions remain open to scholarly debate (Tsonev dated the manuscript on the basis of the watermark: Tsonev 1910, V–IX). There are, however, medieval Bulgarian texts against the *nezhit* from a much earlier date. They are preserved on lead amulets from the tenth to the twelfth centuries (Popkonstantinov and Konstantinova 1998; Popkonstantinov and Kronsteiner 1994). These texts, cited below, are important for the analysis of prayers against the *nezhit*, and are preserved in late medieval Bulgarian manuscripts.

Trebnik № 622 is, in fact, a miscellany, containing different texts in a Serbian redaction of the Old Church Slavonic language. These texts are (in the order of their arrangement in the manuscript):

- the Akathist hymn dedicated to the Mother of God
- fifty-three prayers which are to be read or pronounced at various occasions: celebration of church feasts, giving birth, baptism, marriage, confession, harvest, for curing different illnesses, when building and blessing a new house, when digging a new well, for purifying food vessels, for protection against different illnesses, for protection against the Devil, etc.
- canonical and non-canonical formulae for exorcising the Devil
- blessings for good health
- commemorative lists of people.

In terms of my research, I am particularly interested in the prayers in *Trebnik* № 622. According to the previous scholarship tradition, these texts can be divided into two groups: proper Orthodox Christian prayers, and prayers which deviate from the canon. Concerning the terminology of the second group, some scholars call these texts *apocryphal prayers* or *untrue prayers* (Petkanova 1999, 40; Almazov 1901, 221–340; Iatsimirskii 1913), while other researchers propose a differentiation between *canonical prayer, quasi-canonical prayer, apocryphal prayer, charm with functions of a prayer* and *magical charm* (Shniter 2001, 50–9).[1] In my opinion, two issues must be kept in mind here in connection with this particular *trebnik*. Firstly, there is no distinction between the texts in the manuscript itself. The twelve prayers against the *nezhit* are interspersed among the other prayers, without any notes or comments concerning the canonical or non-canonical character of the texts. Therefore, the later artificial division and classification of the texts is a rather problematic issue.

Secondly, finding a clear and non-misleading Bulgarian and English terminology for designating the medieval Bulgarian non-canonical texts or prayers is very much needed. These texts belong to a mixed genre. They have very specific features in terms of their intermediate position between religious prayer and magical charm, between sacred and prohibited, between popular religion and literature. Consequently, the discussion on the terminology of these texts is definitely a rather urgent scholarly task in general. As much as it requires extensive detailed research, and thus belongs to the future, it is out of the scope of this paper. As the texts are called *молитви* (prayers) in the *trebnik* itself, I will use this term together with the more general term, “texts” in this paper (for a detailed discussion on the terminological issues and also on the problem of including or excluding texts in the category of “prohibited” during the Bulgarian Middle Ages, see Shniter 2001, 50–69).

The above-mentioned twelve prayers concerning the *nezhit* are grouped together in the manuscript, under the title “Prayers about the Cursed Nezhit”. They are preceded by another prayer for a sick person and are followed by a prayer for blessing a new well. For the purpose of convenience in the writing of this paper, I shall enumerate the texts as [Text 1], [Text 2], [Text 3] etc. (Translation is mine, made according to the Old Church Slavonic text in the edition of Tsonev.)

The narrative of the texts

The content of the source material is dedicated exclusively to the illness demon *nezhit*. Texts 1, 2, 4, 5, 6 and 11 tell about the meeting between the

[1] The book is an examination of a series of apocryphal prayers, including ones against the *nezhit*, in terms of philological and stylistic peculiarities of the texts. The author also deals with the manner of transmission and with the reasons for the survival of non-canonical texts.

nezhit and different benevolent supernatural agents: Jesus Christ, Archangels Gabriel, Michael, Uriel and Raphael, St. Cosmas and St. Damian and St. John the Baptist. After declaring its damaging activities, the demon is conjured to stop causing harm and to step away from the sick person. Text 3 tells how Jesus Christ cured Adam of the *nezhit* by placing his hand on Adam's head. Texts 7 and 8 represent direct conjurations, where the demon is commanded in the name of the Creator and of the Archangels to stop its damaging activity and to withdraw to a remote location. Text 9 summons the church saints as helpers against the *nezhit*—it must bow down to them and stop doing harm.

The submission of the *nezhit* to a benevolent supernatural authority, higher and more powerful, constitutes the central motif of the narrative. Only Texts 10 and 12 represent a certain exception. In Text 10, the *nezhit* falls from the sky and is exterminated by the blind shepherds, and in Text 12, it is Adam and Eve who confront the demon.

The purpose of the prayers is to provide protection against the sickness and to expel the demon at a distance, from where it will not be able to do any harm. The texts declare the presence of the demon and the consequences to human health. On one side, the emphasis is on coping with the malefic effects of the *nezhit*. This is pointed out explicitly through strong prohibitive phrases and terms like "expulsion" and "chasing away". On the other hand, as one can read in Text 12, the prayer is supposed to be written on a piece of lead and carried as an amulet, so the prayer also has a preventive function:

> [Text 12] Adam had a nezhit and passed it to Eve. Eve passed the nezhit to the lead, the lead passed it to the sea, the sea passed it to the sand, the sand passed it to the beach, the beach passed it to the grass, the grass passed it to the dew, and the dew passed it to the sun. The sun came up, and the nezhit perished in God's servant (say the name) now, and forever and always.
> Write this prayer on lead.

Here we encounter the problem of orality and literacy. The examples suggest that the magical texts were produced orally (they had to be spoken, pronounced, etc.). At the same time, however, a strong literary component can be seen. (For a recent theoretical discussion on the interaction between oral and written in verbal magic: Smallwood 2004, 12). The prayers have survived in a manuscript, the authorship of which is uncertain, but it is very probable that it was written by a priest or a monk (Petkanova 1999, 24–2). Why would a member of the clergy copy or write down such texts? To some extent, this is connected to the fact that the priests and the monks were virtually the only people literate enough to create such a manuscript.[2]

Additionally, this leads to the question of whether the members of the clergy recognised the canonical or non-canonical character of the texts. And if so, why did they copy a text despite its non-canonical status? This issue is connected to the working hypothesis I have accepted for the purpose of my research:[3] most probably, long oral tradition and usage proved these texts to be very important and very effective and therefore worth being preserved in a more durable form. In this case, the prayers against the *nezhit* appear to be a key medical tool. The question of their canonical or non-canonical features is of less significance, the main concern being their practical effect. On the other hand, the written texts already suggest a certain level of literacy on the part of the user. As we shall see below, the orality/literacy relationship had immediate practical dimensions; the interaction between oral and written emerges again in the sphere of protective amulets.

According to Maria Shniter, the prayers against the *nezhit* have an explicit "magical-devotional-medical" purpose and are among the oldest texts of this type functioning in medieval Bulgaria (Shinter 2001, 53). They went through many transformations, yet they survived as strong magical-medical tools. They were a stable and effective system of protection against the *nezhit*—that was the crucial need and the prayers met this need in a most practical way. They belong to two fields—practical magic and medicine—which are strongly interconnected. This makes them even more effective and applicable. The texts and the amulets are the main components of the protection system, and they secure the

---

[2] Literacy among the clergy has a serious impact on the translation and distribution of apocryphal literature in medieval Bulgaria. Apocryphal texts were mainly translated, written down, copied and distributed by monks and priests: Petkanova 1999, 45.

[3] So far, only Shniter has discussed with some thoroughness this hypothesis in her book *Молитва и магия* [Prayer and magic], connecting the survival of texts (with non-canonical content) with the disintegration of the Bulgarian church authorities during the Ottoman invasion and occupation. She also suggests that a number of texts (including the ones against the *nezhit*) were preserved because of their formal similarities to canonical prayers, with no attention paid to their non-canonical content. In general, it is accepted in the secondary literature that the indexes of prohibited books were not widespread in medieval Bulgaria, therefore many priests did not have guidance as to which texts were permissible and which not: Petkanova 1999, passim; Petkanova 1981, passim.

successful functioning of the mechanism.[4] Pronouncing the texts unlocks their positive curative and protective power; writing them down strengthens the practical effect.

The sickness demon nezhit as a supernatural figure

The *nezhit* is a significant figure in the Slavic supernatural world. It belongs, however, to a long and ancient tradition of demons and bringers of illnesses. But where exactly does it stand among the other demonic figures? In terms of the main characteristics of the *nezhit* and of the health problems it causes, the following supernatural figures should be presented here.

Firstly, the *nezhit* can be related to the primordial malevolent elemental force Lilîtu/Lilith (Barb 1966, 5–8). Originally, Lilith is a Mesopotamian[5] female storm demon, associated with night, wind, illness and death. She represents a demonic paradigm and an operational field, later followed by many malevolent supernatural beings (parallels of Lilith can be found in numerous traditions: Assyrian, Jewish, Arabic, Byzantine, Slavic, etc: Gaster 1900; Winkler 1931, passim). Her activities include attacking pregnant women, kidnapping children, disturbing sleeping people and (which is important here) bringing diseases in general. Although the nature of the illnesses is not specified, it was suggested that Lilith causes fever, various disturbances of the senses and migraine (Barb 1966, passim; Hurwitz 1992, 38–40), which is the exact field of the *nezhit* too. This points towards a parallel between the Slavic demon and another Mesopotamian female demon: Lamashtu. Along with harming pregnant women, slaying children and drinking blood, she is also responsible for infesting the water, causing nightmares and bringing diseases, plague and death (Smith 2002, 84–139).

The *nezhit* is also related to the two other demons known from the Byzantine, Jewish and Slavic traditions[6]—Gyllou (responsible for infertility,

---

[4] For a discussion on the functions of magical texts in crisis situations: Wolf-Knuts 2009, 62–70. On the problem of oral/written transmission in terms of English charms material: Smallwood 2004, 11–31.

[5] The oldest sources regarding Lilith are Sumerian cuneiform inscriptions, circa 4000 BCE. The first pictorial representation of Lilith is circa 1950 BCE. She also appears in Assyrian sources, and later in numerous Jewish texts and in the Bible. (See Barb 1966, 4–5; Hurwitz 1992, 31–84).

[6] For example, Abyzou (under the name Vizusa) appears in a seventeenth-century Bulgarian charm against witches. In this text, Vizusa is one of the names of the

child mortality, sickness, demonic possession and death) and Abyzou (responsible for strangling newborn babies, deafness, blindness, severe pain and madness) (Barb 1966, 5). Its closest parallel, however, can be seen in the face of Antaura, a demon that comes out of the sea and brings migraine, and Abra, a demon that comes out of the sea, eats the bones of the afflicted person and wastes away their flesh. (Known from a Greek inscription, found on a third century CE silver lamella from Carnuntum, Austria. See Barb 1966, passim and especially 2–4; Spier 1993, 33–4. Concerning Abra, Barb redirects to texts, published by O. Janiewitsch, *Archiv für Religionswissenschaft*, 13 1910, 627–30; Barb 1966, 17). The *nezhit* and Antaura/Abra have identical operational fields: headache and body pain.

If we move to Slavic mythology, the *nezhit* can be described as an extremely malevolent supernatural being. Its name means "non-alive", or "non-human". Beyond that, when going into further detail, the different traditions attribute different characteristics to the *nezhit*. For example, the Russian Slavic tradition describes the *nezhit* as an unclean power, without soul and flesh, but with a human visage (Ryan 2005, 38). The *nezhit* is an elemental force, neither a human, nor a spirit. The term is used to designate a group of supernatural beings, namely the *leshii*, the *vodyanoi*, the *rusalka*, the *polevoi*, the *domovoi* and the *kikimora*, but not the supernatural dead (the *upyr'* and the *eretic*), nor the *chort* or the *bies* (Agapkina 2002, 319–21; Zelenin 1995, passim). Furthermore, the term can be used as a name for personified illness and as a synonym of demon (Ryan 2005, 38–9).

The Balkan traditions (Slavic and others) regard the *nezhit* to be an evil spirit, sometimes even the Devil himself. It is an unclean power, the bringer of different illnesses, which makes the affected person "non-alive" (Georgieva 1983, passim; Mitseva 1994, passim). But the *nezhit* can also be a creature, similar to a vampire, "the soul of a dead relative, which attacks sleeping people, sucks out their brain and makes them ill" (Ovcharov 1997). According to the Bulgarian tradition, the *nezhit* appears mainly as a perpetrator of illnesses of the head and of the senses. Interestingly enough, the Bulgarian *nezhit* does not have much of a connection with fever. It is the other key Slavic perpetrators of illnesses, the *tresavitsi,*[7] a group of female demons with a strong connection to the sea, who cause fever in the Bulgarian tradition.

---

witch listed by her in front of the Archangel Michael: Euchologion (NBKM № 273) in Tsonev 1910, 174–5.

[7] "Tresavitsa" means "shaking" or "shaker"; the word has the same stem as "treska" (fever).

As is visible in the examples below, the Bulgarian variant of the demon, however, differs from all these supernatural agents in one important aspect—it lacks the primordial connection with water and the sea, a typical feature of supernatural agents, especially as regards Antaura/Abra. This difference constitutes an important detail in the image of the *nezhit*. While the *tresavitsi* usually originate from the sea, the *nezhit* seems to be detached from this element (Ryan 1999, 42–6 and 217–68; Petkanova 1981, passim). The relation to water as an element of origin is testified to in only one of the texts, preserved on an amulet from the tenth century:

> Dear Lord Christ, triumph! The nezhit was coming from the Red Sea and met Jesus. And Jesus asked him: "Where are you going?" He answered: "I am going to the human, to drink his brain, to shed his blood, to break his bones". Then Jesus said: "I conjure you, nezhit! Do not go to the human, but go to a deserted place…find the deer…enter their [sic!] heads Drink their brains, shed their blood, break their bones and tear their joints, because they can stand any illness. Go there and do not come back!" Now and forever, until the Judgment Day, prepare for him. Fear the Lord, sitting on the cherubic throne, everything visible and invisible is afraid of him. Fear above all the Lord, the glory belongs to him forever. Amen! (Popkonstantinov and Konstantinova 1998, 29; Popkonstantinov and Kronsteiner 1994. The translation is mine, after the Old Church Slavonic text).

This peculiarity is only one of the unstudied aspects of the *nezhit*. For the moment, it remains an open scholarly question closely connected to the problem of the origin of the demon. Was the connection with the sea lost in some stage of the development of the *nezhit*? Or has it never been part of its characteristics? If so, what is the tradition from which the demon originates? Did the *nezhit* lose or acquire other specific features in a later stage of its development?

All these important questions about the *nezhit*'s origin as a malevolent supernatural agent, its thorough earlier development and its historical parallels require separate detailed research.[8] It is important, however, to

---

[8] There is a great need to discover historical parallels of the *nezhit*. Putting this demon in its proper historical and cultural perspective requires serious discussion. Several key books provide valuable materials for comparison. For example, Ohrt provides an opportunity for comparison with Danish material. Also, Pradel provides Greek examples. Spamer gives Western European medieval parallels. Winkler provides an insight into the Arabic tradition. This broader comparison between the Bulgarian texts about the *nezhit* and their parallels is a part of my current research work. Together with the question of continuity, it is also important

point out one fact. If we accept that the *nezhit* is of a rather ancient origin, then the examined late medieval Bulgarian euchologion and the surviving amulets provide an image of the *nezhit* which is a result of a long and complex cultural interaction. Here we can see the demon at a very late stage of its existence as a supernatural figure. For the purposes of this article, it is important to outline the following particular points concerning the Bulgarian late medieval tradition as preserved in the examined manuscript.

Firstly, the *nezhit* preserves most of the features characteristic of older illness demons, in terms of activities and a clearly defined operational sphere. The main differences are: the *nezhit* is a male being and his connection with the sea is rather loose. Also, his image appears to be a combination between the characteristics of Slavic and non-Slavic demonic figures; (on the answered question about the connections between the nezhit and different Slavic pre-Christian supernatural beings, see Ovcharov 1997, 106–107; Ryan 2004, 113–27). Secondly, protection against the *nezhit* exists as a fully developed system: it is provided and supported exclusively through the means of verbal magic. The power of the demon can be opposed most effectively through the power of words. Thirdly, protection against the *nezhit* is additionally very much connected with amulets. Thus, the demon is involved in the field of practical magic. The counteraction to the illness is additionally strengthened by the usage of magical objects. These points show that the figure of the *nezhit* has to be examined not only in the strict terms of demonology, but also in the broader perspective of protective practical magic.

Characteristics of the nezhit according to the Bulgarian source materials

The *nezhit* appears in several medieval and late medieval Bulgarian texts, preserved on amulets and in manuscripts. Up to now, there has been no exact calculation of their number. Such a calculation would be interesting, although will remain open, as new examples may be discovered at any moment. On some occasions, a manuscript contains not only one, but a

---

to examine the details of the medieval environment of the *nezhit*. For the purpose of this study, the book by Spamer is of special value. As is shown further on, Spamer's book provides valuable parallels for one of the most interesting Bulgarian prayers against the *nezhit*, namely Text 10, featuring the enigmatic figures of the blind shepherds (Ohrt 1917–1921; Pradel 1907; Spamer 1958; Winkler 1931).

group of texts about the *nezhit*.[9] The manuscript examined in this article represents probably the biggest surviving group of prayers gathered together in one book. In this respect, *Trebnik* № 622 is especially suitable for research. It provides a longer corpus of texts, thereby providing an opportunity to trace the characteristic features of the demon and its activities in a series of prayers.

The twelve texts in *Trebnik* № 622 do not give a description of the physical outlook of the demon.[10] The source material describes it with such adjectives and phrases as "rabid" and "origin of every illness" (Text 1 and 7), "cursed" (Text 5), "deaf" and "unclean illness" (Text 6), and "menacing" (Text 8). The *nezhit* is usually alone, a single agent, unlike other malevolent figures (like, for example, the *tresavitsi*, which most commonly appear as a group of women).

The demon's place of origin is unspecified as well. In Text 1, Jesus meets the demon somewhere on his way down from the Seventh Heaven. According to Text 5, the *nezhit* falls on humans from above; it is an illness similar to and transmitted by the wind, and attacks in the mornings, at noon and in the evenings. In Text 10, the *nezhit* falls from the sky. In Text 2 and 4, different supernatural agents meet the demon somewhere on the road.[11]

Judging from the pronouns used in the texts, the demon is regarded as male. Not only in *Trebnik* № 622, but also in all the other manuscripts, the *nezhit* is referred to as "him". This is one of the specific features which distinguishes this demon from other perpetrators of illnesses. Unlike most of the other bringers of diseases, the late medieval Bulgarian *nezhit* is a male creature (Barb 1966, 5–6; Ryan 2005, 44–46).

The main activity of the *nezhit* is to bring illnesses connected with the human head and the senses. In Text 1, the demon says:

---

[9] For example, the manuscripts *Sbornik* № 273 from the seventeenth century, containing four prayers against the nezhit and *Trebnik* № 1386 from 1839, containing five prayers against the nezhit. Both manuscripts are kept in the National Library "St. Cyril and Method" in Sofia (Tsonev, 1910, 174–5; Hristova and Karadjova and Vutova 1996, 73–5).

[10] To my knowledge, none of the texts from the other manuscripts provide such descriptions either.

[11] As was mentioned earlier, unlike many other perpetrators of illnesses, the Bulgarian variant of the *nezhit* rarely emerges from the sea. In my opinion, this unusual characteristic feature of the demon deserves serious further research, especially in terms of the *nezhit*'s appearance as a migraine bringer and an elemental force.

> I am going into the human head in order to bemuse the brain, to break the teeth and the jaws, to deafen the ears, to blind the eyes, to distort the mouth, to block up the nose, so there will be headache day and night.

In Text 2, the *nezhit* is conjured: "do not go into the human head, do not devastate the brain, do not distort the eyes!" and a few lines down, the demon itself declares: "I am the *nezhit*, I am going into the human head in order to bemuse the brain and to drink the blood". The same being causes "headache all day and all night long". Text 5 describes a man tortured by a severe pain in the head. In Text 6, the demon is conjured to leave the head and the eyes and not to "bemuse the brain or to blind the eyes", and, in Text 9, not "to shed blood or to twist the joints or to collect pus".

All these examples show that the *nezhit* causes rather serious health problems. The exact diagnosis, however, remains in question. The possibilities suggested so far and related to the Bulgarian variant of the demon differ significantly: teeth and gum afflictions (gingivitis), contagious infections of the bones and the joints, fever, migraine, *meningitis purulenta*, and different mental disorders (Ovcharov 1997, 107. Unfortunately, the author does not give more specific reference to studies dealing with the question of which actual disease(s) is/are presented by the *nezhit*). In comparison, the Romanian tradition also associates the *nezhit* with illnesses like *stomatitis ulcerosa*, catarrh, various skin diseases and purulent wounds (Timotin 2006). Despite its dubious medical character in the strict sense, the *nezhit* undoubtedly remains a significant figure in the realm of the supernatural (Atanassova 2003).

Protection against the nezhit through words

The source material shows that protection against the *nezhit* through words works on two levels.

First comes the level of the magical texts themselves. The purpose of their existence is to shield humans from the demon. Knowing, pronouncing, reading and writing these texts provide healing for those afflicted by the *nezhit* and protection for those who might encounter the demon in the future. Texts 7, 8 and 9 repeat the formula, "I conjure you, nezhit!" followed by commands to the demon. The *nezhit* is repeatedly threatened through the higher authority of benevolent supernatural agents, and banished from humankind into remote locations or into the head of a deer or a ram (for a parallel regarding transferring the illness to an animal, a medieval Greek text from Southern Italy in which Jesus Christ sends the migraine into the desolate mountains and into a bull's head, see Barb 1966, 3).

> [Text 7] I conjure you, nezhit, in the name of the holy Mother of God, holy John the Baptist, the Holy Apostles and all the heavenly powers, cherubim and seraphim, in the name of the holy archangels Michael, Gabriel, Uriel, Raphael and all the church saints. I conjure you, nezhit, not to enter humans, but to go into the forest and into the head of the deer and of the ram, there to wait until Doomsday, when Jesus Christ will judge the entire universe, and you too, nezhit, origin of every illness, be afraid of the Lord, sitting at the cherubic throne. I conjure you, nezhit, in the name of the God of Sabaoth and of the martyrs, stay far from the servant of God, depart from him and do not return, in the name of the Father and the Son.

An important feature here is the triple repetition of the phrase "I conjure you, nezhit!" The third reiteration strengthens even more the impact of the already strong phrase. Further on, the expulsion is extended through sending the demon "into the forest and into the head of the deer and of the ram". This "sending away from humans" motive is combined with an extensive list of benevolent heavenly figures (God, Virgin Mary, the archangels, the saints, etc.). The *nezhit* must obey their celestial superior authority and quit its malefic activities.

In the next example we read:

> [Text 8] I conjure you, nezhit, listen to the prayers and fear the Lord, Creator of everything. He rules over the wind, the sea, the earth, the beasts, the animals, the snakes, the birds, the angels, the archangels, the powers and all the earthly daemons. The abyss is horrible and everything trembles before it. You, menacing, step away from the human head, away from the servant of God, in the name of the Father, the Son and the Holy Ghost.

Here the phrase "I conjure you, nezhit!" appears only once, but in combination with the list of objects and beings under God's rule. This enumeration emphasises the omnipotence of the Lord and the obligation of the *nezhit* to obey the celestial superior authority.

The *nezhit* names and describes itself and its mission. This behaviour of the demon belongs to a rather ancient tradition and reveals another aspect of the usage of words and their power. Through its own speech, the *nezhit* heralds its intentions, but also exercises its power. Speaking out loud and describing its potential, is a usual, indeed almost mandatory feature in the behaviour of the demon.[12]

---

[12] One of the earliest parallels can be seen in the *Testament of Salomon*, where the demons are compelled to declare their activities: Conybeare, 1898. In a medieval Greek text, the Archangel Michael commands Abyzou to tell him her forty names

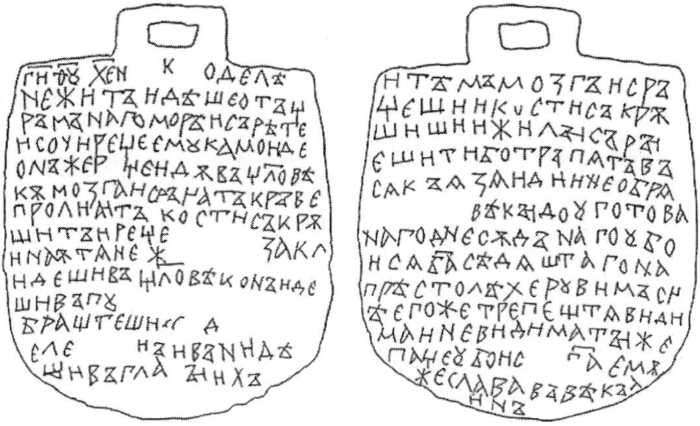

Lead amulet against the *Nezhit* demon from the tenth- and eleventh-century fort in Odarci, North-Eastern Bulgaria. Adapted from Popkonstantinov 2009.

Second is the level of the usage of words presented inside the texts. At their encounter with the demon, the supernatural figures always have a conversation with it. The key element here is the dialogue. It reveals the evil intentions of the *nezhit*, and also gives an opportunity for the benevolent figure to answer and to exercise their power towards the demon. This second level is in an entirely oral sphere. The demon relates its powers and activities, declares its evil intentions, and threatens humans. The benevolent supernatural figures question, conjure and pronounce orders against the *nezhit*. All the characters speak and communicate orally. Their nature and powers are expressed through speech. The conflict between the malevolent and the benevolent figures starts and develops entirely by oral means. Indeed, the result of this battle depends exclusively on the power of words. The dialogue is the key element and the crucial weapon in this verbal duelling (for a series of examples of verbal duelling between Christ and the personified illness, see: Spamer 1958, passim; for a general overview of verbal duelling: Dundes and Leach and Özkök 1970; Mathias 1976). The following text gives an excellent example of such verbal battling:

---

and what she is doing (Pradel 1907, 23–4). The list of activities and especially of names is also very important when confronting Gyllou: Spier 1993, 38.

> [Text 1] Jesus came down from the Seventh Heaven, from his home, met the nezhit and asked it: "Where are you going?" And the nezhit answered: "I am going into the human head, in order to bemuse the brain, to break the teeth and the jaws, to deafen the ears, to blind the eyes, to distort the mouth, to block up the nose, so that there will be headache day and night." And Jesus said to the nezhit: "Go back into the forest and enter the deer's head and the ram's head, because they can bear everything and still survive. And stay there until the end of Heaven and Earth. And fear the Lord who sits on the cherubic throne until He comes to judge the entire universe and you too, rabid nezhit, who are the source of every infirmity. I conjure you, nezhit! Depart from God's servant (say the name) in the name of the Father, the Son and the Holy Ghost."

Here, all the above-mentioned elements (the announcement of the malevolent activity, the list of health problems, the sending away into the head of an animal, the declaration of God's power) are incorporated in the words, pronounced respectively by the demon and by Jesus Christ. We can see a more complex narrative, a dialogue structure, where every character has his fixed set of phrases. (One prominent parallel is Spamer's Berufungssegen (Nr. 10), which contains a dialogue between Christ and the illness demon: Spamer 1958, 48 and 121).

In the next example we read:

> A nezhit was walking, and half a nezhit was walking, and the Archangel Gabriel met him and asked him: "Where are you going, nezhit, and half a nezhit, and a quarter of a nezhit?" [Text 2]

Here, the benevolent figure Archangel Gabriel initiates the dialogue by defining the *nezhit* and giving it certain "impossible" physical parameters. Thus, the impossibility motive provides ways of control over the demon through the definition of its physical existence and through its division and fragmentation.

On both levels, it is the verbal conjuration that is the primary tool for coping with the *nezhit*. The benevolent characters of the prayers speak with the demon, command it and conjure it. The user of the prayers is supposed to pronounce, read or write them. This activity guarantees successful healing or protection. In the case of Texts 7, 8 and 9, the user of the texts has to turn directly to the *nezhit*. Thus, the act of pronouncing the text of the prayer occupies the central position in this particular magical practice.

Protection against the nezhit through objects

As has been shown above, verbal communication has a key role in the interaction with the demon. This method of protection, however, does not stand alone. It is very closely connected with the use of material objects. Protection against the *nezhit* through objects also has two levels.

First, there is the level of the usage of the various objects as described in the prayers themselves. In Text 4, seven archangels are sharpening seven knives and carrying seven candles, with which they will cut and burn the *nezhit*.

> [Text 4] Seven angels were walking, seven archangels were walking, sharpening seven knives, bearing seven candles. Michael and Gabriel met them and asked them, "Where are you going, you seven angels?" And the angels answered, "We are going to slay the nezhit, to burn it with candles, and to remove the blood from the eyes of God's servant (say the name) now, and forever and always."

This text relies on the magical power of the number seven. It has a Bulgarian parallel in a text from the seventeenth-century book of hours № 631, kept in the St. St. Cyril and Methodius National Library in Sofia (Tsonev 1923, 151–2):[13]

> Seven winds and seven fires, each one differently heated, went out. The Holy Mother of the Lord together with the 12 Apostles met them, and asked them: Where are you going, you winds, gales and fires?...

In Text 11, Simon is using a knife to cut out the roots of the illness. In Text 12, Eve receives the *nezhit* and "passes it" to the lead. This is also the text which is explicitly meant to be written on a piece of lead and carried as an amulet, for at the end of Text 12, cited above, we read, "Write this prayer on lead" (about lead amulets: Graf 1997, passim; Faraone 1999, 119–31). Fortunately, the other element of the health-protection system, a lead amulet from the twelfth century, has also survived (Ovcharov 1997, 106. The translation is mine, after the Old Church Slavonic text). It contains the following text:

---

[13] This text contains a number of Slavic words which are difficult to translate. Their interpretation requires separate research beyond the scope of this paper. For comparison, the number seven is important for Lamashtu—she has seven names and often appears as seven witches: Hurwitz 1992, 31–62.

> Adam had a nezhit. He went and gave it to Eve. Eve gave the nezhit to the lead, the lead passed it to the water, the sea passed it to the shores/banks [?],[14] the shores/banks gave it to the grass, the grass gave it to the dew, and the dew gave it to the sun. The sun dried the dew; let the nezhit dry the same way in Marina.

This leads to the second level, where the texts themselves can be transferred into material objects and used as protective amulets. The prayers not only have to be pronounced or read; they also have to be written down. This act puts them into the sphere of material amulets, into the sphere of interaction between purely verbal magical formulae and material magical objects containing certain texts. In this case, the prayers against the *nezhit* become a part of the complex phenomenon of the protective/healing amulet. The creation of a specific magical object probably produced better magical results. As the medieval Bulgarian amulets containing prayers against the *nezhit* are dated from the tenth and eleventh centuries, protection against the demon through a combination of words and objects appears to be of old and stable character (about medieval Bulgarian amulets: Popkonstantinov 1994, 145–67; Popkonstantinov 1996, 243–76). Its effective function is strengthened by the double level of defence: the verbal and the material.

A special case: the nezhit and the shepherds

Text 10 is the most interesting text in the group, a special case worth presenting separately. Here, the blind shepherds encounter the demon and manage to eliminate it:

> [Text 10] The nezhit fell from the sky, the blind shepherds saw it. They chased it without feet, caught it without hands, tied it without a rope, burned it without fire, killed it without a knife, and ate it without mouths. From the bones, the nezhit went into the flesh, into the skin, into the hair, and melted, like salt in water. Let it disappear in the same way from God's servant (say the name) now, and forever and always.

This particular text is interesting not only because it illustrates the usage of magical objects. It also differs from the others in its lack of the usual benevolent supernatural authority. Instead, we can see the mysterious figures of the blind shepherds themselves performing the role usually attributed to Jesus Christ or to different saints. The motif of the shepherds

[14] The original contains an unknown Slavic word. Here I give the translation accepted by scholars as the most probable.

defeating the sickness appears much earlier, for example in the following charm:

> Corce corcedo stagne, pastores te invenerunt, sine manibus collegerunt, sine foco coxerunt, sine dentibus comederunt (Spamer 1958, 323).[15]

And also, in the example:

> Stolpus a coelo cecidit, hunc morbum pastores invenerunt, sine manibus collegerunt, sine igni coxerunt, sine dentibus comederunt.[16]

By way of comparison, this motif can also be connected with a healing charm in Bulgarian folklore from a later period (Georgieva 1990. The author quotes examples from folklore collected in the nineteenth century). There, the three shepherds guard and tend the illness (a certain infection); one of them is deaf, the second one blind, and the third one dumb or crippled. Because of the disabilities of its guardians, the illness escapes and is later eaten by a wolf. This narrative is used in charms against the above-mentioned infection. Here we can see a completely inverted situation. In the texts against the *nezhit,* the strange shepherds are benevolent supernatural agents, successfully defeating the illness. In later folklore tradition, the three shepherds are demonic figures who ensure the success of the evil activity of the illness (ibidem).

On the other hand, the "impossibility" motif of casting away the illness, chasing it without feet, catching it without hands, burning it without fire, etc., represents a special condition for controlling the illness. When put in this "impossible" situation and confronted in "impossible" ways, it becomes possible to defeat the *nezhit*. This motif relates the Bulgarian text to the *Gerichtssegen* presented by Spamer (Spamer 1958, 54 and 317–9). In the German text, the aim of which is to provide good luck and success, we see three dead men, each of them with different physical defects:

> Vor Gericht und Rath zu Recht behalten.
> Jesus Naearenus Rux Judzorum. Zuerst trag diesen Charakter bei dir in der Figur, alsdann sprich folgende Worte: Ich N. N. trete vor des Richtes

[15] This Latin text is a quotation from *De Medicamentis*, XXI, 3 written by Marcellus Empiricus (Marcellus Burdigalensis/Marcel of Bordeaux)—a Gallic medical writer from the fourth/fifth century CE: Stannard 1973.

[16] This is another example by Marcellus Empiricus, quoted by Pócs 2009, 34. The article also discusses the interpretations of the "demon falling from the sky" motif and its parallels.

> Haus, de schauen 3 todte Männer zum Fenster heraus, der eine hat keine Zunge, der andere hat keine Lunge, der dritte erkrankt, erblindt und verstummt. Da ist, wann du vor's Gericht gehest. Oder Amt und eine Rechtsache hast, dagegen dir der Richter nicht günstig ist, so sprich: wenn du gegen ihm gehest, den oben schon stehenden Segen (ibidem).

It is a complex network of positive and negative supernatural figures, exercising their power against each other. The outcome of the struggle has or will have an immediate effect on human health.

Concluding remarks and further considerations

According to the presented source material, the *nezhit* proves to be a crucial malevolent figure in Bulgarian late medieval medicine magic. The ways in which to cope with it give a good example of practical medical magic. It is a case where a supernatural perpetrator of illness attacks a vital aspect of human existence. The means for defence against the demon connect the supernatural sphere with daily life. The prayers can be used as the main means of defence/healing, but they can also be included in the more complex practice of the usage of protective/healing amulets.

Concerning further research, I have recently been working on the incantations against the *nezhit* in terms of putting them into historical context. As is suggested in the secondary literature (Barb 1964, 1–22; Barb 1966, passim; Spier 1993), there are traces of continuity from Babylonian protective incantations against demons of illnesses to Classical Greek and Byzantine ones. The Slavic texts also show similarities with much older examples.[17] Therefore, it is important to trace the connections between the Bulgarian medieval prayers against the *nezhit* and similar texts from other traditions. The primary analysis of previous scholars shows that the incantations against the *nezhit* can be related to Byzantine, Syrian and Egyptian examples in terms of constructive elements of the text, features of the demon, the practice of writing the texts on material supports, and prescriptions for constant everyday usage. I plan to continue with the further analysis of the practical aspects of the texts and their use as tools for immediate magical protection.

---

[17] Ryan 1999, 9–30, where the author on several occasions discusses the connections between Slavic incantations and older examples from Byzantium, Egypt and Asia Minor. The author's focus is mainly on Russian texts, but he also discusses questions concerning Slavic tradition in general. See also Spamer 1958, passim.

Another necessary direction for future research is to examine the medieval Bulgarian sources about the *nezhit* in comparison with later Bulgarian folklore material. Such an interdisciplinary research will provide us with a much broader picture in terms of daily life usage, practicality and effectiveness. It will probably also provide answers to questions concerning the interaction between the oral and written. If we regard "magic as a crossroads, as a crossing-point" between different cultures, but also a complex network of different relationships, interactions, conflicts and forms of perception and transmission of motives and patterns within a certain society in a certain period, it is important to examine and understand how the Bulgarian source material relates to the same (or similar) sources from other Slavic territories as well as to sources from wider geographical and cultural contexts (Graf 1997, 1–19; Kieckhefer 2000, 1–3 and 44–5; Kieckhefer 2002, 2). It is also important, however, to look carefully at the connections between the Bulgarian late medieval texts and other Bulgarian (medieval or other) sources about the *nezhit*. It would be interesting and useful if all the medieval texts and all the folklore material about the *nezhit* were to be examined as a whole corpus, in terms of tracing the development of the demon and determining its context. Such research would certainly reveal other new dimensions to the story of this demonic being. Thus, a key malevolent supernatural figure and perpetrator of illnesses will find its place in the complex context of medical magic.

References

Agapkina, T. A. 2002. *Slavianskaia mifologiia: entsiklopedicheskii slovar* [Slavic Mythology: Encyclopedia]. Moscow: Mezdunarodn'ie otnoshenia.

Almazov, A. I. 1901. *Apokrificheskie molitv'i i zagovor'i* [Apocryphal prayers and charms]. Odessa: Letopis Novorossiikogo Universiteta.

Atanassova, Diana. 2003. "The Prayer-Book of Niketa (№ 646 NBKM): A Case Study." *Scripta & e-Scripta* 1: 187–96.

Barb, A. A. 1966. "Antaura. The Mermaid and the Devil's Grandmother." *Journal of the Warburg and Courtauld Institutes* 29: 1–24.

Conybeare, F. C. 1898. "The Testament of Solomon." *The Jewish Quarterly Review* 11 (1): 1–45.

Dundes, Alan, Jerry W. Leach, and Bora Özkök. 1970. "The Strategy of Turkish Boys' Verbal Dueling Rhymes." *The Journal of American Folklore* 83 (329): 325–49.

Faraone, Christopher A. 1999. *Ancient Greek Love Magic*. Cambridge, Mass.: Harvard University Press.

Gaster, Moses. 1900. "200 Years of a Charm Against the child-stealing Witch." *Folk-Lore* 11: 129–62.
Georgieva, Ivanichka. 1983. *Bălgarska narodna mitologiia* [Bulgarian popular mythology]. Sofia: Nauka i izkustvo.
—. 1990. "Baianiiata kato kosmogonichna kontseptsiia v bălgarskata narodna kultura [Charms as a cosmogonic concept in the Bulgarian popular culture]." *Vekove* 6: 13.
Graf, Fritz. 1997. *Magic in the Ancient World*. Cambridge, Mass., and London: Harvard University Press.
Hristova, B., D. Karadjova, and N. Vutova. 1996. *Opis na slavianskite rukopisi v sofiiskata narodna biblioteka* V [List and description of the Slavic manuscripts in the National Library in Sofia 5]. Sofia: Edition of St. St. Cyril and Methodius National Library.
Hurwitz, Siegmund. 1992. *Lilith, the First Eve: Historical and Psychological Aspects of the Dark Feminine*. Einsiedeln, Switzerland: Daimon.
Iatsimirskii A. I. 1913. "K istorii lozhn'ih molitv v juzhnoslavianskoi pis'menosti [On the history of false prayers in South Slavic literature]." *Izv. ORJAS* 18 (3): 1–102, and 18 (4): 16–126.
Kieckhefer, Richard. 2000. *Magic in the Middle Ages*. Cambridge: Cambridge University Press.
Mathias, Elizabeth. 1976. "La Gara Poetica: Sardinian Shepherds' Verbal Dueling and the Expression of Male Values in an Agro-Pastoral Society." *Ethos* 4 (4): 483–507.
Mitseva, Evgenia. 1994. *Nevidimi notshni gosti* [Invisible night guests]. Sofia: Bălgarski folklore.
Ohrt, Ferdinand Christian Peter. 1917–21. *Danmarks Trylleformler* 1. København: Nordisk Forlag. (FF publications. Northerns series 3.)
Ovcharov, Nikolay. 1997. "Prokletiiat Nezhit" [The cursed nezhit]. *Bălgarska etnologiia* 1–2: 104–8.
Petkanova, D. 1981. *Stara bălgarska literatura v sedem toma 1. Apokrifi* [Old Bulgarian literature in seven volumes 1. Apocrypha]. Sofia: Bălgarska Akademiya na Naukite.
—. 1999. *Starobălgarska literatura—entsiklopediia* [Old Bulgarian Literature-Encyclopedia]. Sofia: Petur Beron.
Pócs, Éva. 2009. "Miracles and Impossibilities in Magic Folk Poetry." In *Charms, Charmers and Charming: International Research on Verbal Magic*, edited by Jonathan Roper, 27–53. New York: Palgrave Macmillan.
Popkonstantinov, Kazimir 1994. "Apokrifna molitva ot X–XI vek vrkhu oloven amulet ot. s. Odurci [Apocryphal prayer from 10–11 century on

a lead amulet from Odurtzi village].” In *Sbornik v čest na akad. Dimităr Angelov* [Festschrift in honour of academician Dimităr Angelov], edited by Velizar Velkov 288-292. Sofia: Bulgarska Akademiya na Naukite.

—. 1996. “Novootkriti epigrafski pametnizi ot X–XI v. (Apokrifni molitvi vurhu olovo) [Recently found epigraphic monuments from 10–11 century (Apocryphal Prayers on Lead)].” In *Trudove na II kongres po strobulgaristika* [Papers from the second congress in Old Church Slavonic Studies], sine editor, 243-276. Sofia: Bălgarska Akademiya na Naukite.

—. 2009. “Zaklinatelnite molitvi varhu olovni amuleti ot srednovekovna Bălgaria i paralelite im v trebnici of srednovekovna Serbia” [Conjurative prayers on lead amulets from medieval Bulgaria and their parallels in euchologia from medieval Serbia].” *Зборник радова Византолошког института,* XLVI /*Recueil des travaux de l'Institut d'études byzantines* XLVI: 341–51.

Popkonstantinov, Kazimir, and V. Konstantinova. 1998. “Za dva olovni amuleta s apokrifni molitvi ot X v [About two lead amulets with apocryphal prayers from tenth century].” *Paleoslavistika i epigrafika. V pamet na Iv. Gulubov*: 28–31.

Popkonstantinov, Kazimir, and O. Kronsteiner. 1994. “Altbulgarische Inschriften.” *Die slavischen Sprachen* 36: 39–40.

Pradel, Fritz. 1907. *Griechische und süditalienische Gebete, Beschwörungen und Rezepte des Mittelalters*. Giessen: A. Töpelmann.

Ryan, W. F. 1999. The *Bathhouse at Midnight: An Historical Survey of Magic and Divination in Russia*. University Park, Pa., and Stroud, UK: Sutton and Pennsylvania State University Press.

—. 2004. “Eclecticism in the Russian Charm Tradition.” In *Charms and Charming in Europe*, edited by Jonathan Roper, 113–27. New York: Palgrave Macmillan.

—. 2005. “Ancient Demons and Russian Fevers.” In *Magic and the Classical Tradition*, edited by Charles Burnett, and W. F. Ryan, 37–58. London: Warburg Colloquia 38.

Shniter, Maria. 2001. *Molitva i magiia* [Prayer and magic]. Sofia: Universitetsko izdatelstvo “Sv. Kliment Ohridski”.

Smallwood, T. M. 2004. “The Transmission of Charms in English, Medieval and Modern.” In *Charms and Charming in Europe*, edited by Jonathan Roper, 11–31. New York: Palgrave Macmillan.

Smith, William Robertson. 2002. *Religion of the Semites*. New Brunswick, N.J.: Transaction Publishers.

Spamer, Adolf. 1958. *Romanusbüchlein: historisch-philologischer Kommentar zu einem deutschen Zauberbuch.* Berlin: Akademie-Verlag.

Spier, Jeffrey. 1993. "Medieval Byzantine Magical Amulets and Their Tradition." *Journal of the Warburg and Courtauld Institutes* 56: 25–62.

Stannard, Jerry. 1973. "Marcellus of Bordeaux and the Beginnings of the Medieval *Materia Medica*." *Pharmacy in History* 15: 48–51.

Timotin, Emanuela. 2006. "*Ieşi, năjite, pricăjite*...de la molitvele minciunoase le descăntece [Get out, bloody *năjit*... From "false prayers" to charms]." *Limba română* 55: 72–83.

Tsonev, B. 1910. *Opis na slaviianskite rukopisis v sofiiskata narodna biblioteka* I. [List and description of the Slavic manuscripts in the National Library in Sofia]. Sofia: Edition of the St. Cyril and Methodius National Library.

—. 1923. *Opis na slaviianskite rukopisis v sofiiskata narodna biblioteka* II. [List and description of the Slavic manuscripts in the National Library in Sofia]. Sofia: Edition of the St. Cyril and Methodius National Library.

Winkler, H. A. 1931. *Salomo und die Karina—Eine orientalische Legende von der Bezwingung einer Kindbettdämonin durch einen heiligen Helden*. Stuttgart: W. Kohlhammer.

Wolf-Knuts, Ulrika. 2009. "Charms as Means of Coping." In *Charms, Charmers and Charming: International Research on Verbal Magic*, edited by Jonathan Roper, 62–70. New York: Palgrave Macmillan.

Zelenin, D. K. 1995. *Izbrannye trudy. Ocherki russkoi mifologii: Umershie neestestvennoio smert'u i rusalki)* [Selected works. Essays on Russian mythology: The dead who died an unnatural death and the *rusalki*]. Moskva: Indrik. [1916].

WORLD VIEW, RELIGION AND DISEASE IN MAGYARFALU

LAURA IANCU

The Bible teaches that the transcendent-immanent ancient cause of the universe, that is, its creator, is a god, or God. According to this world view, those responsible for the suffering of people are the people themselves. Nonetheless, there are sufferings in the world, of natural or other origins, which are not caused by human actions. The religious world view teaches that there are no situations where God—who created and supports the world—would run out of options, not even in the situations where the toolset of human actions does run out (Kessler 2008, 14, 31; Komáromi 1996, 92; Jolly 1996, 91; Nicolescu 2005, 171–2).

The concept of disease is closely linked to the concept of the body within that culture, and to the more or less identifiable origins of the disease, i.e. the cause of it. Knowledge regarding health and how to preserve it is inherent to culture as a whole, coded in the form of belief-like, experience-based practices and elementary rules which help to sort out and explain extraordinary situations.

Local religion in Magyarfalu

In Magyarfalu (Arini; Băcau County, Moldova, Romania), the culture and the institutions engrained in the culture are substantially defined and encompassed by the local religious system. The unity of religious and profane culture results in the fact that its functions cannot be attributed solely to the influence of religion, although it is difficult to separate them from it (cf. Erdélyi 1985, 17–8; Tomka 1990, 156). Doctrinal religion is not materialised and manifested in its full dogmatic excellence. Besides the official elements, magical and rational knowledge function as similar life-leading principles.

Local medicine

In Moldavian communities, the health care institutions of the state were created in the second half of the twentieth century. In Magyarfalu, there is still no doctor's surgery; for medical check-ups, the patients have to travel five kilometres from the settlement to the clinic in Găiceana.

We know little of the nature and function of medicine before our time. Based on the reports of missionaries from the sixteenth to the nineteenth centuries that can be found in the archives of the Vatican, in the course of their activities, the missionary priests applied preventive rules and healing methods necessary to maintain the proper functioning not only of the soul, but of the body as well (see Benda 1989; cf. Spielmann 1979, 42). These historical precedents may be related to the phenomenon whereby, even today, religion and healing connect and sometimes even overlap in the curing of certain diseases.[1]

Popular practices used in local healing procedures mostly include preventive religious and/or magical actions.[2] The healing of some diseases includes the use of sacred and medical tools gathered from the flora and fauna of Magyarfalu and its immediate surroundings (on the use of plants and objects in medical procedures, see Csoma 2000); other diseases are healed with the help of specialists and techniques from outside the village. Among the latter are diseases that are thought to have been occasioned by some kind of spirit or some magical action. Diseases of mental or supernatural origin can be healed via specific procedures belonging to the religious toolset (see Nicolescu 2005, 172). The advent of this type of disease (*fright, epilepsy, depression*) is not strictly related either to age or to gender. There is no rule regarding the order in which they use these healing procedures (popular, magical, priestly, medical, etc.); unless we

---

[1] All this is naturally not a Moldavian specialty. Medical researchers have shown that the tradition of "professionists" has been in operation since the beginning in the context of the common people's knowledge concerning medicine. The holders of "professionist" knowledge (priests, folk healers, less often doctors) disposed of an extra knowledge by (also) being people who were practitioners of religious-magical activities and thus could better establish the psychological atmosphere necessary for the healing process (Gémes 1979, 17). Tünde Komáromi, for instance, calls the Orthodox Romanian priest a "psychosomatic healer" (Komáromi 1996, 91; see also: Pócs 2001, 454; Deáky 2001, 343).

[2] Éva Pócs has shown that folk healing transforms empiric healing methods into beliefs, thus, among the users, the borderlines between magical and "rational" practice are blurred (Pócs 1979, 66). The Transcarpathian parallels of the magical terms used in everyday life can also be found in the publications of Erzsébet Kótyuk (Kótyuk 2005, 235–44).

consider that the people concerned seek out all kinds of methods in order to recover.

There are established patterns followed by the majority as regards which disease requires the activation of which healing system (cf. Keszeg 1997, 7). Spielmann calls most of the folk healing procedures a "finalistic approach", which essentially subordinates the diagnosis and the way of approaching the disease to the therapeutic goal. As he explains, "if a medicine has proved to be effective once, folk medicine will keep on using it without searching the natural cause of its effect" (Speilmann 1979, 36; see also Komáromi 1996, 88).

The complexity of the phenomenon is further increased by the fact that in Magyarfalu, the barriers between health and sickness are very flexible; and the concepts of *disease, malediction, bewitchment,* etc. are intertwined, meaning that it is only possible to heal a disease by applying a special and complex technique.[3]

Local conditions

The everyday life of the Moldavian peasant community is primarily controlled and scheduled by the work that ensures their livelihood; where human life—especially in the case of a disease thought to be incurable—is often judged to be of secondary importance. As Losonczi describes: "a peasant could only fall ill on his own account (…), if he could not work he would perish; he and his family would be in great danger. The constraints of peasant life made health an obligation, and thus a moral standard" (Losonczi 1984, 186). This norm—also prevailing in Magyarfalu—is achieved with a view congruous with the religious beliefs of the locals; namely, that disease can be looked upon as the personal intervention of God.

The reason for seeking the help of religious procedures to heal diseases in Magyarfalu can be described through the intertwining of the following factors: characteristic religious consciousness; religious interpretations complying with the psychosomatic approach to the diseases; the lack of official health institutions; the traditional doctor-patient relationship

[3] According to Tünde Komáromi, "seemingly mysterious, medically un-explained and unaccepted diseases are parts of a completely different world view; which—according to its perspective—describes them within a different system of symbols, and heals them accordingly" (Komáromi 1996, 87; see also: Tánczos 2000, 217, 224).

loaded with stereotypes;[4] the financial condition of the patient (on the financial advantages of a home pharmacy, see Kocsis 2005, 260); the level of fluency in Romanian.[5]

> There were no doctors. It used to be like that. That is why there were more children, and they died sooner, too. In the old days we sometimes buried 10 children a day (Csoma 2000, 17, 87).
>
> I know the herbs well; I'm a *doktorica*! I've grown old, but I've never been to a doctor! (Csoma 2000, 62; for parallels in Aranyosszék, see Komáromi 1996, 87; also see Erdélyi 1976, 139).
>
> I've become weak. There's no use in going to the doctor, so that he can experiment on me, one way or another. I'm just watching as they go, sit and come home! They're all the same. Why should I go see them? (I. L., Magyarfalu, own collection).
>
> My daughter was at home, she said we should call an ambulance; but I didn't want to go, I still had things to do at home (J. C., Magyarfalu, own collection).
>
> When there were no doctors, people healed themselves the best they could. But now that one can go to the hospitals, who would go to the midwives? I wouldn't; not even if I died. Those who don't have money, who believe in this kind of thing, they go to them. Though they have to pay the midwife as well! Moreover, the old diseases no longer exist! We have vaccination now; you don't hear about the plague and other epidemics anymore (I. B., Magyarfalu, own collection).

The doctors themselves assisted in the survival of religious medicine and continue to do so, even today, by encouraging patients to make use of popular, magical practices. Having a mental disorder or a disease of supernatural origin eventually leads to a loss of prestige, which is why in such cases most people seek the help of "secretly public" popular or magical healing methods (on the same issue see Komáromi 2001, 121).

---

[4] According to Mónika Kocsis, who researches Moldavian communities, "in the case of the professional sector, the cultural dimension is dominated by the doctor's knowledge; the healing proceeds based on his body perception (…). The role of the 'patient' and of the 'doctor' are both formalized. The dominant party is the doctor who manifests his power via the language, the terms he uses" (Kocsis 2005, 259).

[5] As the cited examples show, we are dealing with a situation that applies generally to the villages inhabited by Moldavian Hungarians. On the historical dimensions of the intertwined nature of the causes, see Deáky 2001, 343.

Medicina pastoralis

Research has shown that the healing or maledictory activities of the priests were a common phenomenon in medieval Western Christianity. Within the Roman Church, the problems once treated by priestly benediction and exorcism were later assigned to the field of expertise of folk specialists; "in the East, however, [some forms of it] stayed in the hands of priests and monks" (Pócs 2001, 454–7). In peasant societies, the priest was considered an educated person; both his community and his office expected him to provide healing in everyday ailments. Later, medical publications (for more in-depth information on the medicina pastoralis, see Deáky 2001, 345; 2006; 2008) served to widen the priest's medical knowledge, as did courses in medicine taught in the seminaries (Deáky 2001, 353). It is not an incidental circumstance that at that time doctors received a grounding in theology.[6] As a result, the intertwining of the religious and medical traditions not only manifests itself among the common people, but also among intellectuals, and moreover in the literature of the medicina pastoralis, presumably established and sustained by the social circumstances of the time and by this particular world view.[7] According to Éva Pócs, the fact that this once common, European, medieval system—and namely certain elements of it—is still in effect in the Eastern European region can only be justified by "the satisfaction of some kind of compelling need" (Pócs 2001, 455–7). Zita Deáky has shown that the priests who participated in medical education from the eighteenth to the twentieth century "stepped back to the role of the traditional (priestly) healer; even if only on a theoretical level, thus ensuring the continuity of a [...] status maintained over several millennia" (Deáky 2001, 355).

---

[6] Zita Deáky cites a dissertation by the Calvinistic doctor, Alajos Soltra (1826–1891) in which the author claims that in the eighteenth century "theology and medicine belonged together, they were inseparable" (Deáky 2001, 344–345, 350. Cf. Czégényi 2004, 390. On the inseparability of physical and mental healing, see Jolly 1996, 91; Stewart 1991, 212).

[7] In the book *A Book that Helps in Need* written by the Lutheran priest János Kömlei, translated from German and published in 1790, entitled, *Besides the Advice and Instructions for Physical Diseases and Troubles*, there is mention for instance of "enchantment, witches and various natural disasters", etc. (Deáky 2001, 347; cf. Jolly 1996, 66).

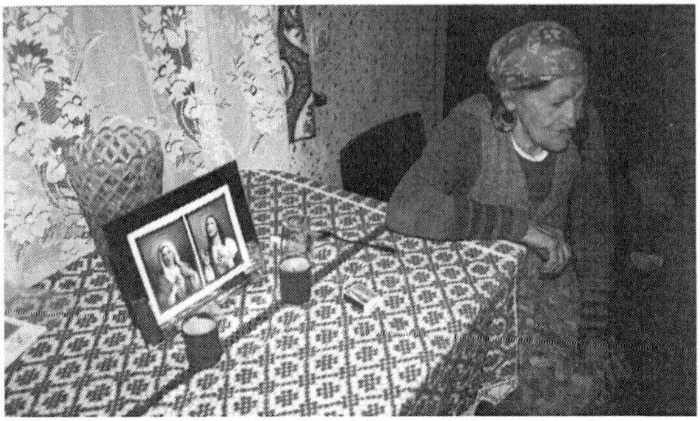

Fig. 1. The patient waits at home for the priest who comes to hear her confession. Table arranged for a home confession. Magyarfalu (*Arini*), Băcau County, Romania, 2005. Photo by Laura Iancu.

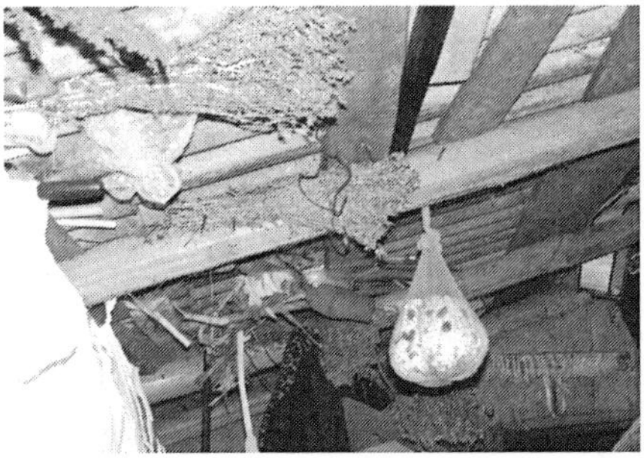

Fig. 2. Dried herbs in the attic. Saint John's wort and yarrow. Magyarfalu (*Arini*), Băcau County, Romania, 2005. Photo by Laura Iancu.

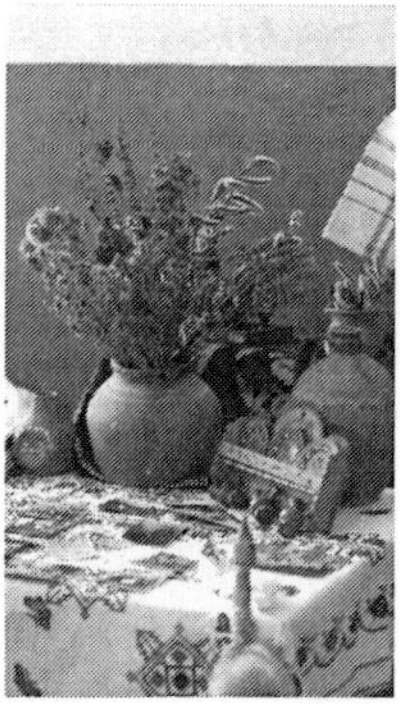

Fig. 3. Consecrated plants in a vase. Magyarfalu (*Arini*), Băcau County, Romania, 2005. Photo by Laura Iancu.

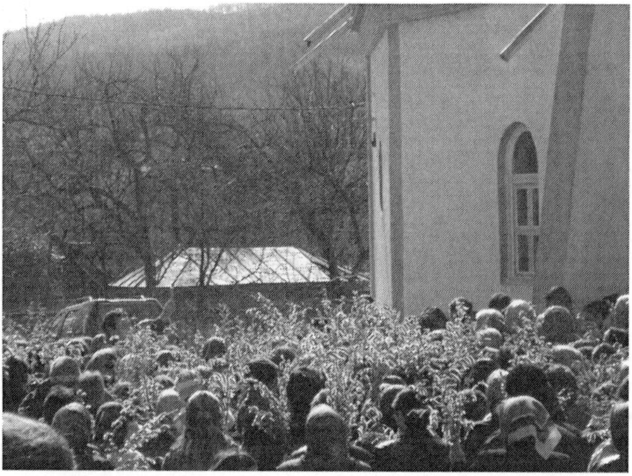

Fig. 4. Catkin consecration on Palm Sunday in the church courtyard. Magyarfalu (*Arini*), Băcau County, Romania, 2005. Photo by Laura Iancu.

Priestly and religious medicine in Magyarfalu

The role the Catholic priests serving in Magyarfalu played in healing was usually manifested in their maintaining and shaping the religious world view mentioned in the introduction, relying upon the tools implied by their status (sermons, teaching, benediction, prayer, etc.); a world view in which the determining role of the spiritual components of the physical diseases remains; in fact, it becomes even more emphatic. In this context, the disease might be related to the adult patient's sins, making an examination of the relation to God and the patient's moral life integral parts of the healing process.

The statement often cited in the literature asserting that the practice of seeking the help of orthodox priestly medicine, namely that the healing power of the priest (or *kaluger*—monk—, nun or other specialist) lies in the fact that he/she is an outsider to the community, language and religion, is not tenable (Györgydeák 2001, 399).[8] My own experience shows that it was not only possible, but necessary to seek out the help of orthodox priestly medicine to cure diseases of magical origin in this religious culture because in such cases, the specialist alloyed one or more traditions, religion and magic, and priestly medicine and psychology, as long as he remained within the borders of the religious sphere, that is, the religious world view (see Gagyi 2008, 380).[9] On the other hand, those who have sought these kinds of healing procedures do not distinguish between the somewhat religious or rather magical or other elements and procedures applied in these priestly techniques. Thus, the functioning of this diverse medicine is sustained not merely and not primarily by the lack of health institutions, but by the particular world view of the community.[10]

---

[8] Orsolya Graf's experiences in Csík resulted in conclusions relevant to the situation in Magyarfalu: "going to the *kaluger* is considered an 'open secret' in the villages. Everyone knows about it, but they prefer not to tell about their experience; or they tell their own experience as if it were someone else's" (Graf 2001, 36).

[9] Dóra Czégényi also establishes that the distance between Catholic and Orthodox piety is minimal, and thus the creatures and the techniques are easily transferred from one system to the other (Czégényi 2004, 383). Éva Pócs has shown in her research in Csík that priestly procedures portrayed the close interlacement of several systems. Furthermore, as she writes: "in Orthodox Eastern Europe the peasant world view, popular beliefs and witchcraft beliefs are closely linked to the devil image of the ecclesiastical demonology" (Pócs 2001a, 451, 453. See also Komáromi 1996, 94).

[10] As Deáky writes, the priests "cannot give up on this activity voluntarily until there is trust and faith in the recovery, in a miracle, which brings the priest together

One example: diseases caused by evil and their remedies

In Magyarfalu, *evil* is the umbrella term for a number of "popular belief figures", a category encompassing the negative features of several supernatural creatures. Its form is a mixture of the Christian notion of the Devil and various types of spirits. A frequently used synonym is *unclean*. In many cases, these two terms (*evil, unclean*) are used to avoid the pronunciation of the word *devil;* (on this phenomenon in the academic literature, see Röhrich 1966, 215; Pócs 2008, 315). The use of all three terms (*evil, unclean, devil*) is followed by reciting a charm and a dedication to God, i.e. a prayer, and sometimes even the mention of an illustrious saint:

> May he go to the barrens, God help us! (I. L., Magyarfalu, own collection).

> Once, one night, I was walking by the Futás.[11] Suddenly a big tuft got between my legs. (…) Hey, is that you, János? Hold up! Stop, so that I can cross myself. (…) I arrived at the flats, and it twirled no more (I. Ir., Magyarfalu, own collection).

According to local beliefs, the *evil one* is a creature that obstructs the regular practice of religion, thereby preventing salvation; its main activity is to challenge Christian qualities (see Keszeg 1999, 90). The consequences of its mischief can be physical harm, damage to health or even disease. The *unclean* is not simply a creature; it is the counterpole to the principle of good, its opposite; thus, it is also suitable for explaining most of the negative happenings that are difficult to interpret. They are often identified with demons or as causes of diseases. (The diseases mentioned are typically demonic disorders. Pócs 2003, 227, 230). For instance, they might cause diseases via *possession*, *sending* (sickness), *fright* or *fear*.

> Our dear János got so frightened, he almost died. He was once frightened by someone in the field, and that fright stayed with him. It was a priest who healed him in the end. But we had to struggle so much, I swear to you, God bless us! (J. T., Magyarfalu, own collection).

---

with his community; and until there is no other, or the people who turn to him cannot see any other alternative" (Deáky 2001, 355. Also see Pócs 2001a, 457; 1979, 71; Graf 2001, 32; Komáromi 2001, 121).

[11] A toponym in Magyarfalu.

> Isti Bácsi was once frightened. First they said it was a ghost, but I know who frightened him [...] he succumbed to the fright [...] and the devil was there, too [...]. When he returned he said: Run off, because the dogs are coming, the dogs will eat you up! We didn't see anything! Only he saw them! And then he said: Look how big they are, and run, and this and that! I swear, may he go to the waste lands! (B. D., Magyarfalu, own collection).

> A heavy sadness fell upon my daughter! She was so sad, that we couldn't console her. Sadness is a terribly bad thing; it blinds you, it kills you. It wipes you off the face of the earth. If the sadness prevails, then the doctors can't do anything about it. It is a truly vile disease. It shrivels you (I. L., Magyarfalu, own collection. Cf. Blum and Blum 1965, 53).[12]

According to belief, the *unclean* operates only in certain places (crossroads, bridges, at the edge of the village, in the forest) at certain times (before midnight, at midnight, at dawn, "at the time of the waning moon"). This is why they protect sacral spaces by offering them to God with the help of certain occasional and cyclically repeated cleansing and preventive rituals.

> A.T.'s parents went to work; they have land beyond the Romanians; and as they went, the old lady sat on the cart, and the old man drove the cattle. At the house of V.F. a goat came out of the pit. [...] A goat appeared and the cattle stopped moving! They started moaning; they saw the evil one and didn't want to move anymore. Well, the old man got off, and started to whip the cattle but they still didn't move. Then he remembered to say: oh my Lord, Jesus Christ, what kind of creature is that? And then the evil one went back to the pit. And so the cattle moved on. Because if the devil hears God's name, he runs off (I. A., Magyarfalu, own collection).

> My neighbor perished there under the bridge. He came with his haversack—it was in the winter—and the evil ones pushed him, pulled him in the water. He didn't die then; they hung his sack to the middle of the bridge where no one could reach it. And then L. and his family heard someone crying in the night. By the time they got there it was too late. They cut the ice, and he was still alive; they took him out; but then he died. The evil ones pushed him in because he didn't believe in God (I. A., Magyarfalu, own collection).

> We bless it with holy water, or fumigate it with consecrated flowers. Or sometimes we burn candles. It drives out evil. The evil thoughts, and the evil things ... and it is very efficient! (G. M., Magyarfalu, own collection).

[12] The Blum author duo also mentions that in the Greek tradition, the main cause of heart disease is sadness and worry (Blum and Blum 1965: 123).

> Earlier we even sprinkled holy water on the crossroads; or others who were afraid fumigated it or prayed there. (I. An., Magyarfalu, own collection).

One of the consequences of the fear, fright and depression linked to the operation of the *unclean* is the urge to commit suicide (see Pócs 2003, 232).

> You see how many people hung themselves this year? They took vows and that vow was not good; when you take it the evil one is there! You've lost your soul. You've given it to the evil one. Those who take vows to the evil one belong to the evil one (B. R., Magyarfalu, own collection).

One of the diseases emanating from the *unclean* is epilepsy. (The local denomination for the disease is "evil disease" or "foul disease" see: Blum and Blum 1965, 124; Kocsis 2005, 243; Pócs 1986, 251).

> My God—may he go to the waste lands, God be with us!—it [i.e. the epileptic seizure] is sent by the evil one! It is from the evil one! The unclean! (T. R., Magyarfalu, own collection).

According to local beliefs, the *unclean* infiltrates the surroundings of the patient in the form of burning charcoal. One way to exorcise it is to bless the surroundings of the patient, or to smear ground pieces of charcoal all over the patient's body.

> When it locks someone down for the first time, if there is a way to dig down in the ground and find the burning charcoal—which were put there by the unclean, when he burrowed himself in—and to crush them and smear it on the patient's body so that the evil one leaves the body, then the patient will no longer be sick (L. Sz., Magyarfalu–Egyházaskozás, own collection).

The subsequent method of recovery is to pray for many long years and to lead a strictly religious life.

> V. has a daughter. She's like a nun. She's smart, she takes communion every day; she used to have the evil diseases as well, but it passed. Because she prayed a lot… it passed (G. M., Magyarfalu, own collection).

One of the remarkable ways of healing epilepsy is to pay for a sermon. (You pay the priest to give a sermon with a specific purpose). It is worth noting that in Magyarfalu, paying for a sermon is a common phenomenon anyway. The most common type of sermon—besides the sermons of various denomination and content commissioned for the dead—aims to procure health and peace within the family. Besides paying for sermons, it is also common practice to fast, often with the purpose of healing.

> I always pay. I go as soon as I have a little money. Here at our church. Well, you can do it with the Vlach priests as well, they are not too bad, it's quite the same, but our priest won't let us! Our priest won't let us go to the Vlach priest! (B. L., Magyarfalu, own collection).

> When I paid [for a sermon] in Bákó when her [daughter's] leg was broken, I paid, and I wanted to ask others how it goes because I didn't know, and there was *la Piața Centrală* [the Central Market] where people discuss things. I signed the register book to show that I had paid. Then the priest told me when he was going to celebrate the mass. It was a Tuesday. He asked me where I lived, and I told him it was another village; they knew our priest; and he told me to go to his [the other priest's] sermon and listen to the sermon on the same day in my village (B. A., Magyarfalu, own collection. Cf. Pócs 2001, 447).

> I was very sick, too. They told me to go see the Vlach priest and ask him to pray for me! So I went, but later I confessed and my priest scolded me! Oh! What was I doing there?! (B. M., Magyarfalu, own collection).

> Some people pay to cause the people they are angry with to die! Oh, the Vlach priests over there as well… they lie! They cheat the world! I've never been there (T. An., Magyarfalu, own collection).

There are many shared elements in the paid sermons of the local or urban Roman Catholic priest or Orthodox priests.[13] According to the locals "there is no difference between the sermons paid to the Catholic or the Orthodox priest". While in other cases, the external formalities of the religion have a determining and dividing power; when it comes to diseases, the differences become subordinate to faith in the same one God.[14] Moreover, they also believe that if a magical or simply a non-Catholic element occurs in the Orthodox practice, the goal itself—for instance, to reveal the truth, punish the guilty or heal a disease—is morally right, religiously accepted, and thus is an act that falls under the scope of sacredness and not that of magic. It can occur that the Orthodox priest requires the patient or the patient's representative to interpret the

---

[13] The sermon itself, the defined amount of money, the specified (time of the) day, the specified number of sermons, the explicit intention and goal, etc.

[14] Such formality is the celibacy of priests, based on which the locals consider their own Catholic religion superior and "more true" than the Orthodox religion.

intervention (for example the exorcism of the spirit causing the disease) correctly; that is, to consider it as a procedure, the aim of which is to solicit God's active intervention.

The healing sermon performed by the Orthodox priest can have no outsider witnesses; what happens during the sermon can only be learned from accounts. If we observe the components of the Orthodox priestly practice closely, we find numerous elements that we know from the Catholic religion, like the Bible, sacramentals (candle, water, etc.), the prayer, the fast, the sermons, etc.

> You pay for a sermon for the sake of the family (*spre binele familiei*), there is no formula to ask for one against evil. Or you say, dear God, take the evil out of this life! And give me goodness instead, and take the evil to the waste lands! And I know that the priest says the same in his prayers when you go to him (B. A., Magyarfalu, own collection).

> My daughter had a friend (*prietena*) who told me about a priest who had performed many miracles (*multe minuni făcut*), and he can tell the origins of my disease, whether it was a bewitchment or not. They used to be here in Adjud, but now they are gone, I don't know where. I don't know where they went. […] The Vlach priest said—after I prepared the writing that my faith was strong (*"am credinţa tare"*), he wrote he was worried (*dar sun indoită*), he asked whether I knew it was like this or that. But with my faith I triumphed over all (*Dar totuşi am credinţă şi prin credinţă am îvnis toate*), and at that time it was enough for me. I didn't need anything else. And he prayed for my health (*pentru sănătatea mea*), too. I didn't bring him money, but I did bring a bottle of wine. He told me to come again, but I don't go to those places anymore. I was trembling with fear. I'd rather go to a hospital! He told me to go to the hospital, too (B. M., Magyarfalu, own collection).[15]

The further elements (e.g. the combination of paper and other unfamiliar objects) which serve to complete the list of shared features are even more significant, as these are the elements that give the patient the impression that they are receiving a treatment, that is, an intervention.

> Well I wouldn't know because I've never been there. […] They say that if you've lost something, or if things go wrong for you or you are sick then […] they give you a piece of paper (*particika*). And if you throw the paper in the water then it will perish in water, if you throw it in the fire, then it will perish in fire. But I wouldn't know (M. M., Magyarfalu, own collection).

[15] On the parallels of the "book opening" in Csík see: Pócs 2001, 443.

> The one who pays has to drink it: if you want it to perish in water, then you have to throw it in water, if you want it to perish in fire, then you have to throw the paper in fire! If you chew on it, then they say that it will suffer or crush itself; [...] and if you eat it then it dies immediately. [...] If someone has an evil sickness they take him/her to pay, it is very efficient! (T. An., Magyarfalu, own collection).

> If someone does wrong to you, or you have an evil kind of a disease then you go and pay. Rather than going to a sorcerer, you would pay for a sermon and fast. For one day, or for nine. And that priest will pray for you, and at the end it will be revealed who did it, what it was. And if the offence is grave, there is a way to make the perpetrator die. But it is only the Orthodox priests who do it (T. L., Magyarfalu, own collection).

The identical elements "warrant" that the patient does not leave the territory of his/her own religion; therefore, the thought that one might be unfaithful to one's particular God does not arise; and the differing elements confirm the presumed or real feeling of being "medically treated" by an intervention. This duality is well expressed in the practice of exorcism and the local healing methods for epilepsy.

> P. was bewitched [...] he turned crazy, he was with the evil one. When he came home in the evening he acted like a rabid person, we couldn't handle him [...] he wanted to kill everyone, he broke everything. [...] They've taught me what to do. I took the journey and went to the priest [the arch priest] and paid him. He then prayed for him, you know, but he kept telling me to bring P. to him, or at least an item of his clothing, so that he could consecrate it. And when I went to see him for the second time, he prayed on the piece of clothing I brought, and sprinkled it with holy water and oil and fumigated it, too. He also gave me some to bring home, and to put it in his food, and to sprinkle on his bed. [...] I had to put candles under his pillow, in the form of a cross. I sewed a cross on his hat and on his shirt as well. [...] It passed. He recovered. But the time we spent on it, God bless us! (B. F., Magyarfalu, own collection).

Among the relatives of the patient, the priestly exorcism of the spirit causing the disease is an intervention that—in this sociocultural milieu—appears as one possible, or even the only possible, cure (for the position of the Church see: Gál, Gál and Pócs 2005, 328; cf. Stewart 1991, 210). Although the priest's prayer is not entirely public (and some of it cannot even be heard), according to the concerned parties, the procedure consists of eliminating and neutralising the evil spirit by invoking God's aid. In this procedure, we can sort of recognise an analogy with baptism, as the executor of the ritual (~ the priest) and the aim of the sacrament (~

offering to God) are identical. The person liberated from the devil (evil spirit) and returned to God can be further protected by the ritualistic and magical use of the sacramental objects.[16]

There is a slight difference between the methods of the Orthodox priest and that of the Orthodox *kaluger* (monk), nun or magical specialist; in the methods of the latter, malediction plays a much stronger role.

> Then he paid at a monastery (*manastirea*); his brother is a Catholic priest, he is praying for him, too! And I'm telling him, well, it is not only you who had to suffer! The things I had to go through with them [i.e. the common enemy]! I burned candles, because that's what they've taught me. When they ring the bells, you have to burn the candle upside down over the threshold and think of the one that you are angry with, the one that harmed you. And you have to say: the way this candle burns should burn my enemy, too; just as the wax drips off the thread, in the same way the meat should melt from his bones. You have to do this while they are ringing the bells. And you have to pray. When one candle goes out, you have to light another and turn that upside down! Nine altogether (I. A., Magyarfalu, own collection. Cf. Pócs 2001, 447).

> She [i.e. the Orthodox nun] is bound to the evil one, she was controlled by the evil one. It is the unclean one that works with those, and it is a great matter! […] she was so bewitched that they carried her to Braila on a broken reed, she woke up in Braila, that is where the evil one killed her (I. R., Magyarfalu, own collection).[17]

> He went to see a midwife to get healed […] the midwife tried to heal him, but the evil one had really overcome him, he was taken by the evil one; he told her that he had been to a shop, that the evil one had given him the power to enter the shop. When he was there, the doors opened up, he took what he wanted and then the doors closed back. That's how strong the evil power was. When the midwife was done with the procedure, his stove broke down. Because of the force of the evil one. We had to give the midwife what she asked for, money, crops, chicken. Whatever she asked for (I. L., Magyarfalu, own collection).

According to Tünde Komáromi, the Romanian priest performs psychotherapy in his procedures: he liberates the patient from the negativity of the

---

[16] Based on the experiences of Charles Stewart, a researcher of Greek exorcism, it is not the elimination of the demon that counts the most in the procedure; the most important thing is to make the demon talk, to reveal his name, since that is how he will become controllable. According to Stewart, the healing is done by the procedure itself, by the ritual (Stewart 1991, 216–217, 218, 221).

[17] On the diabolic reputation of the Romanian priest, see Pócs 2001, 454.

interpersonal efficacy, of its harmful energies. This type of recovery happens, in her words, “mostly as a result of autosuggestion” (Komáromi 1996, 92–97; cf. Stewart 1991, 221).

Furthermore, based on my experiences, the key to the success of ritual healing is that the elements involved in the procedure allow the line between popular belief and doctrinal belief to be crossed; it also makes interaction possible between the clergy and the laity; and it resolves all—essentially contradictory—polarisation, since it provides an experience where one can consider the world in unity; an experience that implements the coherence of the physical and spiritual realities.

There is one more significant factor behind this phenomenon: revealing the true cause of the bewitchment or the disease and punishing the harmful, bewitching person, the creature in this world, in the present. If a patient under a curse is healed by a professional doctor, the case ends with the lesson that the malicious wrongdoer, by using secret knowledge, can unjustly engage in activities endangering the lives of others. The methods employed by priests provide an extra service in that the perpetrator has to suffer punishment for his act; moreover, the victim can keep track of it, and through doing so, can gain public, social rehabilitation.

In this way, the desire to receive evidence of divine retribution is satisfied and at this point, we return to the correlation between world view, religion and medicine outlined in the introduction, and at its social convergence, a phenomenon which can be clearly observed in the culture of Magyarfalu.

References

Benda, Kálmán. 1989. *Moldvai csángó–magyar okmánytár I–II* [Moldavian Csango–Hungarian records I–II]. Budapest: Magyarságkutató Intézet.

Blum Richard and Eva Blum. 1965. *Health and Healing in Rural Greece. A Study of Three Communities.* Stanford, Calif.: Stanford University Press.

Czégényi, Dóra. 2004. “A román pap alakja egy szilágysági közösség hiedelemrendszerében [The character of the Romanian priest in the belief system of a community in Szilágyság].” In *Áldás és átok, csoda és boszorkányság. Vallásetnológiai fogalmak tudományközi megközelítésben* [Blessing and curse, miracle and witchcraft. Religious ethnological concepts in multidisciplinary approach], edited by Éva Pócs, 382–94. Budapest: Balassi. (Tanulmányok a transzcendensről IV.)

Csoma, Gergely. 2000. *Varázslások és gyógyítások a moldvai csángómagyaroknál* [Witchcraft and healing among the Csángós in Moldova]. Pomáz: Kráter Műhely Egyesület.

Deáky, Zita. 2001. "A medicina pastoralis és a papok egészségügyi felvilágosító tevékenysége a XVIII. század végétől a XIX. század közepéig [The medicina pastoralis and the medical education activities of the priests from the end of the eighteenth century until the mid-nineteenth century]." In *Népi vallásosság a Kárpát-medencében II* [Folk religion in the Carpathian basin], edited by Emőke S. Lackovits, and Veronika Mészáros, 343–59. Veszprém: Veszprém Megyei Múzeum Igazgatóság.

—. 2006. *Temetkezési szokások az erdélyi románoknál, 1817* [Burial customs among the Romanians of Transylvania, 1817]. Kolozsvár: Györffy István Néprajzi Egyesület. (Néprajzi Látóhatár Kiskönyvtára 10.)

—, ed. 2008. *Erdély orvosi szemmel a 18–19. században* [Transylvania in a medical perspective in the eighteenth and nineteenth century]. Kolozsvár: Györffy István Néprajzi Egyesület. (Néprajzi Látóhatár Kiskönyvtára 11.)

Erdélyi, Zsuzsanna. 1976. *Hegyet hágék, lőtőt lépék. Archaikus népi imádságok* [I traversed mountains, I went down slopes. Archaic popular prayers]. Budapest: Magvető.

—. 1985. "A Parasztbiblia elé [Preface to the Peasant Bible]." In *Parasztbiblia. Magyar népi biblikus történetek* [Peasant Bible. Hungarian popular biblical stories], edited by Ilona Ilona and Annamária Lammel, 15–35. Budapest: Gondolat.

Gagyi, József. 2008. "'Az egy szent testület…' A kalugerek társadalmi szerepe egy székelyföldi faluban ['It's a holy corporation...' The social role of *kalugers* in a Székelyland village]." In *Démonok, látók, szentek. Vallásetnológiai fogalmak tudományközi megközelítésben* [Demons, seers, saints. Religious ethnological concepts in multidisciplinary approach], edited by Éva Pócs, 380–94. Budapest: Balassi. (Tanulmányok a transzcendensről VI.)

Gál, Péter, Ferenc Gál, and Éva Pócs. 2005. "Ördögűzés [Exorcism]." *Magyar Katolikus Lexikon X,* [Hungarian Catholic encyclopaedia], edited by István Diós, 328–32. Budapest: Szent István Társulat.

Graf, Orsolya. 2001. "A hiedelmek szerepe [The role of beliefs]." In *Két csíki falu néphite a századvégen* [Folk belief of two villages in Csík at the end of the century], edited by Éva Pócs, 13–80. Budapest: Európai Folklór Intézet, and Osiris.

Györgydeák, Anita. 2001. A rontás szociálpszichológiája [The social-psychology of bewitchment] In *Két csíki falu néphite a századvégen* [Folk belief of two villages in Csík at the end of the century], edited by Pócs Éva, 372–418. Budapest: Európai Folklór Intézet and Osiris.

Jolly, Karen Louise. 1996. *Popular religion in late Saxon England*. Chapel Hill and London: The University of North Carolina Press.

Keszeg, Vilmos. 1999. *Mezőségi hiedelmek* [Folkbelief in Mezőség]. Marosvásárhely: Mentor.

Kessler, Hans. 2008. "Hol marad az Isten, amikor teremtményei szenvednek? A természeti csapások és az Isten cselekvését firtató kérdés [Where is God when his creatures are suffering? Natural disasters and the question about God's action]." *Mérleg* 1–2: 13–34.

Kocsis, Mónika. 2005. "Népi gyógyászat Szitáson [Ethnomedicine in Szitás]." In *Adaptáció és modernizáció a moldvai csángó falvakban* [Adaptation and modernisation in villages of the Moldavian Csángós], edited by István Kinda, and Ferenc Pozsony, 235–70. Kolozsvár: Kriza János Néprajzi Társaság.

Komáromi, Tünde. 1996. "Rontásformák Aranyosszéken. A gyógyító román pap [Forms of *maleficium* in Aranyosszék. The Romanian priest as healer]." *Néprajzi Látóhatár* 1–2: 87–98.

—. 2001. "Az ijedség [Fright]." In *Emberek, szövegek, hiedelmek* [People, texts and beliefs], edited by Dóra Czégényi, and Vilmos Keszeg, 112–40. Kolozsvár: Kriza János Néprajzi Társaság.

Losonczi, Ágnes. 1984. "Az egészség és betegség társadalmi szabályozottsága [Social regulation of health and disease]." In *Életmód: modellek és minták* [Way of life: Models and patterns], edited by Mihály Hoppál, and Tamás Szecskő, 181–200. Budapest: Tömegkommunikációs Kutatóközpont.

Nicolescu, Costion. 2005. *Elemente de teologie ţărănească. Chipul creşin ţărănesc al lui Dumnezeu* [Elements of rural theology. The Christian peasantry's notion of God]. Bucureşti: Vremea.

Pócs, Éva. 1986. "A 'gonoszűzés' mágikus és vallásos szövegei. Adatok ráolvasóink egyházi kapcsolataihoz [Magical and religious texts for 'banishing the evil one']." In "*Mert ezt Isten hagyta...*" *Tanulmányok a népi vallásosság köréből* ["Because God let it happen..." Essays on folk piety], edited by Gábor Tüskés, 213–51. Budapest: Magvető.

—. 2001a. "Átok, rontás, divináció: boszorkányság a vallás és mágia határán [Curse, maleficium, divination: Witchcraft on the borderline of religion and magic]." In *Két csíki falu néphite a századvégen* [Folk belief of two villages in Csík at the end of the century], edited by Éva Pócs, 419–59. Budapest: Európai Folklór Intézet and Osiris.

—. 2003. "Megszállottságjelenségek, megszállottságrendszerek. Néhány közép-kelet-európai példa [Possession phenomena, possession-systems. Some East-Central European examples]." *Népi Kultúra—Népi Társadalom* XXI: 211–71.

—. 2008. "'Rajtunk is történt nagy csoda'. Beszélgetések és elbeszélések a természetfelettiről. ['A great miracle has been visited upon us.' Conversations and narratives about the supernatural]." In: *"Vannak csodák, csak észre kell venni...". Helyi vallás, néphit és vallásos folklór Gyimesben* ["Miracles exist, if only you notice them..." Local religion, folk belief and religious folklore in Gyimes], edited by Éva Pócs, 279–351. Budapest: L'Harmattan – PTE Néprajz Tanszék. (Studia Ethnologia Hungarica VIII.)

Röhrich, Lutz. 1966. "Az ördög alakja a népköltészetben [The Devil's figure in folklore]." *Ethnographia* XXVII: 212–28.

Spielmann, József. 1979. "Történelmi reflexiók a népi orvoslás és az orvostudomány viszonyáról [Historical reflections on the relationship of ethnomedicine and medicine]." In *Népi gyógyítás Magyarországon.* Ethnomedicine in Hungary], edited by József Antall, and Géza Buzinkay, 35–50. Budapest: Medicina.

Stewart, Charles. 1991. *Demons and the Devil. Moral imagination in modern Greek culture.* New Jersey: Princenton University Press.

Tomka, Miklós. 1990. "A vallás mint változó rendszer [Religion as a changing system]." *Szociológia* 3–4: 155–85.

MAGICAL CAUSES OF ILLNESSES AND THEIR CURES IN EIGHTEENTH-CENTURY UKRAINE

KATERYNA DYSA

In the modern world of institutionalised medicine, it is hard to grasp how closely medicine was connected to magic in premodern societies. Natural and supernatural causes of sickness and means of healing were intertwined so deeply that it was not easy to separate one from the other. Illnesses, perceived from this perspective, were interpreted as having either natural or supernatural origins. Orthodox Church authorities in Ukraine considered that every sickness had a demonic origin. However, in practice, magical explanation of illness had its limitations. In this study, I would like to touch upon two aspects connecting magic with medicine—first, I will discuss those illnesses allegedly caused by witchcraft and second, I will turn to magical healing used by early modern dwellers of Ukrainian towns and villages.

According to popular early modern beliefs, bewitchment could cause illness and even death. Witches were sometimes accused of causing epidemics (for Ukrainian examples see: no. 30 [1720] and no. 55 [1746] in Antonovich 1877, 73–4 and 105–12). However, the concept of witchcraft as an explanation for misfortune had its limits. Not every kind of sickness and not every death were necessarily connected with witchcraft. People were able to read signs which enabled them to judge the feasible causes of misfortune, and even in situations when misfortune might seem quite mysterious, witchcraft was not among the frequently used explanations (Robisheaux 2001, 198). Witchcraft was not suspected in situations when old people died and "murder was usually just murder and not witchcraft" (ibid., 206). However, the attitude towards the death of young and mature people, and especially children, was quite different—bewitchment was often pronounced as its cause. Yet again, witchcraft was suspected only in specific cases, implicating the existence of someone, "an evil person" or "a witch", who could cause illness or death. Without such a figure with whom the victim of bewitchment or victim's relatives had tensions, the sickness would have been interpreted as being of natural origin, caused "by God's will".

Moreover, there is evidence that bewitchment itself was considered a specific type of illness. The existence of this disease, allegedly caused by witches and so referred to as a "witch disease", even caused some researchers, Leland Estes in particular, to come to the following conclusion: "it was this stereotypical witch disease, and not a witch figure, as has often been supposed, that stimulated the hunt for witches. European civilisation was not really trying to uproot a certain type of human being, but was instead looking for the 'spreaders' of a certain type of illness" (Estes 1983, 274).

Though I do not share this opinion, I do accept that a witch disease could constitute one of the main components of witchcraft mythology. Many Ukrainian sources confirm that bewitchment was perceived as a specific illness. For this, one can find rather compelling evidence. In the eighteenth century, many handwritten books on medical and household recommendations circulated in Ukrainian lands. As a rule, they were re-written from other books of a similar type and were kept by the same family for several generations. These books could be quite chaotic in their organisation but could also be well organised, so that advice on how to preserve milk was separate from recommendations concerning headaches, hernias and diarrhoea. Medical books would usually include some advice concerning diagnosis, recipes for some medicines, useful information about the medical properties of certain substances, for example coffee and vodka, (Naukova Biblioteka L'vivs'koho Derzhavnoho Universutetu. Viddil Rukopysiv [Scientific Library of the Lviv State University. Manuscript Section] (Further: NBLDU VR), no. 396i, ff. 2rev, 6rev.), recommendations about the treatment of the sick and different incantations or "prayers" against various ailments.

Sometimes, these medical books would include information about the treatment of bewitchment. Here is a selection:

> Sagebrush is a good treatment against bewitchment and the one who carries it along is not afraid of witchcraft and is protected from evil women (*Kniga liechebnaia ot mnogikh liekarstv* 1984, 100).

> When someone has been bewitched, one has to take a wooden sliver from a pear or apple tree and has to cook it for quite a long time, then the sick person has to be bathed in this decoction and the one who caused bewitchment will suffer (ibid., 113).

> If one wishes to feel safe from bewitchment, one should leave a little bit from each dish after Shrovetide. All these should be put into one pot and

hidden under the threshold of the house. At Easter one will find a worm in that pot. To keep this worm will aid in recognising all itches (ibid., 110).

One who carries the root of sagebrush is protected from bewitchment (Potebnia 1890).

Although these recommendations are quite simple, they all obviously regard bewitchment as an illness that can be prevented if one follows given advice. Along with these recommendations, some medical books contained incantations that were intoned in order to cure bewitchment (for example, *Kniga liechebnaia ot mnogikh liekarst* 1984, 102).

Trial records also reflect a belief in witchcraft illness. Reading the stories that stood behind the accusations of witchcraft, one can understand what made a witch disease a witch disease. According to Thomas Robisheaux, "What was critical in perceiving witchcraft at work was the conjuncture of several separate cognitive perceptions of the events within their specific contexts" (Robisheaux 2001, 203). There were two essential components that made people suspect that illness or death was caused by witchcraft. These two components should coincide in time and place, and if one was absent, bewitchment was rarely suspected. First, the illness had to be sudden. In most cases, it struck people who were not old and who were healthy, so that the illness seemed to be "for no reason". It could also have strange, unusual symptoms, though not every case has detailed descriptions of these symptoms. Second, a witchcraft illness should be preceded by a quarrel, an open conflict, latent tension, or sometimes, by some mysterious and suspicious event.

There are several examples of how this scheme worked in practice. When the husband of the town-dweller of the Podolian city of Kamianets'-Podil'ski, Katarzyna Głombowiczowa, suddenly fell deadly ill in 1733, she suspected that it was caused by bewitchment. She had good reason since one woman, Helena Kozicka, was angry with her husband because he had used to live with her, but had chosen to marry Katarzyna. Several people testified that they heard Helena cursing Katarzyna's husband, saying that he would repent and would not live long (No. 41 [1733], in Antonovich 1877, 84–5).

In 1747, two children of the miller, Iwan Buteluric from the Volhynian town of Lisniovtsi saw Maruska Iwanicha Petrykowa and Iwanicha Mielniczka doing some strange things (presumably some kind of witchcraft) in a cemetery near a dam. These two women also noticed the children. After some time, other people created a disturbance about these women. They rushed to the cemetery and took them to the castle, whereupon one of Buteluric's sons suddenly fell very ill. His arms and legs ceased to function. Because this sickness was so sudden and it was probably interpreted as revenge meted by the two arrested witches, the parents of the child suspected witchcraft illness (Archiwum Główny Akt Dawnich w Warsawie [Further AGAD], Księga Czarna Krzemienieckie 1747–1777 [mf 18958], 53–5).

In 1732, Daniel Czyźewski, an inhabitant of Vyzhva, another small Volhynian town, had a bitter quarrel with Olianuszka Koladyczewa. During this quarrel, the latter cursed Daniel's children. Shortly afterwards, one of his children "who was absolutely healthy in the evening, fell very ill at night without any obvious reason and in three days the child departed this life" (Tsentral'nyi Derzhavnyi Istorychnyi Arkhiv Ukraiiny u.m. Kyievi [Central State Historical Archive of Ukraine in Kiev] (Further: TDIA [Kiev]), fond 32, op.1, no. 5, f. 229rev). The coincidence of the quarrel, the cursing, sudden illness and death became evident signs for the father that his child had been bewitched.

Childhood ailments and especially childhood deaths were among the main reasons for arousing suspicions of bewitchment (a child's death made people especially sensitive and suspicious, for example, TDIA (Kiev), fond 32, op.1, no. 5, ff. 392rev-393rev [1726]; TDIA [Kiev], fond 1237, op.1, no. 8, ff. 268rev-269 [1730]). These suspicions could grow into resentment against an alleged witch in the case of any mass illness of children, consolidating people in an urge to punish the guilty party. In 1628, four men, Iesko Cieciera, Jacko Koszyn, Karp Krublik and Jasko Rybałka from the town of Oster suspected bewitchment when their children suddenly became ill. They accused their neighbour, Barbara Cierhowa, of causing it and brought collective charges against her in the town court (TDIA [Kiev], fond 1471, op.1, no. 1, f. 23–24). Several members of the furrier's guild of the town of Olyka assigned the sickness of their children to bewitchment in 1727. It followed one event that in the parents' eyes was obviously connected to the problem of their children's health. Sometime before the children fell ill, their parents entered a quarrel with the wife of Maciei Suchowecz, in which most of the guild members were involved. The woman, being upset and angry, cursed the guild members and their children (TDIA [Kiev], fond 1237, op.1, no. 8, ff. 19rev-21).

Yet a quarrel preceding an illness was not a necessary condition for suspecting bewitchment. It was enough to see or even hear from other people that somebody (usually from one's immediate environment, most often one of the neighbours) was doing something strange, inexplicable and cryptic. In 1730, the children of an inhabitant of Olyka, Ihnatovicz fell ill and this illness was assigned to bewitchment since one woman,

Mikitycha Bezpuczka, had seen the wife of Stefan Kaminski taking a handful of soil from under the windows of the Ihnatowicz's house some time before the illness struck. According to local opinion, his strange action was the reason for the children's ailments. (TDIA [Kiev], fond 1237, op.1, no. 8, ff. 346rev-347). In 1739, another woman from Olyka, Anna Szkopilicka, suspected that her child had fallen ill and then died because of bewitchment. She came to this conclusion since Gabriel Lemkiewicz and his wife had told her that Anna Rajska was cooking some charms to bewitch her child (No. 44 [1733], in Antonovich 1877, 88–9).

As trial records show, people believed that not only children but also adults were not immune to illnesses caused by magical means. Ihnat Telepnin from the village of Bereznicza of the Ruthenian palatinate was ill for several years and spent a lot of money in attempts to find a cure. In 1616, he recalled that before he had fallen ill, Iwan Telepianow had poured some magic powder on him, so he decided to accuse Iwan of bewitching him (NBLDU VR, no. 518iii *Akta ekonomji Samborowskiej* [1614–1632], f. 91 (1616)). In 1717, the sickness of the master of Gregori Kruczynski from Kamianets'-Podil'ski was connected to the suspicious actions of Marcin Szczurkowski who left a horse's leg on the furnace of Kruczynski's master's house a few days before the illness struck (TDIA [Kiev], fond 39, op.1, no. 53, f. 309rev). Likewise, Stefan Gębarzowski from the town of Dubno fell ill in 1732. When this illness did not pass after seven weeks, it was assigned to bewitchment because his wife learned that shortly before he became ill, the wife of their neighbour, Andrzej Dęmbski, had put some charms on the fence on the border of their plots. After a brief search, they even managed to find those alleged charms (No. 38 [1732], in Antonovich 1877, 81–2).

Praskevia Ivaniva, mother of the officer Martsev from the village of Gutenivka suffered from a strange and horrible illness in 1759. Finally, she died, allegedly of this illness. Her son considered this illness to be the result of bewitchment since someone had sent her a hare's leg sometime before his mother fell ill (TDIA [Kiev], fond 1819, op.1, no. 132, ff. 1–20).

Sometimes the actions that preceded the illness were more explicit and saturated with danger and menace. In 1767, Karp, a miller from Dubno, became very ill. His legs were paralysed and it was suspected that this had happened as a result of bewitchment. In the course of an investigation that lasted till 1768, it transpired that another miller, Jacko, had used witchcraft against him. In order to bewitch Karp, Jacko had invited two more people, his wife Anna and a practitioner of magic, Tymko Sereda. He asked the latter "to take away" the legs of Karp. Several people testified that they knew that Sereda had prepared different concoctions and that probably one of them was used to bewitch Karp. Jacko's daughter-in-law claimed that she had seen two concoctions in her in-laws' house—they were in flasks, one of which was red and another was ginger. She suspected that these had been prepared to bewitch Karp, for one night, she saw Karp returning home drunk and her mother-in-law giving those concoctions to him. Soon after that, he indeed "lost his legs" (No. 69–70 [1767–1768], in Antonovich 1877, 132–4).

In another part of Ukraine, the Hetmanate, diseases resulting from witchcraft were often seen as being connected with *zakrutki* or "knots" in the fields. *Zakrutki* were specific knots on spikes found in cornfields that were considered to be made by evil people or witches. Finding such a knot in someone's field was taken as a bad sign. People were afraid to untie these knots since it was believed that only the one who had tied the knot, or a mighty healer, could undo it. The entire harvest was thought to be lost and should people dare to use crops from the bewitched field, they were expected to fall ill and soon die. In 1785, it was conveyed in a report to the board of the Kiev vicegerent that several dwellers of the village of Gaturovka had fallen ill with some mysterious sickness. The arms and legs of these people had stopped functioning and eight people had died. It was reported that witchcraft was probably the cause of this illness. Among those who had died was the family of Vasilij Chernoded, who was renowned as a witch. When a knot was found in the cornfield, he said that he was not afraid to undo it, since he had a special power. After he had harvested the crops and his family had eaten bread made from those crops, they fell ill and Vasilij said that they would not recover. Because of such a knot, the family of another villager, Ivan Budila, also died. A trained physician who inspected the corpses announced that the sickness was indeed mysterious and he could not find out the reason for it (TDIA [Kiev], fond 193, op.1, no. 603, ff. 41–42).

These records leave a similar impression about witch disease—it was sudden, long lasting and could well be lethal. Not all the trial records contain explicit, if any, descriptions of the symptoms or specific signs of bewitchment. Nevertheless, one can still find some descriptions. For example, Kośt Łobodziński, a citizen of Kamianets'-Podil'ski who suffered from a bewitchment in 1700, stated that he felt pain which was burning him from inside (No. 1 [1700], in Antonovich 1877, 43). When the child of the above-mentioned Daniel Czyżewski from Vyzhva died in 1732, a Jewish woman, Elowa Syswa, recommended that he should examine the body of the dead infant to find out if his sickness was the result of bewitchment or whether it had happened because it was God's will. The sign of bewitchment would have been a blue spot on the child's back and a white spot somewhere on the abdomen. Since these signs were found, Daniel's suspicions of bewitchment were confirmed (TDIA [Kiev], fond 32, op.1, no. 5, ff. 229rev-230). The mother of the official Martsev mentioned above became unrecognisable after bewitchment—her body swelled and skin burst (TDIA [Kiev], fond 1819, op.1, no. 132, f. 2). Another symptom often attributed to bewitchment was when the victim's arms and/or legs were paralysed (for instance, AGAD, *Księga Czarna Krzemienieckie 1747–1777* (mf 18958), 53–5 [1747]; No. 69–70 [1767–1768], in Antonovich 1877, 132–4; TDIA [Kiev], fond 193, op.1, no. 603, ff. 41–42 [1785]).

If the ailment diagnosed as bewitchment was not grave enough, people might express doubt, even though preceding events indicated that witchcraft could have been at work. For instance, in 1747, the wife of Omelko Jendzeiowicz from the town of Olyka who had previously been accused of witchcraft and of spreading illness was accused for the second time of the same actions—of pouring dirty water onto the street in order to bewitch her neighbours. One of the witnesses in this trial, Jan Szawałkiewicz, testified that sometime earlier, his wife and children had been passing the place where the bewitched water had been poured and that afterwards the children had all become covered with some strange spots. However, the witness claimed that he was not sure if those spots had been the result of bewitchment. One can suspect that most probably in popular opinion spots were not an illness directly associated with bewitchment and that Szawałkiewicz had thought of witchcraft only because he knew for sure that something mysterious and witchcraft-like had happened in the place where his children were passing (No. 62 [1747], in Antonovich 1877, 117).

Reading some of the trial materials, one often comes across references to the witch having "eaten" (*ziadła*) someone. The phrase "has eaten" was used to describe the effect of witchcraft on the victim's health. Probably it was used as a synonym of or variation on "witch disease". If someone was mentioned as having been "eaten" by a witch it meant that this person had fallen ill, that the illness was protracted, that the person's faculties gradually decayed and that the person had faded away. In 1732, while quarrelling with Olexa Koladęcz, the wife of Paweł Ohorelczuk of Vyzhva mentioned among other things that his grandmother, Lomazianka had "eaten" several people and that his mother had also "eaten" one man (TDIA [Kiev], fond 32, op.1, no. 5, ff. 266-266rev). In the materials of the trial concerning Olexa's grandmother, Lomazianka, one finds the same term used by the accusers to describe harm inflicted by Lomazianka.

Lukasz Suproniuk told Lomazianka, “You have already eaten Tokaryk and Chilczuk and now you are going to eat our mother” (No. 21 [1716], in Antonovich 1877, 64). In 1731, the wife of the inhabitant of Olyka, Daniło Szawatkiewicz, accused the wife of Kaspar Koszczei of using witchcraft practices in order “to eat” the wife and daughter of Marko Czuchelewicz (TDIA [Kiev], fond 1237, op.1, no. 8, ff. 394-394rev). Demian Semenowicz, also a dweller inhabitant of Olyka, who was accused of “eating” a man in 1730, managed to find the humorous side of such an accusation and answered that the man was too big to be eaten (TDIA [Kiev], fond 1237, op.1, no. 8, f. 310. Other examples of accusations of “eating” someone can also be found: TDIA (Kiev), fond 32, op.1, no. 5, ff. 14-14rev [1726]; fond 32, op.1, no. 5, ff. 229–230 [1732]).

On the basis of many Ukrainian trial materials, one may conclude that for some reason, people in the eighteenth century were disposed to associate witchcraft with unhygienic behaviour, and either voluntary or involuntary attempts to spread illnesses. It is not clear why people pouring dirty liquids over public ground or on ground belonging to others were accused of attempts to bewitch but this may be additional evidence that witchcraft was associated with various situations representing a danger to health. In 1728, the wife of a Jew, Meusz Leyzorowicz, was beaten by Piotr Pozniewicz, both residents of the town of Olyka. Piotr explained his behaviour by saying that his daughter had fallen ill after Leyzorowicz’s wife had poured dirty water over his land, water in which she had bathed her children (TDIA [Kiev], fond 1237, op.1, no. 8, ff. 80-80rev). A similar story happened in Olyka one year later, when a child of Sytko Olifierowicz fell ill and the infant’s illness was attributed to the evil will of Sytko’s neighbour’s wife who had poured used water in which her child had been bathed under the house of Sytko. The latter even turned to a soothsayer to confirm his suspicions (TDIA [Kiev], fond 1237, op.1, no. 8, f. 163rev). Some people who were constantly creating unhygienic situations in towns excited displeasure on the part of their neighbours, who might have taken this as an attempt at bewitchment of other local inhabitants, and sometimes even evoked the displeasure of the town authorities.

This was the case with the wife of the resident of Olyka, Omelian Jędrzeiowicz, who was involved in several suits during the years 1746–1747. At first, she was accused by Dmitr Ostapowicz of attempts to bewitch his family by pouring some dirty liquid over his territory. Omelian’s wife explained that she did not intend to bewitch anyone; quite the contrary: she was trying to cure her child of a scare. To this end, she had bathed the child and afterwards poured the water over a dog which happened to be lying on a neighbour's ground (No. 59–60 [1746], in Antonovich 1877, 114–6). The next year, the same woman was accused of the same actions—pouring dirty liquid over a neighbour's ground, but this time in the territory of Opanas Moysieiowicz. Although Opanas was not quite sure whether this had been done for good or evil, he still suspected witchcraft, for some people had already fallen ill, so he did not let anyone pass the spot where the unknown liquid had been poured (No. 61–62 [1747], in Antonovich 1877, 116–8). In 1750, the daughter of the town-dweller of Kremenets', Adam Sędkiewicz, was suspected by Paweł Marczenko and his wife of witchcraft and an attempt to spread some contagious disease by pouring dirty water into the street. Adam Sędkiewicz claimed that it was only water used for bathing and that his daughter was ill with rheumatism, an ailment not dangerous to other people. The authorities found both sides to be in the wrong. On the one hand, they claimed that Adam's daughter was endangering the hygienic situation of the city, since no matter what was in that bath, it was not a good idea to pour it into the street where people and animals traversed, while on the other hand, Paweł Marczenko was wrong to state that Adam's daughter was spreading illness if the information was not confirmed (No. 68 [1750], in Antonovich 1877, 132).

Poison was another health-endangering thing associated with witchcraft. An accusation of witchcraft would often include an accusation of poisoning since poisons were often considered magical charms. By the seventeenth century, poison was already under scientific scrutiny by Italian physicians, the knowledge gained constituting a subfield of forensic medicine (Robisheaux 2001, 207). However, the popular mind did not differentiate between chemistry and magic, or poison and charms. In some European countries, even after witches ceased to be persecuted as magic practitioners, they were still tried as poisoners (Levack 1999, 80). One can also find this close association between poisoning and bewitchment in Ukrainian trials. For example, in 1717, Anna Grekowiczycha from Sataniv was accused by her husband, Jacko, of an attempt to bewitch and poison him with some magic charms (TDIA [Kiev], fond 50, op.1, no. 1, ff. 156). In July 1748, Wincent Rużanski was tried and executed for endeavouring to bewitch his master, Michał Zebroszek and his wife with the help of some poison which he had stolen from a shop kept by a Jewish woman (AGAD, *Księga Czarna Krzemienieckie 1747–1777* (mf 18958), 63–8).

After health had been harmed by natural or supernatural means, there was a need to find a cure. Official medicine was still in a poor condition. The situation with the official medicine of the early modern times was best described by Robin Briggs: "The learned medicine of humanist physicians was firmly rooted in this seedbed of error. Its practitioners had no real understanding of reproduction, the digestive system, the function of the blood or the lungs, the nervous system or indeed anything much else. Most of their prescriptions were useless, disgusting or potentially lethal. To preserve the illusion that they were doing something useful, they commonly subjected patients to a regime of emetics, purges and bleeding, the only forms of intervention readily available. It would have taken some ingenuity to devise better methods of undermining strong constitutions and finishing off weak ones; slavish obedience to orthodox medical theory was the quick way to the grave" (Briggs 2002, 57).

Moreover, not everyone could afford the services of a doctor. Consultations were still extremely expensive. An Orthodox preacher of the seventeenth century, Antonij Radyvilovskyi, makes mention of greedy doctors in one of his Sunday sermons: "when doctors work with ill people, they ask a lot of money, and it does not depend on whether they heal them or not: you have to pay them well anyway" (Radyvilovskyi 1688, 340). That is why it is not surprising that most people preferred to go to magic healers. Most information about magic healers originates from trial materials about healings that proved ineffective. Since very little is known about successful healings, it is impossible to estimate how many healings were effective and how many were not. However, even if there were many unsuccessful healings, this did not prevent people from turning to magic healers. As follows from trial materials, some healers kept their practices for many years and had many clients (TDIA [Kiev], fond 35, op. 1, no. 13, ff. 234–6 [1710]; fond 1237, op.1, no. 8, f. 86-86rev [1728]; fond 990, op. 1, no. 535 [1765]). Moreover, when summoned to court, magic healers usually claimed that they were only able to heal certain kinds of illnesses and not others. One can assume that magic healers were prone to taking money from their clients, though one learns about this only from those few cases when the healer took money but did not cure the ill person (for example, TDIA [Kiev], fond 39, op. 1, no. 53, f. 728rev [1721] and fond 35, op. 1, no. 13, ff. 234–236 [1710]). Some healers even managed to kill healthy people with their cures, as did Demko Chaliczow, a healer from the town of Dubno. He claimed that he would cure the infertility of Oryna Michajlukowa. It is not clear what methods he used but after some time he boasted around the town that Oryna would give birth at the beginning of winter. Quite the contrary: soon the woman started to feel ill and her husband turned to other practitioners who said that his wife was not pregnant. Since she was feeling worse, she was taken to an expensive physician in the nearby city of Ostrog: however, the doctor too was useless, and after some time Oryna died (No. 46 [1741], in Antonovich 1877, 90).

Moreover, many people preferred to practise healing on their own without turning to a doctor or healer, becoming, at the least, the doctor for their own family. I have already mentioned medical books used by some families in the Ukrainian territories. Another way of discovering the best method of healing for a sick family member was to take advice from other people. Methods used for healing varied. They included methods that would seem rational from the point of view of the modern observer and in most cases, they would involve the use of different herbs and ointments. Prayers and incantations were other kinds of healing practice. According to the view of the Church, the most effective medicines were prayers and attending church and shrines. However, the way "prayers" were used in popular medicine would not have been approved of by their priests. These were not traditional Christian prayers but specific incantations invoking the names of Christ, the Virgin Mary, the saints and angels.

Finally, there were the magic methods used in popular medicine. However, one can assume that the popular mind did not differentiate between all these methods. People were willing to endeavour in anything that might be effective. John Henry wrote in this respect, "Curing disease by magical means was always popularly regarded as being at least as effective as any other kind of treatment" (Henry 1991, 215. This can be compared with assumptions made by Roper 1994, 184). Methods that would certainly seem strange today were taken quite seriously by contemporaries. Here are several medical recommendations mentioned in medical books:

> If someone has a wound on the lips. Collect several green toads, common ones, those which live in water, put some butter into the mouth of every toad then put those toads into a new pot in which previously you must make several holes, cover this pot and bury it into the soil but leave the top above the ground so that it is possible to pour some oil into it. This is the way to use the oil: collect more toads, dry them in a furnace and make a powder, mix this with the oil when it is ready. It can then be applied to the sick person. However, it is worth being preceded by the use of purging charms (*Liekarstva opisanniie, kotorymi biez miedika v domu vsiak poratovatsia mozhet* 1984, 31).

> If someone has headaches. Take the milk of a woman and mix it with oil and with good vinegar, and apply it to the head (Potebnia 1890, 4).

However, I would suggest that some of these methods were looked at with scepticism even by contemporaries. Some of them appeared plainly superstitious in character. In 1734, three villagers from Chukva in the Ruthenian palatinate were summoned to explain their strange behaviour. During a Christian holiday, they had climbed the bell tower and rang the bell. One of them, Anna, said that they did not mean to do any harm but did it only in the hope that by this she would be cured of infertility (TDIA [(Lviv], fond 142, op. 1, no. 7, 384–6). Many cases demonstrate that quite often the actions of people practising healing were taken by observers as attempts to bewitch someone. This indicates that the methods used for healing and bewitchment were similar and perhaps merged together in popular beliefs.

In 1673, the criminal court of Lviv accused Anna Stanisławowa of witchcraft. She was caught at the time of the Corpus Christi procession as she was collecting soil walked on by the procession. It was suspected that she was going to use that soil for the purpose of carrying out witchcraft. Anna explained in front of the court that she had collected the soil "not to harm people but as a cure for falling sickness from which she suffered each day. She had taken the soil following the advice of an old woman" (TDIA [Lviv], fond 52, op. 2, no. 311, 496). In 1700, two Jews, Abraham Irszeiwicz and Pesia were accused of witchcraft by a citizen of Kovel', Chwedor Andrzeiowicz. He saw Pesia taking a cat to the house of Abraham, where that cat was circumcised, as he assumed, in order to engage in witchcraft. In the court, the accused denied that they were using the cat for witchcraft: quite the opposite, they claimed, they were attempting to use it to heal (TDIA [Kiev], fond 35, op. 1, no. 12, ff. 18rev-19).

In 1710, Hryhory Babiczenko from Kamianets'-Podil'ski was suspected of practising witchcraft by Fedor Jacew because he was seen secretly brewing some suspicious concoction in his house. Hryhory later explained that he was concocting a medicine for his sick child and that no witchcraft was involved (No. 13 [1710], in Antonovich 1877, 57). In 1717, Anna Grekowiczycha was accused by her husband Jacko of immoral behaviour and attempts to bewitch and poison him. To substantiate his claims, Jacko brought a suspicious substance to the town court of Sataniv. Anna defended herself by saying that it was only a medicine. She had some gynaecological problems and a woman had recommended that she prepare a medicine, but Anna was afraid to do so at home. The recipe called for her to burn something and add some herbs. If it were seen, her husband could have suspected some witchcraft (which in the event he actually did). To prove her innocence, it was demanded that Anna drink the suspicious liquid laced with vodka in the court, which she did (TDIA [Kiev], fond 50, op. 1, no. 1, f. 156).

In 1718, a poor Jewish woman, Chajka Szmujlicha, from the town of Dubno was suspected of witchcraft when she was seen on the road burying a pot in the dirt. When asked in the court about the pot and witchcraft, Chajka said that another Jewish woman, Josiowa, had given her money to bury the pot. After this, Josiowa was summoned to the court. She explained that it was not an act of witchcraft but a healing cure. Her daughter had been sick for several days, was getting paler and refused to eat. So, she had consulted with other women about ways of healing her child. One woman recommended that she should mix eggs, wax, flour and poppy seeds and cook them all together. Then she had to put the mixture into a pot and bury it into the ground where no people would walk (No. 27 [1718], in Antonovich 1877, 69. Antonovich by mistake wrote that this case had taken place in Kamianets'-Podil'ski). Łukasz Łasiński, a cooper from Kamianets'-Podil'ski accused Feśka Andrzeiowa Czumakowa in 1729 of attempting to bewitch him. He said that she had taken a knife and a cup of beer from him. After that, he saw her doing something mysterious—dripping the beer over the edge of the knife on the staircase. Feśka confessed that she was doing all those strange things to heal her husband (No. 33 [1729], in Antonovich 1877, 76–7).

To conclude, I would like to emphasise several issues. Natural and supernatural causes of illnesses and their cures were mixed even in learned medicine of the early modern period, not to mention popular medicine. It was true for early modern Ukrainian lands as well. Here, witchcraft was an important factor when it came to diagnosis and remedies. In some cases of mysterious and lethal illness, bewitchment was conceived as a specific ailment in its own right which in most cases was impossible to cure. In other cases, people who were notorious as witches were suspected of causing various illnesses which demanded magical cures. People in Ukraine had a choice—either to turn to a healer or other medical specialist or to search for a remedy on their own. In each case, there was a danger that a person involved in magical healing may be accused of witchcraft because the methods used in taking away people's health and making them recover were so similar that even contemporaries were often unable to distinguish the one from the other.

References

Published Sources

Antonovich, Vladimir B. 1877. *Koldovstvo. Dokumenty—process—izsledovanie* [Witchcraft. Documents—trials—study]. St. Petersburg.

Kniga liechebnaia ot mnogikh liekarstv. 1984. "Kniga liechebnaia ot mnogikh liekarst [The medical book against many ailments]." In *Likars'ki ta hospodars'ki poradnyky XVIII st* [Medical and household manuals of the eighteenth century], edited by Vitalii A. Peredriienko, 92–113. Kiev: Naukova dumka. (Pamiatky ukraïns'koï movy XVIII st. / Seriia naukovoï literatury.)

Liekarstva opisanniie. 1984: "Liekarstva opisanniie, kotorymi biez miedika v domu vsiak poratovatsia mozhet [The description of medicines which everyone can use at home without a doctor]." In *Likars'ki ta hospodars'ki poradnyky XVIII st* [Medical and household manuals of the eighteenth century], edited by Vitalii A. Peredriienko, 19–75. Kiev: Naukova dumka.

Potebnia, Aleksandr. 1890. "Malorusskie domashnie liechebniki XVIII v [Domestic medical books of Malaia Rus of the eighteenth century]." *Kievskaia starina* 28 (1): 91–4.

Radyvilovskyi, Antonii. 1688. *Vieniets Khristov z propoviedii nedelnykh aki z tsvietov rozhanykh na uktrashenie Pravoslavno-katolicheskoi S-toi Vostochnoi Tserkvi spletenyi* [The crown of Christ made of Sunday sermons as if of different flowers to enrich St Eastern Orthodox-Catholic Church]. Kiev.

Literature

Briggs, Robin. 2002. *Witches and Neighbours: The Social and Cultural Context of European Witchcraft*. Oxford: Blackwell Publishers.

Estes, Leland. 1983. "The medical origins of the European witch craze: a hypothesis." *Journal of Social History* 17: 271–84.

Henry, John. 1991. "Doctors and Healers: Popular Culture and the Medical Profession." In *Science, Culture and Popular Belief in Renaissance Europe*, edited by S. Pumfrey, P. L. Rossi, and M. Slawinski, 191–221. Manchester, and New York: Manchester University Press.

Levack, Brian P. 1999. "The Decline and End of Witchcraft Prosecutions." In *The Athlone History of Witchcraft and Magic in Europe. The Eighteenth and Nineteenth Centuries*, edited by S. Clark, and B. Ankarloo, 7–96. London: Athlone.

Robisheux, Thomas. 2001. "Witchcraft and Forensic Medicine in Seventeenth-century Germany." In *Languages of Witchcraft: Narrative, Ideology and Meaning in Early Modern Culture*, edited by Stuart Clark, 197–216. Basingstoke: Macmillan.

Roper, Lyndal. 1994. *Oedipus and the Devil: Witchcraft, Sexuality and Religion in Early Modern Europe.* London and New York: Routledge.

GEORG TALLAR AND THE 1753 VAMPIRE HUNT: ADMINISTRATION, MEDICINE AND THE RETURNING DEAD IN THE HABSBURG BANAT

ÁDÁM MÉZES

Georg Tallar's *Visum repertum* is one of the fundamental eighteenth-century texts dealing with the belief in vampires. Nevertheless, secondary literature has made little effort to uncover the exact context of its generation, which in turn resulted in misconceptions about even very basic data relating to the work. The present article makes an attempt to remedy this situation by analysing the *Visum repertum* in its own historical context of the Habsburg Banat of the 1750s and by comparing the manuscript and the published version of the text. This approach yields a more complete picture of vampirism as an administrative problem, and sheds light on hitherto obscure aspects of the creation of the text: the article offers a new dating to 1753, delineates the members, itinerary and duties of the so-called Kallacsa Commission, as a member of which Tallar carried out his vampire investigations and points out the various textual levels through which he tried to fashion himself as an expert of Vlach culture, a learned surgeon and a humble agent of moral and medical enlightenment.

Vampir, moroi or bloodsucker?

The protagonist of the present essay is Johann Georg Tallar, a German surgeon known for his empirically based medical treatise on vampires. In 1753 Tallar was chosen to join a commission that would carry out investigations about the returning dead. The site was the Habsburg province of the Banat, a region bordered roughly by the rivers Maros (Mureș), Tisza (Tisa) and Danube to the north, west and south and Wallachia to the east. It used to belong to the Hungarian Kingdom until the Ottoman conquest; after the expulsion of the Turks, it was incorporated into the Habsburg Empire in 1718. The provincial government was set up in Temeswar (today Timişoara) and was overseen not by the Hungarian crown, but by the Vienna Aulic Treasury and the Aulic War Council. The reorganisation of life in the Banat was based on a great number and variety of settlers, primarily Vlachs (Romanian), Rascians (Serb) and Germans. The German administration had to face local beliefs in the returning dead early on.

The ethnographic literature on the various types of malicious dead and their related folkloric beings is vast, and the fact that such creatures are known under various names in different areas and that they have changed through history makes classification difficult (see among others: Murgoci 1926; Senn 1982; Barber 1988; Corradi Musi 1995; Pócs 1999, 2001a, 2001b; and for a concise but thorough overview see especially: Kreuter 2001, 45–67). In order to determine what these creatures actually meant to the different inhabitants of the Banat in the eighteenth century, one has to turn to historical sources. A problem is that such sources, by and large, are scarce, occasionally incompatible with each other and essentially translations: the actual holders of such traditions can be read through the filter of a different culture, in this case, that of the German administration. There are three related terms denoting the returning dead that emerge in the sources of the time: *vampir*, *moroi* and *Blutsauger*.

The etymology of the Serbian term *vampir* is contested and is usually traced back either to Slavic or Turkic-through-Slavic origins and would mean "non-flier" or "witch" respectively (Kreuter 2001, 68–9). Based on the few sources so far known to secondary literature, the term *vampir* was strongly present among the Rascians of the eighteenth century. As will be shown below, the creature which it denoted was a corpse that came back to harm the living and that had to be executed in order for the problems to cease. The name or its cognates today are attested all across Eastern, Western and Southern Slavic folklore, and are present in especially diverse forms in Bulgarian. (Kreuter 2001, 69; Afanas'ev 1976, 163, 165).[1] Interestingly enough, in Serbian it became marginalised during the nineteenth century in favour of *vukodlak*, a term originally denoting a

---

[1] In Polish territory, *upior* was a corpse reanimated, basically possessed, by an evil spirit; the term is still there in contemporary Polish and Ukrainian folklore (Betsinger and Scott 2014, 469). In Russian lands, there may have existed the creature *upyr* in medieval times, but it has now disappeared and the malicious dead are called *eretik* (i.e. heretic), which can be either corpses or the ghosts of dead sorcerers who take up the shape of or possess actual corpses; they devour people and cause all sorts of harm (Moszyński 1976, 185; Oinas 1998, 52).

werewolf, i.e. a living person who would periodically transform into a wolf and would mostly attack cattle.[2]

In Romanian, the term "vampire" has apparently never existed. Instead, people talked about the *strigoi* or *moroi* and their female equivalents *strigoica* and *moroica*. However, most eighteenth-century sources call them vampires, for the German language adopted the Rascian name first and used it for the Vlach creature as well. The two creatures are very similar, although today's folklorists distinguish between two related meanings of the *moroi*, the first of which was not part of the make-up of the Rascian vampire. If used for a live person, *moroi* today means "witch" or "wizard"; if on a dead person, it means a malignant, bloodsucking revenant. At the same time, just as in Serbian, its dead meaning became eclipsed by the *vârcolac*, originally denoting a werewolf (Murgoci 1926; Senn 1982).

The history of the terms *moroi* and *vampir* are indicative of the intimate relations between witch, werewolf and the returning dead. Across cultures, the returning dead usually come into existence from those who had something unclean or strange about their birth, life or death. For instance, they were born in a caul or with a tail, lived an unclean life or died unbaptised, were murdered, committed suicide, or some animal jumped through their corpse (Kreuter 2001, 32–7). The witch and the werewolf fit into this pattern due to their abnormal lifestyle and body-soul relations, which can easily be imagined to continue even beyond the grave (Pócs 1999). The concept, today inextricable from the popular image of the vampire, is contagion: those "sucked" by a vampire will themselves necessarily become one after death. While according to Peter Kreuter this idea is not attested in south-east European folklore, in eighteenth-century documents about Rascian and Vlach revenants, it figures emphatically, a phenomenon to be given closer attention later on in the essay (Kreuter 2001, 33. Afanas'ev, however, states that it is part of Serbian folklore. Afanas'ev 1976, 162).

The ways in which the vampire and the *moroi* do harm show great variety, as do the rites to counter them. Usually, their activities involve physical harassment, torturing, pressing on the chest, strangling, sexual intercourse or bloodsucking. Kreuter rightly points out that the sucking is actually rather a taking away of the life force, without biting or puncturing

[2] In 1820, under the Serbian prince Miloš Obrenović, measures were still taken against vampire finders called *vampirdžije*. However, in the middle of the nineteenth century, the ethnographer Vuk Karadžic had already referred to the returning dead as *vukodlak* (Fine 1998, 57–9).

the skin (Kreuter 2001, 170).[3] The first German reports about vampire/*moroi* cases in the 1720s in both Habsburg Serbia and the Banat usually name the creatures "Bloodsuckers".[4] This shows that it was an integral part of the local cultures, even though (as Kreuter suggests) it might have been over-emphasised in the reports by the German officials, who for some reason became fascinated with this specific aspect. The idea that certain measures have to be taken against the malicious dead is widespread across cultures. Skulls severed after death and placed in between the feet, remains of stakes in the chest, corpses placed on their stomachs, limbs tied together and stones wedged into the mouths of corpses have been discovered in archaeological finds in diverse parts of Europe, dating back to various periods of history.[5] Written historical evidence and contemporary folkloric practice also attest to the existence of these practices. Karen Lambrecht cites a number of such sources in her study on the Silesian returning dead (Lambrecht 1994, 53–4), and Georg Tallar also found most of these measures among the Vlachs of the eighteenth century (Tallar 1753, 13r). As will be shown below, on the southern Habsburg borderland of the eighteenth century, the practices of countering the malicious dead included but were not limited to staking, decapitation or burning at the stake. However, archaeologists usually caution against drawing hasty conclusions based solely on archaeological evidence, because possible alternative

---

[3] At the same time, exceptions can be found. In Kashubian tales, there is a puncture on the chest or the nipple of the victim of a vampire (*veshchij*) (Afanas'ev 1976, 163). The Russian "eretik" devours the victims, while in Silesian folklore, certain corpses (the *Nachzehrer*) chew at their shrouds or at their own body and this way cause sicknesses and epidemics without leaving their graves (Schürmann 1990; Lambrecht 1994).

[4] While in Habsburg Serbia the first report of 1725 already gives the name *vampir*, in the Banat, the first instance dates to 1738, Uypalanka (see below); while in the protocol books, this date is 1743, and even then it is secondary (Baróti 1900–1902, 150: "Lugoscher Verwalteramt begleitet ein zur Einsicht ein ärztliches Zeugnis über die Unrichtigkeit der Birnaer Gemeinde-Anklage, dass nämlich dort vor sieben Wochen ein Blutsauger oder Wampir begraben sein solle.").

[5] The relation of pre-Christian ideas about the returning dead to those of Christianity is a complex matter and is dealt with among others by Lecouteux 2009 and Reynolds 2009. The difficulties of interpreting archaeological finds are emphasised by Schaub 2009 and Barrowclough 2014, who cite numerous examples from the early Middle Ages to the eighteenth century. For early medieval Slavic examples, see Krumphanzlová 1961 and 1966; for medieval and early modern Polish examples, see Gardela and Kajkowski 2013 and Betsinger and Scott 2014. Finally, nineteenth-century New England cases are described by Bell 2006.

explanations include homicide, posthumous judicial punishment of criminals or grave robbery.

For the purposes of the present essay, "vampirism" will be understood as a disease-explanatory system consisting of so-called "vampire sickness" and the countermeasures inflicted upon a corpse in order to avert it. The former is a rapidly progressing affliction usually characterised by stomach and chest pains and a general withering away of the victim and is explained by the community as being caused by a vampire. It is contagious in a very peculiar sense: the victims of vampires are likely to become vampires themselves. "Vampires" are returning dead who plague the living in various ways, often by sucking their blood. This definition is based on an eighteenth-century southern Habsburg borderland environment and works well for the eighteenth-century Rascian *vampir*, the Vlach *moroi*, and to a lesser extent for the Silesian returning dead. This is also the sense in which Empress Maria Theresa's personal physician, Gerard van Swieten understood the concept in his manuscript treatise *Remarques sur le Vampyrisme de Sylésie de l'an 1755*.

Using so far largely overlooked sources, the present essay will be able to contribute data to the figure of the *moroi* among the Vlachs of the eighteenth-century Banat. Sources on Rascian vampires still have to be collected, and archival collections from the Ottoman Empire may be especially promising. (For the scarce literature on vampirism in the Ottoman Empire see: Köhbach 1979; Bijedić 2001 and Sariyannis 2013). At the same time, due to the nature of the sources, scholars have to examine the folklore of the time through the filter of the Habsburg administration. During the eighteenth century, the folkloric figure of the vampire became integrated into certain larger discourses, and social, political and cultural processes, and the vampire can be used as a test case for these processes.

Enlightenment, governance and the vampires

The figure of the vampire entered modern European thought through the Habsburg administration of the Southern borderlands in the first half of the eighteenth century.[6] It was a 1725 official report published in the

---

[6] In fact, there was an earlier channel as well, through texts reporting on Polish/Russian folklore (see Vermeir 2011 and Keyworth 2006, 251). A 1693 edition of the French gazette *Mercure Gallant* already gave news from the Russian Empire about "oupires": corpses, or demons that take up the shape of corpses who torment the living (mostly their own family) and suck their blood until they die. In his 1721 *Historia Naturalis Curiosa Regni Poloniae*, the Jesuit Gabriel Rzaczynski also

newspaper *Wienerisches Diarium* that made the "vampire" (spelled "Vampyr") known to the public. (Copia eines Schreibens aus dem Gradisker District in Ungarn. *Wienerisches Diarium* 58, 21.07.1725). The report was sent by the cameral provisor of the Gradiska district in Habsburg Serbia to the Vienna administration about the strange events in the village of Kisilova (today's Kisiljevo).[7] Peter Plogojowitz, a Rascian peasant, returned from the dead and kept tormenting people at night by lying on their chests and sucking their blood, in the end killing nine within a week. The local community requested Johann Frombald, the provisor of Ram-Gradiska district, to visit the village accompanied by an Orthodox priest and oversee the exhumation of Plogojowitz. Frombald consented and to his surprise, the ten-week-old corpse looked fresh: hair, beard and nails had grown, new skin was seen growing under the old that was coming away, and fresh blood was flowing from his orifices. Based on these signs, he was pronounced a *Vampyr*. Locals drove a stake through his heart and saw a copious amount of blood flowing from the wound, as well as other "wild signs" which the provisor did not deem decorous to disclose. He was visibly concerned about having legitimised the rite with his presence and asked his superiors to blame all possible mistakes on the excited mob, for they had threatened him that they would leave the village if they were not granted permission.

The case that catapulted the vampire towards world fame, however, was that of Arnold Paole, a *hayduk* from the village of Medvedia (Medveđa) in the southernmost corner of Habsburg Serbia.[8] The story

---

reported about the Polish belief in the "upier" or female "upierzyca", bloodsucking dead witches. Printed in the Russian Empire in Latin it could reach western audiences as well (Lambrecht 1994. 52).

[7] It is only a copy of the original report that is known today: Copia des vom Herrn Frombald kayserlichen Cameral Provisore […] OESTA - HHSA Turcica I/191, fol. 25–26. Published in: Hamberger 1992, 43–5. The exact location of the village Kisilova is frequently misplaced by scholars to the bank of the Sava river in Slavonia (see: Hamberger 1992, 43; Nowosadtko 2004, 157; Bräunlein 2012, 712). The reason for this mistake is that there was also a Gradiska disctrict. However, according to the report, Kisilova was in the Ram district, opposite Uypalanka, on the right bank of the Danube, in Belgrade-centred Habsburg Serbia (1718–39). Frombald was the provisor of the Ram and the neighbouring Gradiska district as well.

[8] Medvedia is on the left bank of the River Morava and belonged to the district of Iajodina. According to the German terminology of the era, a "Hayduk/Heyduk" was one of the irregular infantry soldiers, mostly (but not exclusively) Orthodox southern Slavs, whose duty in peacetime was border protection, while in times of war they had to join the army. In return for this, they were granted certain self-

started in 1727, when Paole fell off a hay wagon and broke his neck. During his lifetime he used to say that he would surely become a vampire, since he had been plagued by one in Ottoman lands and could only avoid being killed by eating from the soil of its grave. This, however, also meant that he would inevitably turn into a vampire after his death. He indeed returned from the grave, sucking blood and killing several people. The villagers unearthed him as well as his victims and found many of them to be vampires. They were staked, burnt and the ashes were thrown back into the grave. The procedure, however, was not thorough enough: the vampires attacked cattle as well, and anyone eating their meat later on was doomed to become a revenant. This way, four years later, seventeen people died after a rapid illness, complaining that certain dead villagers had tormented them.

The district captain sent Glaser, the physician of the quarantine station of Baragin (today Paraćin), with several military officers to the village to investigate the situation. Glaser examined the sick and decided that they were suffering from tertian and quatrain fever. He also had the bodies exhumed and noted that several corpses had become vampires (*vervampyret*) or were "suspicious". Not willing to make the decision, he had the corpses reburied and sent a report to Belgrade, the provincial centre. The vice governor sent a commission of three military surgeons and several officers to Medvedia. Led by regiment surgeon Flückinger, the surgeons dissected and confirmed Glaser's report: they found certain corpses in a vampire state ("im Vampirstande"); these bodies were decapitated by local Gypsies, burnt at the stake and the ashes thrown into the Morava. It seems that Gypsies were frequently deployed as vampire hunters (see Bijedić 2001, 56–57. For the vampire beliefs of Balkan Gypsies, see Vukanović 1976).

The reason why the Kisilova and Medvedia cases have been presented in greater detail here is that they served as basic sources of later learned discussions on vampirism and had a considerable effect on the development of the vampire-figure in European thought. Moreover, several elements found in these cases, such as the bloody-mouthed, seemingly fresh corpse, the terrified local community threatening to leave the village and the indecisive authorities are recurring features in later stories as well.

---

governing and taxation privileges and allowed to settle with their own community on the military frontier of the Habsburg Empire. For overall relations on the military frontier, see Sokol 1967 and Wessely 1970; for Habsburg Serbia, see Langer 1889; and for the Banat, see Milleker 1937.

Information on the Medvedia case first spread through personal networks and quickly reached the highest circles. Glaser's father published a letter about his son's experiences in the natural philosophy journal *Commercium Litterarium*, provoking a year-long debate. Ensign Kottovitz, stationed in Belgrade at the time, sent a letter to a university professor in Leipzig asking his opinion as to whether there were "sympathetic, devilish or astral spirit-related" effects working in the background. Meanwhile, the reports were published in pamphlets, treatises and university dissertations. (The two reports, alongside several smaller documents are located in OESTA—FHKA Hoffinanz Ungarn, r.Nr. 654, fol. 1131–1136 and 1142–43. The reports are published in: Hamberger 1992, 46–54. For the learned debate on vampirism see among others: Harmening 1983; Klaniczay 2002 and 2004; Hamberger 1992; Magyar 1999 and 2002).

The issue excited the imagination of scholars outside natural philosophy and medicine as well. Among theologians, the most notable contributor to the topic was Dom Augustin Calmet, a French Benedictine abbot (Vidal 2001, 15–22; Keyworth 2010). His 1746 *Traité sur les apparitions de espirits et sur les vampires* had numerous editions in several languages. Calmet took a complex stance. On the one hand, he stated that in general, vampirism was a superstition, but emphasised that the dead might be resurrected through divine miracles. Furthermore, in certain rare cases, the devil might also bring back to life the corpses themselves, and not just their apparitions. Finally, he added that it was also possible that the vampires were actually corpses in a vegetative state, that their soul had not entirely left the body, and that they might be coming out of their graves in search of life-sustaining blood. Pope Benedict XIV also mentions vampires in his *De servorum Dei beatificatione* of 1743; he briefly summarises some of the articles of the *Commercium Litterarium* and states that vampirism is only a superstition born out of fear and ignorance. Contrary to what much of secondary literature holds, this is all he wrote about vampirism; the attribution of a work titled *De vanitate vampyrorum* is entirely unfounded.[9] Meanwhile, the vampire conquered

---

[9] The attribution is based on the misreading of a citation in van Swieten's 1755 *Vampyrismus*: "Vid. Opera de Cannoizatione Sanct. vel Dissertationes Benedicti XIV. P.M. extractas ex dictis operibus. Venet. 1752. Vid Dissert. 5. § 4. Vol.3 ubi de Vanitate Vampyrorum [...]" (Swieten 1768, 23). Here van Swieten refers to two dissertations contained in Benedict's *De servorum Dei beatificatione*. The dissertations (titled *De revocatione mortuorum* and *De nonnullis cadaverum qualitatibus*) analyse the resurrection and lack of decomposition of cadavers in relation to sainthood; the pope mentions vampires only in a single, untitled paragraph in the former dissertation (Benedictus 1743, 198–9). Van Swieten meant

the popular imagination as well and its literary formulation also began (Janion 2006). At the same time, several elements were incorporated into its image, which were alien to the original Rascian creature. These included similar beliefs from other geographic areas, returning dead from ancient literature, and fear of premature burial, bloodsucking plants and bats. (For the entry of other folkloric beliefs, see Hamberger 1992, 65–96; for the phenomenon of bloodsucking in nature, see *Commercium Litterarium* 1732 (Hbd. XXI), 161–162; for premature burial, see Horányi 1997; for historical sources, see Hock 1900, and Harmening 1983).

While the figure of the vampire was being constructed and reconstructed at various levels of European thought, it remained a matter of life and death in various regions of the Habsburg Empire. The Habsburg administration, however, did not take a firm stance on the question until early 1755, when a case in Moravia caused a scandal in Vienna circles. In the village of Hermersdorf, the local council had thirty corpses disinterred and nineteen of them burnt for *magia posthuma*, that is, magic from beyond the grave. The process was especially gruesome, for relatives of the convicted corpses were commanded to drag the corpses through a hole carved into the wall of the cemetery using a hook and a rope. News of this motivated the Viennese court to take steps, for this time it was not a remote Rascian village, but the heart of the empire, and the "executions" were approved by a Catholic bishop. Empress Maria Theresa sent the highest ranked commission ever to investigate vampires to the village: the military physician Dr Wabst and professor of anatomy Dr Gasser (presumably with a suitable entourage). They determined that the lack of decomposition was due to natural causes, while the vampire sickness was a combination of a natural illness causing chest pains and the superstitious fears of the populace. The court in turn decided to deploy Jesuit missionaries and medical experts to fight the sickness with medications and to enlighten the people. Meanwhile, Gerard van Swieten, court physician and *protomedicus* (the head of the empire's medical system) wrote a manuscript treatise for the Empress about the case under the title, *Remarques sur le Vampyrisme de Sylésie de l'an 1755*. The court decided to publish it in German, Italian as well as in Latin.[10]

that the vanity of vampires is the content of this paragraph, not a work on its own. The said paragraph is found first in the 1743 edition of the pope's work and is reprinted in its 1752 edition.

[10] Some of the major sources relating to the Hermersdorf case are the empress's order to the Moravian cameral administration to support Wabst and Gasser (Linzbauer 1852, 722) and the protocols of the collegial body discussing the two physicians' reports (ibid, 722–5). Van Swieten's 1755 manuscript is bilingual, in

The Hermersdorf scandal also prompted Maria Theresa to issue an anti-superstition rescript on 1st March which warned the Catholic Church to report all supernatural phenomena (witchcraft, ghosts, treasure hunting and demonic possession) to the secular authorities, which in turn had to involve investigation of the case by a medical expert (Hamberger 1992, 85–6). From 1755 onwards, the empress engaged in repeated legislation for the decriminalisation of magic and a general fight against superstition. The 1st March rescript became integrated as a section into the empress's famous 1766 act, the *Lex caesaro-regia ad extirpandam superstitionem* that basically ended witchcraft persecutions in the Habsburg Empire by ordering all courts to send any accusations of magic to Vienna (Linzbauer 1852, 776–785. The 1755 rescript is Paragraph 16 (785), but the original introductory references to Moravian returning dead were deleted). As a number of scholars have aptly pointed out, however, the main motivating force behind these processes was not really vampirism but witchcraft and that they went hand in hand with a wide scale medicalisation campaign aimed at reforming public hygiene from the early 1740s onwards (Várkonyi 1991/2, 462–3; Levack 1999, 71–72; Tóth G. 2017).

Nevertheless, vampirism had its own, peculiar place in these processes, for it became formulated at the crux of governmental policies and agendas not relating to witchcraft. It was no accident that the vampire cases of the southern Habsburg borderland alarmed the local administration. The military frontier had been created not only against the Ottomans, but also against epidemics, most prominently the plague (Lesky 1957, 86–8). The threat of epidemics arriving through the military and commercial routes of the Balkans was constant. It was the duty of the civil or military administrative bodies of the borderland to gather information about, investigate and contain epidemics and halt their spread towards the heart of the empire. Since cases of vampirism usually involved sudden, numerous deaths within a community, they demanded the attention of

---

French and German, translated by Antoine Hiltenprand (OENB, Cod. Vindob. 7237 P. I. n. 18, fol. 1–14). The treatise also contains an extract of J.P. de Tournefort's 1718 *Relation d'un voyage du Levant,* a work in which the author, a botanist traveller, relates the measures taken against a Greek *vroucolacas* (a returning dead) which he witnessed in 1701 (see Hamberger 1992, 66–71). Scholarship usually cites the 1768 German printed edition of van Swieten's treatise, which appeared under the title *Vampyrismus,* as an appendix to Andreas Ulrich Mayer's *Abhandlung des Daseyns der Gespenster*. According to the introduction, van Swieten's treatise was printed in French in 1755, followed by a German and an Italian translation, both of them in 1756 (Swieten 1768, a2–a3; Linzbauer 1852, 725–37 also publishes the 1768 version).

local medical and administrative personnel. At the same time, practices related to vampirism also frustrated another facet of the overarching public hygiene project, namely the increasing regulation of cemeteries and dealings with the dead. Cemeteries were moved from churchyards outside the settlements, legislation was passed on the required depths of graves, and certain cultural habits involving physical contact with the dead became prohibited. It was as part of such regulations that in 1784, Joseph II warned the Orthodox Church to take a greater part in the fight against vampirism. (Linzbauer 1853, 122).[11]

A further peculiarity of vampirism is that in its eighteenth-century sense it arose from the cultures of Orthodox settlers in a land regained from Ottoman rule. As Jutta Nowosadtko writes, the issue can be interpreted as a phenomenon of occupation: it was the occupying administrative structure of the Habsburg Empire in the southern borderland which provided the channels for the first cases of revenants to become known (Nowosadtko 2004). Further, based on Gábor Klaniczay's research, Roy Porter remarks that vampirism was a perfect excuse to talk about the need to civilise the empire's inner savages (Klaniczay 2002; Porter 1999, 214–216). Due to the link between vampire beliefs and Orthodox Rascian and Vlach communities, the discourse was also framed in terms of the fight against the ignorant, superstitious Orthodox clergy. Finally, in a more general sense, both the vampire and its victims could be seen as unruly subjects, whose disciplining formed part of more general state measures to gain control over people (see especially Arlaud 2007, 134–5; and based on his work, Danneberg 2010; and Bräunline 2012). This disciplining meant that the vampire disease was medicalised while the seemingly uncorrupted corpses were naturalised and normalised. In these historical narratives of vampirism, the central figure is the Dutch van Swieten, who had a great influence on Maria Theresa's policies from 1743 onwards. Importantly, all these projects are recognised as coming from above and from the West (Klaniczay 1988 and 2002).

The centre-periphery, West-East direction of the spread of medicalisation, enlightenment and social disciplining is a powerful and tenable model in the case of the Habsburg Empire. However, it has the potential to eclipse

[11] "Sepulturae et superstitio de sanguisugis Gr.R.n.U.: Cum consuetudo: mortuos in aperta tumba sepeliendi adhuc in aliquibus locis vigeat, Constitutiones normales, ne in morbis contagionem minantibus demortui in in apertis tumbis circumferantur, denuo publicandae; ac Clerus Graeci Ritus non Uniti, Populi spirituali curae suae concrediti animos a superstitione circa: sanguisugas—Wampier dictos, quibus ultima fata suorum adscribere solent, etiamnum, ut refertur vigente, avertere connitantur."

local relations and render them inert and insignificant. In this sense, the way Georg Tallar is presented in secondary literature on vampirism is indicative. Tallar is frequently seen as a direct instrument in the hands of the Vienna administration, or more specifically van Swieten, who was ordered to carry out enlightenment in practice. Daniel Arlaud presents him as part of a military-medical mission initiated by van Swieten; he supposes that it was he who sent Tallar to the Banat and that he had written his *Vampyrismus* based on the surgeon's report on Vlach vampirism (Arlaud 2007). A blatant problem here is that the said treatise makes no reference whatsoever to Vlach beliefs. Others, like Peter Bräunline or Stéphanie Danneberg suppose that Tallar was "deployed" by Vienna as a second step after the Hermersdorf scandal, and was sent to the Banat to apply Maria Theresa's 1755 rescript in practice (Danneberg 2010, 183–4; Bräunlein 2012, 716). It goes unnoticed that Tallar himself wrote that he had conducted his investigations in 1753, two years before Hermersdorf.

This relation between the Dutch protomedicus and the German surgeon is also true of the way their manuscript treatises on vampirism are dealt with. Van Swieten's and Tallar's works are frequently evoked together as major achievements of medical enlightenment, and while in terms of impact, the protomedicus's work is indeed far more influential,[12] Tallar's work is singled out rather for its empirical foundations (Hamberger 1992, 31; Kreuter 2001, 93). Echoing Gábor Klaniczay's early study, it is lauded for being the most detailed fieldwork-based study on vampirism of the time, and several authors also praise him for his unparalleled interest in Vlach culture and folklore (Klaniczay 2002, 394; Hamberger 1992, 31; Magyar 1999 and 2002; Kreuter 2001, 93; Arlaud 2007; Rauer 2008, 91–2; Danneberg 2010; Bräunlein 2012). While this presentation is fairly accurate, a temporal primacy is also supposed about van Swieten's work. Secondary literature dates the *Vampyrismus* to 1755, while Tallar's *Visum repertum* would follow a year later. As will be shown below, archival records indicate that the *Visum repertum* is falsely dated to 1756 and was in fact written in 1753, which again nuances the Vienna-periphery picture to a small extent.

In general, there is a considerable confusion about even the most basic circumstances of Tallar's work, and this confusion is indicative of secondary literature's obliviousness of local relations. Tallar is variously referred to as Hungarian, German or Austrian, barber surgeon, regimental surgeon or physician, his work having been written at a variety of dates

[12] Van Swieten's *Vampyrismus* was already being widely propagated and published in several languages in the 1750s and 1760s, while Tallar's *Visum repertum* was only published once, as late as 1784.

from 1755 to 1766 and his employer being Maria Theresa, van Swieten, the Habsburg army or the Banat administration.[13] I suggest that the attractiveness of the centre-periphery model distorts the picture of the exact workings of medicalisation, enlightenment and related processes: it fails to give attention and agency either to Tallar himself, or to the local, provincial administration of the Banat. In order to remedy this situation, one has to examine the original environment of the work more closely.

Vampires in the Banat before 1753

The index and protocol books of the Temeswar provincial administration can help to reconstruct the vampire situation in the Banat. These sources provide short descriptions of the documents that were dealt with, and though the documents themselves have mostly been lost, these short descriptions are superb sources of Banatian everyday life.[14] They also offer a glimpse into the heterogeneity of practices and ideas related to vampirism in the era. Between 1718, when the Banat was regained from the Ottomans, and 1766, the year of the publication of the *Lex caesaro-regia*, the protocol books list about thirty cases which altogether claimed a minimum of 230 victims.[15]

The first known case dates to the spring of 1725 and the village of Herinbiesch. On the one hand, it attests to the close connection between witchcraft and vampirism, while on the other, it betrays the general perplexity on the part of the officials. Herr Rácz, the district provisor of Lugos-Faczet was ordered by the provincial administration to exhume the corpse of a witch, who had "got into suspicion". The provisor found that the three-month-old corpse was not decomposed, had its hand by its mouth, and fresh blood could be seen under its head. Rácz could not see any other explanation but that it was a bloodsucker. In his letter to the administration, he asked what should be done with it, and until the answer

[13] The *Visum repertum* has recently been republished for the first time since 1784, which is laudable, the cover text summarising Tallar's life, however, it contains a series of imprecisions, a consequence of secondary literature's lack of attention to the local level (Equiamicus 2013).

[14] MNL-OL E 303: Landesadministration Banat 14–52, 65–96 vols. Lajos Baróti has published a portion of these (14–27. vols.). See Baróti 1893–1907.

[15] The number is in reality much higher: out of the 31 reports, 15 do not mention the number of victims; these cases I counted as 1 or 2 victims. Furthermore, these cases are only those mentioned in the protocol books and do not include those which escaped the attention of the authorities.

arrived, he set guards around the corpse.[16] One can imagine the unbearable tensions in the village at the presence of a disinterred *moroica*. The following year, when news of vampirism from another village reached Rácz, he was a little more confident: he informed the administration that locals had exhumed an old woman suspected of bloodsucking, and that he, based on the recognisable signs, had permitted the decapitation of the body. However, now he wanted to know whether he could allow the burning of the body as well? (Baróti 1900–1902, 136). It seems that in these early years, the provincial administration was willing to permit such anti-vampire measures.

It was not only the provisors who were unsure about the proper procedures. The Serbian Medvedia case of 1732 mentioned above already shows that surgeons and physicians were also puzzled by what they saw. In 1738, during the great plague, a man called Uran (probably a surgeon) gave permission for the exhumation and burning of five corpses in a village in the district of Uypalanka in the Banat. The district provisor, Johann Mayr noted in his report to the Vienna-seated sanitary commission that deaths in the village had ceased after the rite, and that therefore it was unknown whether an epidemic disease or vampires were in the background. The commission, however, did not have doubts. For believing the superstition regarding vampires, and for allowing corpses to be unearthed in plague-stricken times (thereby endangering public health), they ordered Uran to be taken to the plague lazaret of Temeswar, where he had to serve without salary until the epidemic ended (MNL-OL, A 109: Protocolla Commissionis Sanitatis, 1. bundle, 487v–488v and 497v and 504r–505r. The case is cited by Magyary-Kossa 1929–1940, 86. Magyary mistakenly identifies Johann Mayr as a surgeon). There are two more vampire cases prior to Tallar commencing his investigations in 1753 where it is known that medical personnel were present (Baróti 1900–1902, 150; Baróti 1893–1896, 379). A medical examination carried out in 1743 in the district of Orsova decided that locals were wrong to assume that vampires were behind the disease. In 1751, in Kubin (probably today's Opština Kovin), a village of the district of Panczova, however, the physicians found fresh blood in the mouth of the corpse and therefore ("as

[16] Luckily, the letter is preserved in MNL-OL E 303 9. bundle 5–7.fols. See also Baróti 1900–1902, 135. The district provisor (Oberverwalter/Distriktverwalter) was the leading official of the civil (cameral) districts of the Banat, who performed both administrative and judicial duties (Kallbrunner 1958, 25). Even though provisors seem to have been mostly of German origins, it is possible that Joannes Rácz de Mehedia was Rascian. However, based solely on his name, one must be cautious in drawing such a conclusion.

well as in order to calm down the community”), permitted the burning of the corpses.

Apart from the local community, the provisor and the medical experts, the Orthodox clergy also had considerable influence on the development of the vampire cases. Unlike the German authorities, they had been exposed to vampire beliefs for a long time. One can suspect a well-established practice, though it is unclear how unified it was. In 1729, the protopope excommunicated the whole village of Gruin for carrying out vampire killings (Baróti 1900–1902, 140). The excommunication probably only worsened the situation, as denied the proper funerary rite, the dead were most likely to return. In the end, the provincial administration intervened and sent the district provisor to negotiate the revocation of the anathema. Roughly twenty years later, in 1748, the protopope of Caransebes (Caransebeş) participated in a more concerted project to control vampire beliefs. He excommunicated the village of Doppletz (probably today’s Comuna Topleţ) in the Orsova district for executing eleven corpses *without the permission of the church* (Baróti 1900–1902, 206 and 262–4). The corpses were unearthed, some of them burnt at the stake, others scalded with boiling water and then reburied. The Orsova provisor issued a circular prohibiting the exhumation and burning of corpses in the whole district and summoned the perpetrators to court. Nevertheless, the attitude of the church was probably not as unified as it seems. It is a returning cliché in several sources that Orthodox priests and *kalugers* (monks) were contributing to vampire beliefs. Tallar was also of this opinion: in the Temeswar district, a newborn baby suspected of vampirism was exhumed and Tallar argues that the priest had to have known about it, since the stake was set up in the church garden (Tallar 1753, 6v). Others also noted the link between the clergy and vampire beliefs, such as Alberto Fortis, a Venetian naturalist travelling in inner Dalmatia (Fortis 1778, 61–2.); Ignaz von Born, a mineralogist, also refers to it in his letters about Wallachia (born 1774, 14) and Joseph II’s warning to the Orthodox Church can also be cited here.

The military administration of the Banat was exchanged for a civil one in 1751, which within a short period of time had to deal with four cases of vampirism (Baróti 1893–1896, 379, 381; Baróti 1900–1902, 209, 273). As mentioned above, the Panczova district council authorised the burning of the Kubin vampires in 1751. A year later, in the same district, inhabitants of the village of Deliblat (Deliblato) unearthed four corpses, cooked their excised hearts and carried out “various superstitious procedures” with them. As the provisor wrote, the rite was performed without the knowledge of the authorities, so he proceeded against the perpetrators. In the same year, villagers of Slatina (district of Caransebes) disinterred four corpses, removed their intestines and then reburied them.[17] The district council and the church denounced the case and stated that the actions had been carried out in the face of the strictest prohibition. Finally, at the end of 1752, news arrived from Mehedica (Mehadica) in the Orsova district that locals thought that thirty-four people had been killed by vampires. Though the outcome of the case is unknown, probably no permission was granted due to the above-mentioned district prohibition of 1748.

While it seems that by the 1750s the majority of cases were condemned by the authorities, the 1751 event in Kubin and references such as "without the knowledge of the authorities" suggest that it was most of all the arbitrarily performed acts that were denounced. It was possible to justify the rite if it was carried out with official supervision. Regional differences may also be discerned: in the districts of Orsova and Caransebes there seems to have been a stricter rejection of the rites, while at the other end of the Banat, in Panczova, the authorities were more lenient. There are several reasons why a provisor could decide on the authorisation. The first half of the eighteenth century saw the third great wave of witchcraft persecutions in Hungary and it was not an unfamiliar idea that witches might continue their *maleficium* from beyond the grave as well. For instance, in a Transylvanian case of 1723, a dead woman was accused of witchcraft; the town council had the body exhumed, but since it was decaying in an orderly fashion, they reburied it and dropped the charges (Kiss 2004, 161–164; on witchcraft persecutions in Hungary, see Klaniczay 1986). Also, the need to calm the local community could be a seen as a priority. Locals frequently threatened the authorities with leaving the village, a fairly powerful threat, since the Banat was continuously suffering from a lack of settlers. After the expulsion of the Ottomans, the Banat was a sparsely populated, hostile land. Frequent Turkish raids, banditry, epidemics, unhealthy marshlands and disorganised borderland conditions made it a hard place to live. The province even earned the title "the grave of Germans" because of the high mortality rate among settlers (Schwicker 1861. 317.). The ratio of baptisms and deaths among the Germans of Temesvar was indeed dire: between 1726 and 1735, there were 1365 births and 4891 deaths, while in the years 1746–55 this ratio is 1670 to 3954. These numbers are especially striking since they relate to plague-free times (Petri 1988. 45–6). In general, there was plenty of space

[17] Those plagued by vampires sometimes smeared themselves with the "blood" of the unearthed corpse or ate from the soil of its grave (Tallar 1753, 6v; Hamberger 1992, 50). It is possible that the heart and intestines were used in a similar way or destroyed through a further rite.

for the various actors taking part in vampire cases to manoeuver local power dynamics, since neither Vienna nor the provincial administration issued a unified stance regarding the question.

The Kallacsa Commission: the physician, the surgeon and the cleric

This situation, however, was about to change. In 1753, the Banat provincial administration set up a three-member committee in order to investigate vampirism. The main source about the activities of the commission is Johann Georg Tallar's *Visum repertum*, in the preface of which the German surgeon mentions that the commission consisted of himself, the provincial physician of the Banat, and an unknown cleric (Tallar 1753, 3r).[18] The Banat healthcare system was presided over by a single provincial physician, and in 1753, this position was held by the Transylvanian doctor, Paul Adam Kömovesch / Kőműves (Petri 1988, 152 and 157–8).[19] The realisation that Tallar and Kőműves were members of the same vampire-investigating commission allows us to make a link to a source that in secondary literature has so far been considered as separate from Tallar's business: the documentation pertaining to Kőműves's expenses which emerged during his vampire investigations.[20] The other member of the commission, the cleric, is unfortunately as yet unknown. Theoretically, he might even have been an Orthodox priest, but this is

---

[18] "Visum repertum anatomico chyrurgicum oder Unterthänigst gehorsamster Summarischer Bericht, von und über die so genante Vampir oder Bluthsauger; Wallachischer Sprache *Moroi* genant. Welche vermög einer von *Löbl. Kayserl. Königl. Banatischen Landes Administration* ergangenen hohen Verordnung, durch die diesfals abgeschicket *Inquisitions Commission*, bestehend aus einem *Theologo, Cameral* und *Provincial Physico*, dann einem *Chyrurgo* [...]"

[19] Paul Adam Kőműves was born in 1719 in Széplak, Kolozs county in Transylvania and received his doctorate at Vienna University in 1752. Next year he was already nominated to be the provincial physician of the Banat. His rapid career however ended there. Though he requested dislocation from the Banat in 1771 (referring to bad health and the unwholesome air of the region), the treasury only fulfilled his request six years later. He moved to Sopron, then to Vienna and finally to Pressburg (Bratislava), where he died in 1793.

[20] OESTA-FHKA Banater Akten r.Nr.37. 91–92 ff. The documentation consists of the request (dated 23.03.1753) which the Banat provincial administration sent to Vienna asking the ratification of the leasing of the Billiet estate to Kőműves to cover his expenses, and the decision (dated 05.04.1753) of the Vienna cameral authorities signed by the empress. The request is reprinted in: Hamberger 1992, 85–86.

highly unlikely since Tallar's report has a fairly strong anti-Orthodox edge. Most possibly he was a Catholic priest, or (given the lofty expression "*Theologo*"), a monk: both Jesuits and Franciscans had a friary in Temeswar at the time.

According to Tallar, the commission's duties were twofold: to examine the sick and, if possible, to cure them, and to exhume the dead and dissect those who were identified by locals as vampires. It is very likely that the administration sought to take a stance on the question of vampirism based on the work of the commission. The presence of the provincial physician and the fact that unlike earlier commissions, this one had the duty of investigating several villages, not just one, point in this direction. The inclusion of the cleric may further suggest that the administration was not sure whether natural or supernatural causes were in the background.

What secondary literature knows about Tallar's life comes from the introduction he wrote to his treatise. He completed his studies in surgery in Mainz and Strasbourg; after that, he served as a military surgeon in various wars against the French and the Ottomans.[21] It was during these latter campaigns that he witnessed vampire killings four times. Twice he was there only "coincidentally" and was solely an observer; twice, however, he also dissected the supposed vampires. The frequent claim in secondary literature that he was investigating vampires for decades as a military surgeon is, therefore, an exaggeration. In 1728, stationed in Wallachia with the Vetterani regiment, he performed a dissection, but he discloses no further information on this case. Four years before that, the captain of the Transylvanian castle of Déva (Deva), Major Quirin von Pökerer, commissioned him to open up a corpse held by locals to be a bloodsucker. The captain wanted to obtain the magical herbs in its stomach with which Satan is able to bring corpses to life; he explained that he wanted to do "various wonderful things with it". As Tallar notes tauntingly, instead of herbs, the major had to be content with an unbearable stench emanating from the corpse. After the military, he served as a civilian surgeon in various positions: lazarets, spitals and finally in Theresiopolis (Subotica). Here, however, he was dismissed from his position after a year and became poor. Tallar was still in Theresiopolis

[21] The Salzmann College in Strasbourg (where Tallar studied) was a high quality medical academy, where students studied theory as well as practice and were theoretically supposed to visit dissections four times a week (Koenig 2011, 53). His army service included the Jung Wallis infantry regiment (led by Ferdinand von Geyer) in Transylvania in the mid-1720s; the Vetterani cuirassier regiment in Wallachia at the end of the 1720s and the army of J.G Christian Lobkowitz in Transylvania at the end of the 1730s (Tallar 1753, 2v).

when he was contracted by the Banat provincial administration to join the vampire-investigating commission.[22] It can only be conjectured that the reason for his employment was his experience in vampirism (Tallar 1753, 4v, 16r–16v).

The administration certainly needed experience, for in January 1753, the district provisor of Uypalanka sent a letter to Temeswar requesting action because in the adjoining villages of Klein Dikvan (Ticvaniu Mare) and Rakasdia (Răcăşdia), the deaths of no less than fifty people had been attributed by locals to vampires (Baróti 1900–1902, 50). It is quite possible that this was the news that prompted the administration to set up the commission, not least because it touched upon a highly sensitive point. Stéphanie Danneberg rightly suggested that vampirism had financial relevance for Vienna (Danneberg 2010, 186): this is exactly how Tallar explained the graveness of the matter. According to the surgeon, at least one hundred taxpayers were lost annually due to this "vampire"-sickness across the empire (Tallar 1753, 4v). Danneberg further pointed out that the Banat was especially precious for the Habsburg administration because of its mines. While many cases happened far from any mining centres, on the swampy plains of the Banat, Klein Dikvan and Rakasdia were situated at the feet of the ore-mountains, only 7 and 12 kilometres away from the Banat's mining centre, Oravitz (Oraviţa). The two villages were probably linked to the town, with several ties: villagers could work in the mining facilities, while the surrounding fields would most certainly supply the mining towns with food. Deaths in this sensitive region might well have alarmed the provincial authorities. Furthermore, epidemics that emerged in the vicinity of mining centres could result in a quarantine that would totally paralyse production and commerce. Basically, it was in the interest of the mining town to investigate the issue as soon as possible and convince the authorities that there was no longer any need for quarantine. This is exactly what was happening in the same year in the Transylvanian mining town of Kapnik (Cavnic). There, the town administration was happy to send a circular letter to surrounding towns, stating that there was no need to maintain the quarantine, for the deaths had not been caused by an epidemic, but only by the returning dead. These were duly exhumed, subjected to a medical examination which confirmed them to be bloodsuckers and finally were burnt at the stake in the middle of the town square (OESTA-FHKA Münz- und Bergwesen, r.Nr. 90. fols 6–13, 20. Reprinted in: Hamberger 1992, 88–92).

---

[22] In an index book entry about Tallar's monetary compensation for having completed his investigations dated 03.24.1753, he is still referred to as "Tallar Chyrurgo von Theresiopl". MNL-OL E 303 43.vol. (unpaginated) "Tallar"-entry.

Tallar was aware of the importance of his work for the mining industry, since both the dedicatory letter and the epilogue are rife with mining-related metaphors (Tallar 1753, 2r, 20r). In the former section, he likens his own fortunate acceptance into the service of the provincial administration to that of the mineral stone, which is accidentally washed into the way of the chemist, who, cleaning it, finds it useful. In the ending paragraph, he likens vampirism to cobalt. The metaphor is very apt for two reasons. As in the way ignorant people can mistake cobalt for precious ore, so can one confuse natural and supernatural causes; also, both can result in sickness and eventual death. The miner's sickness linked to cobalt had been known for a long time, but the discovery of the metal itself, and its poisonous arsenic content was the recent work of the Swedish mining specialist, Georg Brandt. While he had already referred to cobalt in 1735, he explained it in detail only in his 1748 article in the *Journal of the Royal Scientific Society of Uppsala* (Brandt 1735 and 1748). Tallar's metaphor was therefore not only apt but very topical as well.

The reconstruction of the vampire commission's itinerary is not easy, for the members did not always stick together. According to Tallar, they first visited Klein Dikvan in the south (Uyplanaka district), then on the way back to Temeswar they investigated in Schebell (Jebel) in the Csakova district, and lastly, he went alone north of Temeswar, to Kallacsa (Călacea) (Tallar 1753, 3r, 19r). Interestingly, he does not mention Rakasdia at all; it is possible that the members parted ways and Kőműves went there by himself. Kőműves's remunerations petition claims that the doctor investigated several villages (no names are listed) and that he faced the superstitious mob all alone, an exaggeration in the light of Tallar's assertions. After Schebell, Kőműves stayed south of Temeswar and might have visited vampire cases in Stamora and Wermesch (Vermeş), at least these are the places from which news about vampire killings arrived in Temeswar in January-March, 1753 (Baróti 1893–1896, 486). Meanwhile, Tallar went up north to investigate the disease afflicting the village of Kallacsa; he repeatedly remarked that he was alone there, working only with the community leader (knies) and a council member (Tallar 1753, 6v).[23]

Tallar was writing weekly reports during his work in the commission, which makes it clear why the title of his treatise includes the words, *Summary Report* (Tallar 1753, 11v). According to the protocol books,

[23] "Sie haben zu Kallatsa wohin ich mit dem Oberknies samt einem Beamten zu erst nachgesehend so aber *alleine* verordnet ware […]"; Tallar 1753, 19r. "Observatio 8na: bey allen diesen Kranken, welche *uns* bey dieser Visitation, auch *mihr* zu Kallatsa seind zu handen gekommen […]" (italics mine)

weekly medical reports from Kallacsa indeed arrived in Temeswar from 1st February to 6th March, when the sickness finally stopped (Baróti 1893–1896, 436, 438).[24] The commission's work was finished by the end of March, in line with the usual seasonal pattern of vampire cases in the Banat centring on the winter. The provincial administration handed in Kőműves's and Tallar's remuneration petitions to the Treasury dated 23rd and 24th March. The surviving entry about Tallar's petition explains that Tallar deserves the daily fees for his work in the "Kallacsa commission" and is referred to as a "surgeon from Theresiopolis".[25] This suggests that he was contracted solely for the vampire commission and was not given a stable provincial job. Kőműves's petition is preserved and states that he handed in a report on his findings.[26] Unfortunately, neither Tallar's weekly reports, nor the doctor's report have been found in the archives so far, and whether the anonymous cleric also wrote a report or not is an even greater mystery.

What we do know however, is that the provincial administration handed over Tallar's *Relation (Respu) deren Vampiren*, to a Vienna court commission on 24th December 1753 (MNL-OL E 303 43.vol. (unpaginated), see entries: "Talar" and "Wampirs"; MNL-OL E 303 41.vol. (unpaginated) see entry to the date: 1753.12.24). This commission is probably the Sanitäts Hofcommission which oversaw the sanitary issues of the whole empire, and which was raised to the level of a Hofdeputation in 1753. From January 1753 onwards, the Banat administration was obliged to send in all sanitary-related reports to this commission (Baróti 1893–96, 122).[27] In all likelihood, the *Relation* is, in fact, the *Visum Repertum* and the dating of Tallar's work to 1756 in current secondary literature is mistaken. Nothing is mentioned in the protocol books of later years (including those of 1756) about Tallar or anyone else handing in a report or treatise on vampires. The sole source of the 1756 dating is Johann Georg Mößle, a well-known Vienna publisher, who edited and printed Tallar's work in

[24] None of the entries gives a name for the author of these reports; the first entry mentions the district surgeon of Temeswar. It might be possible that the district surgeon was Tallar himself, but until further sources emerge, the position Tallar held during his investigations remains unclear.

[25] Tallar Chyrurgo von Theresiopl wegen der Galacser commission die diurna zu bezahlen. 1753, Marz. 24. Cameral Zahl Amt'. MNL-OL E 303 43.vol. (unpaginated) see entry: "Tallar".

[26] See note 20. above.

[27] This rescript adds that such reports should also be sent to the Banatisch-Illyrische Hofdeputation, so it is also possible that this was the commission to which the *Visum Repertum* was sent.

1784.[28] Whereas Mößle found the information on the dating unclear, I suggest it is a mistake. The *Visum Repertum* was written and handed in over the Christmas of 1753.

If this is true, why did Tallar write a summary report nine months after the whole vampire issue was over? It is possible that the *Visum Repertum* was Tallar's way of applying for a position of district surgeon. The timing is synchronic with a major change in the leadership of the Banat. On 28th November 1753, Field Marshal von Engelshofen, the earlier military and civilian governor of the Banat, was sent into retirement and was substituted by the first real civilian governor, Francesco Villana-Perlas de Rialpo. Tallar probably intended his treatise to impress the new provincial leadership and he was successful in his attempts, for on 22nd April 1754, he was nominated as the district surgeon of Caransebes, and retained this position until his death in 1762.[29]

In summary, Tallar, Dr Kőműves and a cleric carried out vampire investigations as members of a commission set up by the Banat provincial administration at the beginning of 1753. Tallar compiled the *Visum Repertum* at the end of the same year for the provincial administration; whether it was his own initiative as I suggest here, or he was required to do so, is not entirely clear. The report was handed over to the Vienna sanitary court commission due to a bureaucratic regulation and disappeared from sight for the next three decades; it mysteriously reappeared in 1784 and was published. If this interpretation is correct, it was crucial for Tallar to convince the authorities about his medical skills, his enlightened attitude to superstition as well as his extensive knowledge of Vlach culture and life. In the following chapter, Tallar's manuscript will be examined to see how he attempted to achieve these goals.

---

[28] The *Visum Repertum*'s manuscript version consists of two separate parts: the treatise itself and the two leaves covering it, which have been written by another hand. This cover (Tallar 1753, 1r-v, 22r-v) contains the editorial preface of the 1784 printed version (Tallar 1784, A2–A4), where Mößle notes that the original work was written in 1756. Based on the date in the preface, a third hand (probably an archivist) wrote a note on the cover page saying "Zur Ungarischen Geschichte An: 1756".

[29] MNL-OL E 303 41.vol. (unpaginated) see entry to the date: 1754.04.22.; for his death see: MNL-OL E 303 71.vol. 351v. The entry is dated 1762.12.04. Tallar was also assigned to serve as the quarantine surgeon of Cossova in 1756. See: MNL-OL E 303 65.vol., 224. He left a widow behind, who died in 1771. (MNL-OL E 303 187.vol.) See entry: "Tallarin". Anton Petri lists Tallar among the district surgeons of Caransebes, but under a mistaken name as "Georg Tabar" (Petri 1988, 108).

The Visum Repertum: medicine, culture and demonology

In spite of its title, Tallar's work is not a *visum repertum*, that is, a forensic report. The description of the dissections is less detailed than it should be, given the standards of the time (cf. for instance the *visa reperta* about the Habsburg Serbian vampires, see Hamberger 1992, 46–54). The descriptions of the dissections here only serve as arguments in an overarching natural explanation of the phenomenon of vampirism. The work is, therefore, an empirically based medical treatise. It is neatly structured with explanatory marginal notes and without mistakes or corrections; it is possible that Tallar eventually intended it for publication. He even refers to the "censors" who would read the text (Tallar 1753, 8v, 20r); these might be actual censors or the physicians/officials who would judge his arguments. At the same time, the *Visum Repertum* does not meet the level of contemporary treatises as it lacks references. In the whole course of the work, Tallar makes only two cursory references, one to van Swieten's commentaries on Boerhaave's *Aphorisms* and one to Malpighi (Tallar 1753, 7v, 16v). This blatant lack of references can be explained by the short length of time which Tallar had to compile his treatise and by the fact that he was probably unemployed in Theresiopolis while writing it and simply did not have access to such works.

The treatise seeks to answer the two questions posed to the Kallacsa Commission: what caused the mysterious vampire sickness, and what caused the supposed vampires' lack of bodily decomposition? Tallar approached the question on several levels. First, he gave a medical/naturalistic explanation for the phenomena. Second, as opposed to most writers (including van Swieten), he was not satisfied with giving an alternative, medical explanation: he also sought to test and refute Vlach folkloric ideas about the workings of the demonic world. Finally, he also engaged in moral/demonological discussions about the possibility of satanic influence. These several levels earned him the respect of the provincial administration as well as that of today's scholarship.

Medicine and gastronomy

Tallar determined that there was no connection between the vampire sickness and the undecomposed state of certain corpses: he explained them by unrelated natural causes. Decomposition had not commenced because the cold winter soil and the dry air within the coffins had conserved the bodies. The reason why certain corpses started decomposing earlier than others buried at the same time is due to the different bodily composure people have. Those of sanguine temperament have an abundance of blood, and since blood contains salt, their bodies are conserved longer than those of other temperaments (Tallar 1753, 15r-v, 17r-19v). This is why sanguine corpses were identified as vampires by locals.

He framed the problem of the vampire sickness by stating that among all the peoples of the Banat, it was only Vlachs who suffered from this affliction: German or Rascian settlers, or foreign soldiers never suffered (Tallar 1753, 4r-5v, 19r). The sickness had two major causes. First, the combination of strict Orthodox fasting habits with poor Vlach cuisine. They ate too many vegetables of a cold and wet nature: raw onions, garlic, radish, carrots and sour cabbage. The cold phlegm these create in the stomach can rot and the zealous fasting period can weaken people before the winter sickness set in, eventually killing them. The Rascians presented an anomaly, since they also fasted in the same way and ate the same type of food, and still, according to Tallar, they were never plagued by vampires. This is an awkward statement in the light of the multiple sources attesting to Rascian vampirism. The fact that Tallar did not realise this not only meant that he had not spent much time among Rascians, but also that he had not heard about the vampires of Habsburg Serbia, and that the whole vampire discourse of the 1730s and 40s had escaped him. This again puts him in a different light to his usual portrayal of a persistent investigator of vampires. Tallar's solution to the anomaly was that Rascians were saved by the large amount of hot paprika they used in their cuisine: it neutralised the cold-natured food they ate.

The other major cause of the sickness was the belief that victims of a vampire can only escape immediate death if they smear themselves abundantly with the vampire's blood, that is, the decaying fluids that flow from corpses. This practice multiplied deaths (Tallar 1753, 6v, 13r). By pronouncing the practice of blood smearing to be dangerous, he gave a powerful reason for the authorities not to allow vampire-killing rites to be carried out, even in the presence of officials. On the other hand, Tallar stated that the locals' fear of the dead was extremely strong, and that therefore simply banning the practice could not be successful. Emphasis had to be laid on medical enlightenment and the spread of the usage of medicaments as well (Tallar 1753, 4r-v). By presenting the issue in this way, he skilfully managed to substantiate the utility of his own profession.

Folklore dissected

Tallar also presented himself as a connoisseur of Vlach culture (Tallar 1753, 5r, 10r, 19r, 19v); he stated that without such knowledge, one could not understand the core of the problem. He was proud of his first-hand experiences with Vlachs, emphasising that he had known two of the vampires in person while they were still alive. Furthermore, he underlined that he spoke the Vlach and Hungarian languages fluently, and therefore needed no interpreters. These skills helped him to approach the problem in a direct way.

He subjected local conceptions about vampirism to logical and physical testing, thereby seeking to refute them. In relation to the vampire sickness, he argued that the sick could not have been plagued by bloodsuckers, because if something was indeed sucking their blood, they would have died because of the bloodletting he performed on them; on the contrary, they had been cured. He also tested some of the folkloric ideas related to the corpses. According to locals, a vampire was only in his grave on Saturdays, but Tallar had "vampires" exhumed on other days, and they were always there. Another belief held that one could not lead a black mare across a vampire's grave. Upon trying, he concluded that the horse at first did not want to step over any of the graves (in his opinion because the graves were high and because the horse felt the smell of corpses), but after a little goading, it stepped over all the graves regardless of the inhabitant's nature. On another occasion, he collected the blood found in a vampire's mouth in a small glass and let it stand for a night. The blood separated into two components: a thin, brownish liquid and a brownish residue, and stank horribly. Based on the putrid stench, he concluded that this liquid could not possibly sustain any kind of life. Finally, in Klein Dikvan he also had the opportunity to meet a "living blood sucker", who allegedly had already died twice before and had not eaten or drunk anything for two years. After a two-hour examination (the exact method of which Tallar unfortunately did not disclose), he determined that the person was a fraud (Tallar 1753, 5v, 15r, 16r, 17r, 19v). Whether this peculiar character was a witch, werewolf or living moroi was unclear.

Though Tallar considered all practices carried out against the corpses useless, he described them. He distinguished between the Banatian and the Wallachian rites. In the former province, the decapitated corpse was reburied in some places, while in others it was burnt. In Wallachia, the corpse was taken out of the village on a cart, decapitated, a stone pressed into its mouth, scalded with hot wine, the heart pierced with a stake and left to be preyed upon by birds and dogs (Tallar 1753, 13r). In the Wallachian case, Tallar probably conflated several alternative practices, while it is notable that we have sources attesting to scalding from the Banat as well (Baróti 1900–1902, 206 and 262–4).

Tallar was eager to scrutinise other folkloric creatures as well: he collected six other supernatural disease explanations and ranked them according to the efficacy of their local cures (Tallar 1753, 11r-13v). The "beautiful ones" (*die Schöne*) were groups of witches who cursed the houses which obstructed the route of their night-time flights (for a complex treatment of the belief in Central and South-East European folklore, see Pócs 1989). Such houses either had to have a horse's or oxen's head nailed above the door or had to be demolished and rebuilt elsewhere. Interestingly, Mátyás Bél in his 1735–42 description of Hungary advises similar measures (the hanging of a decaying horse head on the wall) to get rid of bedbugs (Wellmann 1984, 177). If the curse took effect, the patient's sickness was long; wise women were called, who would cast tin into a bowl of water and count the pieces into which it disintegrated, equating it with the number of afflictions the victim had; at other times, she would mix all sorts of "absurd things" and either smear the patient with the mixture or feed it to him or her. They also used incantations, which Tallar did not want to reproduce in the text, partly because they were so foolish and partly because wise women liked to collect them and build them into their repertoire, which Tallar presumably wanted to avoid. He considered all these anti-"beautiful ones" measures to be totally inefficient.

Two other techniques were similarly useless and even dangerous in his opinion. The flying dragon called "smehu" could tread on people, or even have intercourse with them in the way a succubus or accubus [sic] demon would. (Éva Pócs discusses belief in the so-called "lidérc", the Hungarian name for these creatures among Hungarian-speaking Catholics in a Romanian village in Transylvania. See Pócs 2012, 272–80). Such patients according to Tallar were suffering from epilepsy, feverish diseases and hallucinations. The treatment was to shoot an unloaded pistol next to the head of the patient, which in the opinion of the surgeon would only result in convulsions and trembling. Tallar noted that it was difficult to convince Orthodox priests to come and administer the last sacrament to such patients. Another ailment, the witch's binding, referred to when a magical knot (*"coagulum"*) in the vicinity of a person was pulled tight, causing the person to become lame and crooked. In order to deal with this, the victim had to lie on their back on a trough, smeared with oil, the legs tied tight and the body thus stretched. In Tallar's view, the real cause of this condition was fatty clogging in the arteries of the limbs, and that the curative procedure was more harmful than useful.

There were certain treatments, however, which could even be beneficial. Vlachs believed that their enemies could put tiny magical objects into their drinking water, which they would swallow and then fall sick. Tallar supposed this was some sort of love magic and decided that among local cures involving the drinking of honeyed wine or honeyed brandy, the first one could sometimes really work. It was mostly during fasting seasons that people frequently suffered from colicky stomach aches, which according to them, were caused by the sinking of their hearts. The cure consisted of drinking oil from church lamps, which could be efficient if they vomited beforehand. Finally, they thought that certain harmful tumours could develop in their lungs, liver and throats, which they called “schui”. (For this widespread disease name among both Romanians and Hungarians, see Vajkai 1943, 110–1). Tallar diagnosed this as quinsy. The Vlach barber, in this case, would lay the patient on his back, with his legs pointing towards the sun, and then, using an unsophisticated hook manufactured by Gypsies, he would reach into the throat, and cut out the tonsils with a sharp bread knife. Tallar determined that while the procedure could cause copious bleeding, it could be successful, and in the case of sanguine patients, even beneficial. For others, however, it could cause death within 2-3 years, and in this case, not even the Vlach panacea— cabbage soup—could help, Tallar noted biliously.

Morals and the devil

Even though Tallar dismissed all of these Vlach folkloric creatures as imaginary, he could not do so when he came to the possibility of demonic activity. To be more precise, taking the workings of the devil into consideration was a moral and professional requirement throughout the century. Van Swieten hastened to admit this before going on to debunk the belief in vampirism as ignorant superstition, and Maria Theresa’s 1766 *Lex Caesaro-regia* also considered real demonic magic as an existing category to be distinguished from natural causes and fraud. Further, Anton De Haen, the head of the Vienna clinic and pioneer of bedside practice for students of medicine, wrote a whole book on magic in 1774. Finally, Sámuel Rácz, the physiology professor of the University of Buda, included the existence of ghosts, devilish magic, demonic possession and divine miracles into his 1794 university textbook on forensic medicine, but warned students that in most cases the causes were natural (Swieten 1768 [1755]; Linzbauer 1852, 784; Haen 1774; Rácz 1794, 139, 144 and 147–50).

Tallar addressed a peculiar moral problem about vampire sickness at the beginning and end of the treatise. Why does Satan torment Vlachs, who are so zealous in fasting? And why are the German and foreign soldiers left unharmed, if it is precisely they who occasionally commit bloodthirsty acts? In spite of the pun on blood-drinking, this was a real moral dilemma about the motivations behind divine punishment and reward. While posing this question, Tallar inserted a somewhat hazy idea into the text about Satan's this-worldly activity. As he wrote, it would be strange to suppose that Satan distinguished between people on a "political" (i.e. ethnic Vlach vs non-Vlach) basis. And even if we would grant this, Tallar goes on, it would make utterly no sense why Satan continued this distinction after death as well (Tallar 1753, 4r).[30] While it is not easy to interpret this section, it seems that what he is saying is: to suppose that Satan reanimates only Vlach corpses because they are Vlachs goes against the usual way Satan operates; after all, being an instrument of God, he should make his choices based on the moral qualities of people, not their ethnicity.

In an interesting rhetorical move, Tallar asks for the reader's patience and leaves the dilemma unresolved until the very end of the text. Here, he comes back to the issue and gives the following explanation:

"Since the question about the unharmed soldiers and Germans which was posed in the introduction has not been answered satisfactorily, it should be added that the soldiers and the Germans, through their faith, their pastors and through Christian learning are already ripped out of the unhealthy desert of Satanic slavery and faulty superstition in their youths, and are planted into the beloved Land, namely into the healthy garden of knowledge full of herbs, and they laugh at the idle fables and the harms of those corpses; they entrust themselves to the incomprehensibly wonderful aids of their Saviour, and remain uninjured, and even if some of them are gullible, their pastors are apt to teach them" (Tallar 1753, 19v).[31]

---

[30] "Was mag es aber wohl vor eine Beschaffenheit haben, dass die zwahr nur im Fasten so Exemplarische Wallachen von dießem übel so oft und so häufig hin gerißen werden; dahin gegen das Militare Welches doch jederzeit fast mitten unter ihnen Bequartieret, von dem Sattan (wann er jadoch an dießer Menschen freßerey theil haben soll) ganz ohn angefochten, ja ohne ein einziges Exempel zu haben schaadloss gelaßen wird; Wer wollte da nicht schier auf die gedanken verfallen, der Sattan mieße diesfals nebst so vihlen ihme schon zu geeigneten Qualitäten, auch wohl dabey einen Statisten agiren, und sich des Attributi der politic Bedienen; Wann er aber solches in puncto der Krankheit auch thäte, so wüßte ich doch nicht Was er nach dem Tot vor eine Reflection zu machen hette, da sollte wohl billig aller Respect Cessiren; und Wann mann die sache recht Betrachtet so sind sie ja wo es die Noht erfordert, recht zu dem Bluth durst gewidmet."

[31] "Wann die frage in dem vorbericht von dem unbeschädigten Militari und denen Teitschen nicht genugsam beantwortet, so füge hinzu das das Militare, durch den glauben und ihre sehl sorger, samt deren teitschen, schon in der jugend durch

The answer to the dilemma is that Germans and foreigners had a good Christian (i.e. non-Orthodox) education and are therefore impervious to superstitious fables with which Satan could tempt them to make them fear the returning dead.[32] A further interesting aspect of the above quote is its language: it differs markedly from the simple and technical medical discourse of the core text. In fact, it resembles a sermon, crammed with intense expressions and biblical images about Satan's desert (Mt 4:1–11) and the seeds from the sower's parable (Mt 13:1–42). The importance of pastoral work is emphasised at a similar section at the beginning of the text as well. Without well-educated priests, Vlach children learn all sorts of superstitious things from their mothers and from Orthodox monks (*kalugers*). This way, they lose their belief in God and can easily fall into the trap of Satan like a fly in the spider web or the reed which the wind bends in all directions at its liking (Tallar 1753, 3v). Seen in its entirety, this idea involves the moral judgement that Orthodox people in their ignorance of true religion are worse Christians, are more sinful and hence are deservedly tormented by satanic fears and visions.

Finally, there is a point in the text where Tallar actually enters demonological reflections. He writes about the small, round holes found in the soil of the graves which hosted supposed vampires. According to locals, these were the holes through which vampires left their graves at night. Tallar argues however that the holes were, in fact, the results of a burial rite, where men stabbed the grave with their sticks in order to prevent the dead from returning. After this, he adds the following:

"Were Satan able to condense the body so much that it would be able to fit through such a small hole, at the same time not so much that it could penetrate through the loose texture of the soil, then even a single, strong downpour would be able to impede the devilish machination in fitting through the hole" (Tallar 1753, 14v).[33]

---

christen Lehr, aus der irr-aberglaube- und unkraut vollen Wüsten der Sattanischen Sclaverey ausgerißen und in das gelobte Land, nemblich in den heilsamen Kreuter vollen garten der erkantniß vest, gepflanzet, verlachen das nichts Kommende fablern und schaden deren toten, und verlaßen sich auf die anbegreiflich wundervolle hülfsmittel ihres heilands, und bleiben unbeschadigt, und wann schon viele darueber einfältige, so seind ihre sehl sorger sie zu Lehren Aptirt."

[32] Interestingly, whether we look at the medical/gastronomical or the moral explanation of vampirism, the Rascians are anomalies for both. While solving the first with the paprika idea, Tallar is unable to come up with a moral explanation for why they are not tormented by Satan in the same way Vlachs are.

[33] "Solte aber Sattan den Cörper so Compact Condensiren, das er zu einem kleinen runden loch herauß mieße und nicht auch so Extenuiren kennen, das er durch die sehr weite poros der erden herauß penetriren kinne, so möchte ihm wohl ein

In the *Visum Repertum*, these are the only points at which the medical/cultural discussion is interrupted with moral/demonological lines of thinking, which by and large do not fit smoothly into the general argumentation of the text. While the core text bases the explanation of the vampire disease on cultural/ethnic grounds, namely into Vlach gastronomy and the blood smearing practice, the moral discussion goes against it and claims that it would be foolish to think that Satan discriminates on political/ethnic grounds. This and the difference in language make these few instances easily noticeable. In fact, one might even wonder whether these places were really Tallar's idea, or perhaps the suggestions of the unknown cleric.

After having examined vampirism on these three levels, the medical, the folkloric and the moral, Tallar was able to give his conclusion about the matter: in his opinion, there was nothing divine, satanic, magical or even particularly wonderfully natural about the vampire sickness or the corpses of supposed vampires. At the same time, he felt it necessary to yield the ultimate judgement on the issue (especially on Satan's possible involvement) to those whom this decision belonged to (Tallar 1753, 20r).[34]

Vampires after the Visum repertum

The effects of Tallar's treatise on the actual policies of the Banat administration are not easy to determine. For one, it is certain that in 1753, all vampire killings were condemned. The next known news about vampirism came in 1755 from the village of Wermesch in the district of Csakova. The only source pertaining to this case is an index book entry about Tallar's remunerations petition for his expenses (MNL-OL, E 303 81.vol. (unpaginated) See entry: "Tallar"). Even though he was the surgeon of the Caransebes district, it was again Tallar who was called to investigate the case. This attests to his skill in fashioning himself as a vampire-expert and capitalising on it. The same year saw the appearance

einziger starker Plazregen durch zu flößung des Loches das künstliche handwerk verbieten."

[34] "Weilen ich aber mit gewißen nicht ein einzige Spuhr weder einer Himmlisch noch einer Sattanischen erscheinung, weder sonst in der natur der sache segründete artificiente, Magische, prater natürliche operation bey denen kranken so wohl als bey der Toten gefunden habe, so über gebe [ich] es schuldiger maßen denen jenigen, deren es zu Dejudicieren gehört." In a similar vein, see 8v: "Oder ob der Sattan bey dießer krankheit das Dominium führe, will der mahlen nicht in meinem gewalt, sondern bey denen Herrn Censoribus Decidiret zu werden geruhen."

of Maria Theresa's 1st March ordinance, but when this and/or van Swieten's *Vampyrismus* reached the Banat is yet unknown.

According to the testimony of the provincial protocol books, between 1753 and 1766 at least thirteen vampire cases took place in the province, continuing afterwards as well. In the summer of 1756, the villagers of Csepsa (Cebza) were still making a formal appeal to the administration for permission to disinter suspected corpses. This practice, however, probably faded fast. The following year, the communities of Polvaschniza (Bolvaşniţa) and Slatina were condemned for arbitrarily performing the violent practice. Tallar presumably got involved in the cases, since the two villages belonged to his district. Though the official reactions are known in only two other cases, in those the perpetrators were punished in the same way, by physical labour. In 1758 in Peschenova (Csanad d.), they were condemned to eight days of trench work, while inhabitants of the village of Kloschiza (Panczova d.) in 1759 were sentenced to fourteen days of labour (MNL-OL, E 303 65.vol. 303r; 67.vol. 58v; 66.vol. 305.f; 68.vol. 194v; 77.vol. 75v). This might attest to a more unified approach to the question. However, sources are scarce, and at present, the effects of the Kallacsa Commission and the Empress's rescript on how vampire cases were handled in the Banat is difficult to assess. The practice itself did not cease but was probably simply driven underground.

The print version

The *Visum Repertum* lay dormant in Vienna for three decades, and as far as is known, had no effect whatsoever on either van Swieten's *Vampyrismus* or the Habsburg laws against superstition. It re-emerged however in 1784, when Johann Georg Mößle, the Vienna publisher came across the work "by chance" (Tallar 1784, 7). One can only wonder how he could chance upon a thirty-year-old Banatian treatise which probably had been stacked among innumerable other documents of the Habsburg administration. In his own words, Mößle decided to publish it for two reasons. First, because Tallar had shed light on a topic that used to be very popular but still remained a mystery. And second, because such a story was worth remembering. Mößle's publishing house indeed sought to satisfy the wider public's thirst for curiosities: people could hear for instance about the 1683 siege of Vienna, the life of Mohamed or the Styrian Robinson Crusoe's travels to South America (Huhn 1783; Müller 1791; *Leben* 1788). A treatise about vampirism fit into this repertoire perfectly: what at the local level was a matter of life and death, in Vienna, it was not more than one among the many juicy, exciting tabloid news items.

At the same time, Mößle's coincidence story is put into perspective by considering that his publishing house was also fairly diligent in publishing books that served the enlightened absolutist government's agendas or channelled them to the public. Among these, one can find legal collections and handbooks, such as Joseph Kropatschek's illustrious, multi-volume collection of laws issued under Maria Theresa and Joseph II. (Kropatschek 1786; *Von dem Verfahren* 1790; Martini 1799). Books relating to religion are also common: royal religion-related decrees, the collection of Tridentine reforms and an anti-superstition treatise that was published a year before the *Visum Repertum* (Geissau 1786; Schwerdling 1789; Bartholotti 1783). Several other (in a loose sense) enlightening books found their publisher in Mößle: handbooks on what one should think about religion, freemasonry or merchants for instance (Meisel 1783; Sommfels 1783; *Die Freymäurer* 1793). Further, many of the success stories of the enlightenment are also to be found on the list, like publications about the skill and achievements of surgery and chemical medicine (Plenk 1799; Scopoli 1786).

Tallar's treatise was in line with all these agendas; furthermore, it might even be supposed that it was topical to some extent in 1784, at least in the eyes of the Josephine government. The same year, on 2nd November 1784, a rescript was issued addressed to the Orthodox Church in which the king warned the clergy to stop the practice of open coffin burials in times of plague, and to take a greater part in the fight against the belief in vampirism. This rescript is part of a more general series of measures Joseph II took to regulate issues around burial and death (Kropatschek 1785–1790, VI. 530–580). Perhaps someone in court circles remembered Tallar's work, the anti-Orthodox edge of which might have contributed to its publication at this late point in time.

Editorial scissors

The printed version follows the manuscript faithfully, which makes the few changes remarkable. The printed edition does not include Tallar's dedicatory letter in which he expressed his gratitude to the provincial administration for making a contract with him. The last paragraph of the treatise was also cut, where he again thanked the provincial government's trust. In this way, Tallar's mining metaphors linking his treatise to the mining industry were also lost. The first paragraph after the dedicatory letter was removed; here Tallar wrote about the vampire commission, its members and duties. Finally, the title of the work was modified from "summary report", which only made sense in relation to Tallar's earlier, weekly reports, to "thorough report".[35] In this way, the text was lifted out of its original environment and placed at a more general level of the enlightened fight against disease and superstition.

The editor—probably in order to make the treatise easier to read—substituted Tallar's mostly Latin-based technical vocabulary with expressive German wording. This is how for instance *horrend* and *peristaltisch* became *abscheulich* and *wurmähnlich*, while a *Sanguinaeus Temperament* was changed into *Blutreicher Beschaffenheit*, and *Vehemente Convulsiones* and *formula decantationum* were translated into *heftigste Zückungen* and *Seegensprechung*. All in all, the editor was cautious not to modify the original meaning of the expressions.

There was a topic, however, where substantial changes were made. As discussed above, somewhat incongruous with the core medical/gastronomic argumentation, there was a moral/demonological discourse that came up only a few times in the text. The editor cut, modified, or rewrote something in all of these instances. In general, he preserved the moral part of the discussion, but deleted those parts where the manuscript became too entangled in reflections about Satan's behaviour. The demonological discussion about the holes on the graves was entirely cut, and the same happened to the question of Satan's political bias before and beyond the grave (cf: Tallar 1753, 14v, 4r; and Tallar 1784, 63, 12–13). The way the part about the good Christian education of soldiers was modified is especially interesting. The print has a simpler vocabulary that took away much of the sermon-like style so salient in the original text (cf: Tallar 1753, 19v, cited in note 31 above, and Tallar 1784, 83).[36] Finally, a small but telling deletion was made in the medical discussion as well: Tallar quoted the Bible only once, at a place where he was describing the veins and how their malfunction may cause death. Here he added a reference to Ecclesiastes 12:6, which describes death as "before the silver cord is snapped, or the golden bowl is broken, or the pitcher is shattered at the

---

[35] "Visum repertum anatomico-chirurgicum, oder *Gründlicher Bericht* […]" as opposed to the "Visum repertum anatomico chyrurgicum, oder Unterhänigst gehorsamster *Summarischer Bericht* […]" of 1753.

[36] "[…] so füge ich noch hinzu, daß die Soldaten und Deutsche durch den Glauben und getreuen Unterricht ihrer Seelsorger schon von Jugend auf wider die List des Satans und der Irr- und Aberglauben abgehärtet, und in dem heilsamen Kreuter Garten der Erkäntniß fest gepflanzet worden. Sie verlachen alle Märchen, unter was für einen Schein sie sich immer vorstellen, verlassen sich bloß auf die wundervolle Güte ihres Heilandes und bleiben unbeschädigt."

fountain, or the wheel broken at the cistern". This biblical location had been quoted in medical literature several times due to its resonance with William Harvey's discovery of the circulatory system and its collapse (Christianson 2007, 229–30). The editor, however, deemed it unsuitable and cut it.

The modifications made to the *Visum Repertum* attest to a difference in mentality: parts of Tallar's argumentation were simply deemed to be unfit for the milieu of Vienna in the 1780s. His argumentation about Satan's activity, the sermon-like metaphors and biblical references were deemed to be overly baroque. The editor made sure to retain the anti-Orthodox edge of the treatise and its contrast with good Christian education. The moral discourse's contemplations about sin, Satan and vampire disease became more moderate, more presentable and more similar to the core text. Based solely on the printed edition, Tallar's image is a shade more secular, more enlightened and less sensitive to demonological issues than the original.

The editor was not entirely successful in bringing Tallar's work up to date. Some reviews of the time praised him or rendered his arguments without comment (Anonymous 1784; Dionis 1790, 214–220, cited by Petersen 2013). Zacharias Hussty, the author of a book on public health, appreciates Tallar for his first-hand awareness of the question, but he deems his reasoning to be of no consequence, nonmedical and full of obscure hypotheses that taste of the old world (Hussty 1786, 157–65).[37] He received a particularly vitriolic criticism in the *Allgemeine Deutsche Bibliothek.* The anonymous reviewer set the tone by stating that Tallar did not have any command either of the subject matter or of the language. After presenting the main argument about the gastronomical/fasting-related origins of the disease, the reviewer finished Tallar off with a devastating last line: "The rest is wretched reasoning and true nonsense, that tastes of the bloodletting flask" (Anonymous 1786, 103). This mocking reference draws an analogy between the symbolic attribute of the surgeon who (as opposed to the physician) got his hands dirty through his profession, and the superstitious belief in blood-drinking vampires. In essence, Tallar was relegated to the ignorant, nonsensical and gullible culture—the very same one about which he was trying to enlighten the locals and dispel the myths.

[37] "sein Räsonnement ist zu unmedizinisch, mit dunkeln, und nach der Vorwelt schmeckenden Hipothesen zu verwebt, als daß es brauchbar sein könnte."

Conclusion

There is still much research to be done and archives may still be hiding relevant documents that will shed more light on the vampire situation of the Banat in the eighteenth century. However, certain conclusions can already be drawn. For one, the vampire problem seems to have been much larger than previously assumed. During the roughly fifty years investigated here, several hundreds of deaths were attributed by locals to vampires. Even so, the slowness of the provincial administration to react to the problem and to create a unified stance indicates that the administration of the Banat had more serious problems to deal with in the first half of the eighteenth century. During this time, the outcome and adjudication of the cases depended largely on the power dynamics between district authorities, the church and the local community. The situation changed in 1753, when the provincial government set up the Kallacsa Commission, consisting of the new provincial physician of the Banat, Dr Paul Adam Kőműves, the experienced German surgeon, Johann Georg Tallar, and the anonymous cleric. Their investigations in several villages probably helped the administration to formulate a stance towards vampire cases.

The *Visum Repertum*, written at the end of 1753, was Tallar's way of demonstrating his medical expertise, his intimate knowledge of local Vlach culture and his general enlightened disposition to the new civilian governor of the Banat. His empirically based treatise addressed vampirism on multiple levels. For one, he gave a naturalistic explanation to both the lack of decomposition of the vampire corpses and to the vampire sickness. He also provided a good reason (the practice of blood smearing) for prohibiting vampire-killing rites in the province. He also showed off his enlightened mindset by listing the tests to which he subjected local folklore. Finally, he engaged in moral discussions as well, which gave his treatise an anti-Orthodox edge that might have contributed to its print publication in 1784.

The printed version, published by the Vienna-based Johann Georg Mößle, fitted into the profile of the publishing house in several ways. It approached a curious topic related to the empire's inner savages and presented the triumph of enlightened medicine over local superstition. In order to achieve this goal, Mößle made modifications to the original text. He severed many of the roots that linked the treatise to its original birthplace, the Habsburg Banat administration: the information about the commission, the mining metaphors and the reference to the weekly reports in the title were all lost. Furthermore, he sought to make the *Visum Repertum* more palatable for the Vienna audience of the 1780s by editing those parts which ventured too deeply into discussing satanic activity in this world. The Temeswar provincial administration of the 1750s and the Vienna learned public of the 1780s held different expectations towards a medical treatise on the returning dead. Nevertheless, Tallar's first-hand knowledge of Vlach culture remained a constant value: it played a crucial part in earning him the esteem of the Banat administration, was approved of even by the mixed reviews of the 1780s and is still appreciated by today's ethnographers.

Abbreviations

MNL-OL—Magyar Nemzeti Levéltár, Országos Levéltár, Budapest.
OENB—Österreichische National Bibliothek, Wien.
OESTA—Österreichisches Staatsarchiv, Wien.
HHSA: Haus-, Hof- und Staatsarchiv.
KA: Kriegsarchiv.
FHKA: Finanz- und Hofkammerarchiv.

References

Afanas'ev, Alexandr N. 1976. "Poetic views of the Slavs regarding nature." In *Vampires of the Slavs*, edited by Jan L. Perkowski, 160–79. Cambridge: Slavica Publishers.

Anonymous. 1784. "Visum repertum anatomico-chyrurgicum [review]." *Realzeitung für das Jahr 1784*: 101–6. Wien.

—. 1786. "Visum repertum anatomico-chyrurgicum [review]." *Allgemeine Deutsche Bibliothek 1765–96*, 65 (1): 102–3.

Arlaud, Daniel. 2007. "Vampire, Aufklärung und Staat: Eine militärmedizinische Mission in Ungarn, 1755–1756." In *Gespenster und Politik*, edited by Claire Gantet, and Fabrice d' Almeida, 127–41. Berlin: Wilhelm Fink.

Barber, Paul. 1988. *Vampires, burial and death—Folklore and reality*. New Haven, and London: Yale University Press.

Baróti, Lajos, ed. 1893–1907. *Adattár Délmagyarország XVIII. századi történetéhez* 1–4. [Data collection for the 18th century history of Southern Hungary]. Temesvár: Csanád-Egyházmegye Nyomdája.

—, ed. 1893–1896. *Adattár Délmagyarország XVIII. századi történetéhez* 1. [Data collection for the 18th century history of Southern Hungary]. Temesvár: Csanád-Egyházmegye Nyomdája.

—, ed. 1900–1902. *Adattár Délmagyarország XVIII. századi történetéhez* 2. [Data collection for the 18th century history of Southern Hungary]. Temesvár: Csanád-Egyházmegye Nyomdája.

Barrowclough, David 2014. "Time to Slay Vampire Burials? The Archaeological and Historical Evidence for Vampires in Europe". https://www.academia.edu/8854480/Time_to_Slay_Vampire_Burials The_Archaeological_and_Historical_Evidence_for_Vampires_in_Europe, accessed: 28.03.2018.

Bartholotti, Johann Nepomukm and A. Kreil, 1783. *Streitschrift wider die verschiedenen Gattungen des Aberglaubens: Gesammelt aus den görzischen Diktaten*. Wien: Johann Georg Mößle.

Bell, Michael E. 2006. "Vampires and Death in New England, 1784 to 1892." *Anthropology and Humanism* 31 (2): 124–40.

Benedictus XIV. 1743. *De servorum Dei beatificatione et beatorum canonizatione. Liber Quartus & Ultimus, Pars Prima*. Patavii: Typis Seminarii, apud Joannem Manfré.

—. 1752. *Dissertationes in omni doctrinae genere selectissimae ex quatuor ejusdem auctoris De canonizatione sanctorum libris extractae. [...] Volumen tertium continens Tractatum de miraculis*. Venetiis: excudebat Joannes Baptista Aleritius Hier. Fil.

Betsinger, Tracy K., and Amy B. Scott. 2014. "Governing from the Grave: Vampire Burials and Social Order in Post-medieval Poland." *Cambridge Archaeological Journal* 24 (3): 467–76.

Bijedić, Elvira. 2001. "Vampirismus auf dem Balkan zur Zeit der osmanischen Herrschaft." MA Facharbeit, Universität Heidelberg.

Born, Ignaz von. 1774. *Briefe über Mineralogische Gegenstände, auf seiner Reise durch das Temeswarer Bannat, Siebenbürgen, Ober- und Nieder-Ungarn* [...]. Frankfurt, und Leipzig: Johann Jacob Ferber.

Brandt, Georg. 1735. "Dissertatio de semimetallis." *Acta Literaria et Scientiarum Sveciae* 4: 1–10.

—. 1748. "Cobalti nova species examinata et descripta." *Acta Regiae Societatis Scientiarum Upsaliensis* 1 (3): 33–41.

Bräunlein, Peter J. 2012. "The frightening borderlands of Enlightenment: The vampire problem." *Studies in history and philosophy of biological and biomedical sciences* 43 (3): 710–9.

Christianson, Eric S. 2007. *The Ecclesiastes through the centuries*. Malden, Oxford, and Carlton: Blackwell Publishing Ltd.

Corradi Musi, Carla. 1995. *Vampiri europei e vampiri dell'area sciamanica*. Catanzaro: Soveria Mannelli.

Danneberg, Stéphanie. 2010. "'Vampire sind äußerst unordentliche Untertanen'. Überlegungen zur Funktion und Instrumentalisierung des

Vampirphänomens." *Zeitschrift für Siebenbürgische Landeskunde* 2010 (2): 177–92.

Die Freymaurer. 1793. *Die Freymäurer nach ihren verschiedenen Absichten im hellen Lichte dargestellt.* Wien: Mößle.

Dionis, Johann. 1790. *Lexikon der K. K. Medizinalgeseze.* Prag.

Equiamicus, Nicolaus. 2013. *Georg Tallar—Gründlicher Bericht von den sogenannten Blutsaugern, Vampiren, oder in der walachischen Sprache Moroi.* Norderstedt: Books on Demand.

Federmann, Reinhard, and Hermann Schreiber. 1968. *Botschaft aus dem Jenseits.* Basel, und Tübingen: H. Erdmann.

Fine, John V. A. Jr. [1987] 1998. "In defense of vampires." In *The vampire—A casebook,* edited by Alan Dundes, 57–66. Madison, and London: The University of Wisconsin Press.

Fortis, Alberto. [1774] 1778. *Travels into Dalmatia containing general observations on the natural history of that country and the neighbouring islands, the natural productions, arts, manners and customs of the inhabitants* [...] London: J. Robson.

Gardeła, Leszek, and Kamil Kajkowski. 2013. "Vampires, criminals or slaves? Reinterpreting 'deviant burials' in early medieval Poland." *World Archaeology* 45 (5): 780–96.

Geissau, Anton Ferdinand von. 1786. *Des heiligen allgemeinen Kirchenraths zu Trient: Schlüsse und Glaubensregeln welche die Katholische Lehre betreffend.* Wien: Bey Johann Georg Mössle.

Gräf, Rudolf. 1997. "Die Entwicklung des Südbanater Industriegebiets." In *Das Banat als kulturelles Interferenzgebiet. Traditionen und Perspektiven,* edited by Horst Förstler, and Horst Fassel, 79–85. Tübingen: Institut für donauschwäbische Geschichte und Landeskunde.

Haen, Anton de. 1774. *De magia liber.* Lipsiae: I.P. Kravs Bibliopolae Viennensis.

Hamberger, Klaus. 1992. *Mortuus non mordet. Dokumente zur Vampirismus 1689–1791.* Wien: Turia und Kant.

Harmening, Dieter. 1983. *Der Anfang von Dracula—Zur Geschichte der Geschichten.* Würzburg: Königshausen & Neumann.

Hock, Stefan. 1900. *Die Vampyrsagen und ihre Verwertung in der deutschen Literatur.* Berlin: A. Duncker.

Horányi, Ildikó. 1997. "Tetszhalottak, élve eltemetettek—esetleírások a magyarországi tetszhalál-irodalom alapján [Seeming dead, buried alive—case descriptions on the basis of Hungarian literature on the seeming dead]." *Kharón* 1 (1): 1–26.

Huhn, Christian Wilhelm. 1783. *Raritäten oder umständliche Beschreibung, was Anno 1683 vor, bey, und in der denkwürdigen türkischen*

Belagerung Wien, vom 7. Julii bis 12. September täglich vorgelaufen. Wien: Bey Johann Georg Mössle.

Hussty, Zacharias Gottlieb. 1786. *Diskurs über die Medizinische Polizei* 1. Preßburg, and Leipzig: Löwe.

Janion, Maria. 2006. *A vámpír—Szimbolikus biográfia* [The vampire—A symbolic biography]. Budapest: Európa.

Kallbrunner, Josef. 1958. *Das Kaiserliche Banat 1. Einrichtung und Entwicklung des Banats bis 1739.* München: Verlag des Südostdeutschen Kulturwerks.

Keyworth, David G. 2006. "Was the vampire of the eighteenth century a unique type of undead-corpse?" *Folklore* 117: 241–60.

—. 2010. "The Aetiology of Vampires and Revenants: Theological Debate and Popular Belief." *Journal of Religious History* 34 (2): 158–73.

Kiss, András. 2004. *Boszorkányok, kuruzslók, szalmakoszorús paráznák* [Witches, quacks, straw-girdled fornicators]. Kolozsvár: Kriterion.

Klaniczay, Gábor. 1986. "Boszorkányhit, boszorkányvád, boszorkányüldözés a 16–18. században [Witch belief, witch accusation and witchcraft persecution in the 16th and 18th centuries]." *Ethnographia* 97: 257–95.

—. 1988. "Gerard van Swieten und die Anfänge des Kampfes gegen Aberglauben in der Habsburg-Monarchie." *Acta Historica Academiae Scientiarum Hungaricae* 34 (2–3): 225–47.

—. 2002. "Decline of Witches and rise of vampires in 18th-Century Habsburg Monarchy." In *The Witchcraft Reader*, edited by D. Oldridge, 387–98. London: Routledge. [*Ethnologia Europaea* 17 (1987): 165–80.]

—. 2004. "Historische Hintergründe: Der Aufstieg der Vampire im Habsburgerreich des 18. Jahrhunderts." In *Poetische Wiedergänger: Deutschsprachige Vampirismus-Diskurse vom Mittelalter bis zur Gegenwart*, edited by Julia Bertschik, and Christa Agnes Tuczay, 83–112. Tübingen: Francke.

Koenig, Tricia Close. 2011. Betwixt and between. Production and commodification of knowledge in a medical school pathological anatomy laboratory in Strasbourg (mid-19th century to 1939). [Diessertation, Université de Strasbourg].

Köhlbach, Markus. 1979. "Ein Fall von Vampirismus bei den Osmanen." *Balkan Studies* 20: 83–90.

Kreuter, Peter Mario. 2001. *Der Vampirglaube in Südosteuropa. Studien zur Genese, Bedeutung und Funktion. Rumänien und der Balkanraum.* Berlin: Weidler Buchverlag.

—. 2002. *Der Vampyr, ein Fremder? Ethnische Minderheiten im Vampirglauben Südosteuropas. Kakanien Revisited*, cf.

http://www.kakanien.ac.at/beitr/vamp, accessed: 22.03.2014.

Kropatschek, Joseph, ed. 1785–1790. *Handbuch aller unter der Regierung des Kaisers Joseph des II. für die K. K. Erbländer ergangenen Verordnungen und Gesetze in einer Sistematischen Verbindung, 18 Bde*. Wien: Johann Georg Mößle.

—. 1786. *Sammlung aller k. k. Verordnungen und Gesetze vom Jahre 1740 [...] zu dem Handbuche aller unter der Regierung des Kaisers Joseph des II* [...] 1–8. Bände. Wien: Johann Georg Mößle.

Krumphanzlová, Zdeňka. 1961. "Kotázce vampyrismu na slovanských pohřebištích [The issue of vampirism in Slavic burial grounds]." *Památky archeologické* 52 (2): 544–9.

—. 1966. "Der Ritus der slawischen Skelettfriedhöfe der mittleren und jüngeren Burgwallzeit in Böhmen." *Památky archeologické* 57 (1): 277–327.

Lambrecht, Karen. 1994. "Wiedergänger und Vampire in Ostmitteleuropa—Posthume Verbrennung statt Hexenverfolgung?" *Jahrbuch für deutsche und osteuropäische Volkskunde* 37: 49–77.

Langer, Johann. 1889. "Serbien unter der kaiserlichern Regierung 1717–1739." *Mitteilungen des K. K. Kriegs-Archivs*. Neue Folge III: 155–247.

Leben. 1788. *Leben und Geschichte Mohammeds: enthaltend einen vollständigen Abriß der Gründung und Fortpflanzung der von ihm ausgedachten Religion, seiner Kriege und der merkwürdigsten dabey sich ereigneten Vorfallenheiten*. Wien: Mößle.

Lecouteux, Claude. 2009. *The Return of the Dead: Ghosts, Ancestors, and the Transparent Veil of the Pagan Mind.* Rochester: Inner Traditions.

Lesky, Erna. 1957. "Die Österreichische Pestfront an der k. k. Militärgrenze." *Saeculum. Jahrbuch für Universalgeschichte* 8: 82–106.

Levack, Brian. 1999. "The decline and end of witchcraft prosecutions." In *Witchcraft and magic in Europe. The Eighteenth and Nineteenth centuries*, edited by Bengt Ankarloo, and Stuart Clark, 1–94. London: The Athlone.

Linzbauer, Franciscus, Xaver. 1852. *Codex Sanitario-medicinalis Hungariae*. Tom. 1. Budae: Typis Caesareo-Regiae Scientiarum Universitatis.

—. 1853. *Codex Sanitario-medicinalis Hungariae*. Tom. 3, Sect. 1. Budae: Typis Caesareo-Regiae Scientiarum Universitatis.

Magyar, László András. 1999. "Orvosi vita a magyarországi vámpírokról, 1732–1756 [Medical debate on vampires in Hungary]." *Századok* 133 (3): 1247–57.

—. 2002. "Über die siebenbürgische Vampir-Krankheit. Ein Bericht des deutschen Chirurgen Georg Tallar aus dem Jahr 1755." *Zeitschrift für Siebenbürgische Landeskunde* 2: 161–4.

Magyary-Kossa, Gyula. 1929–1940. *Magyar orvosi emlékek* I–V. [Hungarian medical records]. Budapest: Magyar Orvosi Könyvkiadó Társulat.

Martini, Carl Anton von. 1799. *Des Freyherrn Karl von Martini [...]. Allgemeines Recht der Staaten: zum Gebrauch der ö ffentlichen Vorlesungen in den k. k. Staaten.* Wien: bei Joh. Georg Edlen v. Mössle.

Meisel, Reiner. 1783. *Was ist von der Religion, und von den Pflichten gegen Gott &c. zu halten?* Wien: Mößle.

Milleker, Felix. 1937. *Kurze Geschichte der Banater Militärgrenze 1764–1872*. Wrschatz: Kirchner.

Moszyński, Kazimierz. 1976. "Slavic folk culture." In *Vampires of the Slavs*, edited by Jan L. Perkowski, 180–7. Slavica Publishers: Cambridge.

Murgoci, Agnes. 1926. "The vampire in Roumania." *Folklore* 37: 320–49.

Müller, Joseph. 1791. *Der steyerische Robinson oder Reisen und besondere merkwürdige Begebenheiten des Joseph Müller an den Brasilianischen Küsten von Amerika.* Wien: J.G. Mössle.

Nowosadtko, Jutta. 2004. "Der 'Vampyrus Serviensis' und sein Habitat: Impressionen von der österreichischen Militärgrenze." *Militär und Gesellschaft in der Frühen Neuzeit* 8 (2): 151–68.

Oinas, Felix. [1992] 1998. "East European Vampires." In *The vampire—A casebook*, edited by Alan Dundes, 47–56. Madison, and London: The University of Wisconsin Press.

Petri, Anton Peter. 1988. *Beiträge zur Geschichte des Heilwesens im Banat*. Marquartstein: Breit.

Petersen, Niels K. 2013. A surgeon's eyewitness accounts from Transylvania and Wallachia. http://magiaposthuma.blogspot.com/2013_09_01_archive.html, last time accessed May 11, 2015.

Plenk, Joseph Jakob. 1799. *Der Wundarzneykunst Doktors [...]. Lehre von den Augenkrankheiten.* Wien: Bei Joh. Georg Edlen von Mössle.

Pócs, Éva. 1989. *Fairies and witches at the boundary of South-Eastern and Central Europe*. Helsinki: Academia Scientiarum Fennica. (Folklore Fellows' Communications 243).

—. 1999. *Between the Living and the Dead: A Perspective on Witches and Seers in the Early Modern Age*. Budapest: Central European University Press.

—. 2001a. "Démoni megszállottság és ördögűzés Közép-kelet-európai népi hiedelemrendszerekben [Demonic possession and exorcism in Central Eastern European popular belief systems]." In *Demonológia és boszorkányság Európában* [Demonology and witchcraft in Europe], edited by Éva Pócs, 137–98. Budapest, and Pécs: L'Harmattan, and PTE Néprajz Tanszék. (Studia Ethnologica Hungarica I.)

—. 2001b. "Megszálló halottak—halotti megszállottság [Possessing dead—possession of the dead]." In *Lélek, halál, túlvilág. Vallásetnológiai fogalmak tudományközi megközelítésben* [Soul, death, after-life. Religious ethnological concepts in an interdisciplinary approach], edited by Éva Pócs, 121–39. Budapest: Balassi. (Tanulmányok a transzcendensről II.)

—. 2012. "'We, Too, Have Seen a Great Miracle': Conversations and Narratives on the Supernatural Among Hungarian-speaking Catholics in a Romanian Village." In *Vernacular Religion in Everyday Life. Expressions of Belief*, edited by Marion Bowman, and Ülo Valk, 246–80. London, and New York: Routledge.

Porter, Roy. 1999. "Witchcraft and magic in Enlightenment, Romantic and Liberal thought." In *Witchcraft and magic in Europe. The Eighteenth and Nineteenth centuries*, edited by Bengt Ankarloo, and Stuart Clark, 191–282. London: The Athlone.

Rauer, Constantin. 2008. "Von der Aufklärung des Vampirismus zum Vampirismus der Aufklärung: Eine West-Östliche Debatte zwischen Einst und Heute." *Ethica* 7 (1): 87–107.

Rácz, Sámuel. 1794. *A' borbélyi tanításoknak második darabja a' törvényes orvosi tudományról, és az orvosi politziáról...* [The second part of the barbers' education about forensic medicine and medical policing…]. Pest: Trattner.

Reynolds, Andrew. 2009. *Anglo-Saxon Deviant Burial Customs*. Oxford: Oxford University Press.

Sariyannis, Marinos. 2013. "Of Ottoman ghosts, vampires and sorcerers: An old discussion disinterred." *Archivum Ottomanicum* 30: 191–217.

Scopoli, Giovanni Antonio. 1786. *Der Weltweisheit und Arzneikunst Doktors [...]. Anfangsgründe der Chemie: zum Gebrauche seiner Vorlesungen.* Wien, und Leipzig: bei Johann Georg Mössle.

Schaub, Hagen. 2009. *Knochen und Bestattungsriten—Die Bedeutung archäologischer Funde zum Wiedergänger-bzw. Vampirglauben.* Kakanien Revisited, http://www.kakanien.ac.at, last access: March 22, 2014.

Schürmann, Thomas. 1990. *Nachzehrerglauben in Mitteleuropa*. Marburg: N. G. Elwert.

Schwerdling, Johann. 1789. *Practische Anwendung aller k. k. Verordnungen in Gesitlichen Sachen [...] vom Antritte der Regierung weiland Marien Theresien, bis zum Tode weiland Joseph II. nähmlich vom Jahre 1740 bis 1790.* Wien: Mößle.

Schwicker, Johann Heinrich. 1861. *Geschichte des Temeser Banats. Historische Bilder und Skizzen.* Grosz-Becskerek: Verlag von Fr. P. Bettelheim.

Senn, Harry A. 1982. *Werewolf and vampire in Romania*. New York: East European Monographs.

Sokol, Hans. 1967. *Die k. k. Militärgrenze*. Wien: Bergland.

Sommfels, J. 1783. *Was ist vom Bürger, jungen Künstler und Kaufmann zu halten?* Wien: Mößle.

Swieten, Gerard van. 1768. "Vampyrismus." In *Abhandlung des Daseyns der Gespenster, nebst einem Anhange vom Vampyrismus.* Edited by Andreas Ulrich Mayer. Augsburg.

Tallar, Georg. 1753. *Visum repertum anatomico chyrurgicum, oder Unterhänigst gehorsamster Summarischer Bericht. Von und über Die so genannte Vampir oder Blutsauger; Wallachischer Sprache Moroi genant*. OESTA-FHKA, Banater Akten, r. Nr. 53, fol. 1–22.

—. 1784. *Visum repertum anatomico-chirurgicum, oder Gründlicher Bericht von den sogenannten Blutsäugern, VAMPIER, oder in der wallachischen Sprache Moroi in der Wallachen, Siebenbürgen und Banat, welchen eine eigens dahin abgeordnete Untersuchungskommission der löbl. k. k. Administration im Jahre 1756 erstattet hat*. Wien, und Leipzig: Johann Georg Mößle.

Tóth G. Péter. 2017. "The decriminalization of magic and the fight against superstition in Hungary and Transylvania, 1740–1848" In *Witchcraft and Demonology in Hungary and Transylvania*, edited by Gábor Klaniczay and Éva Pócs, 291–317. London: Palgrave Macmillan.

Vajkai, Aurél. 1943. *Népi orvoslás a Borsavölgyében* [Popular medicine in the Borsavalley]. Kolozsvár: Erdélyi Tudományos Intézet.

Várkonyi, Ágnes. 1991/2. "Connections between the cessation of witch trials and the transformation of the social structure related to medicine." *Acta Ethnographica Hungarica* 37: 425–77.

Vermeir, Koen. 2011. "Vampires as Creatures of the Imagination: Theories of Body, Soul and Imagination in Early Modern Vampire Tracts (1659–1755)." In *Diseases of the Imagination and Imaginary Disease in the Early Modern Period*, edited by Yasmin Annabel Haskell, 341–73. Turnout: Brepols Publishers.

Vidal, Franco. 2001. *Extraordinary Bodies and the Physicotheological Imagination*. Berlin: Max Planck Institut für Wissenschaftgeschichte. [Preprint nr. 188.]

Von dem Verfahren. 1790. *Von dem Verfahren wider Kriminalverbrecher: ein Handbuch für Bannrichter, Landgerichtsverwalter und alle die sich in den k. k. Staaten mit der Ausü bung der Kriminalgerichtsbarkeit beschäftigen*. Wien: Bei Johann Georg Edlen von Mössle.

Vukanović, T. P. 1976. "The vampire." In *Vampires of the Slavs*, edited by Jan L. Perkowski, 201–34. Cambridge: Slavica Publishers.

Wellmann, Imre, ed. 1984. *Magyarország népének élete 1730 táján* [The life of the peoples of Hungary around 1730]. Budapest: Gondolat.

Wessely, Kurt. 1970. *Die österreichische Militärgrenze. Rechtstellung, Aufgaben, Bevölkerung. Sonderausdruck aus Volkstum zwischen Moldau Etsch und Donau.* Wien, und Stuttgart: Univeritäts-Verlagsbuchhandlung.

“SHE CONDEMNED ME, SO THAT I DIE…” WRONGDOING, PUNISHMENT, DISEASE: INDIVIDUAL AND COMMUNAL EXPLANATIONS

JÓZSEF GAGYI

During my years of research in the twentieth century, the concept of “getting it done” (*csináltatás*; in the sense of bewitchment) was continuously present in the villages I studied in Székely Land. One of the already explored and presented chapters of this issue is the demand for the magical practices conducted by Orthodox Romanian priests and kalugers (Orthodox monks) and their performances. In my paper on the custom of visiting kalugers (Orthodox monks) (Gagyi 2007; then Gagyi 2010), after describing the practice I observed in the field, I explain the social role of the activities of the kalugers. Having Michel Foucault’s thoughts (Foucault 1975) as a starting point, I try to answer how much the community acknowledges and practises the two basic forms of the cultural mechanisms of truth-seeking: proof and investigation. Moreover, in what situation and why do they not accept the truth constructed by the investigation performed by the institutions of the elite? And under what circumstances and why do they prefer the “eternal” divine truth manifested in the practices of religious-magical specialists, hidden from us but existing and able to be transmitted by the “holy corporation”?

The premise of this present study is that the principle and the practice

1) are of varying intensity, yet are permanently present, and that
2) the general opinion on bewitchment and the relationship with it forms the basis of “reality and truth”; that is, social cohesion and integration, and is thus the fundamental social mechanism for the construction of these.

These same principles serve as a starting point to this study, complemented by the idea that breaching the godly commandments of truth, or put differently, the moral principles of the community, results in one of the forms of punishment (at this point still reversible): illness or its complete, final and irreversible form, death. In certain cases, the "fight" against the illness and the person causing it, as well as the struggle for the reestablishment of physical well-being and of psychic and social integrity, at one and the same time taking place in a medical, magical and social context, can take decades after the diagnosis of the disease. That is, it is a process of diagnosis and therapy (Favret-Saada 1980).

In what follows, I would like to present and interpret the "illnesses" of a man from Szolokma,[1] who was 76 years old at the time of the interview. Our encounter took place in 1996;[2] it was an unusual collecting situation in every sense, and I still think of it as the most puzzling of my field experiences, one that calls for an advanced interpretation.

The integral text of the interview with A.J. and his wife, not overlong but very rich in meaningful content, is enclosed in the Appendix.

…one cannot take the staff out of God's hands…

The popular system of concepts, which also provides the principles defining the practice in terms of seeking truth and doing justice—a system I would name the *culture of proof*—was very accurately resumed by one of my informants at the end of one story.

> [One of my aunts] told me that she went to the Catholic priest to ask him to celebrate a mass for her husband to get better. The priest told her: look, I can very well celebrate a mass for him, but I can't ask for him to get better: it is as the Lord chooses it to be. Because one cannot take the staff out of God's hands; his will must be done; not mine, and not that of others. And then my aunt told the priest that in this case he shouldn't even celebrate a mass, if it was not to make her husband better. But then the priest said that it could only go the way the Lord wanted it to go; he could, nonetheless, ask the Lord to ease his suffering and help him in his illness, but he could not ask him to actually make him get better. For one cannot take the staff out of God's hands, it has to go according to His will. (D.A.T.M.)

[1] Szolokma is a village in Maros County belonging to the Makfalva township and the neighbouring villages of Etéd, Kösmőd and Siklód in the valley of the hills surrounding Kis-Küküllő; before 1918 it belonged to Udvarhely County.

[2] This is when I did my fieldwork in Szolokma. Éva Pócs assigned the collection of belief stories; the collection entitled *Belief narratives from Szolokma* containing 80 studies can be found in the Folk Belief Archives of the HAS Research Centre for the Humanities, Institute of Ethnology.

We cannot know what the Catholic priest actually said. We know that the Romanian (Orthodox) priests and monks (called *kalugers* by the Hungarians of Székely Land) provide magical services (Komáromi 1996; Keszeg 1999; Gagyi 2007). What motivates people to seek their help is the idea that through them, they can turn to God "who knows and imposes the truth". We are dealing here with the concept of a God different from the Western clerical world view, one belonging to the group of phenomena known collectively as folk religion. He is a God who knows and directs the ultimate (moral) order of human society. According to this concept, the power of the highest judge affects both "benediction and malediction". He does not tolerate; he punishes anyone who goes against his will:

> Once there was a hailstorm, a big one, it came and went, and came back, it struck us, and also Makfalva and then Kibéd as well. There was a man who went to see his vegetable garden, he had fine crops, and he saw that every plant was broken. Then he looked up and started threatening the sky! And they say that he suddenly turned black. He stayed like that for three days! This is the truth; it was not long ago, under the collective. He suffered for three days, and then he died. So one must not go against the Lord… That's for certain: if someone opposes the Lord, they might fall victim to strange misfortunes like this one. (D.A.T.M.)

Another feature of this God concept is that it represents an almighty autonomous force. "In popular Christianity, God continuously acts to his children's benefit and in their interests; and this provision (providence) can be influenced by the believers' promises and certain forms of piety", writes Tamás Mohay on folk religion in his book on the pilgrimage of Csíksomlyó (Mohay 2009, 18–9). This direct influence does not concern the God who cannot be addressed directly—in those cases one requires an intermediary. They are not, however, always successful, since the direction of the action is not clear. It occurred that someone was "asking for a bad thing for someone else, but it came back upon him instead". The will of this God—the punishing staff—cannot be modified by human intentions. This Lord (see the denomination below) is the purest of authorities.

The punitive fulfilment of God's will is formulated in numerous narratives in Szolokma. One of the stories is about András Jakab (A.J.), whose illness, that is, his bewitchment, I am about to present in detail in what follows.

…he is sometimes getting better, sometimes worse...

The case I present here is reconstructed on the basis of the conversation I had with the protagonist of the story and his wife, as well as the conversations I had with other members of the village. Fundamentally, I am following the interpretation of my protagonist.

I have divided the interview with A.J. and his wife into seven parts. This division was made according to the information I possessed, that is, the interpretations of outsider witnesses and the content found in the written text which is the interpretation of A.J. himself. This approach indicates the barriers within the interaction forming the conversation; it separates the parts which are different in terms of content and it facilitates the interpretation of the transcribed conversation published in the appendix to this present study.

1. I had never heard of the "diseases" of A.J. until I met him and he started to describe them to me. I only sought the opinion and interpretations of others concerning the issue after I had had the astonishing conversation with him, in an effort to ease my amazement and resolve my incomprehension.

The very first time he mentioned the issue happened under quite unusual circumstances. The researcher collecting narratives of different beliefs usually explores the knowledge of the informant regarding those beliefs question by question, motif by motif; it is rare to have the informant suggest a new topic out of the blue.

> "Don't you want to talk about bewitchment?" asked András Jakab after the warm-up round of questioning. I could not believe my ears, which was clearly apparent from my response: "What?" He explained: "Do you want to know about "doing" (csinálmány), when someone is getting it done to the other?" Then he claimed: "I have already been bewitched. It's been more than 30 years now...", and he continued: "I clarified the issue, and she confessed, that woman who condemned me, so that I die."

In a brief minute we had discovered in-depth connections:

1) it transpired that here we had a case of bewitchment of "effect and power" (Favret-Saada 1980);
2) we also found out that it had been more than thirty years since his life was ruined, since when his greatest misfortunes had fallen upon him, of which he could not free himself;

3) we discovered that he had had doubts, but that he does not have them anymore because he had "clarified" who the agent of the bewitchment was, who it was who had wanted him to die (the reasons for which I will discuss later);
4) that the question of life and death is like a very severe judgement on which everything depends.

The revelation was quite unexpected and very deep: life and death, an "illness" lasting for more than thirty years, it was all included in the simple statement that here, in this village, bewitchment happens when someone "gets it done to the other".

Before I could ask the question, "Was there anything that provoked this?", that is, before I could force him to tell the story, there were two other important "intermezzos". One was the question from his wife: "Wasn't there a wise man in Etéd, or is there one still?" I had mentioned earlier that I had relatives in the neighbouring town of Etéd, and that is why she asked the question—and now that I look back, it was probably also in the hope of discovering a new location and a new person to "heal" her.

The other was when I asked A.J. to tell me what had happened to him ("How did the bewitchment occur?"), which apparently caused him to contemplate who this person was in front of him, what he wanted, and how he could improve or worsen his situation. So, he asked me, "What does it signify if I tell you? Does it mean anything?" I replied, "It means that I would know", which did not put him at ease: "Only that?"

According to my "ex post facto" interpretation, this question was to find out how much of a "wise man" I was; in other words, to find out whether, besides listening to his story, I disposed of any information that would help in undoing what had been done to him and concerning the healing of the disease(s) that I could share with him, and which might raise new hope in him. That is, could he involve me in his struggle, could he count on me being on his side? (see Favret-Saada 1980).

2. Part Two includes the identification of the "wrongdoer" (the "witch"), the primary reason for the bewitchment, and presents the first phase of the disease. It turns out that the enemy is his own sister-in-law and immediate neighbour. Since fresh information is clarified in parts 6 and 7, I will discuss this issue in those sections.

The reason behind his bewitchment can be considered classic in light of the knowledge we have on witch trials: the man sees the woman, his sister-in-law, as she was "philandering" (having sexual intercourse) with someone, and he also lets her know that he has seen the scene by laughing out loud. The reply comes as a threat: "You will regret this!" There is only one exact date attached to the event, and that is when the disease first appears, in 1963; A.J. is 43 years old at that time. The time of the threat is unknown and might not even be important. What is important, however, is that the syndrome first appears as a disease: he goes to a doctor who establishes that he is suffering from "nervous exhaustion, almost of the most severe kind"; he takes medication and undergoes radiation. After ten days of treatment, his condition becomes even worse.

There is a curious circumstance in the story worth consideration: he is not hospitalised but has to undergo the treatments while staying at the lodgings and workplace of the sister-in-law, in Marosvásárhely (Târgu Mureş):

> I slept where that slut went to do her washing, a couple of women used to wash in the city; and she slept next to me, my neighbour, her sister [pointing at his wife].

Thus, for ten nights he had been sleeping in the same bed with the woman that he knew was willing to have casual sexual relations with others. What happened (or what did not happen despite A.J. wanting it) during these nights between them? How could this influence their further relationship or the forming of her role as the one "responsible" for "getting it done to him"? Because we know that during these ten days, the illness alone existed; there was, as yet, no suspicion and therefore no bewitchment either.

The question cannot be answered based on the information gathered. I suspect, however, that the reason for the change in their relationship might have been an eventual rejection.

Turning point: suspicion, assurance

3. Since he is not getting better and he knows that bewitchment is also a possibility, this is when he starts to suspect that his illness cannot be cured by doctors and medical treatments. He has to seek the help of a magical specialist, because "they will tell you if you are a victim of bewitchment". He has to be certain; therefore, he decides to go to a renowned fortune teller in Marosvásárhely.

4. This fortune teller—Mrs Csejdi—used to be a well-known personality in Marosvásárhely in the early 60s. She was mostly visited by maids

serving families in the city.[3] After having spent ten days in Marosvásárhely and getting more and more desperate, A.J. goes to see the fortune teller, but the woman refuses to help him: "She looks me deep in the eye and says: I am not dealing with you!" His second attempt brings the same result; he has no other choice: he has to find another magical specialist.

5. He is advised to go to Gyergyószentmiklós (Gheorgheni), where there is "a Russian woman, who stayed behind after the war of 1944." He agrees with her daughter that they will drive him to the fortune teller. She receives him, makes him draw cards and establishes her diagnosis: he is the victim of bewitchment. She also identifies the date of the wrongdoing, as well as the culprit of the wrongdoing:

> one month, thirty days ago. And who could that person be, who did this wrong? And then she said: the lower neighbour, the blonde woman!

A.J. still considers this moment to be the decisive turning point in the story, the "clarifications" he mentioned in the first part, the enlightenment resetting the order of "cause and effect": the fortune teller "just suddenly told it all. Well, this was more than enough for me."

The fortune teller gave him protective magical objects: "a litre of some kind of medicinal water", and also a thread, on which she tied knots, "more than a hundred, as many as the thread could bear", which he had to tie around his waist, and "told me to wear it until it falls off". A.J. has been wearing this magical object around his waist for years.

The most important feature of this new situation is that it focuses on and interprets the scattered experiences. It builds a confrontational structure upon the system of kin-relations, which explains retrospectively, indeed, some time later as well, situations which could be described in terms of a neutral (scientific) evaluation either as a medically diagnosable and curable disease, or as a misfortune or a stroke of fate.

This situation is at once regressive and reductive, returning to the network of magical explanations and the failure of the rational, alternative explanations.

[3] I can testify to that: when I was little, the maid serving at our house took me to the street next to the main square of Marosvásárhely and showed me where the fortune teller lived and how she could foresee the future.

Turning point: anger

The next step after the "healing": he announces that he has successfully fended off the bewitchment in order to radically alter relations with the sister-in-law. He knows, the man and his wife both know that the sister-in-law is the "owner" of, that is, the one responsible for the bewitchment. She is informed of it as well, and so are the inhabitants of the village. It is at this point that the moral and existential struggle is played out in front of the villagers where each tries to influence their own fate in light of the other's maleficent activity. The imagining of the bewitchment and the awakening of suspicion are the first steps towards publicity; in the announcement of the bewitchment and its healing, their narrative presence is in all respects a reality-generating gesture.

The reality-generating force of publicly speaking about the bewitchment is manifested in the statement, "We are still on bad terms", which brings the storyteller back from the past to the present. According to the definition of Sándor Oláh, "In everyday life, anger is a turning point in the relationship of two individuals. The relation connecting them is transformed; the collective behaviour used before to reinforce their relation is hereafter (from the onset of the anger) suspended; the eventual interactions that occur afterwards are handled differently (with a different "tone" of gestures). We could not establish that all kind of interaction is ceased between the two parties, nonetheless, they continue to coexist in their new roles, as people being on bad terms with one another" (Oláh 1999, 112–13). In this case, they become neighbours who are on bad terms with one another.

From this point on, it is the community that keeps a watch over this relationship, for two reasons. The contentious couple will do anything to externalise their anger on social occasions: they will manifest the nature of their relationship with gestures, in their use of space, in comments referring to the other party. The community cannot ignore this and must evaluate these elements.

Moreover, in a community—especially if it consists of individuals who are interdependent under closed circumstances (in a closed productional and redistributive system)—one cannot violate the laws of solidarity without consequences spreading beyond the individual. The anger cannot mean a complete break-up; there must remain some superficial level of cooperation. As to what degree—this does not concern the other members of the community, but it is the reason why they have to keep an eye on the angry couple, to observe and evaluate any demonstration of willingness to appease, so as to be able to recommend reconciliation at the appropriate moment.

The anger of A.J. had its limits as well. When the "witch" fell ill, his wife, that is, "her sister went to visit her. We were still on bad terms, but in these cases, she still visited her." In the same manner, the "witch" visited A.J. in hospital. However, in consequence, his condition got worse, and according to his own diagnosis, it was as if he had been poisoned, judging from the discharged matter they drained from his stomach, although the reason for his hospitalisation had been a heart attack. Finally, he got out of hospital, and from then on was no longer "ill"—though he was not "healthy" either. His condition is best described in his own words, quoted earlier: he was condemned, so that he dies. In his interpretation, the threat is permanent and the danger is immediate: "I get by as much as I can."

All this caused a great deal of trouble for A.J. in front of his family and the members of the community. As he said: "I get worse, then I get better, first they believe it, then they don't…" His behaviour, the turns in his condition and the explanations presented to the community have weakened his credibility and corroded his moral capital. The story of the wrongdoing was put in different perspectives, and hence the created "patient/victim" role was questioned. Alternative explanations gained ground. The events and their reasons became part of public discussion; finally, it was his well-constructed social status and identity which were challenged.

7. As time passed, the anger faded, which meant that even if the in-laws did not get closer, the sisters did. However, new occasions to revive the old conflict perennially cropped up. Sometimes the mundane events of everyday life: a sickle, spade, pitchfork or hoe was lent to the sister-in-law, never to be returned. Or she asked for some sugar or flour, but never returned it, saying that she could not afford to give it back, and that they had plenty. Or sometimes it was a life-changing event which placed the family of A.J. on the losing end in the competition between the two sisters and their families: when Jakab's son-in-law passed away, their daughter remained a widow with three children, while, conversely, their sister-in-law's son received a big pension on retirement, and since he felt capable of working the land, the question of "land inheritance" arose within the family.

The framework, however, remains the same: if there is any grief or trouble in the family, it is usually judged within the system of relations created by the presumed fate-affecting intentions and machinations of the sister-in-law/neighbour, once initiated and very probably sustained up to the present. "There's nothing to be done about it, this is our fate," A.J.

sighed. They see their lives within the triangle of bewitchment—threat, suspicion and healing. That which becomes inevitable in this coordinate system also becomes their fate.

> A.J.'s moral offence: "…one mustn't do such a thing, to build from tombstones!"

Did the bewitchment, the "condemnation", truly take place?

> The villagers obviously wanted to know the answer to that. They saw that A.J. was wandering around despondently, not even working, because he can't, for "it has been done to him"… he has his place in the cemetery. (N.Á.)

However, this was not the only thing they saw or knew.

There is another plausible, yet very different explanation as well, according to which the illness can be considered a kind of "divine judgement", punishing A.J.'s injurious and "bad" nature. He had committed a moral offence by desecrating the peace and memory of the dead. In this case, there was no need for an intermediary to deliver the punishment, since his crime was so obvious, so atrocious.

This interpretation is determined; the storyteller only allows one valid point of view, and wants to convert the listener to his side:

> Listen closely, darling, let me tell you one thing about this, and then look me in the eye and see if it's true.

Is there any way one could disagree with a representative of the community concerning behaviour which offends the highest of judges? Especially after hearing the following:

> All the tombstones there exist, he took them[4] and built himself a house, and the Lord punished him for it. It was not the wrongdoing of his neighbour! When they were building me this [pointing at his own house], when they were building his, they all read the names, and put the tombstones in the wall; one shouldn't do that, to build a house from the cemetery. He didn't tell you this? How many times have I told him: András! He's my first cousin. I told him: András! Aren't you afraid of God, that he might even punish your children, if you take all the

[4] It is possible to do this in Szolokma: there are many family cemeteries at the end of the gardens and in the adjacent fields, as well as partly abandoned family cemeteries.

> tombstones? They could all read the names carved in the old tombstone.
> …
> Everyone thinks he was punished by the Lord for having carried all those tombstones away to build the house; they were shoving the stones in the foundation so that no one can see. So, there it is, this is what I know, it was some ugly politics… (K.F.GY.M.)

In the opinions of others, as well: "He did this to himself, it was not someone else who had it done to him". Because the more experienced say: "He was a very injurious man" (D.A.T.M.), he robbed others, he destroyed their crops. This was also part of his "ugly politics".

From these voiced opinions, another image of him emerges, circulating within the community. A.J. had used the well-known concept of bewitchment to excuse himself from work and to gain the sympathy of others. This "strange" man is, in other words, someone who is using "ugly politics" to achieve his aim. In my interpretation, here his behaviour is seen as a violation of the village's cooperative system and confrontation with his peers. The village "does not acknowledge" the bewitchment, they rather believe, as was phrased above, that "he was punished by the Lord".

He is ill, yet he is not; people believe it, yet they do not—this is what A.J. said about himself. In this new context, the statement receives a new interpretation. It is especially the second part of the statement that is more emphatic. One has to decide which statement they believe to be true in order to decide how to relate to him. The interpretation, and accordingly the way to relate to him, is decided by what the members of the community believe of him in terms of their valid everyday system of relations based on the dominant interpretations of the community.

Does he belong among those guilty parties who desecrate the memory of the dead, and thus the memory of the community?

The people with whom he had confrontations reply without compunction in the affirmative. In the social space of the village, willingness to cooperate or confront may decide whether any particular person is, in fact, the victim of bewitchment, meaning that they deserve the village's solidarity, or is guilty of offending God and the community, and therefore unworthy of such solidarity. If he is a victim, the community is obliged to sympathise with him and help and support him. If guilty, he deserves the special attention that the necessary punishment for violating the moral principles entails; for he has only got what could be expected based on the valid order of the World, which has inevitably been as valid for him as for anybody else.

There is nothing peculiar in him falling sick, since he has to suffer for his sins. The disease or series of diseases is unfortunate in itself, but in light of the context, it is neither unexpected, nor peculiar. The disease confirms for the inhabitants of the village the moral validity of the cosmic order which is sustaining the community (*communitas*) and is approved by society (*societas*).

References

Favret-Saada, Jeanne. 1980. *Les mots, la mort, les sorts. La sorcellerie dans le Bocage*. Paris: Gallimard.

Foucault, Michel. 1975. Surveiller et punir: Naissance de la prison. Paris: Gallimard.

Gagyi, József. 2007. "'Az egy szent testület...' A kalugerekhez (ortodox szerzetesekhez) járás, a , "próba kultúrája" társadalmi szerepéről ['It's a holy corporation...' On visiting kalugers (Orthodox monks) and on the social role of the 'culture of proof']." *Erdélyi Társadalom* 5 (1): 9–22.

—. 2010 "'Az egy szent testület...' A kalugerekhez (ortodox szerzetesekhez) járás, a "próba kultúrája" társadalmi szerepéről ['It's a holy corporation...' On visiting kalugers (Orthodox monks) and on the social role of the 'culture of proof']." In *Amire vágyunk, amitől félünk, amit remélünk*, 23–39. Marosvásárhely: Mentor.

Keszeg, Vilmos. 1999. "Román pap [Romanian priest]." In *Mezőségi hiedelmek*, 56–67. Marosvásárhely: Mentor.

Komáromi, Tünde. 1996. "A gyógyító román pap [The healing Romanian priest]." *Néprajzi Látóhatár* V (1–2): 87–98.

Mohay, Tamás. 2009. *A csíksomlyói pünkösdi búcsújárás. Történet, eredet, hagyomány* [The Pentecost pilgrimage of Csíksomlyó. History, origin, tradition]. Budapest: Nyitott könyv, and L'Harmattan.

Oláh, Sándor. 1999. "Harag-események [Anger-events]." In *Ismerős terepen. Válogatás csíkszeredai antropológiai írásokból* [In a familiar field. Selections of anthropological studies from Csíkszereda], edited by József Gagyi, 105–125. Csíkszerda: Pro-Print.

Pócs, Éva. 2001. "Átok, rontás, divináció: boszorkányság a vallás és mágia határán [Curse, maleficium, divination: witchcraft on the borderline of religion and magic]." In *Két csíki falu néphite a századvégen* [The popular beliefs of two villages in Csík at the end of the century], edited by Éva Pócs, 419–59. Budapest: Európai Folklór Intézet, and Osiris.

Informants

D.A.T.M.—born in 1919
A.J.—born in 1920
K.F.GY.M.—born in 1924
N.Á.—born in 1913

Appendix

Don't you want to talk about "getting it done"?
What???
Do you want to know about the "getting it done", when someone "gets it done" to someone?
Well, yes, that, too...
It has already been done to me. It's been more than 30 years now since this house...
/Wife: Wasn't there a wise man in Etéd, or is there still one?/
Do you know, if we ask someone... how did it happen?
Should I tell you?
Yes.
I don't know. What does it mean if I tell you? Does it mean anything?
It means that I will know, too.
Only that?
Is there a place, where it is frequent...?
I clarified the issue, and she confessed, that woman, who condemned me, so that I die.
Was there anything that provoked this?
Only that I saw her, because she's a whore, she still is, and I saw her from the garden as she was philandering, and I laughed. Which I came to regret. It cost me dearly, because after this house was finished, in 63, in 1963, I fell so ill that they had to take me to Marosvásárhely. There the doctor didn't want to hospitalise me, he told me to go in for treatment every day for ten days. He prescribed me medication. He told me: you have nervous exhaustion, almost of the most severe kind. So, I stayed there for ten days, I went in every day, they did radiation, I got medications and all, and went in the following day, too. I slept where that slut went to do her washing, a couple of women used to wash in the city; and she slept next to me, my neighbour, her sister [pointing at his wife].
The ten days passed and my condition got only worse. Some people say that there are people who will tell you if you are victim of bewitchment.

So, I went to see one, she had clients, a woman with her daughter, she was disappointed, or whatever, I had to wait for them to finish. So, I went in…
Was it in Marosvásárhely?
In Marosvásárhely. I greeted her, good day…
Which place in Marosvásárhely?
In the main square.
In the main square?
In the main square, not far from the corner, from the market. You know that place?
Isn't it where the movie posters are, across Bolyai street?
A little bit further.
/Wife: Mrs Csejdi./
Csejdi, yes.
Have you heard of her?
Yes, I have.
So, I wanted to say, Madam, please tell me something, because I am very ill. She looks me deep in the eye and says: I'm not dealing with you! Would you tell me, why not? I will pay for it. Do you understand? But she wouldn't deal with me. So, I left; but since I was there for ten days, I had time to go back once more, because I was desperate.
So, I went to see her again; I found her in the main square, sitting on a bench. The lights were on, it was a nice autumn evening; I sat down next to her and asked nicely, please, I am very sick. She looked at me again, and then she said: didn't I tell you? I'm not dealing with you! Yes!
Than at home they told me that in Gyergyószentmiklós there was a Russian woman, who had stayed behind after the war of 1944.
Wasn't it in Gyergyóújfalu (Suseni)?
They said Gyergyószentmiklós, and Vasláb (Voşlăbeni), further away, that's where she used to live, before going to the city. She seduced a young lad, I don't know what she must have done to get married, János was his name, or something. So, I agreed with my daughter that since they have a car, they would take me to her shortly, via the big mountain, and we'd find her.
We only had to wait a little, she was about to return, because they took her on a tour, for she had a great…
/Wife: she had a great talent!/
She had a great talent. When she arrived, she was pale, like I am now, she was over seventy, and she said: János, please give me an Algocalmin, I have a terrible headache. The old lady. And then she got to it right away, or was it only in the morning, I don't remember. When the time came, she called me into the other room, and made me cut the cards. I took the deck

in the middle and cut them. She looked at the card and said: somebody has done it to you. Tell me please, I said, has it been going on for a long time? She said: one month, thirty days ago. And who could that person be, who did this wrong? And then she said: the lower neighbour, the blonde woman! She just suddenly told it all. Well, this was more than enough for me. And then she told me some things. She didn't order me any medication and didn't tell me to come back. But she took a thread and tied as many knots on it, more than a hundred, as many as the thread could bear. She told me to wear it until it fell off. Only for washing, I had to wash it from time to time, because it got sweaty. But I always tied it back on and have been wearing it for years. She also gave me a litre of some kind of medicinal water; that was all the medication I got.

I came home, we'd done it. And then I started to talk about it, because I was getting better and better, and so that the woman would find out that she was the owner of this. I was telling how she slept next to me for ten days, right next to me on the couch. I was moaning, for I was ill, and maybe she was laughing at me.

/Wife: It was this Mrs Csejdi who did this, that's why she didn't receive András, because she knew that he was already bewitched./

You might understand how it is, what I said before. Well she found out…

/Wife: Her talent is so great, she could tell that it was this woman who did it to him…/

And this, this is the biggest question. She told me I was a victim of bewitchment, but she would not deal with me. But I didn't leave it at that, I went to see another, and she was the one who told me off: you're going from one evildoing… to the other…

We are still on bad terms. After we came home, she fell from the attic, right where we sleep, because she went to do the laundry and she went up to the attic to get a pot, and she missed a step and fell, and almost died, she was hospitalised. And this sister of hers went to visit her. We were still on bad terms, but in cases like this, she went to visit. And then when I… when I got better from my disease, then I had a heart attack and I was in hospital. And then they came to visit me, and even brought tulips, one Sunday afternoon, in the two hours of visiting. They came in, smirking; I was lying in bed, alone in a room… but no, at that time there was another Hungarian who also had visitors. And they came up directly to my bed and gave me the flowers, and a kiss, on the mouth, for such a sick person! I was so sick; I haven't been swallowing anything else but the medications for a month.

/Wife: He had a heart attack./

Yes, that. And then, that morning when I had to start eating, I had such a stomach ache, that I couldn't take it. I don't know if it was the food, or if the food transformed into something, other than the medication; I started screaming, and my roommate screamed to get the doctors, and they took me and put me somewhere else, and the people gathered around me, doctors and nurses, and were asking each other, what should we do with him, where does it hurt? They palpated my stomach, there was pain everywhere. Then one of them said they couldn't cut me open because of the heart attack. So, they should do whatever they want, he doesn't know better. Then he suggested draining my stomach, with a rubber tube. And then they put in the tube, and the other end into a jar, which filled up with something black… I didn't even ask what it was, what kind of poison. And it went on for 5 days, and the doctor asked me every day how I was doing. I told him that the pain shifted to only one side, and I had received a perfusion. On one side. And then the day passed, and the next morning he asked me again, how I slept and if my stomach hurt. And it didn't hurt, they could palpate it. "Thank God!" he said. A great doctor saying such a thing, mentioning God, it was a medicine to me that he prays, too.
So that's how I was healed.
I also wanted to tell you, that we were together with these women, well, I wasn't, but they got together. And then she asked for a sickle, and a hoe and a pitchfork, too, that's how she was, but she never returned them without us asking for it. She took the hoe, and we still went hoeing to Szőllőárka, and she left the hoe there in her field, so that she didn't have to carry it the next day. No one took it, though it was a good and new hoe. No one took it, they just told whose it was.
/Wife: Negligent./
And I told her all this, that she takes all our things away and never brings them back, borrowing everything, a sugar and a cup of flour, what will we do about it? And she says: I can't return it. Because she didn't like working, she liked ruling. She was either sleeping or wandering around. Then she tells me: I can't give it back, but you have plenty of it. They have been snatching our wheat with the sister-in-law. Now they started to prosper. Her son grew up, he worked in the mines and was retired…
Which mine? In the Zsil valley?
Yes, he was there. No one knows how much he got, hundreds, thousands. Meanwhile, he married a Romanian, but they didn't get along, so they got a divorce. He paid for it, he even had to go to Bucharest, I remember… He remarried, there are even grandchildren now. Because that woman has a son and a daughter, and they have children, too, so they will inherit the property…

/Wife: Everyone has their own sorrow. So do we; the husband of our daughter died, and she has stayed here with three children, for almost ten years now./
There's nothing to do about it, this is our fate.
/Wife: Our son never got married; he has been paying for the three children since they were little... so much trouble…/

2. PHYSICIANS, MAGICIANS, HEALING PRIESTS

DIVINATION BY SPIRITS AND SPIRIT MEDIUMSHIP IN THE MIDDLE AGES

CHRISTA AGNES TUCZAY

1. Introduction

The ancients, and later the medieval mind, divided divination not according to the content supernormally perceived, but according to the method of perception. They distinguished between "technical" divination or foreboding and "natural" or intuitive divination. Natural divination was supposed to take place in a state of trance but, nevertheless, the medieval thinkers linked the visions of mediums with spirits, angels or demons that appeared and answered the questions. Trance prophesying is a phenomenon widely attested cross-culturally. Especially among women, it is often connected with mediumship or spirit possession. Everywhere, states of possession have been, and still are, viewed with a mixture of fear and religious worship, depending on the physiological symptoms displayed and above all on the belief pattern current in each society. Where the condition is persistent and accompanied by grossly pathological behaviour, the possessing agent is assumed to be an evil spirit and ritual techniques of exorcism are employed—often with the effect of inducing (by suggestion) the symptoms they are intended to cure. When the symptoms are benign, the possessed are highly valued as channels of communication with the supernatural world. Mediumship is deliberately sought, is ritually controlled and channelled, and in many societies, acquires high religious and social value, as was the case with the female medieval mystics.

2. The Delphic Pythia and her reception

The most influential of all Greek religious institutions, the oracle of Delphi, owed her influence entirely to the abilities attributed to an entranced woman, the Pythia (Dodds 1963; Maurizio 2001; Connelly 2007). The belief held by pagans and Christians alike, over a period of more than a millennium, was that through the lips of the Pythia, an alien voice spoke in the first person. The historian, Plutarch, did not keep records about his times and the Delphic oracles, but knew the system from personal experience, having held a priesthood at the oracular shrine at Delphi from 95 CE until his death. He devotes several of his dialogues to the Delphic oracle. In each dialogue, Plutarch treats a specific topic. In his dialogue, *De defectu oraculorum* he relates different points of view on the matter to various dialogue partners such as Lamprias (Pausanias 1913, v. 5; Plutarch 1921). Lamprias rejects the idea that a god is the entity responsible for the oracles, but his point of view presents one of the basic ideas of inspiration among Jews, Christians and Greeks. A spirit enters into a person and speaks through the mouth as would the human spirit under normal conditions.[1]

Three first-century authors reviewed explicitly as Jewish[2] by medieval sources also delineate the communication of spirits through human intermediaries similar to Plutarch. Josephus, Philo and Pseudo-Philo describe the presence and effect of spirits in vivid terms usually considered unique to Greco-Roman as ecstasy and prophetic amnesia (Josephus 1926–1965; Philo of Alexandra 1962)[3]. The possession of both Pythia and pythons was, so far as we know, induced auto-suggestively (Beattie and Middleton 1969, 4).[4] But in the Egyptian papyri, both Greek and Demotic, we find spells by which a magician may induce it. The *Great Magical Papyrus of Paris* gives elaborate instructions for summoning a god to enter into a child or adult and speak through him (Pseudo-Philon 1976; cf. Tibbs 2007, 113–44).

In contrast to the deductive divination (e.g. casting of lots), intuitive divination, or rather prophecy, communicates directly with the divine and does not rely on material means. Therefore M. Weippert's definition applies not only to the Near Eastern territory: "Religious revelatory speech can be described as prophecy if in a cognitive experience vision, audition, audiovisual experience, dream etc. a person encounters the revelation of one or more deities and if this person perceives herself/himself as being

---

[1] Lamprias favours the vapours theory.

[2] These three authors' "Jewishness" in a Hellenistic society shows that the expressions for inspiration available to them would have been typically Greek only from the lexical perspective.

[3] Philo of Alexandria, Werke, vol. I: Leben Mosis book II, 361; Vol. VI: De somniis 269.

[4] It is sometimes asked how much control the subject has over the onset of his trance. The answer is: about the same control as ordinary people have over falling asleep.

able to transmit what was revealed in either verbal (prophecy, prophetic word) or non-verbal communication (symbolic act)" (Weippert 2001).

This offers a model of prophecy as a communicative process. The prophet receives a divine message and communicates it to his or her audience. Although prophecy is mostly oral in character, in many cases, the communication of the message to the audience is achieved in written form (Nissinen 2000). The communication both in antiquity and in early medieval times is not a dialogue but strictly one way: it comes from a divine source and the prophet is the mouthpiece. The prophet merely serves as a communicative facility, an instrument, to the divine, as Jeremiah (XX 7–10) assures. The prophet is overpowered and forced to communicate God's message against his own will.

> O LORD, you deceived me, and I was deceived, you overpowered me and prevailed. I am ridiculed all day long; everyone mocks me. Whenever I speak, I cry out proclaiming violence and destruction. So the word of the LORD has brought me insult and reproach all day long. But if I say, "I will not mention him or speak any more in his name", his word is in my heart like a fire, a fire shut up in my bones. I am weary of holding it in; indeed, I cannot. I hear many whispering, "Terror on every side! Report him! Let's report him!" All my friends are waiting for me to slip, saying, "Perhaps he will be deceived; then we will prevail over him and take our revenge on him."

3. The voice within—ventriloquism

The Pythia of Delphi, the witch of Endor and the young slave girl following the Apostle Paulus (Apostles 16, 16–18) are all named *pythia* or *pythonissae*; all three seem to have an oracular spirit, are prophets and speak with a voice that differs from their "normal" speech and voice. Ventriloquism from late antiquity into the eighteenth century was embedded in Christian discourses about demonic possession, necromancy and pagan idolatry. Many of the discussions on ventriloquy concentrate on the story of the Pythia of Endor recounted in 1 Samuel 28, in which King Saul, who had subdued all magical diviners, disguises himself and visits a sorceress to summon up the ghost of Samuel and discern, with her help, the futures of his battle against the Philistines. Saul then hears the prophet Samuel speak from beyond the grave. This clearly can be interpreted as necromancy, an ill-famed and also forbidden art, but was the whole scene accomplished through devilish powers? (Tropper 1989). Was this apparitional voice of Samuel real and prophetic or only a diabolical illusion created by the sorceress to trick a weak Saul?

As Reginald Scot explained in his *The Discoverie of Witchcraft*, Pythonists or Ventriloqui speak in a "hollowe voice" much different from their usual tone, and "such as take upon them to give oracles" or "to tell where things lost are become" (Reginald Scot 1972). In demonological discussions, such nomenclature referred to one who had "a familiar spirit" who spoke during trances or in an apparently diabolical voice that claimed soothsaying powers. Scot elaborates at length:

> This pythonist being Ventriloqua. That is Speaking as it were from the bottome of hir bellie, did cast hir selfe into a transe, and so aboused Saule answerint to Saule in Samules name in hir counterfeit hollow voice (ibid. 85).

But diabolical as well as prophetic utterances were part of a biblical world of spirits, apparitions and miracles. The term is a Latin translation of the Greek *engastrimythos*, which referred to a form of prophetic speech proceeding from the stomach. Christian writers also localised the oracular voice in the breast and used the expression *sternomatice* to refer to a person who spoke though the chest. This word was used to translate the Hebrew phrase *Baalat Obh* meaning one possessed by a familiar spirit (cf. Vox 1981, 14). The term "familiar spirit" is used by the Holy Office to label the inspirational source of the divining slave in the famous passage in Acts 16, where St Paul mentions a young slave with the gift of divination using her (pythonist's) spirit. When Paul ordered the spirit out of the slave, her masters, who saw in her a source of potential earnings, were distraught:

> Once when we were going to the place of prayer, we were met by a slave girl who had a spirit by which she predicted the future. She earned a great deal of money for her owners by fortune telling. This girl followed Paul and the rest of us, shouting, "These men are servants of the Most High God, who are telling you the way to be saved." She kept this up for many days. Finally, Paul became so troubled that he turned around and said to the spirit, "In the name of Jesus Christ I command you to come out of her!" At that moment the spirit left her. When the owners of the slave girl realized that their hope of making money was gone, they seized Paul and Silas and dragged them into the marketplace to face the authorities. They brought them before the magistrates and said, "These men are Jews, and are throwing our city into an uproar by advocating customs unlawful for us Romans to accept or practise."

This interpretation was a confusing addition to a theological dilemma. The concept of the Latin *familiaris* originally denoting a household servant was applied in the late Middle Ages to a spirit or demon at a witch's command.

It is not the phenomenon of spirit possession alone that is the reason for the noticeable broad reception of Christian theology that gives the *pythonissae* a much greater space than all the other divinations. Both Augustine and Thomas Aquinas made their point about the delusional deceptive feats of the demons on the basis of the slave girl story. The term *python* and the female form *pythonissae* developed from a diviner with an oracular spirit to a diviner who would conjure a spirit. They were known as belly-talkers since they were believed to have a *daemon* in their bellies which spoke through their lips and predicted the future. The medieval theologians were especially fascinated by the *divinatio per pythones* (cf. Harmening 1979, 101, 177, 204, 207–214, 221, 268, 313). The obvious broad interest Christian theology has shown in the matter cannot be explained by the fact that there had been a trance possession phenomenon alone. Quite often, the *pythonissae* were famed to prophesy "the truth". And due to that, they had to find out to what extent the demon's work was involved in the divinatory arts.

In the eighth century, the word *haegtesse* was a synonym for *striga, erynis, eumenis, furia, pythonissa*, and *filia noctis* (Frank, in Hansen 1901, 614–70; Lecouteux 1985, 57–70; Northcott 1991). In the tenth century, *pythonissa helleruna and haegtesse* were apparently applied to any female or male who possessed the spirit of divination. *Haegtesse* as a translation of *striga* and *pythonissa* is interchangeable with human witches (Meaney 1989). Psellos (1018–1078) expresses a general view in his statement that possession may be recognised "when the subject is deprived of all activity [...] but is moved and guided by another spirit, which utters things outside the subject's knowledge and sometimes predicts future events" (On the operation of daemons ed. Stephen Skinner 2010, 38–48; *De operatione daemonum*. ed. J. F. Boissonade 1838, 14).

The medieval German romance authors Conrad of Würzburg, in his *Trojan War* (*Trojanerkrieg*), and Heinrich of the Türlin, in his *Crown* (*Diu Crone*), draw a picture of two different types of prophets. In his portrait of Calcas, Conrad not only changes the character of the Homerian prophet to a trance diviner, a python, but confuses him with the leech or folk healer by calling him a *lachenaere*.

Die brust begunde er villen	he beat his breast with his fists
Vil starke mit der fiuste	
Dur daz daran dû siuste	to enfold the pythonic spirit
Der wâren lâchenîe geist,	and the divine spirit that is necessary
und aller göte volleist,	for the divinatory art.
die nütze wâren zuo der kunst (vv. 27232–237).	

He becomes pale, a spirit possesses him, and he faints:

Âmehteclichen seic er nider,	he swoons and lies there quite
als im geswunden waere.	Still like a piece of wood.

Der alte lâchenaere lac dâ stille sam ein stampf (vv. 27246–49).

He lies there in a state similar to death, his hair stands on end, and finally, he sweats and casts his body around until the spirit is conjured v. 27268–271). (The author informs his readers that it is the ancient art of the lâchenie, he sweats and foams and has to suffer great hardship. His gestures point to the ancient art and follow the ancient behaviour (vv. 27278–287)).

The obviously painful art of divination is performed with the help of a divining spirit that is sent to the diviners (*Swenn in der geist gesendet wart*) when they are deprived of their consciousness. When the spirit possesses the prophet, he becomes weak and unconscious. For his description, Konrad uses the term *lachenaere* and the art of *lachenie.* The Middle High German word *lâchen* means remedy (cf. Gothic: *lêkeis* "medicus") (see Richter 1967, 258–75), the term *lâchenaere* "sorcerer", Old Nordic *laeknari* "medicus"; *lâchenen* "healing with magic"; *lâchenie* "remedy" Ulfila (311) renders medicus with *lêkeis*; Tatian (830) uses *lâchi* as an expression for a physician. The term (with the meaning *medicus*) is only mentioned five times before the thirteenth century. From the mid-thirteenth century, the word is applied to sorcerers and diviners. The German *Bihtebuoch* (Confessional) of the fourteenth century even equates the term with witches and witch: *Vnn ob dv ie gelovbetost an hecse? Vnn an lâchenerin?* ("Have you ever believed in witches and lachnaere?") (*Bihtebuoch* 1784, 46).

The Old High German word *lâchi* is a loanword from Old Irish *liaig* "physician, conjurer". The Gothic word *lêkeis*, Germanic **lekja*, Latin *lego* means "to collect, to pick up runes, to read" (with the additional meaning "to interpret"), and also: somebody who conjures illness by incantations. These incantation-murmuring physicians, soothsayers, conjurers, and prophets soon became mixed up with sorcerers and, in the *Bîhtebuoch*, with witch figures. The magic art of *lâchenie* sorcery "has to be confessed as a sin": *Wan du solt niht geloben an zober/Noch an luppe noch an hess noch an lâchnye.* (You should not believe in magic witchcraft or lachenie).[5]

[5] You shall not believe in sorcery, poisonry, witchcraft or lâchenie (Rieder 1908. Der sogenannte St. Georgener Prediger aus der Freiburger und der Karlsruher Handschrift. 28).

In Lexer's Middle High German Dictionary (Lexer 1992, vol. I col. 1809), another strand of meaning refers to "remedy" deriving from the Old High German lāhhan (Köbler 1995, 236), "cure" or "remedy". *Lāhhi.* Germanic **lēkja-*, **lēkjaz* means male physician, whereas *lāhhida* is the female healer or physician. Significantly enough for our focus, the Latin *pythonissa* is translated as *Lāhhināri* or female physician. The remedy is *lāhhintuom*, the cure *lâchentuom,* while the verb *lâchenen* means to conjure; consequently, *lâchenære* is a conjurer and *lâchenærin* a female conjurer, in the *Bihtebuoch*[6] a synonym for witch. Konrad von Würzburg uses the term with the connotation of the presumably dark "art": *dâ treip diu küneginne ir kunst, lâchenie* (v. 77). The word belongs to the stem *leĝ-, meaning to pick up, collect Greek/Latin *lego* "I count, pick". Between the eighth and the thirteenth centuries, the terms *lāhhi, lâchenære, lâchentuom* are (following Reier's etymological research) general definitions for *medicus*, *remedium medicamentum*, *temperare*. All Latin terms for the physician and his art are translated in the Old High German accounts as *lāhhi*, *lāhhintuom*. However, the magical connection is weaker in the Old High German than in the Anglo-Saxon, which distinguishes between deceptive sorcerer or *scinlaecan drý*, Germanic **drug*, and *laecedom*, the heavenly remedy. Further history of the term proves that it always had a magical connotation that was exploited in the sources. The development starts with *lichen* with the connotation "to heal" and then broadens to a magical connotation thus obscuring the primordial meaning.[7]

Dictionaries of the sixteenth century even contain clearly pejorative meanings. Grimm's Wörterbuch lists *Lachsner* as conjurer, sorcerer and quack, who pretend to help the dead to delude the world. They are called:

> losser und "lachsner der von künfftigen dingen durch das losz weiszsagt" [...], "die lachsner, die tüfels beschwören anezigent, mit diesem oder

---

[6] "Unn ob du ie geloubtestost an hecse? unn an lâchenerin? Unn an segnerin? Unn ob du tete das si dir rieten? Und ob du ie gesegent unn gelâchenet wurde?" [Do You believe in a witch? Or a lachnaerin? And a woman who blesses? And have You followed their advice? Have You ever been blessed or had lachenie?] (*Bihtebuoch* 1784, 46).

[7] *Láchen* n. "remedy", ahd. *láchin, láhhi* "physician, healer", *láhhu* "I heal".—*láchene* swv. "bespeak"—"*ob die ie gesegent und geláchent wurde, oder gemezzen wurde*" If somebody is blessed or bespoken (*Bihtebuoch* 1784, 46).—*láchenaere,* stm. der "bespeaker"– "*zouberer und lachnaere*" (*Deutsche Predigten des 13. Jahrhunderts* 1978. Ed. F.K. Grieshaber 1, 150) *lachenerin* stf. "bespeaker" (*Bihtebuoch* 1784, 46), *lachenie* stf. "bespeak, bewitch" (cf. Reier 1987, 222 and 1976, 19).

jenem werk helfe man den todten […] die thuond nit anders dann daz sy der welt die betrogen will syn, bald darzuo helfend" (Grimm WB 1984, 12: 31).

The female diviner in the romance, *The Crown* has no specific denomination but the description of her behaviour classifies her as a trance diviner. She levitates while prophesying and her oracular spirit is pictured as the wind of inspiration:

Aber schunden sie begunde	the sudden wind did her great harm
Der wint an der stunde	so that the bystanders thought her dead
Und tet ir sô grôze nôt,	the wind raised her quite high
Daz man sie wânde wesen tôt,	
Sô sêre huop er sie ûf:	
Des wart ein michel zuolouf,	many people watched the spectacle in awe
und wânden des, sie wære	believing the hardship had killed her.
Tôt von der swære.	
Dô kam sie wider alsam ê:	but she regained consciousness
Ein wort sie vil lûte schrê:	screamed with a loud voice
Her künec, ir sît verrâten! (vv. 25095f.)	Oh king You are betrayed.

"Evidence" from literary sources does not necessarily mean the depicted material is altogether fictitious. Both authors are renowned for their allusions to everyday life and both describe in detail how the diviners go into a deep trance. The little damsel's trance is described similar to a shaman's deathlike cataleptic state and when she comes round again, she acts like the Greek Pythia or the biblical prophets as the mouthpiece of the spirit whose intermediary she really is.[8]

Centuries later the bishop Olaus Magnus (1450–1523) portrays the Sami shamans in northern Europe:

> If a stranger wants to know how things are back at home they can tell him within 24 hours even if it is 300 miles away or more, and this they do in the following manner: After the magician has performed certain ceremonies and has addressed his hellish gods with certain words, he falls to the ground, like a corpse, from which the soul is gone. And it seems that there is neither movement nor life in him. Then he gives information about the faraway place just as if he has seen it himself.[9]

---

[8] Many mystics were reported to come out of their trance screaming (cf. Weiss 2000, 180).

[9] Anhorn quotes Olaus Magnus in his *Magiologia* 36–57; translation by Behringer 1994, 155.

Another century later, Jean Bodin (1529/30–1596)[10] reports several examples of the witches' and sorcerers' ability to perform trance divination:

> So at Nantes in 1549 seven magi promised to tell what happened within a circuit of 10 miles and at once fell senseless, lying so for three hours, and then related what had happened in Nantes and the vicinity, all of which was verified. They were found guilty of many malefices and were duly burnt (Bodin 1591/1973, 177; cit. Lea 1939, 560).

That this technique belongs to a cross-cultural tradition is demonstrated by another example: when a British field worker in South Africa lost contact with his hunters,[11] he consulted a medicine man (a Kaffir doctor), who opened up the "Gate of Distance" for him.

> He would open the Gate of Distance, and would travel through it, even although his body should lie before me […]. The doctor then made eight little fires—that being the number of my hunters; on each he cast some roots, which emitted a curious sickly odour and thick smoke. Into each he cast a small stone, shouting, as he did so, the name to which the stone was dedicated; then he ate some "medicine" and fell over in what appeared to be a trance for about ten minutes, during all which time his limbs kept moving. Then he seemed to wake, went to one of the fires, raked the ashes about, looked at the stone attentively, described the man faithfully, and said: "This man has died of the fever, and your gut is lost." […] I took a particular note of all this information at the time and to my utter amazement it turned out correct in every particular (cit. Lang 1898, 75sq.)

---

[10] Bodin 1591/1973. In the English translation by Randy A. Scott (Toronto: Centre for Reformation and Renaissance Studies 1995) in Book One, Chapter Four, *On Prophecy and Other Divine Means to Learn Hidden Things* and Book Two, Chapter Five, *On the Ecstasy and Rapture of Witches and the Customary Relations They Have with Demons* are omitted therefore I had to quote from Lea's translation. When the obsessed collector of theologian, demonological and judicial scriptures on witchcraft issued his demonomany, Johann Weyer soon answered with his *De lamiis.* Shortly after Bodin replied with the addenda of a new chapter (*De praestigiis daemonum* 1546, und *De Lamiis* 1580). Cf. Mayer-Tasch 2000. Cf. http://www.historicum net (accessed: 15.02.2006).

[11] The American police occasionally employ the aid of mediums for their crime investigations. http://www.nytimes.com/2011/06/09/us/09psychic.html (accessed: 20.03.2018).

4. Christian prophets—mystics as spirit mediums

Penitentials give good evidence of how important diviners and prophets have been, not only for the so-called superstitious masses but also for the elite. Regardless of the punishment, medieval people seem to have consulted cunning folk, diviners and prophets on a regular basis. Regino of Prüm's[12] treatise was aimed against divination and diviners,[13] and the 1008 penitential of Burkhard of Worms lists countless divinatory practices (cf. Hain 1956). Those practices would not be mentioned so often if the general public had definitely not had a striking affinity with revelatory dreams, visions, omens and prophecy.

According to Luke and Paul, Christian prophecy was a subsequent public declaration of a spontaneous verbal revelation, conceived as a revealed truth and offered to the community on the authority of God or Jesus Christ or the Holy Spirit that might include a prediction of the future. There are three types of Christian prophecy:

1. Wandering prophets who travel from place to place staying for differing periods with Christian groups,
2. Prophets living within congregations,
3. Christians who are not officially considered prophets and who only occasionally prophesy.

The boom time for early Christian prophecy was from AD 29 to AD 100, when it was common in the apostolic period. (Aune 1983, 191-195) The rise of Montanism made these phenomena suspect. After 170 AD prophecies were extremely rare. Before we reach the zenith of medieval prophecy and mysticism, we have to look at the Montanist ecstatic prophecy (Trevett 1996). Eusebius of Caesarea (260–264 in Palaestina; † 337–340), the father of Church history, quotes an unknown opponent of Montanism:

---

[12] The Benedictine Regino of Prüm, abbot of Prüm Monastery in 892. His two treatises *De synodalibus causis et disciplina ecclesisasticis* contain a collection of Church decrees. The flight of the women and the metamorphosis are in Canon 371. Wasserschleben (1851/1958: 354sq.) On Regino of Prüm (ca. 840–915) in general, cf. Schneidmüller (1990: col. 492–495); cf. Maclean (2009: 1–28) Kurze, Friedrich (ed.). *Reginonis abbatis Prumiensis Chronicon cum continuatione Treverensi*. MGH SS rerum Germanicarum in usum scholarum separatim editi 50. Hanover, 1890.

[13] Those who employ the service of diviners and conjurers shall be excluded from the community *De synod. Causis* II can. 357 ibid. 349.

> In Phrygian Mysia there is said to be a village called Ardabau. There they say that a recent convert called Montanus, when Gratius was pronounced of Asia, in unbounded lust of his soul for leadership gave access to himself to the adversary, became obsessed and suddenly fell into frenzy and convulsions. He began to be ecstatic and to speak and to talk strangely, prophesying contrary to the custom which belongs to the tradition and succession of the church from the beginning (Eusebius 1999, 16.6–9; cf. Aune 1983, 313).

The Montanists called their movement the "new prophecy". Indeed, the evidence of Eusebius, who knows of collections of Montanist oracles (and cites the contents of some), reports that these oracles were delivered in plain Greek. Eusebius commented on Montanus that:

> he rose up two more women and filled them with the bastard spirit, so that they spoke madly and improperly and strangely like Montanus (Eusebius 1999, vv. 16.7, 9, 14).

The Montanist concept seems to be a blending of Hellenistic and distinctively Christian ideas and practice.

After the renunciation of Montanism by the mainstream Church, prophecy did not vanish but became a gift available to great saints. By the fourth century, discussions of prophecy by anyone not qualified by Church authorities gave rise to grave doubts. While some[14] believed that charismatic prophecy was a human faculty and therefore available to both men and women, others[15] labelled such claims as heresy. That brings us to the point of disagreement among early Christians and modern scholars alike. There is little consensus concerning the question as to whether prophecy was open to all believers, or more specifically: was prophecy conceived of as the domain of its regular practitioners and to what extent was it conceived as a congregational asset? The apostles Luke and Paul have varying opinions. Luke believes that all Christians are able to speak under the inspiration of the spirit. Paul agrees with Luke about the point that every believer has the Holy Spirit. But Paul has a strong urge to regulate prophecy and demands that:

---

[14] For example, Priscillian of Avila (ca. 340; † 385 in Trier) accepted women as prophets, who were welcomed as men's equals. They were organised into bands of *spirituales* and *abstinentes* (cf. Chadwick 1997).

[15] For example, Priscillian's Italian contemporary Filastrius, bishop of Brescia (ca. 330; † v 397).

> Two or three prophets should speak and the others would weigh carefully what is said [...] For You can all prophesy in turn. So that everyone be instructed and encouraged (1 Cor. 14.29–31).

A very important point concerns Paul's argument of the discernment of spirits and female prophets (cf. Leslie 1976, 125sq.; Wire 1990b, 134–150; and 1990a, 229–232). It is widely agreed that Paul cannot have forbidden female prophets as this would contradict 1 Corinthians 11.5,[16] where permission to prophesy is clearly implied. While the category of demonic possession had an unbroken history from the time of Jesus, serious claims to possession by the Holy Spirit had not been made in the West since the extinction of Montanism. Both the divinely possessed and the demonically possessed were mostly women. These two aspects of the gender were linked in the minds of many medieval contemporaries who commented upon them together. Subsequent writers also explicitly commented on the diffusion of a new and uniquely female strain of religiosity that flourished between the late twelfth and the fifteenth centuries. The new notion of divine possession became a familiar concept by the mid-thirteenth century.

Whereas the Latin terminology for demonic possession is quite elaborate, there are no equivalent words for divine possession. But the permanent character of medieval women's relationship with Christ or the Holy Spirit becomes obvious in the following lines:

> I, Christ, shall place my word in your mouth. Through your speech you will penetrate the hearts of your listeners and they will recognize beyond any doubt that I speak through you (Vita B. Margaritae Faventinae, cit. Caciola 2003, 57).

The danger of being possessed by the wrong spirit is illustrated at length by the Cistercian Caesarius of Heisterbach in the following story:

> There lived a recluse named Bertradis, a holy and religious woman famous for the divine revelations with which she was illuminated. For a long time, this woman mistook an angel of darkness for an angel of light, because she was less than cautious. The devil used to enter her little cell through the window with a fantastic penumbra of light, in order to prophecy the future to her and to instruct her about the things she asked him (Caesarius of Heisterbach 1929, 1: 332).

[16] And every woman who prays or prophesies with her head uncovered dishonours her head—it is just as though her head were shaven (cf. Jensen 1992, 254sq.).

Hildegard of Bingen's greatest fame was based on her visionary writings. Her most important work, *Scivias*, written by divine dictate between 1141 and 1150, recounts 26 visions given to her by the shadow of the living light. Defending both her visions and the divine command she writes in the introduction:

> Again I heard a voice from heaven saying to me: Speak of these marvels and write down what you have learned and say: In the year 1141 of the Incarnation of the Son of God at the age of 452 years and 7 months a flaming light of great brightness from open heaven completely flooded my brain, heart and breast like a flame that does not burn but warms [...] Immediately I was illuminated with a complete understanding and exposition of books like the Psalter and other Catholic tomes [...] (Hildegard of Bingen 1990, 3–6).

She delineates her altered state of consciousness in which she received her vision as high alertness or being wide awake and rejects the term trance (cf. Arbman 1970, 244). Indeed, Hildegard claimed that all her knowledge, including her medical comprehension and herb-lore and her music, was given to her directly from heaven. Hildegard's visions were examined by the archbishop of Mainz and by a papal delegation that feared demonic delusions and possession rather than divine inspiration. Hildegard knew that whoever was inspired by God could also be harassed by demons. From this perspective, her reluctance and disinclination to claim excessive or spectacular divine possession states, like those reported by her younger contemporary Elisabeth of Schönau, seem understandable (Clark, Anne L., ed., Elisabeth of Schönau 2000).

The bridge that enables Elisabeth of Schönau to cross from earth to heaven is her physical suffering. She reports that only after a period of torment and violent struggle would she "relax into ecstasy" and later into a region of light. Once she achieved the trance state, Elisabeth not only sees but also speaks. Some of her prophecies seem to have been transcribed directly from ecstatic elucidations while others were reported to her brother Ekbert or her sisters after the ecstasy. Her brother Ekbert asked Elisabeth what she learned in her visions. She gained information about the otherworldly fate of the deceased, enigmatic parts of scriptural and patristic writings but also about heavenly matters such as angels, Paul's rapture and banal secular affairs. Elisabeth and her brother were, of course, aware of the offensive nature of Elisabeth's divine inspiration and were therefore afraid that her works might be dismissed because of her being female. In his introduction to the second book of vision, Ekbert addresses the critics as follows:

> Indeed [God] is not inhibited by the murmuring of those who think themselves great and disdain whatever they regard as weaker and who do not fear to mock the riches of his goodness in them. They should be afraid that because of their murmuring they will hear the word. […] It scandalizes them that in these days the Lord deigns to magnify his mercy in the weak sex. But why doesn't it occur to them that a similar thing happened in the days of our fathers? When men were given over to negligence holy women were filled with the spirit of God so that they prophesied vigorously, ruled the people of God or triumphed gloriously over the enemies of Israel, as in the case of Hulda, Deborah, Judith, Jael, and others like them? [...] (ibid., 97).

Ekbert defends Elisabeth's claim of divine inspiration by referring to her biblical precedents, as the criticism of their contemporaries was based on gender. First, he links Elisabeth's trances to biblical prophetical women who were also filled with God's spirit. He and Elisabeth herself perceive her as standing in the tradition of the messengers of divine will. The significant distinction between her and the biblical prophetesses is that she is not a passive receptor of the divine message. She interacts and, even more importantly, she deliberately evokes her visions like a diviner. Both Hildegard of Bingen and Elisabeth, her contemporary and friend, were explicitly asked by high Church dignitaries to seek answers for them in their visions. This means a new attitude and a new interpretation of the formula *vidi* "I saw". Now it means "I found". The older theology of vision was the passive pictorial reception of a divine message. Around 1200, the new form came into being and existed alongside the old visionary tradition (cf. Newman 2005; Hamburger 2000; Voaden 1999). Elisabeth of Schönau not only listens to the words she receives in her visions but she answers and speaks, her visions are interactive and have a dialogue structure (for further examples cf. Christensen 2006).

The saving and serving role that mystical women created for themselves in the later Middle Ages was neither an imitation of the clergy nor a rebellion against them. It was a charismatic model that found its parallels in the Greco-Roman and Jewish prophetic tradition but is also a new individual lay model. Women could see themselves as authorised to teach, counsel, prophesy and heal by virtue of their spiritual experience, their spirit mediumship and not by the authorisation of Church offices.

5. Conclusion

The cross-cultural, inter-societal phenomenon of spirit mediumship present in both Greco-Roman culture and Judaism was understood and absorbed as pythonism after the divine Pythia of Delphi and her oracular Spirit, the python. In medieval times, the tradition of prophecy reached a new height in line with the innovative concept of female mysticism. The difference between the Greek Pythia and a medieval spirit medium is the possibility that a deceptive and evil spirit might enter and abuse the prophet. We have traces of a folk tradition of folk healing and folk magic in the term *lachenaere*. Unfortunately, there is only one literary source that applies the word for a healer to a trance diviner. Although we have further evidence that a certain spirit mediumship was employed for the healing procedure, the survey of the medieval sources is too vague to stress the point or provide evidence for a so-called trance healing or faith healing subculture. Nevertheless, I disagree with Brian Levack's statement in his *New Perspectives on Witchcraft, Magic and Demonology* p. 317, that trance healing was not a phenomenon in medieval Europe, because witches and healers practised mechanical magic, not mediumistic magic like a shaman. Better evidence for spirit mediumship, though not often healing, is to be found in the new movement of female spirituality, affective mysticism. Before the new model of mystic sainthood was established, sainthood had been associated with masculinity, noble blood and clerical status. Poor laywomen claiming divine spirit possession were therefore highly suspicious. Demonic possession was a sex-related, gender-specific phenomenon that primarily seemed to afflict women and especially lowly women. Thus, Caciola has elaborated: "The naturalization of these categories as gendered and socially situated—saintliness as essentially masculine, clerical, and noble; demonic possession or delusion as essentially feminine, lay, and lowly—fostered resistance to interpretations of laywomen's spirit possession as divine, rather than demonic in character. Few women claiming to be divinely possessed were accepted as such without contentious struggles" (Caciola 2003, 77).

That is why the method of differentiation, the discernment of spirit, became so important: the ability to discern true and false prophets again was a gift of the Holy Spirit and quite often operated in trance.

References

A. Dictionaries

Grimm, Jacob, and Wilhelm Grimm. 1984. *Deutsches Wörterbuch* 1–16. München: Dtv. [Leipzig: Hirzel 1854–1954.]

Köbler, Gerhard, ed. 1995. *Neuhochdeutsch—Althochdeutsches Wörterbuch*. Gießen an der Lahn: Arbeiten zur Rechts- und Sprachwissenschafts-Verlag.
Lexer, Matthias, ed.1992. *Mittelhochdeutsches Handwörterbuch* 1–3. Stuttgart: Hirzel.

B. Primary Sources

Bihtebuoch. 1784. *Bihtebuoch Dabey die Bezeichenunge der Heiligen Messe*. Edited by Jeremias Oberlin. Straßburg.
Bodin, Jean. 1995. *On the Demon-Mania of Witches*. Translated by R. A. Scott. Toronto: Victoria University Press.
—. 1973. *Vom Außgelaßnen Wütigen Teuffelsheer*. Translated by Johann Fischart. Reprint. Graz: ADEVA. [Straßburg, 1581/1591.]
Caesarius of Heisterbach. 1929. *The dialogue on miracles*. Translated by H. E. Scott, and C. C. Swinton Bland. London: Routledge.
Deutsche Predigten des 13. Jahrhunderts (=Schwarzwälder Predigten). 1978. Edited by F.K. Grieshaber. Abteilung 1.2. Reprint. Hildesheim: Olms. [Stuttgart 1844–46.]
Elisabeth of Schönau. 2000. *The Complete Works*. Edited by Anne L. Clark. New York: Paulist Press.
Eusebius. 1999. *Church History*. Translated by Paul L Maier. Grand Rapids: Kregel Publications.
Heinrich von dem Türlin. 2007. *Diu Crône* 1–2. Edited by Fritz Peter Knapp, and Alfred Ebenbauer. Tübingen: Niemeyer.
Hildegard of Bingen. 1990. *Scivias*. Translated by Mother Columba Hart, and Jane Bishop. Introd.: Barbara J. Newman. Preface: Caroline Walker Bynum. Mahwah, N.Y.: Paulist Press.
Josephus. 1926–1965. *Text and Translation* 1–10. Cambridge, Mass.: Harvard University Press.
Konrad von Würzburg. 1858/1965. *Der Trojanerkrieg*. Edited by Adelbert von Keller. Stuttgart, and Amsterdam: Rodopi.
Pausanias. 1913. *Description of Greece* 1–6. Edited and translated with commentary by Sir James Frazer. London: Biblo and Tannen.
Philo of Alexandria. 1962. *Werke* 1–6. Berlin, Walter de Gruyter & Co.
Plutarch. 1921. *De defectu oraculorum. De Pythiae Oraculis* [On the Decline of Oracles. On the Oracles of the Pythia]. New York: Loeb Library. (Moralia 5.)
Psellos, Michel. 2010. *On the Operation of Daemons*. Edited by Stephen Skinner, translated by Marcus Collison. Singapore: Golden Hoard Press.

—. 1838. *De operatione daemonum*. Edted by J. F. Boissonade. Norimberga: Campe.
Pseudo-Philon. 1976. *Les Antiquités bibliques*. Paris: Ed. Du Cerf.
Reginald Scot. 1972. *The discoverie of witchcraft*. New York: Dover.
Regino von Prüm. 2004. *Das Sendhandbuch des Regino von Prüm*. Edited and translated by Wilfried Hartmann. Darmstadt: Wissenschaftliche Buchgesellschaft. [*Reginonis abbatis Prumiensis libro duo De synodalibus causis et disciplinis ecclesiasticis*. Edited by F. G. A. Wasserschleben. Leipzig: Hirzel 1840.]

C. Secondary sources

Arbman, Ernst. 1970. *Ecstasy or religious Trance*. Stockholm: Svenska Bokförl.
Aune, David. 1983. *Prophecy in Early Christianity and the Ancient Mediterranean World.* Grand Rapids: Eerdmans.
Beattie, John, and John Middleton. 1969. *Spirit Mediumship and Society in Africa*. London: Routledge & Kegan.
Behringer, Wolfgang. 1994. *Shaman of Oberstdorf: Chonrad Stoecklin and the Phantoms of the Night.* Charlottesville: University Press of Virginia.
Caciola, Nancy. 2003. *Discerning spirits. Divine and demonic possession in the Middle Ages.* Ithaca: Cornell University Press.
Chadwick, Henry. 1997. *Priscillian of Avila. The Occult and the Charismatic in the Early Church.* Oxford: Clarendon Press.
Christensen, Kirsten M. 2006. "Unsichtbare Visionen sichtbarer Frauen. Visualisierungsstrategien in den Texten mittelalterlicher Mystikerinnen nach 1200." In *Visualisierungsstrategien in mittelalterlichen Bildern und Texten*, edited by Horst Wenzel et al., 213–25. Berlin: Schmidt.
Connelly, Joan Breton. 2007. *Portrait of a Priestess: Women and Ritual in Ancient Greece*. Princeton: Princeton University Press.
Dodds, Eric Robertson. 1963. *The Greeks and the Irrational* Berkeley: University of California Press.
Hain, Mathilde. 1956. "Burchard von Worms (+1025) und der Volksglaube seiner Zeit." *Hessische Blätter für Volkskunde* 47: 39–50.
Hamburger, Jeffrey, F. 2000. "Speculation on speculation. Vision on Perception in the Theory and Practise of Mystical Devotion." In *Deutsche Mystik im abendländischen Zusammenhang. Neu erschlossenen Texte, neue methodische Ansätze, neue Theoretische Konzepte. Kolloquium Kloster Fischingen 1998*, edited by Walter Haug, and Wolfram Schneider-Lastin, 353–408. Tübingen: Niemeyer.

Hansen, Josef. 1901. *Quellen und Untersuchungen zur Geschichte des Hexenwahns und der Hexenverfolgung im Mittelalter*. Bonn: Hanstein.

Harmening, Dieter. 1979. *Superstitio. Überlieferungs- und theoriegeschichtliche Untersuchungen zur kirchlich-theologischen Aberglaubensliteratur des Mittelalters.* Berlin: Schmidt.

Jensen, Anne. 1992. *Gottes selbstbewusste Töchter. Frauenemanzipation im frühen Christentum?* Freiburg: Herder.

Lang, Andrew. 1898. *The Making of Religion.* London: Longmans, Green & Co.

Lea, Charles. 1939. *Materials toward a history of Witchcraft.* Philadelphia: University of Philadelphia Press.

Lecouteux, Claude. 1985. "Hagazussa–Striga–Hexe." *Hessische Blätter für Volkskunde* NF 18: 57–70.

Leslie, William H. 1976. "The Concept of Woman in the Pauline Corpus in the light of the Social and Religious Environment of the First Century." Thesis Northwestern University Press.

Levison, John R. 1995. "The prophetic spirit as an angel according to Philo." *Harvard Theological Review* 88 (2): 189–207.

—. 1995. "Inspiration and the divine Spirit in the writings of Philo Judaeus." *Journal for the Study of Judaism* 26 (3): 271–323.

—. 2009. *Filled with the Spirit*. Grand Rapids, Mich.: Eerdmans.

Maclean, Simon. 2009. "Insinuation, Censorship and the Struggle for Late Carolingian Lotharingia in Regino of Prüm's Chronicle." *English Historical Review* 74 (February): 1–28.

Maurizio, Lisa. 2001. "The Voice at the Centre of the World: The Pythia's Ambiguity and Authority." In *Making Silence Speak: Women's Voices in Greek Literature and Society*, edited by Andre Lardinois, and Laura McClure, 46–50. Princeton: Princeton University Press.

Mayer-Tasch, P. C. 2000. *Jean Bodin: eine Einführung in sein Leben, sein Werk und seine Wirkung; mit einer Bibliographie zum geistes- und sozialwissenschaftlichen Schrifttum über Bodin zwischen dem Jahr 1800 und dem Jahr 2000*. Düsseldorf: Parerga.

Meaney, Audrey. 1989. "Women, Witchcraft and Magic in Anglo-Saxon England." In *Superstition and Popular Medicine in Anglo-Saxon England*, edited by Donald G. Scragg, 9–41. Manchester: University of Manchester Press.

Newman, Barbara. 2005. "What Does it mean to say, 'I saw'? The Clash between Theory and Practice in Medieval Visionary culture." *Speculum* 80 (1): 1–43.

Nissinen, Martti. 2000. "Spoken Written Quoted and Invented: Orality and Writtenness in Ancient Near Eastern Prophecy." In *Writings and*

Speech in Israelite and Ancient Near Eastern Prophecy (SBL Symposium Series 10), Ehud Ben Zvi, and Michael H. Floyd, 235–71. Atlanta: Society of Biblical Literature.

Northcott, Michael et al., eds. 1991. *Vision and prophecy: the tasks of social theology today*: *Conference: Papers*. Edinburgh: University of Edinburgh Press.

Reier, Herbert. 1976. *Heilkunde im mittelalterlichen Skandinavien* I–II. Kiel: Universitäts Habil.Schrift.

—. 1987. *Leben, Krankheiten und Heilungen im Mittelalter* (800–1400). Kiel: H. Reier Verlag.

Richter, Gerlinde. 1966. "Bezeichnungen für den Heilkundigen." *Beiträge für deutsche Sprache und Literatur* 88: 258-75.

Schneidmüller, Bernd. 1990. "*Regino von Prüm*." In *Handwörterbuch zur deutschen Rechtsgeschichte* IV, edited by Adalbert Erler, and Ekkehard Kaufmann, 492–5 Berlin: Schmidt.

Smith, Daniel B. 2007. *Muses, Madmen, and Prophets: Hearing voices and the borders of Sanity*. New York: Penguin Books.

Tibbs, Clint. 2007. *Religious Experience of the Pneuma. Communication with the Spirit World in Corinthians 12 and 14*. Tübingen: Mohr Siebeck.

Trevett, Christine. 1996. *Montanism: Gender, Authority and the New Prophecy*. Cambridge: Cambridge University Press.

Tropper, Josef. 1989. *Nekromantie. Totenbefragung im alten Orient und im Alten Testament.* Neukirchen-Vluyn: Neukirchener Verlag.

Voaden, Rosalynn. 1999. *God's Words, Women's Voices: The Discernment of Spirits in the Writings of Late Medieval Women Visionaries.* Woodbridge: York Medieval Press.

Vox; Valentine. 1981. *I see Your Lips Moving. The History and Art of Ventriloquism*. Tadworth: Kaye & Ward.

Wasserschleben, Friedrich Wilhelm. 1958. *Die Bussordnungen der abendländischen Kirche, nebst einer rechtsgeschichtlichen Einleitung.* Reprint. Graz: ADEVA. [Halle, 1851.]

Weippert, M. 2001. "Prophetie im alten Orient." *Neues Bibel Lexikon* 3: 196–200.

Weiss, Bardo. 2000. *Ekstase und Liebe*. Paderborn: Schöningh.

Whitlock, Jonathan. 2002. *Schrift und Inspiration. Studien zur Vorstellung von inspirierter Schrift und inspirierter Schriftauslegung im antiken Judentum und in den paulinischen Briefen*. Neukirchen: Neukirchener Verlag.

Wire, Antoinette Clark. 1990a. *The Corinthian Women Prophets: a Reconstruction Through Paul's Rhetoric*. Minneapolis: Fortress Press.

—. 1990b. “Prophecy and Women Prophets in Corinth.” In *Gospel and Christian Beginnings. In Honor of James M. Robinson*, edited by James E. Goehring, et al., 134–50. Sonoma: Polebridge Press.

Understanding Medical Knowledge and Practice: Strategies for the Reading of Early Modern Norwegian Manuscripts

ANE OHRVIK

In the traditional view of historians of medicine, folk medicine has been regarded as "… unscientific, irrational, superstitious, and simply bad…" (Lindemann 1999, 4). Folk medicine has, in this sense, become the opposite of scientific and rational school medicine, and the history of medicine, which in earlier decades was mostly written by physicians and historians, has been written as a story of progress (see also Lindemann 2010, 3–4). Ethnologists and folklorists have often accepted and adopted these polarities by using similar concepts to describe early modern practices of medicine, or by simply labelling it magic. The latter solution consequently places folk medicine as non-scientific. Later historians have managed to gain a "monopoly" in defining the medical reality of everyday life in early modern Europe. One way, and maybe the most important way, of managing this has been to define, label and describe practitioners who throughout history have offered their services in the medical sphere. In the history of medicine, we find both physicians, surgeons and apothecaries, quacks, empirics, wise men and women, charlatans and mountebanks. Historians and physicians have, in seeking to come to terms with this variety, also attempted to categorise these groups into various polarities such as learned and unlearned, orthodox and unorthodox, elite and popular, professional and lay. Consequently, one of the most common features in the writings of medical history by twentieth-century scholars is the story of medical diversity alongside a construction of professional medical power and hierarchy (cf. Jenner and Wallis 2007, 1).

The emergence of the new social history of medicine makes room for new and refreshing interdisciplinary perspectives (see de Blécourt and Usborne 2004b; Elmer 2004; Gijswijt-Hofstra, Marland and de Waardt 1997). Scholars show new interest in studying "history from below" where patients' experience of health and sickness is as important as the experience of practitioners in the field, where the study of medical education covers all brands of knowledge regimes, and where investigations into influential factors such as religion play an important role in the understanding of the history of medicine (De Renzi 2004, 29; Lindemann 2010 [1999], 7–8; de Blécourt and Usborne 2004a, 1–9). Another perspective is simply to avoid the polarities used in describing medical practices, such as scientific and unscientific, learned and unlearned, and recognise that the boundaries may have been more fluid. Even though the emerging scientific world view in the early modern period gave one branch of medical practitioners both privileges and political power, in Norway, as in most European states, there was a simultaneous demand for a great variety of practitioners, who continued to practise their medicine. I share the view of the historian Silvia de Renzi who states that the labels and polarities traditionally used by writers of the history of medicine are not justified by the reality on the ground and how people practised medicine and used medical practitioners in early modern Europe. What this suggests—from what I can see—is the need for more studies into the knowledge and practice of medicine; in the broadest sense of the term.

In this article, I want to draw attention to the knowledge and practice of medicine in eighteenth- and nineteenth-century Norway. My article will not offer prepared conclusions, rather it will suggest two ways of analysing material in the process of better understanding specific parts of the history of medicine. The material on which I base my arguments comes from Norwegian black books (magic books) from the eighteenth and nineteenth centuries.[1] Before presenting some suggestions as to how one can read these books to improve the understanding of medical knowledge and practice in early modern Norway, I will start by describing essential features of the Norwegian black books.

Norwegian black books as medical books

The most comprehensive compilation of Norwegian *svartebøker* (black books) is the book *Norske Hexeformularer og magiske opskrifter* (Norwegian witch formulas and magic recipes) edited and published by the Norwegian church historian Anton Christian Bang (1840–1913) in 1901–1902 (Bang 1901–1902. For more on Bang's work on Norwegian

[1] In this study, black books will be characterised as books, works or manuscripts, even though I acknowledge that the meanings of these concepts differ and could be perceived as contradictions.

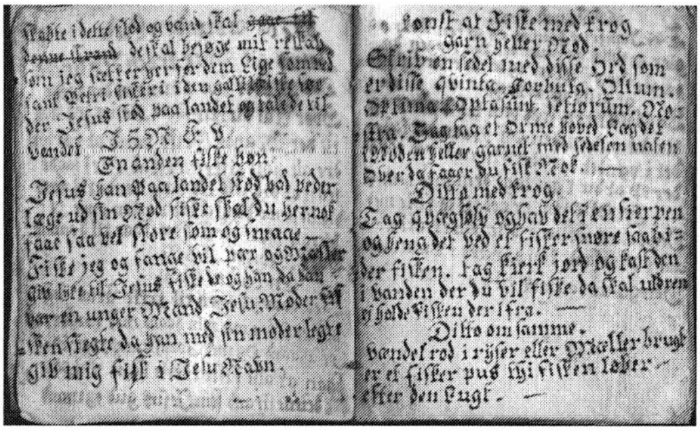

Fig. 1: Eighteenth-century black book from Ringebu, Norway. Black book collection at The Norwegian Folklore Archive, University of Oslo. Photo by the Norwegian Folklore Archive

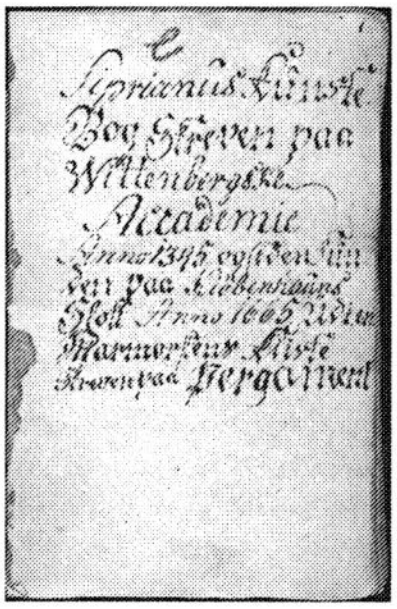

Fig. 2: Cover of a black book in the black book collection at The Norwegian Folklore Archive, University of Oslo. In addition to being attributed to Cyprian, black books are often said to originate from the Academy of Wittenberg, notoriously known for being the great school of magic art, or other famous places of learning. Furthermore, the books are given a false dating back in time and are often said to have been found in central locations, like this title page, at the royal castle in Copenhagen. These elements contribute to the authorizing and legitimizing of the black books. Photo by the Norwegian Folklore Archive.

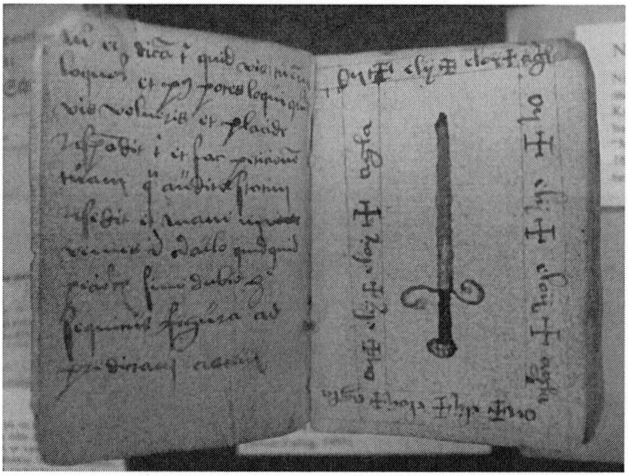

Fig. 3. *The Vinje book* c. 1480, the oldest known magic book in Norway. In 1796, a very interesting discovery was made in Vinje in Telemark, Norway. Workers, whose job was to tear down the decayed stave church, found a tiny book hidden underneath the wooden panel in the choir near the altar. The book was handwritten, consisted of 108 pages of text, illustrations and symbols and was the size of a small matchstick box (4.8x7.0 cm). The content of the book is a mixture of recipes, formulas, chants and prayers for curing ailments and injuries in people and animals. Photo by Ane Ohrvik.

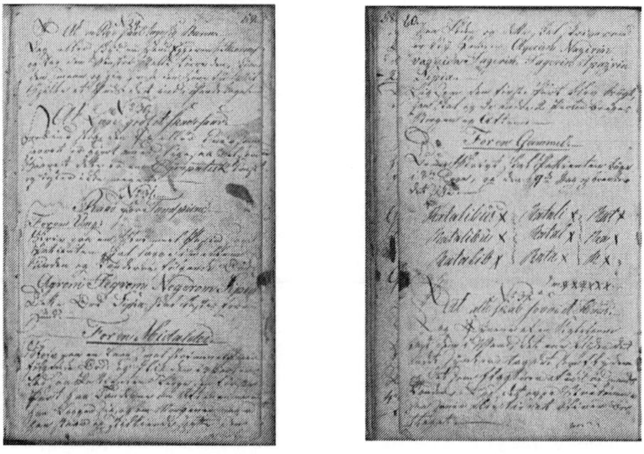

Fig. 4-5. The recipes for curing toothache from *Cÿprianus Konstbok*. Photo by the Norwegian Folklore Archive.

charms, see Amundsen 2013). In his book, Bang refers to nearly 50 black books that he uses, among other sources, as material for the book.

The National Library in Oslo, which received some of Bang's material subsequent to the book being published, holds, together with the Norwegian Folklore Archive, the majority of black books preserved, totalling more than one hundred original manuscripts.[2] Additionally, number of other libraries and archive institutions around Norway also hold single or small collections of manuscripts. Only a few of the manuscripts are properly dated by their authors, but by examining the written style and content, most of known manuscripts can be dated to the period between 1700 and 1850 (Ohrvik 2012).

It is important to stress that the collective name *svartebok* (black book) is younger than many of the books. We first find the term used at the beginning of the eighteenth century, as a title or explanation in the introductions of the books, and during the nineteenth century, the term came into use more frequently. Furthermore, in the compilation of Norwegian legends, collected and published during the nineteenth century, we find several where the term *svartebok* is a common reference to the written tradition. It is safe to assume that the influence of written and oral tradition has gone both ways in this case.

Alongside common titles such as *Konst Bog* (Art Book), *Lacker Bog* (Lacquer Book) and *Læge Bog* (Leech Book), the Norwegian black books are frequently given the title *Cyprianus* (Cyprian) or *Cyprianus Konst Bog* (Cyprian Art Book). The name Cyprian most probably has a double origin. An ancient legend from the third century tells us of the powerful magician Cyprian of Antioch. After having experienced the piousness of a Christian woman named Justina who rejects him, Cyprian releases himself from his diabolic pact with the Devil and becomes a Christian. The church receives him and later he becomes a bishop but suffers martyrdom with Justina (Butler 1993; Stokker 2007, 100). Cyprian of Antioch was confused with one of the early Church fathers, the actual Cyprian of Carthage, who suffered martyrdom in AD 258. We find the conflation of the two Cyprians in Christian writing as early as the late fourth century (Davies 2009, 32-3; Ohrvik 2018, 112-20). While Cyprian of Carthage was a

[2] During the past decade, *Norsk Folkeminnesamling* (the Norwegian Folklore Archive) has worked on digitising and making fully accessible key sources from its collection. Among the collection of legends, fairy tales, autobiographies and a comprehensive transcript of 650 out of 900 witch trials held in Norway there is also a selection of black books from the archive, see http://www.hf.uio.no/ikos/tjenester/kunnskap/samlinger/norsk-folkeminnesamling/ (accessed 27 April 2017). Unfortunately, this website is not available in English.

historical person, it is doubtful whether Cyprian of Antioch ever lived. Nevertheless, during the medieval period, several books about the conversion, confession and martyrdom of the magician Cyprian of Antioch circulated widely in manuscripts written in several languages in Europe and the Middle East.

It comes as no surprise that Norwegian black books are attributed to Cyprian. Attributing books to both mythical and real doctors and magicians was an integral part of the European grimoire tradition. Even though many of the "authors" were associated with sinful, magical practices, their knowledge, wisdom and Christian piety made them attractive as authors as they contributed to the authorisation of the books and legitimisation of the knowledge they presented (cf. ibid.; Kavey 2007, 34; Clegg 2005). During the Middle Ages and the early modern period, names like Zoroaster, Moses, Solomon, Hermes Trismegistus, Albertus Magnus (c. 1193–1280), Peter d'Abano and several popes appear in lists of authors. Some of the books attributed to them appear as late as the seventeenth or eighteenth century, as is the case with Cyprian books in Norway. The very first known black book, *Sybrianus,* printed in 1771, may very well have reinforced this practice (Rosenlund 1771). The titles of the black books give us a good clue as to the content of the books, even though each individual book is unique and primarily reflects the interests and practical needs of the person who wrote it. Recipes for luck in cards and games, love and battle are typical for black books that can be credited to men with a military profession or background (see for example Amundsen 1987). Furthermore, recipes for increasing one's luck in hunting and fishing in addition to advice on protection against and treatment of ailments in humans and livestock indicate peasant writings. A few books, where the writer uses Latin systematically and the content refers to learned traditions, reflect clerical writers, which is the case with the oldest black book in Norway, *The Vinje book*, which can be dated to 1480 (Garstein 1993). In this book, we can identify 12 different writers, who wrote the book over a span of several decades or possibly centuries. However, in many of the books, the influence of European magic and medical literature is evident, even though it is coloured in line with the authors' tastes and interests.

There is no doubt that printing, in general, had an influence on the Norwegian tradition. Still, it is not necessarily clear in what ways, except as obvious sources of medical and magical advice. If we look to Europe, literary magic experienced democratisation after the introduction of the printing press. *Grimoires* became bestsellers on the market, with France as one of the most significant exponents. These and other books probably also reached the Nordic countries. As such, the Norwegian manuscripts and the printed grimoires might have been a result of a two-sided influence and reciprocity, collecting information and materials from each other, as Owen Davies points out:

> While print drained power from the grimoire in terms of its magical integrity, it also empowered it through growing access and social influence. Furthermore, print did not usurp the role of manuscript; the magic latent in the words contained in print grimoires could be reactivated through transcription (Davies 2009, 5).

The idea that printing did not put an end to writing by hand has been put forward by Don Skemer, who points to the fact that while late medieval western Europe was introduced to batch production of broadside amulets, handwritten amulets continued to circulate (Skemer 2006, 283). The role of writing is an interesting point that might serve as part of an explanation as to why the number of manuscripts is greater than that of printed grimoires in Norway.

There has been a long tradition in Scandinavia for connecting the act of writing itself with a magical and seemingly essential and important part of the making of a black book, influencing the power and effect of the very medical knowledge it held (see also Skemer 2006, 116–24). Just as important when it comes to the Nordic tradition is the personal touch a manuscript was given in the writing of the book and the value it was given by its owner. As a result, the vast majority of Norwegian black books are individually designed and hardly ever a result of direct copying.

The Norwegian legend tied by tradition to ownership and transmission of black books tells us that only a selected few could learn the art of healing and magic and consequently own a book. Even though in reality this must have been subject to wide interpretation by people who wrote and owned black books, still the popular beliefs and customs connected with the black books must be paid serious attention. In this respect, it is understandable that a printed grimoire would have trouble competing with a manuscript.

Reading strategy 1: Medical texts as speech acts

As already pointed out, the black books are an important source of medical knowledge and treatment practices in early modern Norway. They represent the medical advice of writers and those who carried out the treatment, the "specialists". This makes the manuscripts unique because they provide access to a universe of knowledge that otherwise was most often transmitted orally and hence has left few written sources. Through a close reading of the texts, we can improve our understanding of *which* knowledge the black books represented, and *how* this knowledge came into use when treating ailments.

Schematically, the medical content of Norwegian black books may be divided into two categories: a) chants, charms and formulas and b) practical instructions. The chants and formulas are epic and poetic prayers with religious themes as well as illogical words. They are intended either to be spoken or written down on paper to have an effect, and they belong together with the practical instructions describing the actions that must be carried out in connection with the recitation of the written words. Hence, black book texts and practices are indivisible and only give the assumed effect *together*. A typical example of this is the following nineteenth-century prayer against rheumatism collected from Jostedalen in western Norway, which follows practical instructions and descriptions of the elements in the treatment:

> Rheumatism prayer
> Jesus stepped ashore
> Met rheumatism on sand
> What do you want asked Jesus
> Suck blood and broken bone.
> Jesus said: I shall address you
> You shall address you
> Harm no man.-

> These words to be read in tar or liquor, whereupon to spit three times and rub it on the sick spot.—He who carries "rheumatism cures" on him may not speak to any person. If he must speak to any person, he must first set down the "cure" (NFS: S. Tillier II, 75).

The text indicates which prayer is to be spoken by the specialist, the actions that should follow the recitation of the prayer and the objects or elements that were part of the treatment. The sick person acted according to specific instructions as to what to do and not to do during the treatment process if it was to have an effect. The speech and actions ascribed to Christ also bring a time dimension into the treatment process, where Christ "chants" the rheumatism (the sickness) away. The text thus introduces four actors on both actual and symbolic levels: the sick person who needs treatment, the persons administering the treatment, Jesus and the sickness (the rheumatism). As demonstrated by the example here, one possible way to study the black book text focuses on the relation between speech and action in the text.

There are sliding transitions between the levels of speech, acts and actors in the text, and different actors are introduced on the different levels. To understand these complex relations, one way of reading the text might be to use the construct *speech act* as a point of departure, a construct inspired by language philosopher John L. Austin. A speech act is an utterance that *does something* to reality (Austin 1971 [1962]). The aspect of truth is not important here, but the utterances must be assessed based on the degree to which they achieve their end. To this end, Austin also introduced the terms *constatives* and *performatives* which refer, respectively, to descriptive statements about the world which have a truth value, and to utterances which perform actions. According to Austin, a speech act consists of three levels of action, which he calls *locutionary*, *illocutionary* and *perlocutionary* acts. These are separate, but related. In a locutionary speech act, a meaningful sentence is stated, while an illocutionary speech act gives the content of the meaning a special force, an intended understanding of the words (Gilje 1987, 72). The perlocutionary act refers to the effect that the words have.

Austin's constructs are useful as a reading strategy for the black book texts, because they point out what the text *does* and not merely what it says. Black books are not written as texts for external contemporary readers, but are rather knowledge manifestations for the folk medicine expert and designed to be applied at the time the text was used. Only when it was spoken out loud did the actors in fact act and encompass power, and the words and their meaning receive their intended effect (cf. Ilomäki 2004, 56). Hence, the speech act construct is useful as a gateway to understanding the black book texts as *historical* texts (cf. Skinner 1969).

Studying the locutionary, illocutionary and perlocutionary acts in a black book text is nevertheless not sufficient if we are to understand the scope of the meaning and the context of the texts. The following sentence from a black book from 1732 containing a recipe for how to stop bleeding illustrates this: "Write these words on a piece of paper that is clean: 'Burig', 'Berto', 'Berig', and put in the nose this helps" (Amundsen 1987, 21). The speech acts of this text clearly illustrate what most texts of this kind recognise, namely that they depend on physical acts (rituals) for the words to gain meaning, power and effect. Thus, the black book text cannot be interpreted alone, but rather requires (the ritual) acts for the words "to work". Austin's speech act construct has a shortcoming in that it disregards the relation between words and acts in a communication situation. Nonetheless, the speech act construct is useful because it allows for a more functional approach to the black book texts and because the construct makes it possible to return the words in the text to their specific context or the situation in which they were applied (cf. Jordheim 2001, 216).

As stated, the speech acts in the black book texts must be placed in relation to the situations where the speech acts were applied or practised. This means that the speech acts in these texts only convey meaning if considered part of a physical practice. It is precisely *within* this practice that the words become actual speech acts (cf. Telste 2006, 105). It is also through this practice, where words become knowledge and so relevant, that the black book texts themselves become texts about sickness and treatment. Hence, the concept of rituals, which generally include stylistic and formal characteristics, and also the dimension of the meaning of the practice can be applied here. The content of black book texts may be described as what Catherine Bell calls *textualised* rituals. This is because these texts represent authoritative guidelines for how the treatment of sickness was to be carried out (cf. Bell 1997, 204). Such literary elements, which closely connect to and prescribe the ritual acts, help to create a special liturgical language. The descriptions of how the treatment of sickness was to be carried out vary in scope in the texts, but common to them all is that the frame, order and content of the acts to be carried out are clear. Treatment of sickness thus differs from other acts, and it is precisely this differentiation that renders the treatment powerful. It is also within this context that the speech acts "work" and the words transform into meaning, power and effect.

Reading strategy 2: Healing practices as embodiment

Following the idea of treatments as acts and how they work in specific situations, the next reading strategy involves the performative interplay between senses, movement and embodiment in the execution of medical knowledge in the black books—here exemplified through the treatment of toothache. How is the body used or transformed into an instrument in the performative treatment situation? How can we understand the eating of words as part of a medical treatment? Let us take a closer look at three examples from the Norwegian black book *Cÿprianus Konstbog* from the second half of the eighteenth century, which provide cures for toothache.

> No 31./ Cure for toothache
> For a youth
> Write the following words on a strip of paper that the patient must put between the cheek and the teeth: Agroni Jegrom Negerom Sipia. The word Sipia must be thrown to a dog.

> For a middle-aged person
> Write the words below on a long strip of paper. Cut it into three parts, then let the patient put the first part on his teeth at night when he goes to bed, and the following morning as he gets up he should while maintaining silence spit it onto the fire—and this must be written with a new pen. Algerien Nagirin vagerien Iagerin Ipazerin Sipia. The next two parts must be used in the same way as the first strip both morning and night.
>
> For an old person
> This writing the patient must use for eight days and on the ninth day burn the last one. Batalibus X Batali X Bat X Batalibu X Batal X Ba X Batalib X Bata X B X (NB Ms 4 1819).

As we can see from these examples, artefacts, bodily movements and senses are in play in the execution of the treatments. Of artefacts, we detect paper, of movements we can identify specific actions executed according to a scheme, and of senses, we find taste as an implicit factor in the treatment. Moreover, the treatment act also relies on time and place as decisive factors for the treatment to be a success. Lastly, partly identified as an artefact, partly as a symbolic feature, words constitute a crucial part of the treatment. These different features constitute specific roles, functions and meaning in the treatment.

At first glance, the paper primarily appears as a practical tool whose function is to make present and reify the words, something which appears to be of vital importance in this context. However, the instruction of writing the words on *a strip of paper* indicates that its form is far from indifferent to its function. By using a strip of paper the patient can split it into parts, thus separating the words according to the instructions given and destroying them in succession.

However, when reaching the process of paper destruction, neither the paper nor the words written on it are merely that—words on paper—but embody the actual toothache itself. When placed between the cheek and the painful tooth, the idea of *transference* or *transmission* has been put into play—and processed by time. During the time when the paper has been in contact with the actual source of the pain, the pain has *moved* from tooth to paper. When the paper, then, is thrown to a dog, spat out or thrown into the fire, a symbolic demolition of the toothache itself is conducted. From being a mere tool in the treatment process, the paper ends up embodying the actual illness itself. Whether this embodiment is factual—in the sense that the patient regarded the strip of paper as holding the ache—or whether it was viewed as a *symbolic* embodiment, is hard to say. The irrevocable destruction by fire might support the first notion. It is not, however, crucial for our understanding of the treatment process. Here

I believe that the most important element is the transformation process to which the paper is subject. From an artefact, it turns into the subject—factual or symbolical—of the toothache, the illness itself.

Crucial to the healing process are the bodily movements that must be performed in specific ways. The fairly detailed descriptions of how to shape the paper, how to write the specific words on the paper strip, when to use the paper strip "at night when he goes to bed until the following morning when he gets up", or "use for eight days and on the ninth day burn the last one", and how to demolish the paper strip by throwing it to the dog or into the fire all testify to the crucial role of movement. These descriptions can be seen as ritual scripts tied to the healing process and crucial components for the treatment to be a success. The body turns into an instrument that in this context serves equally in the healing act as do the artefacts and the words. Furthermore, the bodily movements closely connect to time and place, adding additional dimensions to movements that are more than mere physical acts. The body acts in a specific dimension of time and space that equally contributes to making the healing process happen. As such, the treatment act makes use of qualities connected to time and place (in terms of night and day and the fireplace)—qualities we may assume to hold specific significance and power in the healing act.

A central element in the treatment process are the words written on the strip of paper. The words reveal a particularly common feature of this type of advised treatment, namely the absence—at least explicitly—of references to a Christian context by way of naming God, Jesus, the Holy Spirit or other biblical persons and figures or, for that matter, demons or devils. Instead, the words appear to be without any immediate semantic meaning. This, however, does not mean that they are without meaning; for their power lies precisely in their seeming meaninglessness.

In his book *Binding Words*, published in 2006, Don Skemer analyses textual amulets in the Middle Ages and focuses on their fundamental apotropaic function. They were thought to protect the bearer against known or unknown enemies, to drive away or exorcise evil spirits, to heal specific afflictions caused by demonic invasions of the protected person and to bring people good fortune, even at the expense of others. The various different writings on amulets included what were called cryptic writings, either comprising regular words with no apparent semantic meaning or signs and symbols often referred to as characters which in practice implied secret writing. We can detect both ways of writing in Norwegian black books: the use of characters called *lønnskrift* (hidden writing) and cryptic writing, which often goes by the term *noaord* (words without any apparent meaning). In both cases, however, the use of this form of writing indicates ideas of magic and power as lying embedded in the words. As such, the very words are potent. Often, these ways of writing are activated when recited and spoken aloud, but in this case, the opposite is explicitly stressed. They were to be written down and placed in the mouth accordingly and destroyed *in silence*.

Even though I label these wordings as *noaord,* it is worth mentioning that for all the words here, the resemblance to Latin phrases is striking. The use of Latin phrases is very common in the black books. In all likelihood, they partly contribute to giving the overall text and particular phrases the impression of being learned, and partly play on the medieval sacred language used in church services. As such, we can assume they seek to benefit from the sacred power inhabiting the words. Either way, we can assume that these particular words gave meaning to their users.

However, what happens when the words are put into play? When placed between the cheek and the painful tooth, the power of the words activates the transference or transmission process of the pain/ailment. From being "mere" words or signs, their embedded power processes the healing of the patient. When the strip of paper is thrown away, the toothache itself is destroyed. As such, the words on the strip of paper become one of the most central healing agents in the healing process.

Final remarks

A close reading of the black books based on Austin's construct of speech acts in addition to performative healing acts as embodiments are only two possible ways of seeking a better understanding of the medical texts. The most important thing is to recognise the inseparable tie between text and practice in the black books. Only when when we do so and move beyond categorising, labelling and the use of political and ideological concepts can we understand the complexity of the healing process. My intentions here have been to present a traditional field and traditional material for folklorists and ethnologists that requires new attention and fresh questions. Further studies of medical knowledge and practice in the early modern black books would reveal interesting knowledge about how human individuals have adopted, produced and transmitted medical skills that have had an impact not only on individuals but also on society and how we view medical knowledge and practice today.

References

Amundsen, Arne Bugge. 1987. *Svarteboken fra Borge* [The black book of Borge]. Sarpsborg: Borgarsyssel Museum.

—. 2013. "A Genre in the Making. The First Study of Charms in Norway." In *The Power of Words. Studies on Charms and Charming in Europe*, edited by James Kapalo, Éva Pócs, and William Ryan, 15–26. Budapest, and New York: Central European University Press.

Austin, John Langshaw. 1971 [1962]. *How to do things with words. The William James Lectures delivered at Harvard University in 1955.* London, Oxford, and New York: Oxford University Press.

Bang, Anton Christian. 1901–1902. *Norske Hexeformularer og Magiske Opskrifter* [Norwegian witch formulas and magic recipes]. Kristiania: I commission hos Jacob Dybwad.

Bell, Catherine. 1997. *Ritual. Perspectives and Dimensions.* New York, and Oxford: Oxford University Press.

Blécourt, Willem de, and Cornelie Usborne. 2004a. "Medicine, Mediation and Meaning." In *Cultural Approaches to the History of Medicine. Mediating Medicine in Early Modern and Modern Europe*, edited by Willem de Blécourt, and Cornelie Usborne, 1–10. New York: Palgrave Macmillan.

—, eds. 2004b. *Cultural Approaches to the History of Medicine. Mediating Medicine in Early Modern and Modern Europe.* New York: Palgrave Macmillan.

Butler, Elisabeth M. 1993. *The Myth of the Magus*. Cambridge: Cambridge University Press.

Clegg, Cyndia Susan. 2005. "'The Author of This Book': Attributing Authorship, 1580–1640." *Pacific Coast Philology* 40 (2): 27–37.

Davies, Owen. 2009. *Grimoires. A History of Magic Books*. Oxford, and New York: Oxford University Press.

De Renzi, Silvia. 2004. "The sick and their healers." In *The Healing Arts: Health, Disease and Society in Europe 1500–1800*, edited by Peter Elmer, 27–58. Manchester: Manchester University Press.

Elmer, Peter, ed. 2004. *The Healing Arts: Health, Disease and Society in Europe 1500–1800*. Manchester: Manchester University Press.

Garstein, Oscar. 1993. *Vinjeboka: Den eldste svartebok fra norsk middelalder* [The Vinje Book: The oldest black book from the Norwegian middle ages]. Oslo: Solum.

Gijswijt-Hofstra, Marijke, Hilary Marland, and Hans de Waardt, eds. 1997. "Illness and Healing Alternatives in Western Europe." *Studies in the Social History of Medicine Series*. London, and New York: Routledge.

Gilje, Nils. 1987. *Hermeneutikk i vitenskapsteoretisk perspektiv* [Hermeneutics from a scientific perspective]. Bergen: Universitetet i Bergen. (Skriftserien / Universitetet i Bergen, Vitskapsteoretisk forum 6.)

Ilomäki, Henni. 2004. "The Self of a Charm." In *Charms and Charming in Europe*, edited by Jonathan Roper, 47–58. Houndmills, Basingstoke, Hampshire, and New York: Palgrave Macmillan.

Jenner, Mark S. R., and Patrick Wallis. 2007. "The Medical Marketplace." In *Medicine and the Market in England and Its Colonies, c. 1450–c. 1850*, edited by Mark S. R. Jenner, and Patrick Wallis, 1–23. Basingstoke, and New York: Palgrave Macmillan.

Jordheim, Helge. 2001. *Lesningens vitenskap. Utkast til en ny filologi* [The science of reading: Draft for a new philology]. Oslo: Universitetsforlaget.

Kavey, Allison. 2007. *Books of Secrets: Natural Philosophy in England, 1550–1600*. Urbana, and Chicago: University of Illinois Press.

Lindemann, Mary. 1999. *Medicine and Society in Early Modern Europe*. Cambridge: Cambridge University Press.

—. 2010 [1999]. *Medicine and Society in Early Modern Europe*. Cambridge: Cambridge University Press.

Ohrvik, Ane. 2012. "Conceptualizing Knowledge in Early Modern Norway: A Study of Paratexts in Norwegian Black Books." Doctoral thesis, Faculty of Humanities, University of Oslo.

—. 2018: *Medicine, Magic and Art in Early Modern Norway. Conseptualising Knowledge*. London: Palgrave Macmillan.

Rosenlund, Søren. 1771. *Sybrianus. P.P.P., paa nye oplagt efter Originalen* [Cyprian. P.P.P. Published after the original]. Malmøe: Henrich Smed.

Skemer, Don C. 2006. *Binding words. Textual amulets in the Middle Ages*. University Park, Pa.: Pennsylvania State University Press.

Skinner, Quentin. 1969. "Meaning and Understanding in the History of Ideas." *History and Theory. Studies in the Philosophy of History* 8: 3–53.

Stokker, Kathleen. 2007. *Remedies and Rituals: Folk Medicine in Norway and the New Land*. St. Paul, Minn.: Minnesota Historical Society Press.

Telste, Kari. 2006. "Et bryllup i Bergen. Ekteskapsløftets poetikk og politick [A wedding in Bergen. The poetics and politics of the marriage vow]." In *Ritualer. Kulturhistoriske studier* [Rituals. Studies in cultural history], edited by Arne Bugge Amundsen, Bjarne Hodne, and Ane Ohrvik, 93–117. Oslo: Universitetsforlaget.

Sources

NFS S. Tillier II (Norwegian Folk Archive).
NB Ms 4 1819 (National Library).
www.folkeminne.uio.no, downloaded February 1, 2014.

TALKING TO VEPSIAN *TEDAI*: DIFFERENT ROLES, CONCEPTS, WORLDS[95]

MADIS ARUKASK

1.

Today, the biggest group of Vepsian villages lies in the eastern part of Leningrad oblast, Russia where—particularly in the settlements situated along the Oyat river—it is still possible to hear Vepsian as a living language spoken by members of the older and middle generations. (For more detail about Vepsians see Kolga et al. 2001; Kurs 2001; Strogalschikova 2014). Those regions, articulated by great forests, marshes and lakes, are also the place where animistic beliefs still survive in spite of a modernising world, thanks primarily to the natural environment and to the fact that subsistence activities connected with forests, lakes and rivers are continuously practised there. Thus, it may be said that regardless of the spread of satellite television or modern education, traditional practices of magic and healing have survived, too. Apparently, the manifestations of New Age spirituality currently spreading via popular books or the Internet do not play too great a role, at least not for the older generation. People are still aware that those cognisant of traditional verbal magic may do both good and evil; they also have detailed memories of magically induced harm done by certain persons in the past, and all in all, they remain rather reserved concerning such activities.

Yet it would seem that the time of famous seers (*tedai* in Vepsian, "the-one-who-knows") of wider renown is coming to an end. It is quite common to hear people remark on famous healers who still lived a few years ago, and express their regret that no persons of such powers are left among the living. Such statements may, of course, be folkloric stereotypes aimed at researchers, or reflect a conscious desire to mislead them. Still, it

[95] This research was supported by the Estonian Ministry of Education and Research (Institutional Research Project IUT2–43).

is obvious that in spite of everything, folk magic displays no signs of being on the wane in the Vepsian villages. In order to approach this issue, the researcher must be patient, systematic, and most importantly, develop a relationship of trust with one informant or another—a task, however, that requires time and the fruits of which are not to be reaped before two or three years.

The present article intends to describe—or attempt to describe—a dialogue of that kind with a remarkable representative of the local traditional society; a dialogue stemming from the researcher's desire to grasp and interpret such traditionality as is still extant, as well as to demonstrate how our contemporary modern world view addresses the traditional—both in the practical consciousness of the informant, and in the activities and influence of the researcher standing outside the traditional society. The traditional and the modern or, to put it more simply, the continuously extant different cultural forms, are obviously never totally dissociated from each other. Dialogue can be powered by the will of the participants, but even better by mental models, familiarity or at least acquaintance with which is (in addition to daily communication) of great help in research work.

2.

The present article focuses on the individual as the embodiment of a traditional way of living and the carrier of it. In view of the scope and purpose of the paper, as well as the amount of data gathered so far, it is emphatically not attempted to achieve any system building conclusiveness. It is also hoped that work in this area will go on. What we have here is a person whose status and variety of roles in her environment depart from the usual—a seer, healer, and ritual specialist. An extraordinary status is, no doubt, a factor that may rather distance a person from any traditional "average" than draw her closer to it. In the given case, however, the Central Vepsian *tedai* we observed can rather be said to constitute a quintessence of the traditional Vepsian oral culture. Thus, we have here an informant whose synchronic being has preserved, both in memory and in practice, a great deal of the primevally authentic that remains in close contact with the society and community surrounding her, modernising as best it can.

The material presented here has been recorded during fieldwork carried out together with two of my colleagues in the summers of 2007–2009 in Vepsian villages situated along the Oyat river. All in all, we held seven or eight interviewing sessions, of a few hours' length each, both in the *tedai*'s home and occasionally outside of it (while visiting the local cemetery, for instance). So far, the dialogue between us and these people of different cultures has been richly informative, although at the same time somewhat enigmatic. The complex set of roles surrounding a person of extraordinary status clearly does not always afford easy access to everything that might be of interest. Thus, it may be that at present, the fieldwork has not yet advanced far enough to allow for exhaustive acquaintance with the informant.

During our first stay in the Vepsian villages by the Oyat river (the Podporozhye region of Leningrad oblast, Russia) in July 2007, in Vidl (Rus. Vinnitsy) settlement we found lodgings in the riverside household of a local schoolteacher and Vepsian activist. In the course of our lengthy conversations with our hostess, we learned among many other things that in the near vicinity, in a part of Vidl known by the name of Veliky Dvor and located almost directly across the river, there lived and worked the seer and healer, Tatiana Arsentievna.[96] Speaking about her, our hostess used the Russian word *znakharka* which caught our attention and signified Tatiana's special status in the community. Although a magical world view complete with its practices and elements of animism always surfaced quite as expected in our conversations with other Vepsian informants, too, their attitude towards Tatiana nevertheless spoke of something more profound, causing us to feel rather thoughtful when we set out to visit her for the first time.

Regardless of the attitude his or her community may have developed, no informant is a static object (unless "worn" into such a state by repeated boring visits), and their personality and the information obtained take shape in mutual cooperation (see, for instance, Vasenkari and Pekkala 2000). Indeed, we had no reason to doubt Tatiana's social status when we began our communication with her—at least as far as concerns the aspect of a traditional society. Tatiana's demeanour, her behaviour and communication, did not lead us to doubt her really being a seer, unlike many other colourful Vepsian elderly women who, while having a knowledge of charms or healing practices, did not set them in primary place in their daily activities. Accordingly, we were happy to accept her more special position both in the immediate neighbourhood and further

[96] I am using in this article her forename and patronym. It may be useful to know that the seer was also known by the names of Taisia and Taska, as well as Natalia and Natasha sometimes—sobriquets which we had the chance to hear and which are not variants of one and the same name. This might possibly be considered proof that the seer belongs to more than one narrow target group, being known under different names according to the distance separating her from each group.

away, since this also opened up a route towards the information we were interested in.

At the same time, we obviously did not qualify as common visitors or patients (who indeed visited Tatiana) either; our different interests, roots and language use also led Tatiana to adopt a behaviour that diverged from her more usual role and opened herself from a social aspect in ways other than that of a mere helper. Traditional society also consists of individuals, even though there may be reason to presume that the proportion of modern egocentrism in it is incomparably smaller and that collective beliefs play a far greater role in maintaining consensual balance, from which persons of extraordinary status, primarily, may perhaps find it possible to diverge. Tatiana increasingly opened to us as precisely such an individual in her social dynamics, a person with her own story and personal world view.

At the same time, we were fascinated primarily by the seer as a carrier and practiser of a traditional religious world picture; after all, it was this kind of interest that had brought us to her, in the first place. As Tatiana's religious world view was opened to us, it raised questions as to whether we were capable of understanding its systematics—whether people like us were able to explain it and associate it with earlier knowledge of other aspects of the Finnic traditional vernacular religion. It may be said here that, predictably, contact between our worlds was perhaps easier to achieve on common human grounds, as it were. Our research into the more special information attributed to a seer's role in traditional society, however, on several occasions made us ask whether the modern and the traditional can ever enter into a dialogue of any form desirable to us, or whether the dialogue rather becomes entangled into communication noise, leaving the parties separated in the end—separated regardless of their sincere desire to obtain an understanding of the cultural Other and its organisation.

3.

Tatiana Arsentievna, a childless widow, was born in 1931 in the village of Rebagj (Rus. Rebov Konets) in the southern part of Central Vepsia, a territory situated along the lakes which has now been abandoned and made inaccessible. Both the region itself and the people who come from there seemed to have some special significance for the populace living along the Oyat river; in any case, such origins were cited more than once for one informant or another. According to Tatiana herself, she was already "seeing" at the age of three, which means that she had acquired a seer's powers and self-consciousness not only through traditional learning but also through traditionally acceptable "supernatural" channels. (On acquiring supernatural knowledge among seers in North Russia, see also Dobrovolskaia 2001, 97 ff). Being the fifth born in her family, she was endowed with the knowledge to be handed down—a fifth-generation seer unfortunately destined, because of her childlessness, to remain the last one. As a material sign of her hereditary seer's status, she showed us a pentagon formed of hand lines in her palm—a sign that, in her view, obviously constituted the most easily demonstrable argument in support of this claim, probably for all possible doubters.

Tatiana's mother tongue was Vepsian. In the modern social environment, it was, of course, inevitable that she spoke Russian, especially as many of her patients were either arrivals from elsewhere or younger people unable to speak Vepsian. Fortunately, however, she did not always resort to Russian like many other people both of her own age and younger, when she sometimes sensed our inadequate resources of self-expression in Vepsian while talking to us.

Tatiana's extraordinary descent was complemented by—something perhaps even rarer—her almost complete illiteracy. We did have a chance to see her guessing at the capital letters printed on pillboxes; she also claimed she was able to pen the letters necessary to write her signature. Nevertheless, since she had never attended school, this had to be taken rather as a craftsman's skill than participation in a literate culture complete with its impact on the ways of looking for information, on the memorising and structuring of things. Since a literate culture is more than just written oral culture, involving a far greater tendency towards system building and all kinds of subordination and classification (that is, scientific thinking, see Goody 1977; Ong 2002), our dialogue sometimes proceeded incoherently, as regards content, requiring a fair amount of guesswork from both parties. Sitting in Tatiana's kitchen and "testing" her knowledge by the various accounts of the folk religion of Finnic peoples, precisely the kind of a local form of the vernacular religion of an oral culture that she doubtlessly felt most at home in, we were forced to admit that concepts or schemes familiar to us from theory did not necessarily behave similarly in the consciousness of a real seer and healer whose familiarity with them stemmed rather from practical life than theoretical speculations.

4.

In what follows, I would like to try to bring out some characteristic aspects of the personal reflections of Tatiana's traditional world view. Again, I can only do so fragmentarily, based on the existing information that the seer conceded to share with us. Undoubtedly, Tatiana's world was alive in the animistic sense, a fact proven best of all by her phrases referring to the concept of power, for instance: *vsjakajad silad omma* [Veps. "All sorts of powers exist"]. In that world imbued with powers, there also existed in recognisable form some kind of a dualistic principle, apparently Christian in origin: *Kaikille om sila. Nečistaja sila om, i čistaja sila om; i nečistõi duh i čistõi duh om…* [Veps. "Everything has power. There is unclean power and clean power, and unclean spirit and clean spirit."] At the same time, Tatiana did not seem to stand in particularly close connection with Christian-ecclesiastical authority and its representatives in the shape of God or the saints. The ecclesiastical existed in her world as one religious *locus* among others, whereas people's relevant behavioural practices were, in her view, connected rather to moral than to narrowly religious aspects. What she did criticise was the relaxation of manners upon attending church in the present day (men and women standing unseparated during services, wearing inappropriate clothes for the service), and ritual observances by priests in Petersburg or Moscow (which she had recently visited for the first time) which apparently differed from what she was used to. Thus, it would seem that a hypothetical Christian God and the Church as an institution were rather loosely interconnected in her consciousness, the one relating to a world of powers and spiritual beings, the other to human issues of morality.

Through her illiteracy, Tatiana had also developed a characteristic relationship with literacy. That issue arose when she mentioned an old "Bible deriving from the sixth year", which had recently been pilfered and sold by a neighbour. In Tatiana's imagination, the book had really been almost as old as mankind itself ("from the sixth year" here signifying "from the beginning of time"), containing antiquated manuscript texts "in Latin and Vepsian", the latter of which, as she claimed, she had been able to read herself. It is difficult to guess what kind of a source this may have been exactly; in any case, Tatiana narrated some apocryphal folkloric stories about the beginning of time in connection with it—about how the originally hairy first humans lost their fur,[97] or how earlier, each blade of corn had grown several ears and been much bigger. That lost book, which had been handed down from one generation to the next (by the time of speaking, it had already gone missing), was part of the authoritative

[97] It is worth checking whether this statement may be a peculiar apocryphal parallel developed by the forest zone peoples to the story of the original Fall and the man and the woman finding themselves naked, losing the "robes of glory" after Adam's sin.

evidence demonstrating her connection with a kind of supernatural—the literate—world that Tatiana presented to us.[98]

Several features provided proof of her higher morality, especially important for a seer in her profession. Although illiterate, Tatiana knew through television about events in the wider world and uttered global prophecies about the fate of humankind and the Russian state. Among other things, she mentioned the destruction, by the year 2010, of three major cities of the world in cataclysms. In 2008, she already saw things moving in that direction; one of the doomed regions was to be the flood-ridden Florida, another was China with its flood that shocked the world in June of the same year, before the Beijing Olympics. Next, it would soon be Moscow's turn. People getting killed in military conflicts constituted, in Tatiana's eyes, another sign firmly located within her framework of prognosticative concepts through which the future of all things was to be interpreted.

The line separating the ethical from the unethical ran, in her view, right across ecclesiastical religious life too, although she herself seemed to stand autonomously outside of it or at least not to participate in it as zealously as is characteristic of orthodox village Christianity in general, and of post-soviet Russia in particular. As a seer, Tatiana was as self-conscious and self-sufficient as one would expect. The state, the church, literary culture, official medicine and other phenomena of the modern world were issues of which the seer was more or less informed but felt no obvious attraction towards—again unlike general members of the community who must constantly carry on some kind of a dialogue in order to anticipate unexpected events, as well as maintain a mutual controlling consensus concerning everything official and therefore apparently occupying a higher position in the hierarchy—that is, primarily modernity perceived as high culture.

Probably, she really didn't always have time to follow the futilities of contemporary life, due to her work and the issues of the spiritual world. Various spiritual beings and Tatiana's relationship with them was one of the issues that most interested us—but it was also the field where our science-based quest for a system and her (oral) organisation of the material need not have found common ground. A world inhabited by spirits, "masters and mistresses", as well as the relevant invocations, are at present still common knowledge among the whole of the older generation of Vepsians (cf. also Salve 1995, 415 ff). As expected, Tatiana had had

[98] In precisely the way the ownership of the *Seven Books of Moses* or any written material whatsoever has, in oral culture, served as evidence of the owner's special status and position.

several experiences with such creatures: spiritual beings had repeatedly appeared to her, and she was also able to describe them. It is worth noting that in her descriptions of the spirits of the forest, she never mentioned such obligatory characteristics as a remarkably rich growth of hair or some other type of shagginess (cf. also ibid. 428), a common feature in corresponding accounts of the religion and mythologies of the Finno-Ugric peoples, noting instead their diversity. While the appearance of spiritual beings was largely a matter of their own choice—fairies allow men to see them only when they themselves deem it necessary for the person—, Tatiana was nevertheless able to describe our own familiar house spirits, mentioning their size, gender and looks.

Besides the house spirit, the *domovik* (Rus.) or *pertižandaine* (Veps.), mention was made in our conversations also of the *mecižandaine* (Veps. "master of the forest"), *maižandaine* (Veps. "master of the earth"), and *pöüdan ižänd* (Veps. "master of the field"). From the interviews conducted so far, the master of the earth would seem to be associated with Tatiana's gardening and potato cultivation, whereas the master of the field appears to be some kind of more general and, according to one of her statements, even the most powerful of all spiritual beings.[99] The domain of the master of the forest is, in practical life and in Tatiana's activities, connected with getting lost or disappearing, although these events need not have taken place in forests. During our visit of summer 2008, we were present during a phone call from Podporozhye, the regional centre, in which Tatiana was asked to help find a pet cat that had gone missing in the city, tens of kilometres away—a procedure the seer undertook that same evening in her own neighbourhood, at the crossing of three roads, when it was indeed precisely the master of the forest she invoked.[100]

In the summer of 2009, we again attempted during our fieldwork to clarify the possibly hierarchical nature of Tatiana's belief system. This time, when we asked who was the most powerful of all gods (resp. masters-mistresses), she answered, "Allah". The answer seemed to be quite serious since she explained that in order to fend off hail and rain, it was precisely Allah she had taken to invoking (apparently already for quite some time). Such an incursion of a remote deity into the sphere of Orthodox village Christianity testifies to the continuing vitality of

[99] Could this be explained by the fact that in charms, it is often the open field that figures as one of the places reflecting the original potentiality, the place where, in texts, people go in order to try and deliver themselves from some trouble?

[100] About the seers' "talking to the forest" in the Vepsian tradition, see Salve 1995: 416 ff. We later learned from Tatiana that the cat had actually been run over by a car (meaning that the invoking of the forest spirits had been pointless).

syncretic phenomena even in the contemporary world. In all likelihood, Tatiana will have learned about Allah via television. Problems related to the assault of Islam are topical not only in the Western world, but—with their own specific nuances—also in the domestic politics of Russia. Tatiana's relations with Allah, however, were clearly not ideological, but practical/pragmatic. Of course, it would have been enormously interesting to record a charm of that kind.

As a real seer and healer, Tatiana naturally had no intention of giving us an exhaustive overview of her secret knowledge and spiritual world, which may be the reason why we learned only a casual and superficial part of her knowledge about the spiritual beings we were interested in. It also remained unclear whether Tatiana had any closer helping spirits, perhaps embodied in the material form of some amulet or other magical object—a phenomenon also known in Finnic witchcraft beliefs (see, for instance, Siikala 2002, 195 ff). We certainly got no direct affirmation of anything of the sort. What she did say, however, was that "God spoke to her" (Veps. *min'i jumaл sanob*), and it seemed that it was from this talk that she obtained her knowledge about future events and possibly other supernatural issues, too.

What struck us as somewhat peculiar, however, was Tatiana's relationship with her old dog. For the dog seemed to be not so much a pet as a creature capable of sharing something with its mistress. Tatiana was childless and thus unable, according to her own conviction, to pass on her secret knowledge to anybody. A widely distributed folk belief states that a witch that cannot pass on her knowledge must die a particularly harrowing death. In Tatiana's view, however, this was not a motif from a story but actual reality awaiting her, and about which she told us without any prompting on our part. Yet, in connection with that, she remarked that she could pass on her knowledge to her dog if she so pleased. Thus, the dog Pirat was in that respect more thoroughly initiated than Tatiana's own relatives, neighbours or any other human beings. By the summer of 2008, however, Pirat had died.

The fieldwork of 2009 brought further clarity to the issues of permutations of supernatural information over generations, and of its mediators. Tatiana mentioned that she had acquired her seer's knowledge directly from her mother, but also from God. Her mother had also passed some of her knowledge on to a dog who subsequently "howled it up into the heavens". From there, it was passed on, this time "through the mediation of God", to Tatiana. Quite obviously, here (and in Vepsian folklore in general), the concept of God is not merely reduced to the Orthodox Christian God, even if it is strongly influenced by it.

Tatiana absolutely refused to reveal her charms to us. When we inquired about them, she answered only: *i sa* [Veps. "I can't (say)"]. Yet over the same period, many old Vepsian women would recite to us various charms which seemed to be circulating almost publicly in traditional practice. On some occasions, charms for snakes or blood seem to have been acquired in a manner similar to learning a practical skill or folk song through observing an example. Due to Tatiana's status, however, the situation was different with her. On just the one occasion, she did, nevertheless, recite (or rather retell) a few lines of a charm. This was when we asked how the words for stopping blood worked. In broad outline, it emerged that the words were recited onto the wounded place, but that at the same time, the healer maintained a dialogue with "a black man sitting on the bank of the river, beneath a birch tree, who hears the healer and stitches up the wound with a red thread" (Veps. *mužt-verne rissit(u), ižtub koivun all jogen randal i ruskeil nitil ombleb necen ranan*).

From the aspect of the phenomenology of the soul, it is worth noting that Tatiana did not recognise blood as the seat and carrier of the soul—or else she did not understand what our question was about. But she knew that upon the slaughtering of animals, blood had been drunk. The most powerful meat of all was in her view that of an ox. Life had also brought her into frequent contact with wild animals—primarily while herding domestic animals and making hay, as well as through her husband's hunting. Her father had killed several bears, some of them in a quite unbelievable manner (essentially with his bare hands). Tatiana considered bear's meat to be sweet and similar to that of humans, which she also associated with the totemistic(?) knowledge that men had sprung from the bear (while women came from the frog). In connection with the spirit of the house or the cattle shed, she found the colour of domestic animals to be important—her own animals had bred (that is, her *domovik* had favoured) offspring of reddish or white colour. She thought that all living beings had souls, which were equal in size to the relevant creature's fist, hoof or cloven foot. The ancient notion that it was possible to have many souls was not known to her in that form.

Nevertheless, she did not regard the relationship of man and animal as one between equals. It was possible, according to her knowledge, to talk to a wild animal, but animals themselves could not speak. Unlike humans, animals were able to see spiritual beings. The names of humans could not be given to animals, because it was not good for the animal to be taken for a human. Her own pig had been called Borya, and when we remarked that this was a human's name too, she responded that it was not the same as Boris. Pig keeping had rewarded her in 2007 with 54 three-litre jars of meat preserve, and on a number of occasions, she treated us, too, to the delicious soup made from it.

Interesting, too, was Tatiana's attitude towards birds who—especially the migratory species—have, according to a widespread view, been held in rather an ambivalent regard (cf. Vinokurova 2006, 47). The notion of the "bird-cheat", pretty widespread in Finnic folklore, was at any rate quite unknown to her—or else she did not accept it. She considered birds to be creatures harmless to man. When I asked her about bird flu as a disease deadly to humans, which she must have been aware of through the media, she also found that notion unrealistic.

The questions and discussions of problems concerning the animistic world and the phenomenology of the soul demonstrated clearly that our views on these issues, mainly learned through folklore publications and in a way systematic, needn't in specific cases overlap with the systems, or rather creeds, circulating and practised in living tradition. Questions concerning some ethnocultural or areal belief system—like the Finno-Ugric or Proto-Uralic original religion or world picture, discussed in one way or another by several scholars (see, for instance, Napolskikh 1992; Siikala 2000 and many others)—become unrealistic, too idealistic in practice. The living and practised religion in its vernacular shape is so place-, experience- and tradition-specific that here, scientific theorising and system building may well begin to distance us from reality.

5.

First and foremost, however, it was Tatiana's role, profession and destiny to be a healer. As such, she was known far beyond the boundaries of her own community. People had been coming to her with their various complaints from Siberia, the Carpathians, and Central Asia, and naturally from the more immediate vicinity. She knew the cures of several illnesses, and in addition to lighter ailments, people came to her with asthma, polio or AIDS, all of which she claimed to be able to cure. She had apparently very successfully cured slowly healing post operational wounds, for which purpose, she said, even professors from St. Petersburg had sent their patients to her. Although it was not our aim to study folk medicine or to give an "adequate" estimation of Tatiana's healing activities, we could see that she suffered from no lack of work or patients.

Tatiana knew her herbs and also used elements of massage and acupuncture in her treatment. Where needed, she seemed to also make use of products of the pharmaceutical industry. Thus, she recommended analgine dissolved in Troinoi eau-de-cologne for gastritis which, when administered internally, was supposed to banish the illness. Undeniably, Tatiana's most important instrument, however, was healing charms, which she recited at various substances—during our visits, mainly at vodka. For this purpose, she withdrew behind a curtain, although occasionally she might recite the words in the patient's presence, too. In addition to food or drink meant for later consumption, she could also recite her words straight at the ailing place or wound. Manifold recitals were always concluded by spittings three times onto the place or substance being recited at. Upon reciting, what seemed to be important was to get into as immediate physical contact as possible with the target of the words. Tatiana declined to recite at vodka contained in a modern bottle furnished with a plastic device to facilitate pouring; apparently, the device prevented the power of the words from entering the liquid. Thus, for her, the recital was by no means a symbolic act or mystification, but an essential part of the cure comparable perhaps to a lancet in the surgeon's hand.

Apparently, then, in the eyes of a traditional healer, a verbally operative cure also constitutes a mechanical mechanism, not a psychological procedure working through suggestion. A key question to be answered in order to understand this kind of "unofficial" treatment, is how patients have taken it in traditional cultures, and how they take it in the modern world. On the basis of certain symptoms, Tatiana would classify rheumatic pains caused by the cold or wind, as *gryzha/purend* (cf. Rus. *gryzt′*, Veps. *purda*—"to chew, gnaw"). In such cases, articular matter was supposedly being eaten away by a corresponding supernatural creature—the personified disease *gryzha/purend*—the "gnawer" or "chewer", to whom the words were addressed. On one occasion, we managed to discern among the words recited at the diseased place in a muffled voice, the descriptive names of various types of *gryzha/purend* who were to be named—that is, recognised, cast a charm on—in the respective universal incantation.[101] Thus, the healer's activity seemed to consist not so much in dealing with the ailing place or with the patient, but primarily in communication (or, in the beginning, the quest for contact, establishing a relationship) with the spirit of the disease.

---

[101] By way of illustration, I add here the beginning of a different Vepsian healing charm which reflects the same idea: "Deliver me, the slave of the God from *purend* of head, *purend* of back, *purend* of navel, *purend* of bollock, *purend* of joints... (Veps. *Pästän minä netsen raban pän purondas, rungun purondas, naban purondas, muinaižen purondas, niveлoiden purondas*..."; Setälä et al. 1951, 150–1). From what we could hear, Tatiana's charm for *gryzha* seemed to be at least partially in Russian.

But people also sought Tatiana out because of curses, their love life, or other personal problems. In the summer of 2008, the seer herself demonstrated to us her belief in the power of the evil word. She showed us the patch of potatoes planted by her kitchen window, part of which had lost all their stems in a section delineated so sharply as if a line had been drawn with a ruler. The phenomenon could not be explained by a night frost or by a selective attack, as it were, of vermin; if there was any rational explanation at all, it could only be associated with different potato varieties planted in consecutive furrows. Tatiana herself thought it was the revenge of a former neighbour, motivated by envy.

We had the chance to personally witness the visit of a young woman who, after a failed relationship, had experienced long-term problems in making contact with the opposite sex. Here, too, Tatiana was able to recognise the evil influence brought about by some ill-wishers and to offer help. From what we heard during our fieldwork, it seems that in Central Vepsia, love magic performed by a witch or a seer has traditionally been quite recommended and welcome during weddings, too, where the seer has again played an important role. At any rate, we did not meet the view that the results of love magic should be of a temporary nature. Tatiana, too, regarded love magic as a natural part of her profession. She also engaged in finding lost people or setting out destinies. She described a case where she had known that a local young man was presumably lost by drowning but had actually met a violent death—a judgement later confirmed by forensic expertise. In summer 2008, however, it became evident that her power of finding lost people had receded... since she had no teeth of her own left in her mouth.

Among Tatiana's social roles were those of midwife and baptiser. She herself confessed to having baptised 160 people and received 180 babies, mostly in the Soviet period. The range of her roles can be described as uncommonly extensive even for a traditional society, in a way resembling the functions of a shaman in time when more specific social specialisation had not yet taken place (cf. e.g. Honko 1969, 47–51).

6.

Even though Tatiana was a famed, highly esteemed and respected seer and fulfilled her role very successfully in the eyes of her community, she was, typically of a healer, unable to help herself. She had survived two heart attacks and four difficult operations that had left the formerly buxom woman grey-haired and skinny. Therefore, she had developed a personal relationship with official medicine, the production of which, as materialised in the shape of expensive medication, she partly disdained, yet was partly also inevitably dependent on. Our acquaintance with Tatiana began at a time when she was already alone and, although esteemed as a healer, still a lonely woman shunned as a person. This may have been the reason why we were treated to her hospitality, her table, but also to her rather personal self-revelations on three consecutive summers.

A particularly close view of her twofold nature and destiny opened up to us in the summer of 2008, when we happened to arrive right at the time of one of her health crises. On the previous day, Tatiana had slaughtered a pig with the help of a local man, and then had laboured on alone to gut and clean the carcass, cut up the meat and portion it out into jars to make preserves. Lifting the heavy water containers had left her in great pain, and she believed she would die right in front of us. We overheard her telephone call to the doctor on duty in the local hospital, who scolded her not as the esteemed healer that she was in her own role, but as a bad patient. Armed conflict had just broken out in Southern Ossetia, and when the doctor inquired for whom Tatiana had made such a quantity of meat preserve, the seer had angrily retorted it was for the state. A war had broken out, she said, and like in the old days, so now, too, we would have to pay a tithe for it out of our supplies. The response was obviously more than a mere burst of sarcasm from an old woman suffering from great pain; rather, it seemed to reflect Tatiana's experience as a person and a seer in which a past full of misfortunes, ill luck in personal life, separation from her place of birth and the kinsmen buried there, and solitude ahead of a tormenting death were entwined, all of this framed by a global cataclysm known from prophecies and indeed looming imminently.

Our communication offered many intimate moments revealing a sense of the tragic which seems to be universally shared both by people inhabiting the modern world and those living in the traditional world. Unlike common members of the traditional society whose self-identification changes in the course of vital experiences without establishing links with former identities (on such changes as associated with the experience of grief see Adonieva 2004, 216–39), Tatiana was capable of (auto-) biography. From the traditional aspect, it was probably her very early awareness of herself as a seer that had facilitated the development of such an ability: as far as her present-day sense of the biographic was concerned, it was apparently fostered by her severance from her home in Rebagj—its landscapes, the home she had built there, the graves of her kinfolk. Thus, we came to hear a lot of personal information falling beyond the seer's professional behavioural role.

Tatiana had been fated to become a healer. For various reasons, she had missed out on many other roles important for a woman that she enumerated to us. Both as a seer and as a human being, Tatiana would have loved to be a mother, too. When asked what had now become of her, with things standing as they did, she on one occasion retorted, full of embitterment: "A devil" (Rus. *čert*), a response that, in view of her status and background, sounded particularly ambiguous at that moment—or perhaps, on the contrary, quite unambiguous. A self-reflection of such generalising power from a person quite untouched by the linearity of literacy can in a traditional society be explained only by the special status of a seer, but also by a longing for simple human happiness. Tatiana appeared similar to the "eternal bride" of folk songs who in her liminal phase compares, in poetic language and from a personal angle, her life before and after the wedding, giving clear preference to the circumstances and attitudes that had prevailed in her father's home.[102]

Tatiana had a keen desire to visit the cemetery of her old home village, in order to meet her loved ones there for one more time. Unfortunately, this did not prove possible during our stay there, since getting there would have required special transport over roads that had already become practically non-existent. Like the inhabitants of several other Vepsian villages situated in the same region, Tatiana had relocated from Rebagj at the end of the seventies as a result of geological prospecting. Since that time, Tatiana had also lodged a dislike in her heart for Mikhail Gorbachev, the leader of the Soviet Union from 1985 to 1991.

We could, however, visit the graves of Tatiana's husband and one of her sisters in Vidl, commemorating them according to the customs. Tatiana was no longer able to lament in full voice, but she did seem to know the appropriate words. Her conception of the afterworld also felt somewhat archaic and pre-Christian. She knew that life after death meant a peaceful stay underground as the deceased. She did not associate life after death with Heaven; rather, it seemed that heaven signified for her mere thin air together with the clouds sailing around it and occasionally coming down. In connection with lamenting for her dead, Tatiana revealed a probably very ancient element of her views—she did not think it proper as his wife to lament for her husband. She said point blank that the husband—unlike the mother, the father or a child—is not a blood relation and that ritual weeping on the husband's grave would be like a cow's lowing for a bull. A hint at the one-time matrilinearity among the Finno-

[102] I believe this has been practised in traditional society, by performance of relevant songs, mainly in order to facilitate the adoption of a new status as wedded wife, not as a sign of wilfully becoming mired in past maidenhood.

Ugric peoples could possibly be read into this statement—a hypothesis that requires further information and investigation.

In the spring of 2009, Tatiana's health had again deteriorated into a critical state, as a result of which she had spent four days lying, unconscious, in the local hospital under the doctors' care. She herself said that during that time, she had visited the aforementioned afterworld and met its inhabitants. Among them, she mentioned the people from her remote and extinct home, the village of Rebagj, beginning with her closest deceased relatives. Life in the underworld had, according to her, been a habitual continuation of life on earth, a kind of existence which could, on the basis of what she told us, be compared to the underworld notions of Kalevala-metric songs and laments describing communal life in the afterworld, *Toonela/Manala*, full of work and care just like life on this side of the grave. In the summer of 2009, just as we were about to leave the region, Tatiana had been hospitalised once again. We went to visit her there, to say goodbye. When another old woman lying in the same ward ventured to say that it was time for all of them to die, Tatiana responded in her characteristic manner that first one must recover and only then can one begin to think about dying—sick people are not welcome in the afterworld.

It is the seer's role and destiny to be in all situations like one swimming up against the current. This is what Tatiana has demonstrated to us, both in her deeds and in her words. Were we to try and define our roles in our dialogical relationship with Tatiana, we should probably be identified as her missing relatives, perhaps (though barely) even as the children she never had. Probably this is a role we have also played before when communicating with elderly informants in their mother tongue.

Tatiana quite evidently opened up to us in a manner different from the way she opened to the other people in her daily life. This did not merely involve a desperate or melancholy sense of chaos: her emotional dynamics covered the whole range up to robust and vital sociability when she hosted us, offered us tea and vodka and recited chastushkas both in Vepsian and in Russian. The latter, however, just like Tatiana's observations about people's relationships and sexual habits, were not mere entertaining gossip but deeply felt vital reality—in keeping with the fact that traditional culture seems to lack what is known as obscenity in contemporary polite discourse, and that even seemingly indecent wording is actually fulfilling its function in reflecting reality. Let one of Tatiana's chastushkas be quoted here:

Koto män(d)o sures koivus kägi kukkob kerta viž.	On the way home, in a tall birch tree the cuckoo calls five times.

Čoma neidiš—rusked roza kerdän andab, toižen i.	A bonny maid with a healthy face gives herself once but not for a second time.

Upon comleting a chastushka of this kind, Tatiana often asked: *Proud om?* [Veps. "That's true, isn't it?"], or *Muga?* [Veps. "Isn't it right?"]; or else commented: *Tože byvaet* [Rus. "That may also come to pass."] Here, the chastushkas constitute a telling illustration of the synergetics characteristic of a traditional culture, combining entertainment, education, sarcasm and fun.

7.

The encounter with a person enjoying a special status in her community is indicative of traditional information obtained with a peculiar stamp. This is not mere folklore as improvisational, vital and variable "collective creation", but rather the heady stuff of a tradition of which its carrier is aware in a manner different from common awareness, and for the handing down of which she seems to take personal responsibility. The study of a person of special social status living and practising in a preliterate and partly premodern culture is a problematic undertaking. It is easy to rephrase a culturally different individual world view in words that, either by conceptualising or poeticising it, satisfy the student himself. The student's problem, however, lies in his inability to always adequately grasp the reality of the informant—precisely because he carries a different world view himself.

In this respect, the example of Tatiana Arsentievna is a characteristic one. Our dialogue has been comprehensible and even open to compromise on the human plane; how much we really could comprehend the reality of her different world view, is a question that must remain unanswered. The close connection with contemporary Vepsian folk culture and its traditional past is very much evident, even when observing the customs and attitudes reflecting the world view of common community members. A nuanced understanding of the innermost, and for the most, part hidden values of that culture requires further contacts and interviews. Undoubtedly, people of extraordinary status are important information sources here; yet because of the specifically non-public-oriented character of their profession, they are sources which are difficult to open up. "Changes in non-material culture are thus events which are neither mechanical nor straightforward, but rather complex or random, processes in which progressive and conservative tendencies tend to function as a mutually interactive balance of forces" (Siikala 2002, 32). The placing of one individual with his/her unique world view—the only kind a seer can have—into the focus of these events creates a characteristic dimension in a culture. Frequently, the role of the extraordinary individual is one that both values and organises the habitual "average", and at the same time, introduces and generates change and innovation by breaking the rules.

P.S. Tatiana Arsentievna, the great Vepsian healer and specialist of verbal magic, passed away in early spring 2010. She died alone at her home.

References

Adonieva, S. B. 2004. *Pragmatika fol'klora* [The pragmatic of folklore]. Sankt Peterburg: Sankt Peterburgskii universitet.

Dobrovolskaia, V. E. 2001. "Narodnye predstavleniia o koldunakh v neskazochnoi proze [Folk beliefs about sorcerers in the realistic prose]." In *Muzhskoi sbornik.* Vysh. 1. *Muzhshchina v traditsionnoi kul'ture* [Male collection. Part 1. Man in traditional culture], 95–105. Moskva: Labirint.

Goody, Jack. 1977. *The Domestication of the Savage Mind.* Cambridge: University Press.

Honko, Lauri. 1969. "Role-Taking of the Shaman." *Temenos* 4: 26–55.

Kolga, Margus, Igor Tõnurist, Vaba Lembit, and Jüri Viikberg. 2001. "The Veps." In *The Red Book of the Peoples of the Russian Empire*, 351–5. Tallinn: NGO Red Book. http://www.eki.ee/books/redbook/veps.shtml.

Kurs, Ott. 2001. "The Vepsians: An Administratively Divided Nationality." *Nationalities Papers* 29: 69–83.

Napolskikh, Vladimir. 1992. "Proto-Uralic World Picture: A Reconstruction." In *Northern Religions and Shamanism*, edited by Mihály Hoppál, and Juha Pentikäinen, 3–20. Budapest and Helsinki: Akadémiai and Finnish Literature Society.

Ong, Walter. J. 2002. *Orality and Literacy: The Technologizing of the Word.* New York: Routledge.

Salve, Kristi. 1995. "Forest Fairies in the Vepsian Folk Tradition." In *Folk Belief Today*, edited by Mare Kõiva, and Vassiljeva Kai, 413–34. Tartu: Institute of the Estonian Language and Estonian Museum of Literature.

Setälä, E. N., and J. H. Kala. 1951. *Näytteitä äänis-ja keskivepsän murteista. Julkaissut ja suomentanut E. A. Tunkelo apuaan Reino Peltola* [Samples of sounds and medieval dialects. Edited and translated by E. A. Tunkelo, and Reino Peltola]. Helsinki: Suomalais-ugrilainen Seura. (Suomalais-ugrilaisen Seuran Toimituksia 100.)

Siikala, Anna-Leena. 2000. "What Myths Tell about Past Finno-Ugric Models of Thinking." In *Congressus Nonus Internationalis Fenno-Ugristarum 7–13. 8. 2000 Tartu. Pars I. Orationes plenariae & Orationes publicae*, edited by Anu Nurk, and Triinu Palo, 127–40. Tartu: Tartu Eesti Fennougristide Komitee.

—. 2002. *Mythic Images and Shamanism. A Perspective on Kalevala Poetry*. Helsinki: Academia Scientarum Fennica. (FF Communications 280.)

Strogalschikova Z. I. 2014. Vepsy. Ocherki istorii i kul'tury [Vepsians. Essays on history and culture]. Sankt Peterburg: Inkeri.

Vasenkari, Maria and Armi Pekkala. 2000. "Dialogic Methodology." In *Thick Corpus, Organic Variation and Textuality in Oral Tradition*, edited by Lauri Honko, 243–54. Helsinki: Finnish Literature Society. (Studia Fennica Folkloristica 7.)

Vinokurova I. Iu. 2006. *Zhivotnye v traditsionnom mirovozzrenii vepsov (opyt rekonstruktsii)* [Animals in the traditional world view of Vepsians (attempt of reconstruction)]. Petrozavodsk: Izd-vo PetrGU.

Magic and Counter-Magic and the Social Position of the Bru Shaman-sorcerer (Central Vietnamese Highlands)

Gábor Vargyas

According to traditional conceptions in ethnography, the history of religion, the sociology of religion, phenomenology and other related disciplines, not to speak of New Age ideology, the Eurasian and/or American shaman is a highly positive figure who is considered to be a "healer" working unselfishly for the benefit of his fellow humans, curing illnesses and warding off supernatural malefices. A huge body of literature running from Eliade to Harner and from Hultkrantz to Hoppál repeats and recreates this benevolent and peaceful image of shamans and shamanism (Eliade 1974; Harner 1980; Hultkrantz 1984; Hoppál 1994). For instance, Eliade, while dealing with the different functions of the shaman in his influential pioneering study on shamanism, states that "all through Asia and North America, and elsewhere as well [...] the shaman performs the function of doctor and healer" (Eliade 1974, 182) and writing about North American shamanism specifically, he underlines the "*positive* function" of the shaman (Eliade 1974, 299, italics in original). In his voluminous work, one finds only one passing hint as to the ambivalence of shamanic power: "it is not one of the shaman's specialties to harm his clients' enemies, although sometimes he will undertake to do so" (Eliade 1974, 184); in his index, no mention is made of sorcery, harm or violence. A quarter of a century later, in his last words on the theme, he gives an appraisal of the religious and cultural importance of the shamans as follows: "shamans have played an essential role in the defence of the psychic integrity of the community. They are pre-eminently the antidemonic champions; they combat not only demons and disease, but also the 'black' magicians. In a general way, it can be said that shamanism defends life, health, fertility, and the world of 'light', against death, disease, sterility, disasters, and the world of 'darkness'" (Eliade 2005, 8273). Two decades later, in the second edition of the same

Encyclopedia of Religion, this scope is further enlarged: "As a biologically based spiritual and healing system that played a significant role in human survival, social relations, and cosmology, shamanism was humanity's original neurotheology" (Winkelman 2005, 8279).

Founder of the New Age neoshamanic movement, "shamanthropologist" M. Harner argues along the same lines. In his guide "for power and healing" i.e. for people outside traditional shamanistic cultures to learn shamanic methods, he writes: "Shamans—whom we in the 'civilised' world have called 'medicine men' and 'witch doctors'—are the keepers of a remarkable body of ancient techniques that they use to achieve and maintain well-being and healing for themselves and members of their communities" (Harner 1980, XVII). And a page later, he promises to his readers that "by employing the methods described in this book, you will have an opportunity to acquire the experience of shamanic power and *to help yourself and others*" (Harner 1980, XVIII, italics added). The positive, healing function of the shaman, and the help he renders his community are clear enough from what has been said; there is no need to multiply the examples.

And yet in sociocultural anthropology, it is almost plain that violence and shamanism *may be* (and in fact often *are*) linked. To take Elkin, a classic amply but selectively used by Eliade, the Australian Aboriginal medicine men, or as Elkin calls them the "Aboriginal men of high degree" are just as much "*leeches*, in that they use objective means for the curing of illnesses and wounds. They are [also, G.V.] *magical practitioners*, for they cure some sicknesses by magical rituals and spells. In many parts they are *sorcerers* as well; they know how to, and may, insert evil magic, extract 'human fat', or cause the soul to leave the victim's body, bringing about sickness and death. And finally, they also possess, in many cases, *occult powers*: they can commune with the dead [...]. They therefore partake of the character of witches, clairvoyants, mediums and psychic experts" (Elkin 1977, XX. Italics added). As for sorcery or black magic, which concerns us here, it "provides the explanation of illnesses, pains and deaths, the causes of which are not known, or are not obvious" (Elkin 1977, 38.). And since not knowing "the causes of illness and death [...] by which the solidarity and efficiency of the community are weakened, is a disturbing factor in psychological and social life", Elkin sees the positive function of black magic in the fact that "to have an accepted explanation and to have acted on that explanation, enables the community to readjust itself to events and to go about its business" (Elkin 1977, 38.). His work is consequently full of examples of shamanic black magic, violence, extraction of "human fat", use of "pointing bones" and the like, bringing about sickness and death.

A more modern source, Vitebsky, echoes very closely Elkin's position: "Many traditional societies see sorcery as integrally related to healing" (Vitebsky 1995, 112). Taking the Achuar living on the Peru-Ecuador frontier as an example, he elaborates on the theme as follows: "Spirits which appear helpful to some people may seem to be hostile to others. The link between shamans and violence is most apparent when communities are at war" (Vitebsky 1995, 110). At the Achuar "there is no cause of illness or misfortune except someone else's aggression, usually in the form of magical darts: even someone who drowns in rapids is believed to have been dragged under by an anaconda sent by a hostile shaman. *Here the power to heal depends on the power to kill.* A cure can be effected only by a shaman who possesses an identical kind of dart to that used by the aggressor [...]" (Vitebsky 1995, 110–1). It follows that "as a person with extraordinary powers, the shaman may need to be held in check by the society he or she serves. Both Baruya [an ethnic group living in the Highlands of Papua New Guinea, G.V.] and Achuar shamans are considered unreliable. *More Achuar shamans are murdered by their neighbours than killed by rivals' darts* [...] *In both societies, a shaman could not avoid attacking people because this would also amount to a refusal to heal"* (Vitebsky 1995, 111–2).

To sum up this kind of argumentation, a third author, Seymour-Smith points out that "shamanism is also similar in certain respects to witchcraft in that it may involve the use of mystical powers to attack enemies and cause disease. The South American shaman, for example, is both a curer and a sorcerer, and the patterns of accusations and interpretations of sorcery reveal social tensions and structural features in the same manner as in the classic social anthropological studies of witchcraft in African settings." And: "students of South American shamanism have noted [...] the fundamental ambiguity of the shaman's role as curer and sorcerer..." (Seymour-Smith 1986, 256).

In what follows, I shall proceed along the same line and argue that counter-magic and magic are two interconnected things that presuppose each other: they are two sides of the same coin. In order to counteract a magical offence, one also has to know how to cause magical harm since both go back to the same principles. Thus, in Bru society, the dividing line between an anti-social shaman-sorcerer and a social shaman-healer is very thin—shamans constantly have to balance on a razor-edge. The supernatural power at their disposal makes them suspicious to common people: they are often charged with black magic. Black magic or witchcraft accusations[1] and the resulting public ordeals in order to prove *pro* or *contra* the truth are consequently not an uncommon feature in Bru and, generally speaking, in the Southeast Asian Highlanders' religious life (see Ner 1935). Departing from the symbolism of some attributes on Bru shamanic headdresses and referring to this ambiguous power that can be both used and misused, I shall examine in the following the social position of the Bru shaman and illustrate through a concrete case study some social mechanisms that cope with the ambiguity inherent in this "profession".

***

In an earlier paper in Hungarian (Vargyas 2004; see also Vargyas 2008) I analysed in detail a Bru folk story, in "anthropological" terms an origin myth, relating to some of the attributes of a shamanic headdress: a claw of a flying-fox, a pangolin scale and a canine of a civet-cat. The story is far too long to be presented here in detail. Its protagonists are the three above-mentioned animals, two of whom, in mythic times, acted as a shaman (the flying-fox) and the shaman's assistant (the pangolin): their friend (the civet-cat) helped them only by carrying their baskets. One day, by command of the ruler of the upper world, they rob the soul of a beautiful fairy-woman turned into a human, and the wife of an orphelin; that is to say they kill her by black magic so that the ruler may receive her as a concubine in his realm. The husband of the deceased woman goes up into the sky in order to find her. He is informed about the misdeeds of the three protagonists. He convinces the ruler to hand them over to him; he carries them down to Earth in a cage. Arriving at his home, he forces them to make a counter-magic and revive his wife. At the end of the story, he punishes them and that is how they acquire their present-day characteristics: the tongue of the flying-fox is cut out so that he cannot perform a singing ceremony any more—this is why this animal is "mute"; the teeth of the pangolin are hit out so that he cannot hold the idioglott clarinet, the *pĩ* (the par excellence musical instrument of the shaman's assistant) in his mouth and blow it—this is why the pangolin does not have teeth today. As for the civet-cat, he is released since he has not done any particular harm—he simply helped them by carrying their basket...

The lesson of this story is obvious. The anti-social mythical shamans-sorcerers are severely punished while their harmless friend is mildly rebuked. The claw of the flying-fox, the pangolin scale and the canine of

---

[1] Throughout this paper I use these two terms as synonyms.

the civet-cat in the shamanic headdress thus remind all the time their wearer, the shaman, that he cannot misuse his supernatural power for anti-social purposes and go unpunished!

This takes us to one of the key problems of Bru and, in fact, any shamanism: to the relationship of the supernatural power and human society, or, more specifically, to the ambivalence of supernatural power. As I have mentioned above, supernatural power, just as any other power, can be both used and misused. Magic and counter-magic only differ from each other in intention: what is harmful to one person or one group is beneficial to the other; black magic performed for attacking someone is negative, while for protecting the attacked, it is positive, even if it necessarily means killing or eliminating the aggressor. What is true for the Achuar and countless other ethnic groups is also true for the Bru: "the power to heal depends on the power to kill" (Vitebsky 1995, 111). Suspicion hovers, therefore, about the activity of the shaman from the beginning onwards: shamans are often accused of witchcraft or sorcery, while counteracting this activity means fighting with (the deeds of) their congeners.

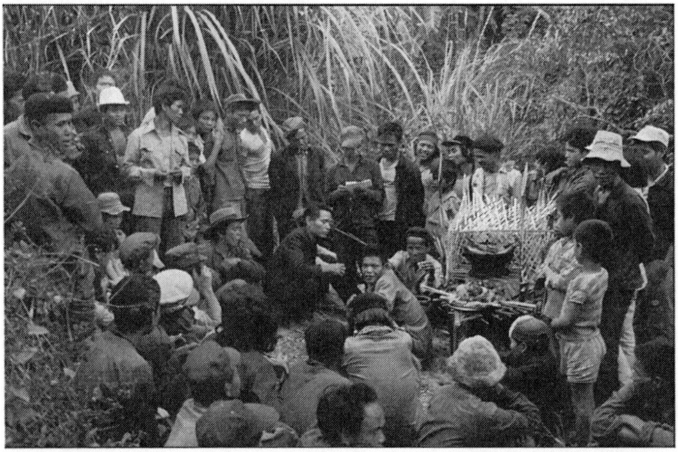

Fig. 1. The scene of the oath taking and the participants. Crouching before the altar is *achuaih* H., holding the straw of the rice-beer jar; behind him is a man with the list of the participants. 17 February, 1988. Photo by Gábor Vargyas.

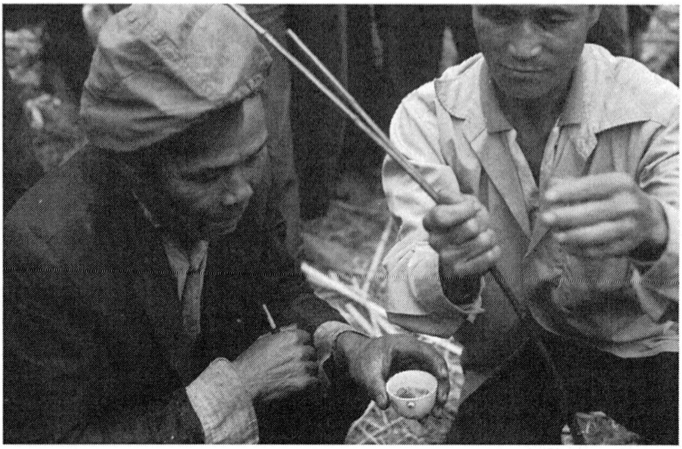

Fig. 2. *Achuaih* B., the accused shaman, holding a cup containing rice-beer mixed with the blood of the sacrificial animal reciting the text of the oath. Next to him is *achuaih* H., holding the straw of a rice-beer jar. 17 February, 1988. Photo by Gábor Vargyas.

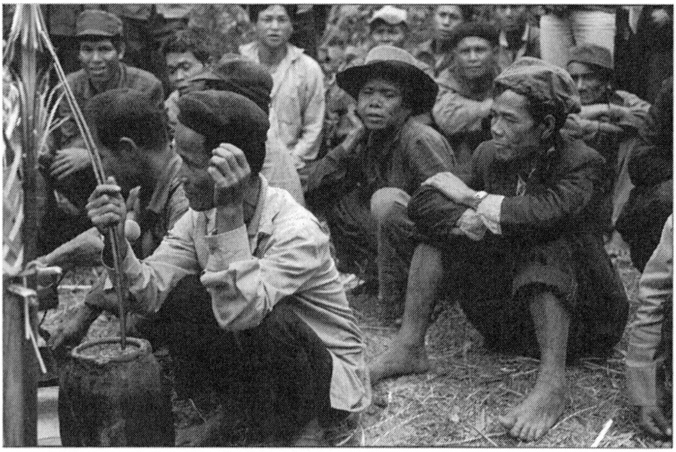

Fig. 3. *Achuaih* H., "guarding" or "keeping down" *yĩang Sorsĩ* during the ritual by holding the straw of a rice-beer jar. Behind him, on the right, is *achuaih* B., the accused shaman. 17 February, 1988. Photo by Gábor Vargyas.

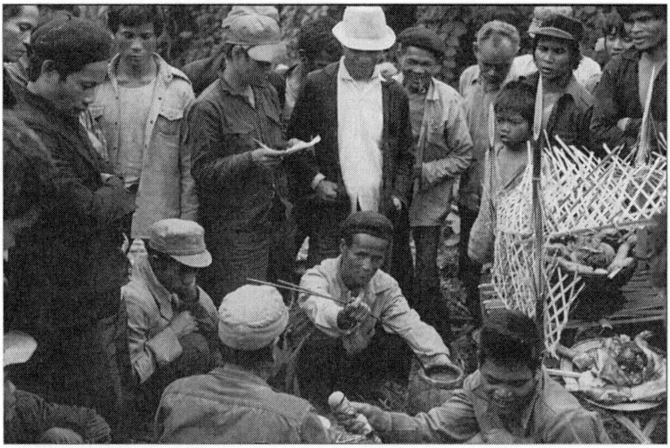

Fig. 4. The villagers waiting for their turn listen to the oath of one of the participants. In the background, a man checks off the names of the men who had already taken the oath from the list containing the names of all the heads of family. In the foreground, a praying man turns his back; next to him, a man is recording the oath with the anthropologist's tape recorder; across from them is *achuaih* H., holding the straw of a rice-beer jar. 17 February, 1988. Photo by Gábor Vargyas.

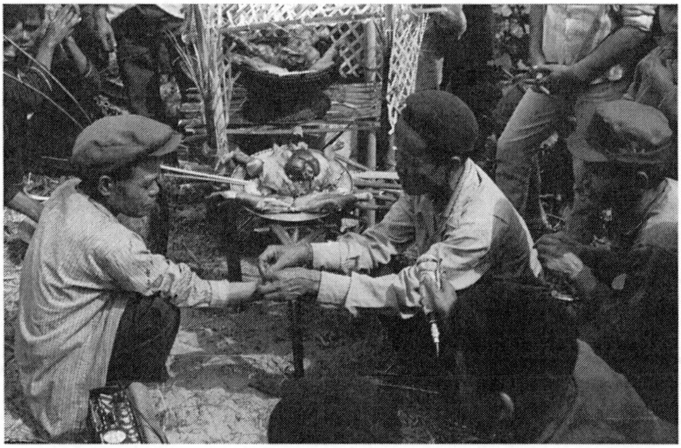

Fig. 5. *Achuaih* H. ties the thread around the wrist of one of the participants at the end of the "recall of the soul" *(arô ruviêi)*. In the background is the altar with the sacrificial platter. 17 February, 1988. Photo by Gábor Vargyas.

It is by no means sheer accident then that Bru shamans are in a way "reluctant" to perform their séances. At the beginning, they ritually pronounce a speech in which they decline any responsibility for whatever has happened and will happen; they publicly understate and underestimate their power and emphasise that they act only out of urgent need and of compassion towards their "fellow humans" (the Bru expression being that "they like people and/or friends" *[ayo͘oq yo͘u]*), and because they were "hired out" *(mian)* and solicited to perform the "work" *(táq ranáq).*

In connection with all this, one has to know that Bru shamans *get paid* for their services, even if in most cases this means a payment in kind (e.g. a prescribed part of the sacrificed animal, a living chicken "for his helping spirit", alcohol etc.); in some cases, however, they also receive money or valuables (silver bracelets, bronze or brass cooking pots etc.). If we add to all this that a shamanic ceremony necessarily implies a huge amount of sacrificial meat and drink, i.e. it means consuming a lot of meat and alcohol, and if we are aware of what kind of preconceived ideas and associations all this may bring forth in a constrained vegetarian society, we may understand that the playground for the Bru shamans is very limited.[2] A sword of Damocles always hangs above their head; they may be accused at any time of misusing their supernatural power, to use it for illegitimate purposes, for black magic or witchcraft. As we have seen: unselfish

---

[2] In order to clearly assess the importance of this question, one has to know that in the everyday nutrition of the Bru—as in that of any tropical cultivator—animal protein is conspicuously missing. Meat (except for wild animals) is not consumed for ordinary purposes, killing a domestic animal is imaginable only in a sacred context and for sacrificial purposes. It is very telling that on a linguistic level, "sacrifice" and "meat eating" are synonymous: an invitation to a buffalo sacrifice runs as follows: "the lineage of X and Y is going to eat a buffalo tomorrow".

In the same way, the consumption of alcohol is also regulated by strict prescriptions and taboos. To the Bru mind, alcohol is of sacred origin; opening a jar of rice-beer or a bottle of spirit implies concomitant prayers; in a non-sacred context, alcohol consumption is practically non-existent. The origin of rice and rice-beer or rice spirit made from it is the theme of one of the most popular epic cycles *(nsũar tâng sanõ͘t)* sung to the accompaniment of a flute, which, in turn, is performed again only in ritual circumstances.

Shamans have consequently to be aware that their activity recalling the land of milk and honey may give rise to jealousy and envy, and that their behaviour is watched with the eyes of a lynx. I myself have heard several times comments like "shamans have a great time, they eat as much meat and drink as much alcohol as they want", or "X or Y has become a shaman only because he likes eating and drinking".

counter-magic and selfish black magic are within a hair's breadth of each other.

It is then in the Bru shamans' elementary interest to communicate an ideal picture of themselves, to emphasise the charitable character of their work, to persuade their clients that they are performing not through greediness, nor for the sheer pleasure of eating and drinking, but as a result of philanthropic compassion. At the end of the séances, they never eat of the meat of the sacrificed animals, but share it around so that they cannot be blamed for "being hungry of meat" which could be one of the reasons for committing anti-social acts—since later they would harvest the fruits as a repayment for the damages caused by themselves. Visibly, Bru shamans are keen on emphasising the positive sides of their dangerous profession. All this is accentuated by their modest behaviour, by their words and gestures: they are reluctant to perform and require much soliciting, they stress the fact that they are compelled to work against their wish and that they obey circumstances beyond their control. In short: it is *not they who want* the ceremony—*they are wanted/required* for the ceremony. And still! If the news is spread about a "sorcerer", an avalanche is launched. I know of a few old cases when Bru society rejected and/or eliminated an unsociable, quarrelsome, bullying, greedy, evil shaman. A shaman is consequently just as much a fallible figure at the mercy of his group as an envied religious specialist within society.

The question may be raised then whether the reason for and meaning of the universal shamanic conception according to which shamans are *chosen and called by the spirit world against their will* is not to be looked for in this context: that of the ambivalence of supernatural power. The parallel between the call and the behaviour of the Bru shaman is, at any rate, obvious. Just as the shaman has become a shaman because he was chosen by the representatives of the spirit world and because he could not escape that call, he is now performing the séance not of his own will but because human society, a power transcending him, compels him to do so and he cannot escape this call either. It seems as if this *external pressure* or force would be the razor-edge balancing upon which he could dissipate the dark shades cast on his supernatural power; as if this psychological motif alone would be enough to decide the sense or tone of the judgement on his activity between the poles of good and bad, benevolence and harm, healing and bewitchment.

***

Let us now turn our attention to the social mechanisms that cope with the ambiguity inherent in the shamanic "profession" by examining a concrete case of witchcraft accusation and the resulting public oath or ordeal. On 15th February, 1988, I received a sudden unexpected visit from a very good friend of mine from a neighbouring village[3]: the old *achuaih*[4] H., the traditional village chief and representative of the land-owning lineage[5] of that locality. He came to invite me to a unique event that was to be organised within two days in his village: a ceremony called *nguaiq dõq thễ kóp yĩang Sorsĩ*[6]—"to drink the water of oath with *yĩang Sorsĩ*". Surprised as I was, I found out the following: one of the shamans (*mo yao*) of the village, *achuaih* B., a quiet old man in his sixties, had been denounced by some unknown village people to the police of the provincial headquarters in Khe Sanh as being a sorcerer and to have bewitched some of his neighbours through black magic. The accusation was taken seriously and after an official interrogation (the gun of the policeman being pointed at *achuaih* B.'s head!), he had no choice other than to "admit" having committed these sins. To put it in Bru terms, he admitted that he *táq kũai, bữn rahâu, pánh kũai, kachĩt kũai,* i.e. "he harmed people, he had magic substances for committing black magic, he shot them into his victims/hunted for people, he killed people". As a consequence, his shamanic headdress, symbol and essential paraphernalia of the shamanic "profession" were taken from him and burnt by the policeman, and he was publicly humiliated. Being stigmatised as a sorcerer or witch, he was not only unable to perform shamanic séances but was also officially prohibited from doing so. Claiming his innocence and wanting to repair the injustice against him, some time later he turned to *achuaih* H., the traditional or religious head of the village, asking him to organise for him this most important and rare ceremony—a kind of solemn and public oath or ordeal taking the mightiest of all the divinities, *yĩang Sorsĩ*, as a testimony in a sacrifice of two pigs and with the participation of the whole community, proving his innocence and reinforcing social solidarity.

I cannot go into the details here of black magic itself. Suffice it to say that although Bru society seems to be very peaceful and harmonious, sorcery or witchcraft is latently omnipresent. I stress the word *latently*, as apart from this case and a few stories about the past referred to above

---

3 This village was a one day walk from the village I lived in.

4 *Achuaih* = "grandfather", a title also used for old men.

5 "Master of land": first inhabitant or first comer, having a religious relationship with the divinity of the Earth.

6 *Nguaiq* = to drink; *dõq* = water; *thễ* (< viet: *thề*) to swear, to make an oath; *kóp* = with; *yĩang* = divinity, spirit; *Sorsĩ* = personal name of the Bru Deus Otiosus

when suspected or inculpated sorcerers were chased from the village or simply killed as revenge in secret, I do not know of any concrete evidence of sorcery *in practice*. However, my informants seemed to agree about its existence, methods, occasions and reasons, even if in the everyday practice there was not much discourse about it. Out of fear of spreading malevolent gossip that could backfire against them, local people were very careful about discussing witchcraft accusations, even in private. Only occasional remarks, timid questions and tender warnings caused me to realise the existence of this problem in the field.[7] Its special occasions were said to be the great festivals involving marriage or funeral ceremonies when several hundreds of people from different and potentially hostile (because they were "foreign") villages came together. But any other occasion may do. Its methods are manifold. Some of the most frequent ones are shooting magical projectiles (a small piece of bone, wood, crystals, grains of sand etc.) into the victims (*pánh kutrien,* to shoot a magical substance); "tying" or "twisting" their intestines, causing them great pain and a slow death; putting *rahâu* (medicine, poison, magical substance) under one's fingernails and dripping it into the drinking cup of the other person, etc. As for the reasons behind black magic, the most frequent explanations were greed, jealousy and envy. As many Bru people put it: "sorcerers are jealous because others *do* have rice, meat and fish, but they do not receive from it". Another possible reason is rivalry between shamans: one is more solicited than the other, thus receiving more payments in kind or cash. There are only two ways of counteracting this dreadful practice: a) to call a shaman and let him cure the sick patient by removing the magical projectile, untying the intestines, giving amulets to counterbalance the negative effects or to exorcise the harmful divinity out of the patient's body; b) more radically, to eliminate the ultimate cause of the sorcery, i.e. the person suspected of practising it. Besides the traditional methods of killing, as mentioned above, there is a more modern way: to denounce them to the local police, which then leads them to court and prison. This is what partly happened in this case. The action of the policeman described above was a preliminary to this solution, a "last warning". We shall come

[7] I remember vividly when, before departing for a three-day-long secondary burial feast in a faraway village, my landlord's wife, first among the Bru, warned me "in motherly fashion" of the potential threat the great number of "strangers" gathering at such occasions may pose. Also, at one unique occasion, under the effect of alcohol consumed in great quantity, the otherwise very shy *achuaih* H. explained to me in great secrecy the Bru concepts of the ways and means of poisoning somebody with "magic".

back later to this point, the interference of modern criminal law with traditional methods of jurisprudence.

Now let us turn our attention to the ritual of oath or ordeal. The expression "to drink the water of oath with *yĩang Sorsĩ"*, refers to a type of ceremony which is known in this part of the world in different socio-political contexts, for expressing loyalty and fidelity to a superior power. As we know from an early French source on the Bru, the expanding Siamese empire in the nineteenth century used to oblige subjugated populations, among them hill tribes including the Bru, to make an oath of allegiance twice a year in the Siamese town of Ubon,[8] or "to make this oath at their respective localities by *drinking the consecrated water of oath* brought there by the heads of Siamese posts..." (Lemire, 1894, 42, *my translation, italics added*). According to the same source, this trip to Ubon and back was a lengthy and expensive one: altogether it lasted 25 days, of which the journey itself took 18 days of walking. But people "attach to this oath a superstitious fear because of the splendour that surrounds it". I quote: "The Siamese functionaries and soldiers are gathered in a pagoda. The chiefs who will take the oath are brought here. The bonzes recite prayers. A secretary or a bonze reads the formula of the oath. The chiefs repeat it and, passing in front of the Siamese commissary, they dip their hands into a cup full of water from the river, in which weapons and gunpowder had been immersed and onto which spells of malediction had been pronounced by the bonzes for all those who would not observe the sworn submission. Then the chiefs bow in front of the portrait of the king and all of them drink a cup of sacred water while the bonzes recite Pali sentences. The Khâ-Luong (= the Siamese commissary), or his deputy, advise fidelity to the king, the power and goodness of whom is praised. Finally, the commissary distributes tin betel containers decorated with painted portraits of the king and the queen of Siam" (Lemire 1894, 42; *my translation*).

To come back to our case, "drinking the water of oath with *yĩang Sorsĩ"*, means something very similar, but here the character of the ceremony is not so much socio-political as magico-religious. The highest instance that "presides" the events and that is taken as a testimony is the Bru *deus otiosus, yĩang* Sorsĩ. This in itself is a unique phenomenon. In the very complex Bru pantheon where everything, animate and inanimate alike, has (or may have) a spirit or divinity influencing the fate of that thing and also that of the humans and where all these divinities are the object of frequent sacrifices, *yĩang* Sorsĩ does not figure practically at all.

---

[8] Today Ubon Ratchathani, on the Mae Nam Mun river, an affluent of the Mekong.

Being a true *deus otiosus* as he is, after an ill-defined mythical period during which he reigned as a supreme god or divinity, he withdrew himself from the world of humans. Though his name is known and people agree that he is to be considered the mightiest of all the *yĩang,*[9] he or his name is never evoked during rituals and, especially, no sacrifices are made to him. This is the only (type of) ritual I have witnessed or know of where *yĩang* Sorsĩ played an important role, where he was invited to come down and partake in the sacrificial meal as is usual for all the other divinities, and where he was explicitly called upon to interfere in human matters. "Drinking the water of oath with *yĩang Sorsĩ"* is thus an exceptionally rare event, so much so that even the organisers had never witnessed one before! *Achuaih* H. himself had to inquire after it, the model being a similar event held in another far-off village, R., a few months earlier—in itself said to be an exceptional occasion.[10]

Now we may return to our concrete case. The day following the visit of *achuaih* H. at our place, we went together to his village. The first surprise came in the course of that occasion. On our way, we called in to village X to see and inform the secretary of the local Communist Party cell and the policeman of the district of our arrival. The president of the district council, who was my host, had by then been formally informed in our village. As it transpired, the district leaders had had to be advised in written form about the events and give their consent to its organisation since such cases of witchcraft or sorcery, being highly disruptive to the social order, are considered as falling under their responsibility, a matter of "internal affairs" to be supervised by the state apparatus.

The permission obtained, one day later, on 17th February, 1988, the ceremony took place in village L. Essentially, it consisted of a sacrifice of two pigs; one offered to the most important "divinity in the bush" (i.e. the non-civilised, uninhabited zone; nature), *yĩang* Sũ, the divinity of the earth or soil, supervising the whole district. A second pig was destined for a very important and relatively frequent ceremony called *arô ruviêi*, "calling back the soul" (of the participant/s). This rite, usually considered a typical thai/lao ceremony (see Zago, 1972, 129–70), aims in general to spiritually reinforce an individual and, in case of illness, to cure him by reintegrating

---

9 This is why during evangelisation his name was chosen as denoting the God-father. (See *Parnai O* 1981).

10 Given the fact that in a relatively short period of time there were two such occurrences in a comparatively small territory, one may wonder whether these occasions are truly so "exceptional". If yes, the question may be raised, too, what kinds of special circumstances or eventual new forms of socio-political stresses may have played a role in their more frequent occurrence.

the soul(s) that left his body, thereby causing his sickness. As during such rituals, the soul(s) not only of the person in question but of all the participants are called back one after the other and fastened symbolically to their wrists, these *arô ruviêi* function as the *par excellence* ritual method of reaffirming social solidarity (see Vargyas 1998).

As for *yĩang* Sorsĩ himself, he did not receive a sacrifice, but he was invited and "present" during the whole ceremony. It was the special task of the head of the land-owning lineage "master of land" and traditional village chief, *achuaih* H., to secure him, holding without interruption throughout the full length of the ceremony the drinking straw of the jar containing rice-beer mixed with the blood of the sacrificed pigs and consecrated for the event. *Yĩang* Sorsĩ was thus supposed to assist in and preside over the ceremony from the jar in front of the sacrificial altar built for the purpose. The direct physical contact with this mightiest divinity made such a terrible impression on *achuaih* H. that he was literally shaking for many minutes;[11] a few days after the ceremony, he felt inevitable the organisation for himself of a second, personal *arô ruviêi,* recalling his soul, and thus reinforcing his mental and physical state.

Beyond the presence of *yĩang* Sorsĩ, two other circumstances gave a special overtone to the whole ceremony, during which first *achuaih* B., the alleged sorcerer and then the representatives of each of the 53 houses of the village (among them five rival shamans!), one after the other in a row, had to swear solemnly, in front of the whole community and taking *yĩang* Sorsĩ to testify that "they were not sorcerers", that "they had never committed such acts", and "if they should ever do so, they should die immediately", on the spot, due to his intervention. Some of the participants, while reciting the formula of the oath and drinking from the sacred liquid, even enacted the punishment they were to suffer in case they were lying and/or disobeying *yĩang* Sorsĩ: they fell down on the ground, rolling there in their "great pain". Moreover, the expected punishment transcended the present: it went down through four generations, to the sons', the grandsons', the great grandsons' and the great-great grandsons' generations—thus putting at risk the existence of the whole lineage. Who would dare to sin against one's descendants?

I hesitate as to how to name this ritual. Is it an oath or an ordeal? More than the former and less than the latter. True ordeals with trials of hot lead, boiling water and the like were not uncommon among the hill tribes of the Vietnamese Cordilleras (see Ner 1935). The Bru, however, do not seem to

[11] I was next to him and could well observe it, but he also told me later in detail about his feelings.

have practised them or, in any event, they have never talked about it. According to the literature, such cases of black magic or witchcraft accusations were typical occasions for traditional jurisprudence by ordeal. In his unique testimony on the topic, Ner explicitly states that the two go hand in hand and that such accusations are "the cause of almost all murders" since "any mortal accident, any illness is considered to be the result of the action of sorcerers" (Ner 1935, 14). In our case, the malediction formulae pronounced on all who would breach the norms of social solidarity point to the fact that even if this event was not a true ordeal in the strict sense of the word, the eventual possibility of an immediate supernatural repression exerted the same effect as is usual in the case of an ordeal having a strong refraining force. I shall come back to this point soon.

There is a second circumstance that makes this story so exceptional and fascinating. It is the fact that the representatives of the state machinery (policemen, secretaries of local communist party cells, presidents of local councils etc.), themselves ordinary Bru people, but perhaps a bit more learned and under stronger Vietnamese influence than is the average case, had to participate, or rather, to supervise it. I have photos of one of the local policemen crossing out the names, one after the other, from a list containing all the names of the family heads of the village, and we have also seen the preliminaries of the ceremony, the necessary "state" authorisation for its organisation.

This takes me to my last point. How is it possible that in a "communist" state, in a "rational" and "modern" legal system, witchcraft and sorcery accusations find acceptance? How are we to explain all the cases when in Khe Sanh, in the local headquarters, more or less learned representatives of the Vietnamese state imprison for several months some suspected or accused witches following an interrogation recorded with the help of a tape recorder hidden under the floor? How is it possible that while claiming not to be superstitious, they legitimatise "superstition"?

In my opinion, there is only one answer to this question. Vietnamese authorities know by practice what generations of anthropologists have pointed out since Evans-Pritchard's influential monograph on Azande witchcraft (Evans-Pritchard 1937); namely, that in many traditional and small-scale societies, witchcraft and sorcery are mechanisms of social control and expressions and resolutions of real social tensions and of interpersonal and/or intergroup conflicts.[12] Even if since then the other

[12] One-time French administrator, Mr Ner (1935, 14), who observed the ordeals resulting from witchcraft and magic accusations with the eyes of a civil servant whose task was to maintain social harmony, goes as far as to claim the *positive*

side of the coin has also been pointed out, and by now we are well aware of the fact that these accusations are just as much the *causes* of social tensions as the *resolutions* of them, that view could help us in understanding our case. Oath or ordeal, the aim of the ceremony was to re-establish social solidarity through the menace of superhuman jurisprudence.

However, when social cohesion is irrevocably broken, even measures such as these are inappropriate—fission in society is inevitable. As I found out later, many people feared *achuaih* B., *achuaih* H. himself included. Whatever the reason for this, and here, unfortunately, my data are far from sufficiently complete to indulge in any thorough sociological analysis, the fear was so pronounced that by the time of the oath/ordeal, a few families from the vicinity of *achuaih* B.'s house had moved out of the village. Though after the ceremony described above he recommenced shamanic practice, he was not really solicited any more. And, as I understood, the events went on along these lines later, too. Soon afterwards some more families left L. village, and the stigma of the sorcerer remained with the old man forever—notwithstanding the unique and very costly face-saving ceremony he had financed.

References

Eliade, Mircea. 1974. *Shamanism. Archaic techniques of Ecstasy.* New York, and London: Routledge and Kegan Paul. [Le chamanisme et les techniques archaïques de l'extase. Paris, Payot, 1951].

—. 2005. "Shamanism: An Overview (First Edition)." In *Encyclopedia of Religion.* (Second ed.), edited by Lindsay Jones, 8269–8274. New York: Macmillan. [1987].

Elkin, Adolphus Peter. 1977. *Aboriginal Men of High Degree.* Second ed. Reprinted, 1980. St. Lucia, Q.: University of Queensland Press. [Sydney: Australasian Pub. 1945].

Evans-Pritchard, Edward Evan. 1937. *Magic, Witchcraft and Oracle among the Azande.* Oxford: Clarendon Press.

---

effect of the ordeals, emphasising their great refraining force. I quote: "its menace alone is enough for the guilty to admit his sin or for the calumniator to take back his slander. It enables thus the involved parties to settle things and conclude discussions that would otherwise never end…" This is because "it is not the ordeal in itself which is harmful: it plays its normal role ending disputes since its results are accepted by both parties. *It is rather the belief in sorcerers that is the true and deep reason of social troubles which, in turn, is attenuated by the ordeals themselves…*" (Ner 1935, 14, italics added).

Harner, Michael. 1980. *The way of the shaman: A Guide to Power and Healing*. New York: Harper & Row Publishers.
Hoppál, Mihály 1994. *Sámánok. Lelkek és jelképek* [Shamans. Souls and symbols]. Budapest: Helikon.
Hultkrantz, Åke. 1984. "Shamanism and Soul Ideology." In *Shamanism in Eurasia* I., edited by Mihály Hoppál, 28–36. Göttingen: Herodot.
Charles. 1894. "Le pays des Tiem et des Moïs entre l'Annam Central et le Mékong. Région restituée par le traité de Bangkok du 3 octobre 1893." In *Le Laos Annamite,* 1–54. Plaquette de 86 pages. Paris: Callamet.
Ner, M. 1935. "Les ordalies en pay moï." *Cahiers d'EFEO* 4: 13–15.
Seymour-Smith, Charlotte. 1986. "Shamanism" In *Macmillan Dictionary of Anthropology,* London and Basingstoke: Macmillan Press Ltd.
Parnai O 1981. *Parnai O Tễ Yiang Sursĩ: Pún Atỡng Tễ Ngê Yê-su Crĩt* [The Bru Bible]. Tiếng Brũ. Vietnam: Kinh-Thánh Tân-Ước.
Vargyas, Gábor. 1998. Conjurer l'inéluctable. *Péninsule. Etudes interdisciplinaires sur l'Asie du Sud-Est Péninsulaire.* XXIXème année (37): 99–156.
—. 2004. "A brú sámánfejdísz [The Bru shamanic headdress]." In *Az idő rostájában. Tanulmányok Vargyas Lajos 90. születésnapjára* I–III., edited by Bertalan Andrásfalvy, Mária Domokos, and Ilona Nagy, II. 395–436. Budapest: L'Harmattan.
—. 2008. *Dacolva az elkerülhetetlennel. Egy közép-vietnami hegyi törzs, a brúk kultúrája és vallása. (Válogatott tanulmányok)* [Fighting with the ineluctable. Bru religion and culture. (Selected writings)]. Budapest: L'Harmattan.
Vitebsky, Piers. 1995. *The Shaman. Voyages of the Soul, Trance, Ecstasy and Healing from Siberia to the Amazon.* London: Macmillan in association with Duncan Baird Publishers. ("Living Wisdom").
Winkelmann, M. 2005. "Shamanism: An Overview (Further Considerations)." In *Encyclopedia of Religion*, edited by Lindsay Jones, 8274–8280. (Second Edition). New York: Macmillan Reference USA, Thomson Gale, 12. [1987].
Zago, Marcel. 1972. *Rites et cérémonies en milieu bouddhistes Lao.* Roma: Universitá Gregoriana Editrice.

THE QURAN, SPIRITS AND BIOENERGY: ON RELIGIOUS HEALING IN UZBEKISTAN

KRISZTINA KEHL-BODROGI

According to the renowned American psychiatrist and anthropologist, Arthur Kleinman, the various actions taken to restore health constitute a special health care system for each society, which will include concepts of diseases and their causes and the social norms that in turn guide the choice and evaluation of the appropriate therapy as well as the whole gamut of individuals and institutions participating in the healing process (Kleinman 1980, 24). Kleinman distinguishes three, co-existing and overlapping sectors in the health care systems of complex societies, which he calls (1) popular, (2) professional and (3) folk or traditional sectors of healing (Kleinman 1980, 49–60). In Kleinman's model, the popular sector encompasses the "management of the disease" within the family and the wider community; that is, the area of health care where the malady is first identified and the first steps of treatment are taken. The professional sector, on the other hand, refers to an officially approved and institutionalised health care system of a given society, today primarily based on Western type scientific medicine. Finally, the folk or traditional healing sector refers to non-institutionalised, unorganised areas of health care where knowledge of the disease and the measures to heal the disease are directly embedded in the local culture.

In the technologically and economically developed societies of the world, modern medicine has almost everywhere marginalised the traditional healing sectors, even if it has not eliminated them completely. That notwithstanding, under certain conditions, an upswing of interest in folk medicine and various "alternative" healing methods can be observed, the reasons for which can be found, among others, in dissatisfaction with the methods of modern medicine, in the eventual high costs of public health care services or in changes concerning the ideological orientation of the society in question.

The present study explores folk medicine based on the above-mentioned model, and its recent recovery in Uzbekistan in the period after the dissolution of the Soviet Union and the country's independence. The basis for the study is the data gathered during a total of nine months' anthropological fieldwork between 2004 and 2007 in the province of Khorezm, in the North-West of Uzbekistan. My research, supported by the Max Planck Research Institute for Social Anthropology in Halle, aimed to explore the religious life of Muslims in the light of post-socialist developments. Therefore, within the folk healing sector, the research focused on religious healing. By this term, I mean—in the footsteps of Doumato—all therapeutic practices which "are based on religious knowledge and performance and are acting concurrently", in order to restore any physical or mental state considered as illness (Doumato 2000, 36). Thus, healing practices such as herbal or osteopathic medicine, considered by the literature as the secular branch of folk medicine, fall out of the scope of this study. Nonetheless, we must mention that in Khorezm, as in many other parts of the world, the dividing line between secular and religious folk medicine is blurred, and methods used by healers classified in various categories in practice often overlap (cf. Kleinman 1980, 59).

Health care: Soviet and Post-Soviet developments

If we take Kleinman's model, until the first quarter of the twentieth century, the health care systems of Central Asia[1] were based almost exclusively on the popular and folk sectors. The development of the professional healing sector in the region started after the seizure of power by the Bolsheviks. In a very short time, the Soviet authorities had established a close network of hospitals, clinics and health centres in the countryside, functioning exclusively on the principles of modern medicine and providing the population with free medical care. This resulted in a significant increase in life expectancy and the general health of the population (Feshbach 1984, 82–84). The development of the health care system served also as a propaganda tool for the communists to advertise the ideology of Socialist modernisation in Central Asia (Michaels 2003). Propaganda campaigns encouraging the use of modern health care services involved the disparagement and repression of the traditional healing sector, claiming it to be a cluster of reactionary, superstitious and often dangerous practices and beliefs. In the Soviet Union, the only officially approved and permitted healing sector was the health care sector based on scientific medicine.

[1] I use the term to refer to the region including today's Kazakhstan, Kirgizstan, Uzbekistan, Turkmenistan and Tadzhikistan.

The population of Central Asia appreciated the achievements of modern medicine, and widely used the services of the official healthcare sector. Nevertheless, the negative judgement of the religious folk medicine by the official ideology was not uniformly accepted among the local population. Besides the various anti-religious propaganda leaflets and the reports within the Party, the ethnographic literature also provides ample evidence proving that when there was illness, the people often sought the help of folk healers, some of whom—even if secretly—continued their activities (Michaels 2003, 67; Ro'i 2000, 359; Saksonov 1984, 49–50).

The transformation processes following the dissolution of the Soviet Union and the independence of the Central Asian socialist republics[2] brought about the revival of the traditional healing sector and especially that of religious healing. As Pelkmans pertinently remarks, besides the existential uncertainty resulting from the severe economic crisis, the fact that many have lost their faith in the secular ideologies after the fall of Socialism contributed largely to the newfound popularity of religious healing (Pelkmans 2006, 21). All this was reinforced by the general decline of the professional health care sector. During my fieldwork, I had the chance to personally experience the shockingly bad conditions of the medical care in Uzbekistan. Here, as in the other new Central Asian states, the state-administered health care system introduced by the Soviet regime had remained basically intact; however, the infrastructure of the institutions and the quality of the services have severely deteriorated. It is a serious problem today that the standards of medical training are rapidly declining and the acquisition of medical degrees in exchange for money has become common practice. Technical equipment in hospitals and clinics is obsolete, and the supply of pharmaceuticals is extremely limited. The families of the patients have to buy their medications in the pharmacies or on the black market, and they also have to pay for the medical services despite the medical care allegedly being free. Remunerating medical care with illegal gratuities was already common practice in the Soviet era. Considering, however, the fact that since independence the economic situation of the population's majority has drastically deteriorated, today this practice means a much greater burden on the patient and the patient's family. Financial considerations often play a crucial part in the decision on the part of patients and their families to seek help from the folk healer rather than from the official health sector. As one of my informants, a seventy-three-year-old healer woman,

[2] Kazakhstan, Kirgizstan, Uzbekistan, Turkmenistan and Tadzhikistan gained their independence in 1991.

emphasised: "Many can't afford the doctors. They turn to me because I take what they can offer."

Since independence, there has been a significant change in behaviour towards the traditional health sector of the new states. Today, those of the political elite who want to prove their radical break from the Soviet ideology generally have a positive attitude towards all the religious and cultural traditions which had been judged and often banned by their predecessors. In Kazakhstan, for instance, the traditional healing methods, especially "shaman healing" that involves the help of spirits, have gained official recognition as parts of the cultural national heritage; moreover, today "Kazakh folk healing" has a prominent place on the curriculum of the capital's Centre for Medicine (Penkala-Gawęçka i. p.). Even though in Uzbekistan they do not invest in the traditional healing sector, and it is not regarded as an aspect of national identity, the authorities do accept the activities of the healers and do not disturb their practice.

To add to these factors, in the past two decades, the growing interest in religion has also contributed to the appreciation of religious healing, which can also be traced in the significant increase in the number of both the healers and their clients. For example, of the 22 healers I have come in closer contact with, only two practised their profession during the Soviet era, while the others only started their healing activities in the 1990s. Nevertheless, there are significant differences between the various kinds of religious healing in terms of the extent of the upsurge, just as the specialists working in each category do not enjoy the same unanimous recognition. The reputation of each healer is not permanent; it is a constant subject of evaluation among the other healers, the clients and the members of the wider social environment. Relatives and acquaintances pass on and discuss their experiences of the healers they have consulted; these personal accounts form the basis of the reputation and the credibility of any given healer; or in some cases, the disrepute of being a quack.

Religious healing and healers in Khorezm

Among the mostly Uzbek and Muslim population[3] of Khorezm, it is a widely accepted view that diseases can be of "natural" origin, but they can also occur due to supernatural interventions, like the evil eye *(yomon*

[3] Approximately 95% of the Khorezmian population claims to be Uzbek. Besides them, among others, there is a relatively low number of Turkmens, Russians, Tatars and "Uzbekicized" Persians; these last are the descendants of slaves seized from Iran in the nineteenth century.

go'z), bewitchment *(dava)* or possession by spirits *(jillilik)*.[4] According to this model, "natural" diseases are cured by professional doctors, and disorders arising from supernatural interference fall under the scope of healers. To know whether a certain condition belongs to one category or the other can often only be decided after having engaged both healing sectors. It is also common practice to seek the services of a fortune teller who has expertise in diagnostics. The fortune teller tries to tell by using various methods to ascertain whether a certain health problem falls within the area of expertise of the doctors or that of the healers. Most fortune tellers make their diagnosis by palpating the patient's pulse. As one of them explained to us, "if the pulse throbs backwards, the patient is certainly possessed by evil spirits." Others try to establish the source of the disease by randomly opening the *Quran* and interpreting the paragraphs on the page. The most famous fortune tellers are said to be able to make a diagnosis merely by looking at the patient.

Among my Khorezmian acquaintances, there were several who, in the event of a health problem, always went first to see a fortune teller or a healer. Most of them, however, only sought the help of the folk healing sector if the medical treatment turned out to be unsuccessful. It is especially common with chronic diseases that, in order to maximise the results, the patient visits the doctors at the clinic and the healers in parallel.

Nevertheless, before a family decision is made regarding which health sector to turn to, many people resort to a simple ritual anyone can perform, and which is meant to neutralise the effect of the supernatural forces that might have played a role in one of the family member's falling ill. It consists of taking a bunch of dry herbs known for their protective powers (*isvat*), which they light up in a specially designed frying pan exclusively used for this purpose and fumigating the patient with it while repeating religious formulae.[5] During my fieldwork, whenever I fell ill, my hosts performed the same ritual on me, saying that it didn't hurt, even if my symptoms were not caused by the evil eye or bewitchment, but only by a viral infection.

In Khorezm, the representatives of the folk healing sector can be categorised into different groups according to the therapeutic methods and legitimacy strategies they use; although in many cases the demarcation line between the different categories is blurred and the methods of the

---

[4] The words in parenthesis are in the official Latin spelling, which was introduced into Uzbekistan in 2005, after the abolition of the Cyrillic alphabet.

[5] Fumigation against the evil eye and bewitchment is a common defence method among the Arabs as well, see Spooner 1970, 317–8.

different healers overlap. The Khorezmians have only an exclusive term for the *spirit healers*, all the other healers are called *tabib.*

Most Khorezmians consider healing activity to be a vocation which cannot be voluntarily chosen, just as they believe that the knowledge necessary for the job cannot be learned through individual efforts. On the contrary, they consider the ability to heal a gift from God, or from supernatural creatures acting on God's commission (spirits, long deceased Muslim saints), only bestowed upon chosen people. This gift—of which the chosen person is informed during a dream vision—cannot be refused without getting into serious, often mortal danger.

One of the culturally acknowledged ways of becoming a healer is the "initiation sickness". Most of the healers I questioned emphasised that when the "calling" reached them in their dreams, they were suffering from some kind of a disease themselves that the doctors were unable to cure. The symptoms usually appeared as frequent fainting and partial paralysis, which all disappeared at once as soon the patient accepted his/her status as a healer. Looking back, my informants described their sicknesses as a coercive force that ensured that they accept their vocation. They also underlined that they could not give up their profession without falling sick again. Being called upon in a dream and the sickness preceding the acceptance of the vocation was considered indispensable even if the profession was inherited from an ancestor.[6] In this case, it is the spirit of the ancestor who calls on the chosen descendant to follow the vocation of healing in a dream vision experienced during a sickness.

The initiation sickness, which can only be overcome by accepting the vocation of healing, is a common trait of the profession of healing with the help of spirits in all of Central Asia and Siberia, and which is mostly referred to as "shaman healing" in the literature. The fact that in Central Asia, and thus in Khorezm as well, it is not only the spirit healers, but also members of other folk healing categories who follow this cultural pattern only confirms the overlapping between the healing traditions of the region (cf. Bellér-Hann 2008, 404).

---

[6] Among the twenty-two healers, the narratives of whom I have recorded, ten claimed their vocation to be a family heritage.

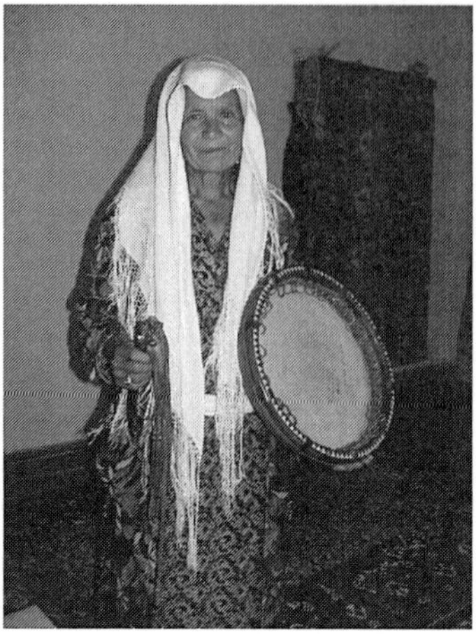

Fig. 1. *Folbin* with a drum and a whip, 2005. Photo by Krisztina Kehl-Bodrogi.

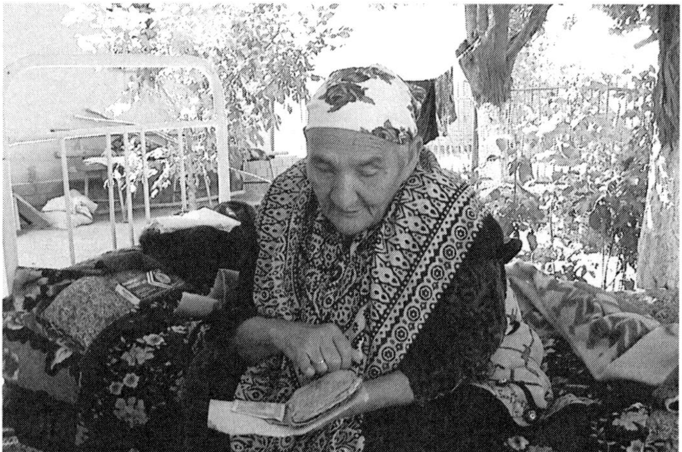

Fig. 2. *Folbin* during divination, 2004.
Photo by Krisztina Kehl-Bodrogi.

The spirit healers

In Khorezm, the spirit healers, that is, the specialists who seek the services of spirits in their therapeutic practice, are usually called *folbin*s.[7] The word is formed from the contraction of the Arabic *fal* ("fate") and the Persian *bin* (etymon of the verb "to see") and means *fortune teller*; the term is an exclusive denotation of people who practise divination. In the northern parts of the province, the spirit healers are called *parixon*, a term used also among the neighbouring Turkmens. The word, of Persian origin, denotes people who, during the healing ritual, invoke the help of a special group of spirits, the *pari*.[8] In Khorezm, as is usual in Central Asia, the services of spirit healers are mostly sought in cases of psychological or mental disorders, but people also turn to them to heal barrenness and other health problems blamed on evil spirits or black magic. Furthermore, some *folbin*s are also fortune tellers: this activity includes diagnostic prediction, but also the tracing of lost objects or predicting the outcome of a planned business venture.

According to popular beliefs, the *folbin*s are in personal contact with the spirits, who support them in their healing and in their predictions, and in return, they ask for obedience. Nineteenth- and twentieth-century ethnographic literature provides numerous examples of the widespread idea in Central Asia that the *pari* (or in the Islamic demonology the *djinni*) often have sexual relations with the men and women who were chosen by them and whom they invest with healing powers in return for obedience and faithfulness.[9] While it is still an accepted view that the chosen people cannot refuse the relationship, the sexual factor is currently barely part of the healers' narratives or of the general concepts of them. Among my informants, only one *folbin* referred to this detail, as in calling her helping spirit her husband and life partner, emphasising that she cannot do anything without his approval. Besides the *pari,* the Muslim saints also play an important role in healing; which shows the strong influence of Islam on spirit healing in past centuries.

The most typical healing ritual of the *folbin*s is the *o'yin*, the "game" or "dance", during which "the healer forces the evil spirit to dance and to immediately leave the body of the possessed patient" (Bellér-Hann 2000, 643). I witnessed during an *o'yin* in the summer of 2005 the workings of a

---

[7] Outside of Khorezm the spirit healers are usually called *baxshi.*

[8] The *pari* are well-known characters in Persian mythology; outside Central Asia they also play a role in the beliefs of the Muslim population of Asia Minor.

[9] Regarding the *folbin*s Snesarev (2003, 25, 36–7) had already recorded similar ideas in the 1940s.

healer in her fifties, Malika, who solicited her helping spirits by singing and drumming, calling upon the *pari* and the Muslim saints by name.[10] While chanting, she was circling faster and faster around the patient who was sitting on the ground under a white veil. After a while, the other participants in the ritual—the female relatives of the patient, six people altogether—also joined the "dance": they started to circle around the patient as well, holding hands, while rhythmically yelling to Allah and leaning back and forth to the rhythm of the drum. Meanwhile, Malika continued her "game" walking round the outer circle. From time to time, she held her drum close to the women's chests and lightly patted them with it. An hour later, Malika pulled the veil off the woman suffering from psychological disorders, and by yelling "Go away!" she asked the spirits possessing her to leave. As Malika later explained, the spirits leaving the body of the patient at the end of the "game" are caught and tied up by her helping spirits and taken to the desert where they let them go. According to other healers, the *pari* deliver the evil spirits to a Muslim saint who disables them. In Khorezm, it is Yusuf Hamadani—whose alleged grave is the most popular pilgrimage site of the province—who has the reputation of being the most efficient ghost exterminator.

According to my informants, the *o'yin* is only performed in case of severe psychological and mental disorders. For the sake of the recovery from being possessed, they repeat the ritual three or four times within a forty-day period, during which the patient cannot leave the house. If they consider the patient to be liable to hurt himself/herself or others they tie him/her up for the ritual, but sometimes they keep the patient chained down for 40 days. They say that if the exorcism is successful, the chains come off by themselves on the fortieth day.[11]

In the first half of the twentieth century, it often happened that the healers, as a proof of their supernatural powers, exercised ecstatic performances during the *o'yin*. The ethnographic data confirm that the Khorezmian *folbin*s sometimes walked on hot cinders, licked hot iron or stood on the blade of a sword without showing any sign of pain (Snesarev 2003, 42; Zadykhina 1952, 413). All this, however, is now in the past, just as "making the spirits dance" is also a rarity nowadays. Today there are

[10] For a detailed description of the *o'yin* and the texts of the spirit-invoking songs, see Kehl-Bodrogi (2008, 199–208).

[11] A similar procedure is still applied at the graves of saints. At some pilgrimage sites, the "frantic" patient is chained down for forty days in a windowless room, in the hope that on the intervention of the saint, they will recover and the chains will fall off. Shortly before my first visit to Khorezm, a similar case at the pilgrimage site dedicated to the saint Yusuf Hamadani ended in the death of the patient.

relatively few *folbin*s who have the necessary knowledge to perform an *o'yin.* During my fieldwork, I only met six *folbin*s who were able to "make the spirits dance" in the above-described manner. The information they provided also leads to the conclusion that the number of *folbin*s who can heal in the traditional way is very limited in Khorezm.

Nowadays, the *folbin*s resort mostly to simpler rituals in their practice, like the *alas*, during which they try to exorcise the spirits with fire, or to neutralise the assumed bewitchment on the patient. The healer takes a piece of cloth soaked in gasoline attached to a stick (the "flag") and sets it on fire which the healer carries around the patient while repeating magic formulae, thumping the back of the patient three times every now and then and demanding the maleficent forces to leave. Finally, the patient has to jump three times over the burning "flag" thrown to the ground.

There is also a ritual in the *folbin*s' repertoire in which the healer pours the blood of a freshly killed animal (chicken or lamb) on the patient. This gesture is based on the idea that the spirits leave the patient at the smell of blood, which provides an opportunity for the helping spirits of the healer to catch the possessor spirits and obliterate them. On other occasions, the *folbin,* while chanting spirit-invoking songs, strikes the patient's body with a whip in order to drive out the spirits. Moreover, most of the *folbin*s apply a series of treatment methods which public opinion rather relates to the activities of the *tabib*s, presented below.

In Khorezm, as in many other places of the world, the social situation of the individuals renowned for having relations with supernatural creatures is quite controversial. Thus, if someone turns to a certain *folbin* to cast off a presumed bewitchment, one can never be sure that it was not, in fact, the healer himself who sent the bewitchment on the request of another client. The connection between healing and bewitchment is based on the conviction that "possessing the knowledge of the proper healing solution already implies the maleficent use of the same knowledge" (Lambek 1993, 237). Since the *folbin*s I consulted were all aware of the suspicions surrounding their personas, they all insisted on establishing at our first encounter that they never used their connections to the universe of spirits to do wrong to others. The decline of the profession's prestige also shows in the fact that, while in the past there were both women and men to be found among the *folbin*s in Khorezm, today it is almost exclusively women who work in the field (cf. Snesarev 2003, 36; Zadykhina 1952, 413).

The tabibs

The term *tabib,* meaning "doctor" in Arabic, is used in a very wide sense in Khorezm. This, similar to the observations made by Bruce Privratsky in Kazakhstan, "reveals the diffusive nature of the Muslim healers' profession" (Privratsky 2001, 193). A specialist, for instance, who is labelled as a *tabib,* can be an osteopath or a naturopath. Furthermore, the Khorezmians put everyone in the category of *tabib*s who heal by the laying on of hands and/or by reciting the *Quran*. Islamic religious law also recognises the method of reciting the *Quran* as a legitimate treatment for the evil eye, bewitchment and possession; therefore, it might also be applied by the official representatives of the religion. Thus, the healers who in their therapeutic practices (also) involve the *Quran* are often called *molla*, regardless of whether they fulfil the religious responsibilities inherent to this title or not. Moreover, some of the healers known as *tabib*s provide handmade amulets for the people who turn to them, and they too often work as fortune tellers.

The "laying on of hands" is a relatively recent method in local healing, which spread in Khorezm through the influence of the "transcendent" healing which became particularly popular after the dissolution of the Soviet Union. This method is nowadays often part of the therapeutic practices of the *folbin*s. According to my acquaintances, the explanation for the effectiveness of the laying on of hands is that certain healers possess the power of *bioenergy (biotok)*, a term which entered the Uzbek language from the vocabulary of Russian parapsychology. Some of the healers also tried to convince me during our discussions that the bioenergy in their possession had also been demonstrated with scientific experiments. Apparently, the bioenergy of one *tabib* was detected by a delegation of doctors sent by UNESCO with the help of sensitive instruments. According to another healer, she underwent the same examination on behalf of the delegation of the Tashkent Health Ministry, also with positive results.

It is obvious that the bioenergy concept is used by the healers and their clients as a modernising etiquette, the task of which is to confirm the scientific nature of the therapies applied. Nevertheless, the ideas concerning the nature of the bioenergy all stem from traditional healing concepts. Instead of interpreting the phenomenon in the usual (pseudo-)scientific way as the connection of energy transfer and magnetic fields, for my Khorezmian acquaintances, the *biotok* is nothing other than the "divine power" the healers were invested with in their dreams by the supernatural creatures.

In most cases, however, the healers known as *tabib*s use different combinations of methods, while it is hard to find two specialists who would have an identical way of performing each element. These healers use variations of the traditional methods according to their skills and personal attitudes, as is well illustrated in the exemplary cases presented below.

Abdullah: fortune teller and Quran healer

Abdullah was known as a "powerful" healer even outside of his village, and was around 45 years old when I went to see him in the summer of 2005 with an acquaintance of mine who had already sought his services on several occasions. According to my acquaintance, Abdullah earned his reputation by successfully casting off bewitchments, and healing fevers and epilepsy. The *tabib* received us in one of the rooms in his home reserved for healing. According to Uzbek custom, he was sitting on the floor, a little table in front of him with his healing instruments: a copy of the *Quran* covered with a cloth, a stack of blank pieces of paper and a pen. As he told us, and as my acquaintance later confirmed based on his personal experience, Abdullah usually first takes the *Quran* in his hands. With his eyes closed, he points at a section on a randomly opened page of the Holy Book, from which he establishes the nature of his visitor's problem without their having said a word. In order to cure the thus diagnosed problem, Abdullah recites a couple of suras from the *Quran* by heart; then he blows three times onto the patient to reinforce the healing effect of his words.[12] Next, he takes one of the stacks of papers and writes a magical formula in Arabic upon it, which, according to the instructions, the patient has to burn as soon as he/she get home and to drink the ashes of it mixed in water. The locals also turn to Abdullah to find lost or stolen objects. As many of my acquaintances in the village confirmed, in these cases too the *tabib* reaches out to the *Quran*, while the magic words he writes on the piece of paper are meant to help to find the lost objects.

Yusup: naturopath and exorcist

Besides healing "natural" diseases with herbs, Yusup, a man in his fifties, also performed spirit exorcism. Since, as he claimed, he does not possess the gift of diagnostic prediction, he works together with a fortune teller

[12] The healing power of the saliva spat out after having recited the *Quran* is generally acknowledged in Islam. See Doumato 2000, 131–46.

woman, who is able to establish the cause of the disease. If the diagnosis implies spirit possession, Yusup first circles the patient in the presence of his/her relatives. He draws up a magical circle, through which he prevents the spirits from leaving that circle and thus harming the people present. Then Yusup steps next to the patient lying on the floor and starts reciting suras from the *Quran*. Meanwhile, he flicks both of his palms with force over the patient's body, downwards from the head, as if he was pulling the spirits out of it, shaking them off his hands each time at the feet of the patient. He repeats these gestures until a shrilling pain in his arms signals that the spirits have left the body and moved into his. After a short while, the spirits—in Yusup's words—leave him through his mouth with a hissing sound and fly off in the air.

Yusup, like most of the healers, practises his profession either at home, or—in severe cases—at the home of the patient; besides the healer and the patient, a few relatives of the latter are also usually present at the event. Like everywhere in Central Asia, it used to be customary in Khorezm as well for the healer to receive the patients next to the tombs of healing saints, basically in public.[13] With folk healing forced into illegality, this practice disappeared almost entirely in the Soviet era. Since the dissolution of the Soviet Union, however, parallel to the spectacular revival of pilgrimages,[14] this tradition has also slowly been on the rise. Besides the fortune tellers at the Holy sites, the healers have also reappeared, who try to help the people who turn to them with simple, short practices (laying on of hands, prayer).

The most famous and most charismatic healer of Khorezm, To'xtavoy, also keeps up the tradition of healing at the holy graves. In only a couple of years, this former truck driver managed to establish a healing centre next to the tomb of a long-forgotten saint that patients visit from all around Uzbekistan. During my repeated visits between 2004 and 2007, I had the opportunity to observe this healing complex in operation.

To'xtavoy: a new saint?

The story of how To'xtavoy became a healer follows more or less the patterns of what the tradition requires from *tabib*s. According to his own

[13] According to popular belief, the healing power attributed to Muslim saints continues its effectiveness at the graves of the saints. Thus, the legitimacy of healing at pilgrimage sites is further increased by the proximity of the saints buried near the site.

[14] Regarding the post-Soviet revival of the tradition of pilgrimages to holy graves in Uzbekistan, see Kehl-Bodrogi 2006.

account and those of his followers, one night, To'xtavoy got stuck in the sand with his truck near to an abandoned cemetery; they could not get him out of there, not even with the tractor sent to help him. In his dream, a saint came to him, who told him to build a new tomb instead of the old which had already disappeared without a trace. If he promised to do so, the saint would give him the gift of healing powers. To'xtavoy reassured him that as soon as his financial situation allowed, he would fulfil his request. To'xtavoy was from there on under the protection of the saint, which was confirmed the following morning when he managed to free his truck from the desert sand without any difficulty. They did not have to wait long for the subsequent miracle. Not long after the dream experience, a paralysed man started to walk and a mentally confused person regained his sanity at the bare touch of To'xtavoy's hand.

As the reputation of his healing powers spread, more and more people came to visit him. To'xtavoy gave up his former job and dedicated himself completely to his new vocation. In two years, he was able to gather enough money to raise a majestic mausoleum for the saint. The marble imbedded building decorated with gilded ornaments shortly became the most visited pilgrimage site in Khorezm, which further increased the popularity of the healer. After a while, To'xtavoy and his family moved permanently to the premises of the cemetery, far from any populated area, where in a few years he established a huge "health centre". In 1998 he extended the existing complex with a monumental mosque; the establishment included, besides the *türbe* and a building serving the purpose of mass healing, the healing residence, an office building and two "hospitals" providing accommodation for over a hundred people. The kitchen providing for the patients is under the supervision of To'xtavoy's female relatives, but the resident patients also help with the everyday tasks related to the maintenance of the centre. All in all, the complex, with its buildings and its wooded parks, exuberant flowerbeds and artificial lake, gives the impression of a sanatorium for the visitors.

With the increase in the number of patients, To'xtavoy soon switched to group healing. During my visits, he held "séances" (a term used by him and his clients) twice on weekdays and three times on weekends. In the summer, there are often three or four hundred people present at the weekend séances, many accompanied by their relatives. During my visits, I met several former patients, carpenters, locksmiths and whittlers among them, who, as a sign of gratitude for their recovery, come back every year to To'xtavoy for a shorter or longer period of time to help out in the continuous expansion. This work is considered as a good deed in God's eye (*savop*), which will positively influence their judgement on the Day of Resurrection.

The séance, the duration of which is two to three hours depending on the number of participants, consists of two major parts and the procedure is as follows: To'xtavoy enters the building reserved for the séance at a given moment, where the participants have already taken their seats on the floor on the pillows placed in rows. He sits behind the small table facing the rows of participants and starts reciting. For one hour, the only thing we hear in the big hall with a capacity to seat up to four hundred people is the healer's voice reciting with short interruptions the same one short text (according to general belief, it is a sura from the *Quran*) over and over again. Then To'xtavoy steps up to the patients and puts his hands on their heads, one after the other; he strokes their body with his hands while mumbling incomprehensible words, and finally thumps them hard on the back. Meanwhile, he stops from time to time to deliver a short sermon in which he usually calls upon the participants to keep to religious requirements and abstain from sorcery, which in Islam is considered to be a sin.

These sermons are to confirm that the healer is a good Muslim and to divert any suspicion of To'xtavoy using his powers to harm others. To'xtavoy places a particular emphasis on demonstrating his pious Muslim side, which is also shown by the mosque added to the complex, and by the fact that the healer has also financed the construction of another mosque at a pilgrimage site a few kilometres further away. As a legacy to To'xtavoy, the mosque finished in 2007 is named after him. Moreover, To'xtavoy is also careful to hold ritual prayers five times a day and to follow Muslim eating restrictions, something which he explicitly emphasised during our discussions. He also expects his patients to perform the ritual cleaning required by Islam before the séances. These efforts can (also) be interpreted as a legitimation strategy to fend off attacks by Islamic "fundamentalists" in the religious healing sector of independent Uzbekistan.

The success of this strategy is shown by the fact that contrary to most representatives of the religious healing sector, the Khorezmian religious elite recognises To'xtavoy as a "proper" Islamic healer. Among his patients, there are many who claim that they would never turn to *folbin*s or *tabib*s because, unlike To'xtavoy, they apply methods that are against Islamic law. According to them, the success of To'xtavoy's healing is due to the *Quran*'s healing power and not his. Many of the visitors, however, see some kind of medium in To'xtavoy, through whom the healing power of the nearby resting saint takes effect. For them, the fact that he practises his profession on the premises of a sanctuary—which folk belief considers to possess healing powers *per se*—strengthens the effectiveness of his therapeutic practices. Others believe that To'xtavoy is a saint himself who is capable of healing thanks to the miracle-working power (*karamat*) he possesses as a divine gift. I have also spoken to people who are convinced that To'xtavoy is assisted by helping spirits; moreover, some even claim to have seen these spirits during the séances.

As far as he is concerned, the source of his healing power is the saint appearing in a dream vision, and the fact that he practises his vocation next to a holy grave shows that To'xtavoy is unequivocally relying on models rooted in the local culture. His healing séances, however, draw upon various traditions. While reciting the *Quran* is one of the most important elements in classical religious healing, transmitting the healing power via the touch of the hand is a typical component of folk religion, especially of the cult of saints, which is nonetheless rejected by the normative branch of Islam. Regarding their form, the séances reflect the influence of the transcendent healing performances, which are currently highly popular in Russia, and which, via media broadcast, are widely known in Uzbekistan as well. Besides his charismatic personality, the extraordinary popularity of To'xtavoy lies above all in the combination of traditional and modern elements applied in his séances, which help him to engage and serve individuals of different needs and of different world views.

Religious healing: revival and rejection

In Khorezm, like everywhere in Uzbekistan, the revival of religious healing after the dissolution of the Soviet Union is taking place amidst contradictory ideological processes. On the one hand, the rupture with Soviet ideology and the new nation-building politics lead to the valorisation of a series of traditions considered as part of the national cultural heritage, including the local forms of religious healing. In Khorezm for instance, the practice of fending off harmful supernatural forces with fire and drums is considered by the local cultural and political elite as the heritage of the old Iranian religion, Zoroastrianism, prevailing before the rise of Islam.[15] On the other hand, one of the most characteristic phenomena accompanying the post-socialist transformations was the remarkable resurgence in the interest in Islam. During the dissolution of

[15] Khorezm is usually considered as the place of creation of the *Avesta.* As the regional heritage of Khorezm, they have dedicated an entire museum to the *Avesta* in the capital of the province.

the Soviet Union, some of the movements and trends gained strength, launching a fight against popular Islam in the name of a universal Islam which exclusively acknowledges the *Quran* and the prophetic traditions. The age-old characteristics of the local religious life, like the cult of the saints, the domestic rituals aiming to neutralise the harmful supernatural forces, and above-described various forms of religious healing (with the exception of reciting the *Quran*) are all considered by these puritan protectors of Islam as pagan elements which have to be purged from the Islamic religion.

In Khorezm, contrary to some other provinces of Uzbekistan, the doctrines of normative Islam in the narrow sense have found relatively few followers. Even today, the vast majority of Khorezmians do not keep strictly to religious regulations. Nevertheless, in the first years of independence, under the influence of a particularly active Islamic propaganda, a part of the population had a critical attitude towards certain traditions, which was also manifested in the general opinion of the various forms of religious healing. There were many among my acquaintances who judged negatively the activities of the *folbin*s, arguing that cooperating with spirits is considered a sin in Islam. Contrary to these arguments, those who have sought the services of spirit healers, or who hoped to gain recovery at the holy sites, all referred to the traditions, emphasising that it is an integral part of their Muslim identity, that is, of the Muslim lifestyle rooted in traditions. Nonetheless, the form of healing exercised by the *folbin*s shows a significantly lower upswing than the healing methods based on reciting the *Quran*. As To'xtavoy's example well illustrates, the religious healers can best earn unanimous recognition if they manage to convincingly create an aura of a "correct" Islam without giving up the ways of the traditional legitimacy.

In conclusion, the contemporary upswing of religious healing cannot be regarded as the mere revival of traditions under post-socialist circumstances. Nowadays in Khorezm, as the adaptation of mass healing with the laying on of hands and of the concept of bioenergy demonstrates, religious healing includes both reconstructed traditions and new methods and interpretations.

References

Bellér-Hann, Ildikó. 2000. "Uyghur-healers." In *An Encyclopedia of World Beliefs, Practices, and Culture Shamanism*, edited by Mariko N. Walter, and Eva J. N. Fridman, 642–6. Oxford: ABC-Clio.

—. 2008. *Community Matters in Xinjiang 1880–1949. Towards a historical anthropology of the Uyghur*. Leiden: Brill.
Doumato, Eleanor Abdella. 2000. *Getting God's Ear. Women, Islam, and Healing in Saudi Arabia and the Gulf.* New York: Columbia University Press.
Feshbach, Murray. 1984. "Soviet Health Problems." *Proceedings of the Academy of Political Science* 35: 81–97.
Kehl-Bodrogi, Krisztina. 2006. "Who owns the shrine? Competing meanings and Authorities at a Pilgrimage Site in Khorezm." *Central Asia Survey* 25 (3): 235–50.
—. 2008: *"Religion is not so strong here". Muslim Religious Life in Khorezm after Socialism*. Berlin: LIT Verlag.
Kleinman, Arthur. 1980. *Patients and Healers in the Context of Culture. An Exploration of the Borderland between Anthropology, Medicine, and Psychiatry*. Berkeley: University of California Press.
Lambek, Michael. 1993. *Knowledge and Practice in Mayotte. Local Discourses of Islam, Sorcery, and Spirit Possession*. Toronto, Buffalo, and London: University of Toronto Press.
Michaels, Paula. 2003. *Curative Powers: Medicine and Empire in Stalin's Central Asia.* Pittsburgh: University of Pittsburgh Press.
Pelkmans, Mathijs. 2006. "Establishing Credibility: Secular legacies and new spiritual realities in post-Soviet Kyrgyzstan." Paper presented at the conference "The social dimensions of understanding illness and healing: Islamic societies from Africa to Central Asia", Orientwissenschaftliches Zentrum der Martin-Luther Universität, Halle/S, 31 March–1 April.
Penkala-Gaweçka, Danuta. [i. p.]: "Rebirth of Tradition: Recruitment of Spiritual Healers in Contemporary Kazakhstan." Manuscript (by courtesy of the author).

BENEDICTIONS SERVING EARLY MODERN BENEDICTINE MEDICINE

DÁNIEL BÁRTH

The aim of the medieval and early modern benediction practices was basically to satisfy the everyday needs of believers with some kind of special tool set (Franz 1909; Thomas 1971, 25–50; Kieckhefer 1989, 69–75; Pócs 2002; Jensen 2007). It was the expressed needs of the believers that formed the circumstances of offering benedictions, most of them of agricultural character (Veit 1936, 164; Scribner 1987, 6). Besides the benedictions related to agricultural work, from the beginning, the sacramentals targeting people and their physical problems were also present (Franz 1909, II. 399–513). Among these, the most considerable in terms of recognition, significance and spectacular use is the exorcism performed to expel demonic possession (Franz 1909, II. 514–615; Bárth 2008).[1] Other than the great exorcisms, however, there is little mention in the literature of the Church's medicinal practices with regard to the treatment of specific diseases not necessarily of demonic origin along with the performing of smaller rituals.[2] In the following, we intend to shed light on the contours of these practices by presenting the relevant data of an extremely significant, though so far unprocessed, Hungarian source.

The variety and thematic diversity of benedictions in the centuries preceding clerical Enlightenment at the end of the eighteenth century testify to the regular use of a veritable "arsenal of benedictions" within the Western (Catholic) Church. Even though with the publication of the *Rituale Romanum* (ROM 1614), after the Council of Trent (1545–1563), one could, on the one hand, observe on an official, diocesan level, the

[1] The most significant early modern exorcist handbooks contain numerous short benedictions. These sacramentals could be applied at exorcisms or independently. To illustrate the assertions in my study I have used the following manuals: FD 1697; FuD 1697; Stampa 1605; Eynatten 1626.

[2] In the respective chapter of Franz's work he discusses in detail the benedictions against fever, eye disease and epilepsy. Furthermore, he briefly mentions the clerical treatments to cure gout and bleeding, Franz 1909, II. 467–513.

partial restriction of benediction practices and the strengthening of central supervision. On the other, one could expect the "semi-official" survival or even improvement of such activities, especially as part of monastic pastoral practices. These cases of survival in typically Catholic parts of Europe are dated from different time periods. These early modern books of benedictions, which were at most "tolerated" on an official level, but definitely not supported, overlap significantly in terms of content; the mechanism of these collections can be mostly considered as a compilation with regards to local characteristics (Bárth 2007).[3]

When assembling the early modern Hungarian sources of benediction practices, it was a felicitous turn of events when after having found, mostly printed, Jesuit and Franciscan collections, we unexpectedly came upon a manuscript of a Benedictine collection, also written in Hungary (for the different stages of the research, see Bárth 2004; 2006; 2007; the most significant printed benediction books of Hungarian origin: FT 1739; FB 1749; AD 1774).[4] Besides a few rituals of the order, the liturgical book from the end of the seventeenth century entitled *Sacra arca benedictionum magni fundatoris religionum patriarchae Benedicti* mostly contains benedictions. The detailed presentation and the analysis of the book's content is the task of another, considerably larger study. In this present study—relating to the theme of this book—we only explore the benedictions which refer directly to medicinal practice. Before beginning, however, it seems necessary to outline the content of the manuscript and the history of its making.

* * *

The liturgical book was written and is currently kept at the Benedictine Pannonhalma Archabbey[5] where one of the monks—shrouded in

---

[3] The early modern European "alternative" benediction handbooks processed during the research and applied for the comparative perspective of this present study are the following: FRA 1685; MB 1685; Cochem 1692; Nucleus 1706; LT 1709.

[4] Here I would like to thank my friend Tamás Dénesi who as an archivist in Pannonhalma has brought this very important source—highly relevant to my research topic—to my attention. I am also grateful to the prior of Pannonhalma, Cirill T. Hortobágyi for letting me examine the benediction book and for lending me his notes on the source, which were especially useful during the biological identification of certain plants. Finally, I would like to thank Archabbot Asztrik Várszegi for giving his consent to the publication of the photocopies of the source.

[5] Pannonhalmi Főapátsági Könyvtár (Library of Pannonhalma Archabbey, hereafter: PFK) BKA 6.

anonymity—transcribed it into a book of 59 folios, 297x194 mm in size (Szabó 1981, 22). He finished his work on April 3, 1697. Since the hand transcribing the text did not write cursively, it would be hard to identify the author. There were approximately twenty monks living that year in the abbey under the leadership of Archabbot Placid Lendvay.[6] Many of them left written traces for posterity; the monk especially productive in Pannonhalma in this regard was Bonifác Lancsics (1674–1737) (on the personality and the works of Lancsics, see Gulyás 2006). It is interesting to note that Lancsics started to write his book for medical purposes (*Libellus Medicinalis pro diversis morbis curandis vel vitandis*...), also a manuscript, in the same year, 1697.[7]

Besides the uncertainty concerning the identity of the author, and a not very informative note in the text ("*Haec collecta sunt ex auctoribus orthodoxis...per quemdam fratrem professum ad S. Martinum Sacri Montis Pannoniae*"), the manuscript also fails to reveal the direct sources of the book of benedictions. As regards the rituals related to the life of monks, they mention just once (f. 12v) that it is based on the book of rituals of the order ("*ex Monastico Coeremoniali Ordinis S. P. N. Benedicti desumpta*"). There is also another ritual concerning the profession of a vow (f. 15v)—irrelevant to our topic—which is obviously the copy of an earlier *ordo* written in 1675; moreover, the petition formula mentions the name of the then archabbot Egyed Gencsy (1630–1684). In the matter of the origins of the benediction and exorcist texts, we can only rely on assumptions and present late medieval and early modern analogies.

Regarding the use of the liturgical book, it is the sections from the later eighteenth century on the last two folios of the book (58r–59v) that tell us the most. On the one hand, they continue the text without any transition and explanation; on the other hand, they engage in polemics with the previous sections (especially concerning the "new" ritual of rosary blessing). The last entry of benediction was in 1778. These late entries, however, provide convincing arguments proving that the liturgical book of our study was in use in the eighteenth century—presumably until the 1786 dissolution of the order.

---

[6] I estimated the approximate number based on the list of names of the old order history, Molnár Sz. 1906, 677–81. The same assumption is made by Hervay 2003, 341. Regarding the Archabbey under the direction of Placid Lendvay (1693–1699), see the history of the Order of Pannonhalma and the comprehensive summaries of the era: Szakály 1996; Molnár A. 1996.

[7] The medicinal book (current register number: PFK BK^{+} 13/3.) was undiscovered at the beginning of the twentieth century, therefore the author of the order's history could only infer its content: Molnár Sz. 1906: 605.

The content outline of the manuscript is as follows:

1. ff. 2r–4v. Forma induendi infantes pro voto
1. a. f. 2v. Benedictio cinguli
2. ff. 4v–5v. Benedictio ad exuendum puerum vel puellam completo tempore voti
3. ff. 5v–6r. Benedictio rosariorum
4. ff. 6r–12v. Benedictio numismatum et crucum sanctissimi patris nostri Benedicti
4. a. ff. 9r–9v. Benedictio olei simplicis
5. ff. 12v–15r. Formula renovationis votorum in festo Circumcisionis domini nostri Jesu Christi ex monastic coeremoniali ordinis sanctissimi patris nostri Benedicti desumpta
6. ff. 15v–19v. Forma profitendi sub beatissimi patris nostri Benedicti regula
7. ff. 19v–21r. Ordo generaliter absolvendi fratres in capitulo feria secunda post dominicam primam Quadragesimae
8. ff. 21r–21v. Ordo observandus caeremoni(alis)…(excommunicationis)
9. ff. 21v–22r. Benedictio incensi
10. ff. 22r–22v. Benedictio ruttae (sic!) contra veneficia doemoniaca
11. f. 22v. Benedictio herbarum in festo et octava Assumptionis B. V. Mariae
12. ff. 22v–23r. Benedictio animalium tempore pestis
13. ff. 23r–23v. Benedictio salis qui datur animalibus
14. ff. 23v–24r. Benedictio avenae vel hordei in festo sancti Stephani protomartyris quod datur animalibus
15. f. 24r. Benedictio novi fontis
16. f. 24v. Benedictio ad quodcunque comestibile
17. ff. 24v–25r. Benedictio quarumcunque rerum
18. f. 25r. Benedictio communis ad omnia
19. ff. 25r–27v. Exorcismus domus a malis spiritibus vexatae
20. ff. 28r–32v. Exorcismus contra imminentem tempestatem fulgurum et grandinum
21. f. 32v. Benedictio candelarum extra solemnitatem beatissimae virginis Mariae purificationem
22. ff. 32v–36v. Benedictio salis et aquae
23. ff. 36v–37r. Benedictio vini ad sanandum maleficiatos et venefic[iat]os
24. ff. 37r–37v. Benedictio rutae et salviae
25. ff. 37v–38r. Benedictio olei, camphorae et cardi pro potione
26. f. 38r. Sequitur benedictio suffitus circa maleficiatos
26. a. f. 38v. Benedictio sulphuris
26. b. ff. 38v–39r. Benedictio myrhae
26. c. ff. 39r–39v. Benedictio thuris
26. d. f. 39v. Benedictio camphorae
26. e. ff. 39v–40r. Benedictio lavendularum, rosarum, cariophilorum

26. f. f. 40r. Benedictio rutae, cardi et salviae
27. ff. 40r–41r. Benedictio ignis ad comburenda instrumenta maleficialia
28. f. 41r. Benedictio auri contra regium morbum
29. ff. 41r–41v. Alia benedictio auri, thuris et myrhae adversus incubos et succubos et contra insultus maleficorum
30. f. 41v. Contra febres
31. ff. 41v–42v. Contra morbum caducum
32. ff. 42v–43r. Contra dolores calculi
33. ff. 43r–43v. Contra frenesim infantium
34. ff. 43v–44r. Contra praesuras praegnantium
35. ff. 44r–51r. Exorcismus potentissimus mirabilisque efficaciae ad expellendas omnes facturas, maleficia, praestigia, ligaturas, et opus nefarium diaboli ab hominibus
36. ff. 51r–56v. Exorcismus mirabilis efficatiae, qui in matrimonio a doemonibus vel maleficiis au tarte diabolica impediuntur seu maleficiantur
37. ff. 56v–57v. Benedictio aquae contra maleficium taciturnitatis

* * *

The *Sacra arca benedictionum*... shows traces of the Benedictine background and its Hungarian origin. There are rituals which can be interpreted in terms of the Benedictine horizon, and which were included in the selection as special rituals of the order despite the fact that they contain practically no benedictions (ordo 5, 6, 7). The ritual concerning excommunication (8) is closer to the intention designated by the title of the manuscript, which is a special expression of benediction/malediction practice with negative connotations. At the beginning of the collection, there are the benedictions driven by the needs of the Order (1, 1a, 2, 4), the texts of which—if we substitute the names of the referred saints—can be put in parallel with the practices of many other religious orders.

For the purposes of our research, the core material of the collection can be divided into four larger thematic groups. To form these groups, we have used the results of our longer study, including the comparative analysis of certain rituals.

a) In the first group, including most ordines, belong rituals with numerous Hungarian and European analogies for blessing various things. As the rubric of the ninth ordo states: "*Sequuntur benedictiones rerum variarum*" (f. 21v). These include the blessing of the rosary as an amulet (3), that of the rue plant which has exorcist powers (10) and also most of the benedictions (4a, 11, 12, 13, 14, 15, 16, 17, 18, 21).

b) We separated the exorcisms which have a specific maledictory character and which obviously bear in their titles this type of orientation.

Thus "the house tormented by demons" (19), the "exorcism against a storm" (20), "the great, festive exorcism of the victims of bewitchment" (35) and the healing of the "victims of marital bewitchment" (36) all belong to the same group.

c) The third group consists of rituals aiming to cast off bewitchment, usually referred to as *maleficium* (22, 23, 24, 25, 26a–f, 29, 37). Many among them contain only remotely parallel elements or no analogy whatsoever. The introductory rubrics of this type of benediction express precisely the aim they want to reach: "*Sequuntur benedictiones contra maleficia et veneficia*" (f. 32v).

d) Last but not least, there are the actual medical rituals against illnesses (28, 30, 31, 32, 33, 34), which are connected to the others but also constitute a separate group and which make our source truly special. As the author of the liturgical book says at the end of the manuscript (f. 57v), presumably regarding the entire collection, these ordines were assembled in this book to benefit the ill and the bewitched (*"in gratiam langventium et maleficiatorum"*).

After having established these premises, let us discuss the rituals in the d) group one by one.

28. Blessing gold against jaundice

f. 41r. Benedictio auri contra regium morbum

V. Adjutorium nostrum in nomine Domini
R. Qui fecit coelum et terram
V. Dominus vobiscum
R. Et cum spiritu tuo

Oremus

Bene+dic itaque domine Jesu Christe in titulum omnipotentiae tuae et spem salutis fidelium utentium hanc creaturam auri, ut quidquid a nobis in tuo nomine digne ac perfecte agitur, a te fieri credatur. Adesto quaesumus nostro officio servitutis, et bene+dicere ac sancti+ficare digneris hanc creaturam auri, quam in tuo nomine sancto gloriae tuae bene+dicere confidimus. Qui vivis et regnas cum Patre et Spiritu Sancto Deus per omnia saecula saeculorum. Amen.

Aspergat aqua benedicta; instruat infirmum, ut aurum imponat ad poculum, ex illo semper summat haustum.

As yet, we have found no analogies[8] for medicinal benedictions based on the idea of homeopathic magic.[9] The short oration of the unique benediction does not even refer to the actual medical purpose, which we know solely from the title. According to the instructions, it is the priest who tells the patient to put the blessed gold in the cup and to only drink from the cup with the gold.

30. Against shivers (fever)
f. 41v. Contra febres
Amygdala et nuccleos persicorum bene siccos conterat in pulveres. Deinde benedicat hoc modo.

V. Adjutorium nostrum in nomine Domini
R. Qui fecit coelum et terram
V. Dominus vobiscum
R. Et cum spiritu tuo

Oremus

Bene+dic Domine creaturam istam pulverum, ut sit remedium salutare generi humano, et praesta per invocationem sancti tui nominis, ut quicunque ex his pulveribus sumpserint vel gustaverint, liberentur a febribus tertianis, quartanis, quotidianis et continuis. Per Christum dominum nostrum. Amen.

Aspergat aqua benedicta.

Deinde dicat infirmo, ut in cuspide cultri (neque enim manu tangat) ter injiciat in poculum, bene comisceat in vino vel in aqua, quandoque febres invadunt, tunc summat bene se cooperiendo et se calide servando, schedulam febricitantem etiam collo alligando.

---

[8] In the vast, summarising collection of medieval benediction practices, Franz does not even mention this type of disease (Franz 1909).

[9] See Frazer's well-known and oft-quoted example of the Hindu healing procedure against jaundice: Frazer 1995, 26–28. The same idea appears in a Hungarian medicinal book from the early seventeenth century: "On the matter of jaundice. If a man with jaundice sees a bird called *sternadel* (also called a yellow sparrow) and watches the bird intensely until it lands and until it dies, and then the patient is healed." ("*Az sargasagrul. Az sternadel neveo madarra (sarga uerebnekis hijak) sarghasagu ember ha kemenjen nezj mind adigh, migh le szal az madar, megh hal az madar, az patiens megh giogiul.*") MBM 1989, 73. Hungarian peasant incantations often mention methods involving the use of egg-yolk: Pócs 1985–1986, 66, 68, 72.

The proper subject of the benediction against fever is a powder made of crushed dry almonds and peach kernel, upon which the priest asked God's blessing, so that the consumer of the powder is delivered of the "third day, fourth day, everyday and continuous" fever (for its medicinal use at the time, see Melius 1979, 142–3). The priest had to explain to the patient to put, without making contact with their hands, three pinches of the powder in a cup, to mix with wine or water and, when the fever attacks, to drink of the liquid, under covers and in the warm, with the slip of paper against fever placed around their neck.

We know of numerous incantations against the shivers, and only slightly fewer benedictions with the same aim.[10] So far, we have not been able to confirm any definite parallel between the text and the procedure.

31. Against falling sickness (epilepsy)
    ff. 41v–42v. Contra morbum caducum
    Jecur testudinum et conchas inferiores bene exsicet et conterat in pulveres, benedicat hoc modo.

    Exorcismus

    Exorcizo te creatura pulverum in nomine Pa+tris, et Fi +lii et Spiritus +Sancti, ut per hanc invocationem individuae trinitatis, ac unius virtute deitatis, omnis nequissima virtus adversarii, omnis inveterata malitia deaboli, omnis violenta incursio, omne confusum et coecum phantasma eradicetur, fugetur et discedat ab his pulveribus, et omnes, qui ex eis biberint vel sumpserint, fiat sanitas super eos ab omni maleficio diabolico, ut non possit latere ulla malignorum spirituum

[10] AD 1774, 162: Under the title "Benedictio S. Salvatoris ab horta Franciscani contra febres", a benediction was published against shivers with a different text (although mentioning the "third day, fourth day, everyday and continuous" fever). The prayer of the sixteenth-century Franciscan Saint Salvator of Horta ("*Potentia Dei Patris + Sapientia Dei Filii + Virtus Spiritus + Sancti liberet te ab omni febre tertiana, quartana et continua, B. Salvatore orante pro te famulo suo, vel famula sua. + Dominus te N. benedicat, + ab infirmitate et ab omni malo te semper defendat, Amen.*") was usually written on a slip of paper and hung around the neck of the patient. It is demonstrative of the popularity of the benediction in the seventeenth and eighteenth centuries that it also figures in Sannig's collection: FRA 1685, 290–1; moreover, it is also included in a "medicinal booklet", written around 1665: MBM 1989, 266. For similar benedictions see also: LT 1709, 220–7: "Remedium contra febres ex S. Ambrosio". Regarding the matter in general, see Franz (1909: II. 467–484). Regarding the sixteenth and seventeenth century texts on the borderline of incantations and benedictions, see Magyary-Kossa 1929–1940, III. 289; Pócs 1985–1986, II. 424; Sávai 1997, 215–8.

nequitia. Per eundem dominum nostrum Jesum Christum, qui cum Deo Patre, et Filio et Spiritu Sancto vivit et regnat in saecula saeculorum. Amen.

De cenomano Libori sancte patrone magne invocamus te, tu qui Deo gratus extitisti, eamque gratiam meruisti, ut adjuves, quos morbus caducus excruciat, quaesumus nos famuli, Deum pro nobis pius exora, ut hos pulveres bene+dicere et sancti+ficare dignetur, et ne ob scelera nostra in vita nos puniat morbo caduco, sed clemens liberet hoc saeculo; nobis quoque chorus angelorum succurrat in valle lachrymarum, ut post hanc vitae miseriam ducat nos omnes in coeli patriam. Amen.

V. Adjutorium nostrum in nomine Domini
R. Qui fecit coelum et terram
V. Dominus vobiscum
R. Et cum spiritu tuo

Oremus

Deus, qui sanctum miraculis clarum episcopum Liborium, profligatorem morbi caduci singulari gratia et privilegio donasti: quaesumus, ut per ejus merita et intercessionem hos pulveres bene+dicas et sancti+fices contra morbum et ab omni liberemur, ejusque gloriae in coelis participes esse mereamur. Per Christum dominum nostrum. Amen.

Deinde aspergat aqua benedicta, post hoc ad poculum fundat recentam aquam, ter ponat in illam aquam ex pulveribus et ex benedicta ruta, bene commisceat, bibat infirmum et hoc frequentius usque dum vigorem sentiat corporis.

A powder that had been blessed was also used to heal patients with falling sickness (St. John's evil, grand mal, epilepsy). (Regarding the history of the disease and its healing treatments, see Magyary-Kossa 1929–1940, III. 26–7). Turtle liver[11] and clams had to be dried[12] and crushed, and after the

[11] On the similar use of this peculiar "medicine", we have various Hungarian data from this period: *"Contra caducum morbum... Az tekenős békának az máját vegyed, aszald meg, terd meg, fejér borba add meginnya az kórságos embernek."* ["take the liver of the turtle, dry it, crush it, mix it with white wine and give it to the sick person"] (mid-sixteenth century) Magyary-Kossa (1929–1940: III. 281); *"Az tekenös bekanak mayat ueöd ki, es teörd megh, ad megh innia, mikor rea esik."* [take the liver of the turtle, crush it, and make the patient drink it when having an attack] (beginning of seventeenth century) (MBM 1989, 87, 104).

powder had been blessed, three portions of it were mixed in fresh water with a piece of blessed rue. The patient had to drink this mixture until they got better. There is no known parallel to this treatment. The special feature of this ritual, besides the benedictions, lies in the exorcism of the object of the ritual, for the text explicitly refers to the illness as being considered the result of diabolical intervention (bewitchment). (There is an excellent liturgical history monograph on the exorcism of objects based primarily on medieval sources: Bartsch 1967). The texts of the two prayers about Saint Liborius are also included in one of the important Hungarian Franciscan benediction collections where they recommend them as orations (and not benedictions) against falling sickness and bladder stone problems (AD 1774, 106–7).

32. Against bladder stone pain
ff. 42v–43r. Contra dolores calculi
Accipe ex rubo granorum semina, enulae campanae radicem bene exsices et conteras in pulveres, benedicas hoc modo.

V. Adjutorium nostrum in nomine Domini
R. Qui fecit coelum et terram
V. Dominus vobiscum
R. Et cum spiritu tuo

Descendat quaesumus domine sancte pater omnipotens aeterne Deus, per amorem unigeniti filii tui, virtus Spiritus Sancti, quae ita istos pulveres bene+dicat, inflammet et exorcizet, ut quicunque ex eis biberint vel gustaverint in nomine tuo et filii tui dilectissimi et Spiritus Sancti, ab omnibus infirmitatibus morbis calculi et epidimiae sanentur et salvent. Da domine sancte pater omnipotens aeterne Deus, ut quod rogamus et exoramus, obtineamus in nomine tuo et dilecti filii tui et Spiritus Sancti. Amen.

Oremus

Veni Sancte Spiritus, et clementi bonitate bene+dic, sancti+fica hos pulveres contra morbum calculi et epidimiae, ut omnes, qui sumpserint vel gustaverint, ab omni morbo curentur et salventur, in nomine domini nostri Jesu Christi, qui cum Patre et Spiritu Sancto eodem vivit et regnat in saecula saeculorum. Amen.

---

[12] Regarding the medicinal use (against shivers) of the "shelled snail", see MBM 1989, 64–5. A medical book from the beginning of the seventeenth century recommends aquatic snails against the falling sickness: MBM 1989, 199.

> Deinde aspergat aqua benedicta, post hoc in distillata aqua petrosolii bene conmiscens, ter injiciat cuspide cultri ex illis pulveribus, mane et vesperi summat, proficit.

Here, too, the priest blesses a powder. Through the use of his procedure, bladder stone problems could be healed by mixing dried and crushed blackberry seeds and elecampane root (*enula campana*) blessed in an ecclesiastical ritual. (Regarding its medicinal use in the sixteenth century, see Melius 1979, 126–7 and 284–6). One had to add three pinches of the powder to water dripped from parsley and take the mix in the morning and at noon. "It works"—adds the author of the liturgical manuscript in his recipe-like phrasing.

3. Against children's *frenesis* (frenzy)

> *ff. 43r–43v. Contra frenesim infantium*
> Supercilia carpionum vel oculos cancrorum colligat, bene exsiccet, et conterat in pulveres, benedicat hoc modo.
>
> V. Adjutorium nostrum in nomine Domini
> R. Qui fecit coelum et terram
> V. Dominus vobiscum
> R. Et cum spiritu tuo
>
> Descendat quaesumus domine sancte pater omnipotens aeterne Deus in hos pulveres virtus Spiritus Sancti, et per hoc signum + crucis fugiant omnes doemones, sive phantasmata vel quodcunque opus diabolicum ab omnibus famulis tuis, quicunque gustaverint vel biberint ex his pulveribus, omnis omnino virtus diaboli extingvatur et annihiletur in eis ad honorem excelsae majestatis tuae, et omnis creatura facta ad imaginem et similitudinem tuam per horum pulverum medicamen ab omnibus spiritibus immundis ac illusionibus eorum sanetur et salvetur. In nomine domini nostri Jesu Christi, qui cum Patre et Spiritu Sancto vivit et regnat per omnia saecula saeculorum. Amen.
>
> Deinde aspergat aqua benedicta, ex post infantis parentes instruat, quomodo utendum fore his pulveribus.
> Accipiat lac calidum in cochliari, in cuspide cultri modice injiciat, bene comisceat quando laborat frenesi, et det ad bibendum, sic permittat infantem dormire.
> Quando infantes tremunt, pro suffitu ipsis adbibeantur herbae benedictae, salvia, ruta, cum cera et thure benedicto.

This benediction was also employed in an attempt to provide transcendent help against *prhenesis*, a children's disease characterised by convulsive, epileptic seizures (briefly on the disease, see Magyary-Kossa 1929–1940, III. 26 and 153). The eyebrows of a carp and the eyes of a shrimp were dried[13] and then crushed to a powder which was mixed and then blessed. A pinch of the powder was added to a spoonful of warm milk and the medicine given to the sick child before going to sleep. For the fumigation of children trembling from a seizure, blessed herbs, sage, rue, holy incense and wax were recommended. The latter procedure and the explicit reference to it in the oration ("ab omnibus spiritibus immundis ac illusionibus eorum") confirms that, just as in the case of the falling sickness (morbus caducus), demonic powers were suspected to lie behind the sickness, evidently due to the epileptic symptoms of the condition.

Even though, in general, there are examples for the benediction of a sick child, we do not know of analogies expressly for this kind of liturgical action.

34. Against the pressures of women in labour
ff. 43v–44r. Contra praesuras praegnantium
conficiat candellam ex cera, salvia, ruta, hysopo, thure, myrha. Deinde benedicat hoc modo

V. Adjutorium nostrum in nomine Domini
R. Qui fecit coelum et terram
V. Dominus vobiscum
R. Et cum spiritu tuo

Bene+dic domine hanc creaturam candelae, quam educi mandasti in remedium salutare generi humano, et praesta per invocationem sancti tui nominis, ut quicunque ea fumigati fuerint, dolores et praesurae ab eis expellantur, et corporis sanitatem animaeque tutelam recipiant. Per Christum dominum nostrum. Amen.

Deinde aspergat aqua benedicta.

Potest adhiberi iste suffitus parturientibus etiam et quae fluxum sangvinis patiuntur, iis bibere ex grano Sancti Joannis vel cruce S. P. N. Benedicti aquam recentem fontanam, bene autem notet sibi pater spiritualis praegnantibus, quae habent fluxum sangvinis, potum ex salvia et ruta benedicta, nec amittant foetum, sed bene re examinata concedere potest in calido vino vel jusculo, de die autem semel

---

[13] The eye of the shrimp was usually used "against stone" according to the medicinal books of the time. One recipe from the beginning of the seventeenth century explicitly recommends the powder made from it for children suffering from bladder stones ("*az mely giermeket keo bant*"): (MBM 1989, 199 and 257).

> summant ad captum modice cuspidis cultri, suffitu autem frequentius uti possunt dum modo in calido se servent.

This ritual consists of the benediction of a special candle made of wax, sage, rue, hyssop, incense and myrrh. Its purpose was to ease the pain at childbirth. As parallels, we can only mention general benedictions,[14] while for analogies of the text and the candle for fumigation, we can find no trace whatsoever. In the closing rubric, the same fumigation recipe as in the previous (33) ordo is recommended to a similar end. Here, a medicinal drink for women's bleeding is also mentioned; this was supposed to be drunk as fresh spring water off the seeds of Saint John's wort[15] or the cross of Saint Benedict. Likewise, it was considered helpful to take holy sage and rue consumed (strictly in a small dosage[16]) mixed with mulled wine or soup. (On the healing procedure of drinking off a cross (especially to treat fever) there are numerous medieval data in Franz 1909, II. 468–84).

* * *

Summarising the presentation of the six medicinal sacramentals of the Pannonhalma liturgical book, we can establish that the relevant medieval and early modern analogies are far from reflecting a similar, explicit medicinal practice. Our source in this regard—in terms of the Western Church[17]—can undoubtedly be considered unique. It is not surprising that these types of rituals are completely missing from the official diocesan liturgical books. It is even more noteworthy that among the "alternative" benedictions offered by the large European benediction selections, we only rarely find rituals that explicitly aim to fight diseases; they usually merely

---

[14] (Blessing women in labour, with a completely different text: MBP 1845, 180–2; VIEN 1889, II. 36–8; LT 1709, 163–6; on blessing women in labour in general: Franz 1909, II. 186–208; this ritual also figures in the Pray codex: Zalán 1927).

[15] Here, presumably they meant the plant called *hypericon* (S. Johanneskraut), which was mentioned in several sixteenth and seventeenth century sources for effectively stopping the blood flow: Melius 1979, 277–8; MBM 1989, 19. For identification, see the instructions of the early seventeenth century recipes related to the Herbarium of Melius: "Collige gemmas florum de hipericon, sive fuga demonum…" (MBM 1989, 25).

[16] This restriction can be explained presumably by the effect of the rue plant causing barrenness: Melius 1979, 275.

[17] As for the orthodox practices of this kind, we still have to conduct further analyses to reveal the sources. Goar's classic work includes significantly fewer benedictions than expected (and than actually used): Goar 1647.

describe a few general benedictions to bless the sick or the medicine.[18] As for the illnesses related to bewitchment (*maleficium*) (e.g. impotence), the contemporary European analogies are more traceable. The texts of the early modern benediction books are full of this type of manifestation of the clerical and secular mentalities and beliefs of the era, although their deeper analysis should be the subject of another study. Hence, in this present study, we do not discuss in detail the forms of ecclesiastical protection against maleficium (see above Group C of the rituals), despite the fact that bewitchment naturally might often have had health-related consequences.

How could it be explained that among the rituals of the Pannonhalma benediction book from the end of the seventeenth century there are so many explicitly medicinal benedictions? Perhaps it would be easier to answer this question if we knew the identity of the author of the manuscript. The uniqueness of the benedictions in the manuscript suggests that their creation might have been an individual invention. Around the time when the manuscript was written, the most inventive and also the most graphomaniac monk in Pannonhalma was the above-mentioned Bonifác Lancsics, who is also known for writing the manuscript of the book of recipes in 1697, the *Libellus medicinalis*. This perfect coincidence cannot be an accident, and hopefully does not contribute to unwittingly misleading posterity! Unfortunately, such scholarly literature of medical history with which we are familiar has not yet analysed the sources of Lancsics's medicinal booklet, the content and the significance of its recipes. In the absence of these analyses, we have to give up on our endeavour—however significant the conclusions we may have drawn from it—to concretise the overlapping of the secular (profane) and ecclesiastical (sacral) medicinal practices appearing at the same time in the same place.[19] For now, all we can do is document the obvious existence of this

[18] On the medieval practices, see Franz 1909, II. 399–513; my assertion is based on the representative sample of the early modern collections quoted in footnotes 4, 7 and 8.

[19] The preliminary overview of the *Libellus medicinalis* (PFK BK^{+} 13/3.) shows that from the six rituals we mention there are four (morbus regius, febres, caducus morbus, calculus) which also figure in the manuscript booklet as medical procedures. The central elements of these show minimal overlapping with the blessed vegetal and animal derivatives of the benedictions. For instance, the central ingredients in healing jaundice are alabaster and celandine root; in the treatment of the falling disease, raven, crow, black cherry, lavender, incense and the bladder of a wild boar were applied, while in the treatments healing bladder stones, carp bile, blackthorn, elder juice, rose mushrooms, strawberry juice, chickpeas and incense were used. The two sources faintly overlap in that in the medicinal practice, both use parsley (root) against bladder stones and almonds to treat fever.

dichotomy in the practices of the Benedictine monks of Pannonhalma at the end of the seventeenth century, and presumably all of the eighteenth century. The intertwining of the two types of practice is unequivocally based on the published liturgies. The blessing of the church and the occasional exorcism established the sacramental character of the produced medicine, the need for which presumably stemmed from the inseparability of the material and spiritual sides of healing, and from the idea that the joint employment of the two sides had an increased effectiveness.

References

AD 1774: *Arca Domini, selectam Deum, Divosque precandi, confitendi et communicandi methodum continens, olim ad usum et commoditatem Sacerdotum altissimi ad S. Aras litantium erecta, nunc denuo ad eorum spirituale solamen renovata, et multiplicibus absolutionum, benedictionum, et exorcismorum formulis locupletata omnium fidelium devotioni patet reserata.* Posonii: Typis et impensis Joannis Michaelis Landerer.

Bartsch, Elmar. 1967. *Die Sachbeschwörungen der Römischen Liturgie. Eine liturgiegeschichtliche und liturgietheologische Studie.* Münster: Aschendorff.

Bárth, Dániel. 2004. "Egyházi benedikciós gyakorlat a kora újkori Magyarországon [Clerical benediction practices in early modern Hungary]." In *Áldás és átok, csoda és boszorkányság. Vallásetnológiai fogalmak tudományközi megközelítésben* [Blessing and curse, miracle and witchcraft. Interdisciplinary approach to concepts in ethnology of religion], edited by Éva Pócs, 30–46 Budapest: Balassi. (Tanulmányok a transzcendensről IV.)

—. 2006. "Kirchliche Benediktionspraxis im frühneuzeitlichen Ungarn." In *Religion und Magie in Ostmitteleuropa. Spielräume theologischer Normierungsprozesse in Spätmittelalter und Früher Neuzeit*, edited by Thomas Wünsch, 301–20. Berlin: Lit Verlag. (Religions- und Kulturgeschichte in Ostmittel- und Südosteuropa 8.)

—. 2007. "Földi bajok transzcendens gyógyítása: benedikció és exorcizmus a kora újkori Magyarországon [Transcendent healing of earthly troubles: benediction and exorcism in early modern Hungary]." In *Előadások a vallásról* [Lectures on religion], edited by Bulcsú Hoppál Kál, 89–97. Budapest: Mozaik. (Vallástudományi Tanulmányok 7–8.)

—. 2008: "Papok és démonok viadala: exorcizmus a kora újkori Magyarországon [Duel of priests and demons: exorcism in early modern Hungary]." In *Démonok, látók, szentek. Vallásetnológiai fogalmak tudományközi megközelítésben* [Demons, seers, saints. Concepts of ethnology of religion from an interdisciplinary approach], edited by Éva Pócs, 59–68. Budapest: Balassi. (Tanulmányok a transzcendensről VI.)

Cochem, Martin von. 1692. *Libellus benedictionum et exorcismorum, in quo efficacissimae benedictiones tam sacrarum, quam profanarum rerum et terribiles exorcismi ad varia maleficia tam ab hominibus, quam pecoribus et locis infestis depellenda continentur.* Francofurti ad Moenum.

Eynatten, Maximilian von. 1626. *Manuale exorcismorum, continens instructiones et exorcismos ad ejiciendos e corporibus obsessis spiritus malignos, et ad quaevis maleficia depellenda, et ad quascumque infestationes daemonum reprimendas*. Antverpiae.

FB 1749: *Fasciculus benedictionum, exorcismorum, et validissimarum conjurationum ad effugandas aëreas tempestates. Ex approbatis libris a S. R. E. collectus. Litaniae quoque et duodecim evangelia cum suis orationibus pro benedicendis agris et fructibus terrae. Praeterea benedictiones super cruces, quae in triviu collocantur, ac contra vermes, locistas et alia animalia fruges vastantia etc.* Reimpressum in Typographia Csik Somlyoviensi.

FD 1697: *Flagellum daemonum, exorcismos terribiles, potentissimos, et efficaces, remediaque probatissima, ac doctrinam singularem in malignos spiritus expellendos, facturasque et maleficia fuganda de obsessis corporibus complectens, cum suis benedictionibus, et omnibus requisitis ad eorum expulsionem. Accessit postremo pars secunda, quae Fustis daemonum inscribitur. Quibus novi exorcismi et alia nonnulla, quae prius desiderabantur, superaddita fuerunt. Auctore R. P. F. Hieronymo Mengo Vitellianensi, Ord. Min. Reg. Observantiae.* Venetiis: Apud Paulum Balleonium.

FRA 1685: *Rituale Franciscanum continens varias Absolutiones, Benedictiones, Conjurationes, Exorcizmos, Ritus, ac alias Caeremonias Ecclesiasticas, ad utilitatem Christi Fidelium, et praxim Sacerdotum, maxime Ordinis S. Francisci; ex variis Ritualibus coordinatum a Fr. Bernardo Sannig, Ord. S. Francisci Reform Provinciae Bohemiae S. Wenceslai D. et M. Sacerdote, et Iterato Ministro Provinciali dictae Provinciae.* Neo-Pragae.

Franz, Adolph. 1909. *Die kirchlichen Benediktionen im Mittelalter* I–II. Freiburg im Breisgau: Herder.

Frazer, James George. 1995. *Az Aranyág* [The Golden Bough]. Translated by Tibor Bodrogi, and György Bónis. Budapest: Osiris. [*The golden bough: a study in magic and religion.* London: Macmillan, 1890.]

FT 1739: *Fasciculus triplex exorcismorum et benedictionum in Romano-Catholica Ecclesia usitatorum, ex variis authoribus approbatis collectus, et historiis ac exemplis subinde illustratus, cum adnexo tractatu de indulgentiis et jubilaeo, ac resolutionibus moralibus, in gratiam curatorum ecclesiae, ac priorum fidelium utilitatem luci publicae datus.* Tyrnaviae: Typis Academicis.

FuD 1697: *Fustis daemonum, adjurationes formidabiles, potentissimas et efficaces in malignos spiritus fugandos de opressis corporibus humanis. Ex sacrae apocalypsis fonte, variisque sanctorum patrum auctoritatibus haustus complectens. Auctore R. P. F. Hieronymo Mengo Vitellanensi, Ord. Min. Reg. Observantiae. Opus sane ad maximam exorcistarum commoditatem nunc in locum editum.* Venetiis: Apud Paulum Balleonium.

Goar, Jacobus. 1647. *Eucholigion sive Rituale Graecorum complectens Ritus et Ordines Divinae Liturgiae, officiorum, Sacrramentorum Consecrationum, Benedictionum, Funerum, Orationum, etc. cuilibet personae, statui, vel tempori congruos, iusta usum orientalis ecclesiae.* Paris.

Gulyás, Borbála. 2006. "Lancsics Bonifác [Bonifác Lancsics]." In *Magyar Művelődéstörténeti Lexikon* VI. [Encyclopaedia of Hungarian cultural history], edited by Péter Kőszeghy, 383–4. Budapest: Balassi.

Hervay, Ferenc Levente. 2003. "Bencések [Benedictines]." In *Magyar Művelődéstörténeti Lexikon* I. [Encyclopaedia of Hungarian cultural history], edited by Péter Kőszeghy, 337–41. Budapest: Balassi.

Jensen, Jürgen. 2007. *Kirchliche Rituale als Waffen gegen Dämonenwirken und Zauberei. Ein Beitrag zu einem Komplex von Schutz- und Abwehrritualen der Katholischen Kirche des 17. und 18. Jahrhunderts in Italien unter besonderer Berücksichtigung systematisch-ethnologischer Gesichtspunkte.* Berlin: Lit Verlag. (Interethnische Beziehungen und Kulturwandel 60.)

Kieckhefer, Richard. 1989. *Magic in the Middle Ages*. Cambridge: University Press.

LT 1709: *Locupletissimus thesaurus, continens varias et selectissimas benedictiones, conjurationes, exorcismos, absolutiones, ritus, administrationem sacramentorum, aliorumque munerum pastoralium ad utilitatem Christi fidelium, et commodiorem usum parochorum, omniumque sacerdotum tam saecularium, quam religiosorum. Ex diversis ritualibus et probatissimis authoribus collectus a Gelasio di Cilia.* Vohburgi.

Magyary-Kossa, Gyula. 1929–1940. *Magyar orvosi emlékek. Értekezések a magyar orvostörténelem köréből* I–IV. [Medical monuments of

Hungary. Studies in the history of Hungarian medicine]. Budapest: Magyar Orvosi Könyvkiadó Társulat.

MB 1685: *Manuale benedictionum, rituumque ecclesiasticorum tam intra, quam extra Ecclesias occurrentium. Ex ritualibus, Romano, Constantiensi, aliarumque Dioecesium. Pro parochorum et sacerdotum omnium commodiore usu collectum.* Editio tertia. Typis monasterii Einsidlensis.

MBM 1989: *Medicusi és borbélyi mesterség. Régi magyar ember- és állatrovosló könyvek Radvánszky Béla gyűjtéséből* [The professions of medics and barbers. Old Hungarian books on healing people and animals collected by Béla Radvánszky]. Edited by Gizella Hoffmann. Budapest: MTA ITI.

MBP 1845: *Manuale benedictionum. Accedunt processiones variae publicis necessitatibus congruentes. Commodo animarum pastorum usui adaptavit Severinus Lueg, dioeceseos Passaviensis presbyter.* Passavii.

Melius, Péter. 1979. *Herbárium. Az fáknak, füveknek nevekről, természetekről és hasznairól* [Herbarium. On the names, natures and uses of trees and grasses]. Edited by Attila Szabó. Bucharest: Kriterion.

Molnár, Antal. 1996. "Karner Egyed kora (1699–1708) [The age of Egyed Karner (1699–1708)]." In *Mons Sacer 996–1996. Pannonhalma 1000 éve* I–III. [The 1000 years of Pannonhalma], edited by Imre Takács, II. 49–58. Pannonhalma: Pannonhalmi Főapátság.

Molnár, Szulpicz. 1906. *A Pannonhalmi Főapátság története. Negyedik korszak (1535–1708)* [History of the Pannonhalma Archabbey. Fourth period (1535–1708)]. Budapest: Stephaneum. (A pannonhalmi Szent Benedek-rend története IV.)

Nucleus 1706: *Nucleus continens benedictiones rerum diversarum, item exorcismos ad varia maleficia depellenda, conjurationes item ad fugandas a daemonibus eorumque excitatas aereas tempestates. Collectus tam ex Romano, quam diversarum dioecesium ritualibus in cleri ruralis usum.* Viennae Austriae.

Pócs, Éva. 1985–1986. *Magyar ráolvasások* I–II. [Hungarian incantations]. Budapest: MTA Könyvtára.

—. 2002. "'Én vagyok mindennél nagyobb orvos, te vagy mindennél nagyobb bájos': egyházi benedikció—paraszti ráolvasás ['I am a doctor the greatest of all, you are a charmer the greatest of all': Church benediction—peasant incantation]." In *Magyar néphit Közép- és Kelet-Európa határán* [Hungarian folk belief on the border of Central and

Eastern Europe], 173–211. Budapest: L'Harmattan. (Válogatott tanulmányok I.)

Reifenberg, Hermann. 1971–1972. *Sakramente, Sakramentalien und Ritualien im Bistum Mainz seit dem Spätmittelalter* I–II. Münster.

ROM 1614: *Rituale Romanum Pauli V. Pont. Max. jussu editum.* Romae [Reprint edition: Rituale Romanum. Editio Princeps (1614). Edizione anastatica, Introduzione e Appendice a cura di Manlio Sodi—Juan Javier Flores Arcas. Città del Vaticano, 2004.]

Sávai, János. 1997. *Missziók, mesterek, licenciátusok* [Missions, masters, licentiates]. Szeged: Agapé. (Missziós dokumentumok Magyarországról és a hódoltságról II/I.)

Scribner, Robert W. 1987. *Popular Culture and Popular Movements in Reformation Germany.* London and Ronceverte: The Hambledon Press.

Stampa, Petrus Antonius. 1605. *Fuga Satanae exorcismus. Ex sacrarum litterarum fontibus, pioque S. Ecclesiae instituto exhaustus.* Venetiis.

Szabó, Flóris. 1981. *A Pannonhalmi Főapátsági Könyvtár kéziratkatalógusa. 1850 előtti kéziratok* [Catalogue of manuscripts of the Pannonhalma Archabbey Library. Manuscripts before 1850]. Budapest: OSZK. (Magyarországi egyházi könyvtárak kéziratkatalógusai 2.)

Szakály, Ferenc. 1996. "Pannonhalma a török időkben [Pannonhalma in the Turkish era]." In *Mons Sacer 996–1996. Pannonhalma 1000 éve* I–III., edited by Imre Takács, II. 13–24. Pannonhalma: Pannonhalmi Főapátság.

Thomas, Keith. 1971. *Religion and the Decline of Magic.* London: Routledge, and Kegan Paul.

Veit, Ludwig Andreas. 1936. *Volksfrommes Brauchtum und Kirche im deutschen Mittelalter.* Freiburg im Breisgau: Herder.

VIEN 1889: *Collectio Rituum Archidioeceseos Viennensis ex Venia Sanctae Sedis Retinendorum in administratione Sacramentorum, in Benedictionibus et Exorcismus, in Processionibus aliisque ecclesiasticis functionibus jussu et auctoritate ordinarii edita I–III.* Viennae.

Zalán, Menyhért. 1927. "A Pray-kódex benedictiói [The benedictions of the Pray codex]." *Magyar Könyvszemle* XXXIV: 44–66.

EXORCISM IN THE TRINITY-SERGIUS LAVRA

TÜNDE KOMÁROMI

The Trinity-Sergius Lavra *(Troitse-Sergieva Lavra)* is located in the small town of Sergiev Posad[1] in the vicinity of Moscow. I conducted fieldwork in the city over a period of fourteen months.[2] Over the course of my research, I studied the religious life of the city and its surroundings, the institutional system and the publications of the Russian Orthodox Church, and contemporary demonology in its wider sense. What follows is based on the experiences acquired during this time.

The aim of my study is to describe and analyse the exorcisms that take place regularly in the Gate Church of the Nativity of John the Baptist in the Trinity-Sergius Lavra. The vast majority of the people participating in the exorcism are pilgrims, but it is important to note that only a certain fraction of all pilgrims is interested in these rituals. In the introduction, I will briefly discuss the historical significance of the monastery and of its great figures, living or dead, who attract the pilgrims to go there. This will be followed by the main part of the study, in which I describe and analyse the exorcism performed by Father Herman.[3] In the closing section of the article, I will draw conclusions about possession *(oderzhimost', besnovanie)* and exorcism *(otchitka, egzortsizm)* in the context of the

---

[1] In Soviet times it was known as Zagorsk.

[2] The research leading to these results has received funding from the European Research Council under the European Union's Seventh Framework Programme (FP7/2007–2013) / ERC grant agreement № 324214. I conducted the fieldwork as a postdoctoral fellow of the Max Planck Institute for Social Anthropology in Halle, in the framework of the *Religion and morality* research project between 2006 and 2009. Cf. Komáromi 2010. I am grateful for the comments of Alexander Agadjanian, Detelina Tocheva and Christine Worobec on the manuscript.

[3] In light of his renown, I left the name of archimadrite Herman (German) Chesnokov unchanged. There are articles about him in both the electronic and printed press. His sermons were published in several languages. The original Russian version can be purchased at the monastery and in several bookstores of the Russian Orthodox Church's book distribution network. A movie has also been made about exorcism, which can be purchased as well.

literature related to Orthodoxy.

The monastery, Saint Sergius and contemporary charismatic monks

In past centuries, the Trinity-Sergius Lavra has been a very important ecclesiastical and cultural centre. Besides the beautiful church buildings and the monastic cells, the monastery hosts numerous institutions, such as the Moscow Theological Academy and Seminary (*Moskovskaia dukhovnaia akademia i seminariia*), a publishing house, a valuable library, two museums, a centre for organising pilgrimages and several offices, as well as a hospital, a few refectories (for monks, theology students, pilgrims), the palace of the patriarch, a hotel,[4] several dozen shops and a café. There are five churches on the premises of the monastery where people come from the city every day to attend services, or simply to pray. Services are held at various times in different churches, basically covering the entire day. The earliest service is the prayers of the monks at five in the morning in the Trinity Cathedral, which is the oldest church in the monastery, and this is where they keep the relics of Saint Sergius.[5] The largest church with the capacity to hold the most people is the Assumption Cathedral or *Uspenskii sobor* ("Dormition of Mary"), which was built on the orders of Ivan the Terrible in the sixteenth century. The smaller church of the Theological Academy is also popular, mostly attracting the relatives of priests and theology teachers living in the city. Pilgrims usually visit the central churches of the monastery and also go to the sacred fountains in the courtyard and in the vicinity of the monastery. One of the fountains outside the walls of the monastery is indoors and masses of pilgrims come here all year long to bathe in the water in the hope of recovery.

According to Victor and Edith Turner, there is always a hierarchy among the places of worship within a given country (Turner and Turner 1978, 6).[6] In the times of Muscovite Russia, Trinity-Sergius Lavra was the

---

[4] It is a very representative hotel. There are two other hotels suitable for hosting guests in the immediate proximity, but outside the monastery, they have a capacity for several hundred, in various price ranges. In the city, there are two further establishments hosting guests near two churches.

[5] The Holy Trinity mural by Andrei Rubliov, currently kept at the Tretiakov Gallery, was originally at the Trinity Cathedral.

[6] In an international context, the central role of Jerusalem is indisputable, as is the symbolic significance of Kiev Monastery of the Caves from the time of the Kievan Rus' (*Kiev Pechersk Lavra*, established around the middle of the eleventh century by monk Antonii after his return from Mount Athos).

most important monastery and the spiritual centre of the country.[7] Orthodox Russians make pilgrimages abroad if their financial situation allows them, but they mostly go to places of worship within the country. It has been a custom of every social stratum since early modern times to make the pilgrimage on foot, trusting to divine providence, whenever they could (or in case they were lacking financial means). Today, there are people who take the cheapest local trains from station to station to get to holy places.

Even though there once existed earlier monasteries, established by rulers and boyars, that subsequently fell victim to the Mongol invasion, the Trinity-Sergius Lavra is considered to be the "first" monastery of Muscovite Russia. There is a reason for this: its establishment marks a new era in the history of Russian monasteries and, according to ecclesiastical historians, in the history of Russia as well. It was founded by Sergius of Radonezh (1314–1392; canonised in 1452) and his brother in the fourteenth century; from 1354, on an episcopal request, he became the abbot of the monastery (Kenworthy 2010). The figure of Saint Sergius contributed to the monastery becoming a centre for two reasons. Contrary to the founder of the Lavra in Kiev, he started a movement. In European Russia, the establishment of an entire series of monasteries is linked to the names of his disciples and followers. These monasteries were "cenobitic" monasteries[8] that wished to become centres of religious contemplation, far

[7] In accordance with local terminology, I will refer to the monastery by its Russian name in my study. The *Lavra* is a privileged monastery directly subordinated to the patriarch. It is ruled by the bishop, who acts as patriarchal vicar; beside him there is always an *ot'ets blagochinnyi,* a priest responsible for the monks. During my fieldwork, this position was filled by a thirty-eight-year-old, relatively young monk.

[8] There are two basic types of Christian monasticism: eremitical and cenobitic. In the case of the latter, which is also our case, the emphasis is on the communal prayer and the humble obedience to one's superior. The life of a monk or a nun (prayer, work, eating and sleeping) is led according to a strict order; the emphasis is not on an extreme asceticism. The fruit of the work is reaped by the community; the monk cannot keep any personal belonging. This is mostly important as opposed to the monasteries established by the princes and the *boyars*, since they exclusively accepted monks to the monastery from the aristocracy, who, not least, were important because of their donated possessions. And the founder had a considerable influence on the life in the monastery. Moreover, they were usually established in unpopulated areas, often in the wilderness, as opposed to the monasteries of the aristocracy established in cities, cf. Kenworthy 2010, 12–14. The Trinity Lavra was independent; yet later, it became a monastery having great influence and a considerable capital.

from the noise of the world. The reputation of Saint Sergius is also linked to defeating the Mongols in the battle of Kulikovo,[9] which is also when Muscovite Russia was established; therefore, he is worshipped as a national patron saint.[10] But the historical significance of Saint Sergius also lies in the fact that the princes (*kniazy*) respected him and listened to him regardless of any political conflict of interest.

He is still a very popular saint among the people; the locals and the pilgrims all believe that there is practically no human trouble to which his assistance could not come. Whether someone is seriously ill or merely a—not even religious—student before a difficult exam, anyone can attend and bow down in prayer in front of his earthly remains. Within the framework offered by the Church, thousands of people who seek a solution to their problems in religion come here. They come from all over the country, from the post-Soviet states and even from other countries. Meanwhile, an abundance of foreign tourists visits the monastery; they come on organised trips to admire the beauty of the building complex, the church murals and icons and the museums with their displays of extremely valuable collections. Their curiosity extends to the residents of the monastery, the monks, the theologians, and even the praying believers who, on the contrary, try to dissociate themselves from the worldly visitors. In general, the tourists are only in touch with their travel guides, among whom some are students in theology and speak a foreign language. The pilgrims, on the other hand, usually confess and ask for advice from the monks of the Lavra.

As a result of the flourishing cult of saints, Saint Sergius is also a living figure in popular culture. Local legends claim that snakes and even lizards avoid the Trinity monastery in a hundred-kilometre radius; the bells chase away the dangerous reptiles. Locals tell the story that in his silver coffin, Saint Sergius dons his clothes again every year and his shoes always get worn out because he walks so much in order to help those who pray to him. The miracle stories we hear today are evidently related to the stories noted in the hagiography; however, I will not discuss this aspect in detail.

---

[9] He gave his blessing to the Grand Prince of Vladimir, Dmitrii Ivanovich (Saint Dimitrii Donskoi) to fight the Tatar, which was followed by the victory of Kulikovo in 1380. Furthermore, it was Saint Sergius who encouraged the Russian princes to join forces and unite, which is why his name is associated with the establishment of Russia, cf. Kenworthy 2010, 16–7.

[10] In accordance with the classification of Turner and Turner, the Lavra is a medieval shrine and its history (and implicitly the history of the miracles) is strongly linked to national history. Cf. Turner and Turner 1978, 17–8.

Popular imagination invests the "living saints" with equally miraculous characteristics. There is, for instance, Father Herman, the exorcist monk from Sergiev Posad, whose helpers and acquaintances relate myriads of visions and miracles. Father Herman is not the only charismatic monk of the Lavra who attracts large crowds; undoubtedly, however, he is the most important person in the Lavra's contemporary life; he attracts the greatest number of pilgrims to the Lavra after Saint Sergius. Besides him, there are two other important and widely known figures in the Lavra. One of them is archimandrite Naum, an elderly monk respected as a *starets* who in the past decades has revived and established numerous monasteries all across Russia through a basically invisible network of connections. His name is also associated with legends.[11] Another important person whose circle of activities and "spiritual children" can be found all over Russia is Father Cyprian, a teacher at the Academy of Theology in Moscow, head of the Department of Pedagogy. He organises one-week training sessions twice a year for future theology teachers; he also lobbies for the introduction of theology in public education.[12]

Evidently, a simple believer only has free access to two great figures in the monastery and its surroundings: Saint Sergius and Father Herman. It is very difficult to meet Father Naum.[13] He has too many "spiritual children"; moreover, theologians, aspirant monks and women contemplating sisterhood also turn to him to find help in making this big life decision. Father Cyprian is "specialised" in the matter of education; in this sense, he has a mission. Since hundreds of people come to attend all of his training, the number of his followers has grown to thousands over the course of the years. Taking all this into consideration, we can establish that the three significant monks living today in the Lavra all have their different "fields" (and their followers do not overlap): one encourages religious education in the secular environment and thus tries to proselytise among atheists and

[11] Again, I will not go into detail regarding Father Naum. He is mentioned in detail in the monograph by Nikolai Mitrokhin (Mitrokhin 2004, 99–101) and he is also usually known in religious circles in the Moscow province. Archimandrite Kirill, another famous *starets* of the Lavra, who during my fieldwork lived at the residence of Aleksii II, is mentioned as well in the book of Mitrokhin (2004, 101–2) along with other famous spiriual fathers.

[12] Father Cyprian lived in a Siberian city before the perestroika and was a researcher in pedagogy at the Research Institute of the Academy (private communication by Father Cyprian). After that he came to the Lavra and was soon initiated as a monk, and a teacher monk (which is one of the optional lifestyles at the monastery only given to a few).

[13] On the 13th of October 2017, archimandrite Naum (Baiborodin) died.

negligent Christians; the other affects the number of those taking holy orders and the quality of monastic communities. Father Herman fights Evil, he helps large crowds to tackle those problems of the modern world which cause personal troubles, crises and illnesses in an individual's life.

In today's Russia, in the wide region of Moscow, there are three very popular saints: besides Saint Sergius, there is Matrionushka (Matrona Moskovskaya, 1885–1952) in Moscow, and *Seraphim of Sarov* (1759–1833) in Diveevo, around Nizhny Novgorod. Orthodox pilgrims come to visit all three saints from Russia and from the former Soviet territories. (On Saint Matrona of Moscow, see Kormina 2013).[14] It is characteristic of the movement of religious renewal over the past two and a half decades that pilgrimage corresponds to a quest in a wider sense. For many, it is the start of a new way of life, often at a new place. It is a migration phenomenon related to religious conversion, which might not affect huge crowds, but plays an important role in the life of the place of worship. Those who settle will make a useful workforce, and also propagate knowledge on miracles attracting new pilgrims (cf. Tarabukina 2000). This phenomenon is of key importance in the case of Father Herman and the exorcisms we shall discuss in this study.[15]

The exorcisms I have chosen as the subject of my discussion take place in the most significant Orthodox monastery of modern Russia. The place of worship and the cult of saints, as well as the service of the monks dealing with the problems of our age, with the personal troubles and illnesses of our contemporaries, and the cult surrounding them mutually complement and bolster one another, sustaining the high number of visitors. In what follows, I will examine the institutional framework and

---

[14] Similar in significance of the cult of Saint Matrona of Moscow is that of Xenia Petersburgskaya (born 1719–1730—died 1803; year of canonisation 1978 and 1988, Russian Orthodox Church Abroad), see for instance Kormina and Shtyrkov 2007.

[15] On a local level, there are still a few individuals who have an extraordinary charisma among the believers and are worshipped as living saints; there are priests who recently passed away and are worshipped as a saint and people take pilgrimages to their graves. During my fieldwork, I observed the cult of a priest from Sergiev Posad and another who passed away in a neighbouring village, in Semkhoz, the famous Father Aleksander Men. It is very interesting how the local priest motivated the simple people and a part of the local clergy, while the cult of father Men inspired the intelligentsia of Moscow to whom he gave lectures and sermons in his life. They have commemorations at the grave of the priest from Sergiev Posad, but for Father Men, who is considered a martyr because of the circumstances of his death, they have even built a church in Semkhoz (the patron saint of which is Saint Sergius).

the human relations under which Father Herman's exorcisms have been conducted over the past two and a half decades; I will analyse the procedure of the exorcism ritual, its social milieu and its reception at various religious forums.

Exorcism in the Gate Church of John the Baptist

The following description and analysis are based upon my own observations, narratives and conversations with local priests, monks, the students of the Moscow Academy and Faculty of Theology, with the people working at the local parish church directed by Father Herman and at the guesthouse and school operating next to it. I also used interviews made with pilgrims and locals who have participated in exorcisms more than once, and the Russian ecclesiastical publications and articles published in the press on exorcism. It was from such sources that I learned that Father Herman was not the only exorcist monk in Russia, but that he was undoubtedly the most famous.[16]

There are various attitudes towards exorcism within the Church. The ecclesiastical elite is rather reserved in this matter. They believe that Satan only rules sinners and non-believers; although in the history of the Church and of Christian monasticism, it is also admitted that diabolical temptation does not spare monks either. The people who come to the exorcisms with all kinds of sicknesses and troubles are mostly not practising their religion (*nevotserkovlennye*). In this sense, exorcism is a phenomenon that only involves believers peripherally. Regarding the special situation of the Church in the period following perestroika, however, exorcism is of great significance and the number of people it attracts to church and convinces to become converted is also relatively high.

Nonetheless, the students of the Academy and the Seminary who live on the premises of the Monastery rarely go to the rituals of Father Herman

---

16 There are well-known exorcists in any region; for instance, at the Pskov monastery and in the region of Pskov, around Saint Petersburg, etc. Another monk from the Lavra recently did an exorcism near Sergiev Posad, in Radonezh, where the parents of Saint Sergius used to live after moving here from Rostov. Although his exorcism attracted fewer people, he is also a charismatic individual. Members of the local clergy believe he was distanced because of the competition, but he continues his healing activity in another *oblast*. Based on *underground* ecclesiastical sources from the Soviet times, it is believed that Father Herman learned to exorcise from an exorcist from Pskov. The relatives of Father Herman say he lived for a while in the *dacha* of patriarch Pimen, and he first started exorcising in the chapel there (a small number of possessed at the time).

and are also mostly reluctant as regards the type of ecclesiastical literature on demonology which address a wider audience. I have never seen the monks of the monastery at the exorcisms; neither have my informants met them there. Among local priests, who also never attend exorcisms, it is a frequent opinion that the patriarch and the bishop turn a blind eye to the phenomenon because of the substantial financial gain; since, even though they do not ask for money from the participants, usually everyone donates some amount, and in my experience, a substantial sum. The believers from Sergiev Posad know about the exorcisms, they know Father Herman and are more tolerant towards them than the clerics and the students in general. Many have felt the need over the course of their lives to participate in an exorcism, here or at some other place; some people have been regular attendees of exorcisms over a longer period of time.

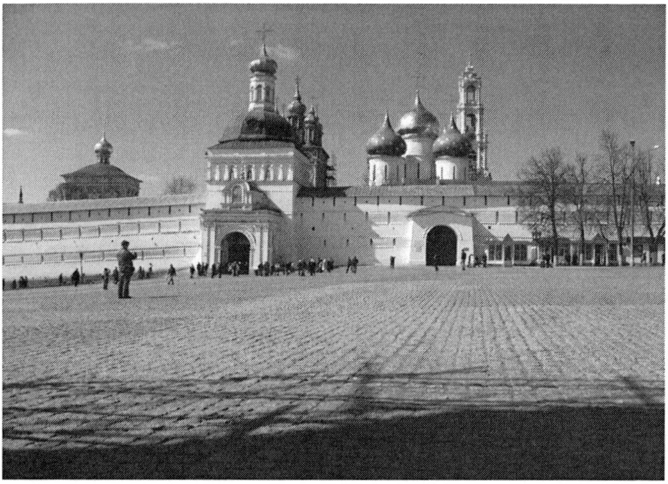

Fig. 1. Monastery of the Trinity-Saint Sergius Lavra (Sergiev Posad, Moscow region). The marketplace in front of the monastery and the monastery's main gate: behind the gatehouse is the Gate Church of John the Baptist; on the right, the towers of the Assumption Cathedral; and in the background, the bell tower, 2007. Photo by Tünde Komáromi.

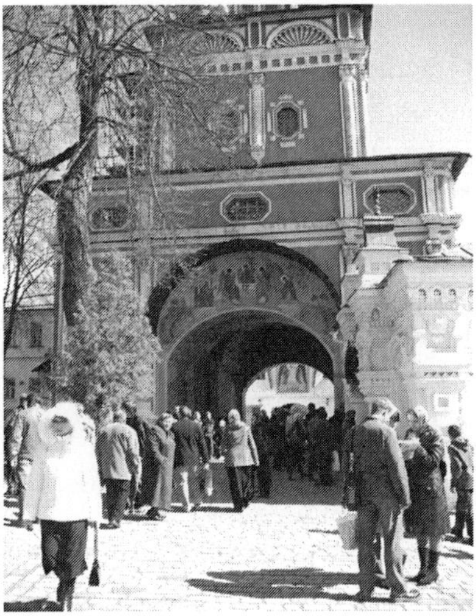

Fig. 2. Gate Church of Saint John the Baptist; the arch with pilgrims, Sunday morning, 2007. Photo by Tünde Komáromi.

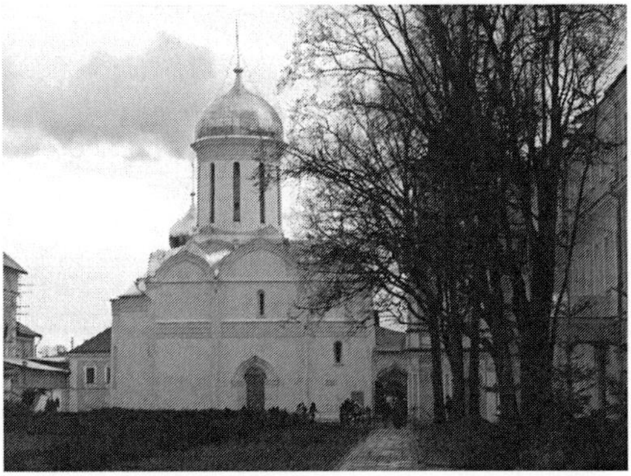

Fig. 3. The Trinity Cathedral, 2007. Photo by Tünde Komáromi.

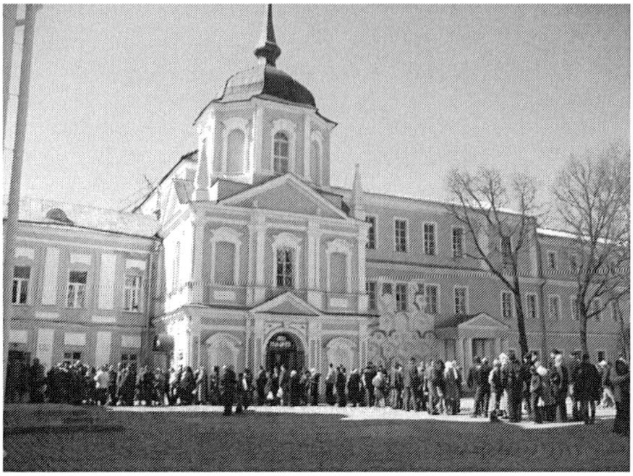

Fig. 4. Series of pilgrims standing in line at the relics of Saint Sergius on a Sunday in April, 2007. Photo by Tünde Komáromi.

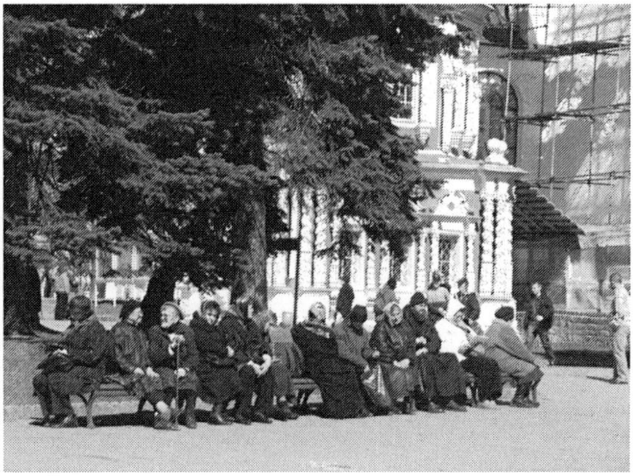

Fig. 5. Pilgrims sitting on a bench in the courtyard of the Lavra with a monk. 2007. Photo by Tünde Komáromi.

In the Orthodox Church, exorcisms can only be carried out with the permission of the bishop and exclusively by members of the black clergy, i.e. the monk-priests. In the Russian Orthodox Church[17], the ceremony is usually conducted according to the service book of the seventeenth-century metropolitan bishop of Kiev, Piotr Mogyla, by reading the prayer of exorcism from it.[18] It is also this approximately twenty-minute long prayer that Father Herman reads out loud during his ceremony. According to the articles published in the ecclesiastical press (an opinion shared by several members of the clergy), the ability to exorcise is a mighty blessing from God and also an extremely difficult service. In the history of Christianity, it is known from its beginnings and its original model is provided by the exorcisms performed by Jesus. It is believed that there are few people who are capable of exorcism; nowadays, on the other hand, there are too many possessed, because people are susceptible to give in to demons and are living a godless life. In the online ecclesiastical press, one can often read about the exorcisms of Father Herman and others. Father Rodion wrote a book about demonic phenomena in the 1990s entitled *People and Demons* (Rodion 2005); he also described in an interview the forms in which the Devil exits the possessed body (as snakes or as a small dark cloud coming out of the mouth).

If people decide to travel to the Lavra to participate in an exorcism, they have to ask for the advice of their confessor, spiritual father or simply the local priest. Similarly, in cases where there is a sick family member, they have to consult with the priest over whether it is advisable to take the sick to an exorcism. Father Herman advises everyone to confess their sins before exorcism and to obtain absolution so that they show up to the ceremony with a purged soul and in hope of a new life. The number of pilgrims turning to them for help is so high that Father Herman no longer has the possibility to speak with each one of them personally. Before the ritual, a few initiated helpers are present in the church to detect the mentally ill among the possessed in order to avoid their participation, for it

---

[17] An acquaintance from Sergiev Posad, who used to go to Kishinev for exorcism twenty years earlier, told me that the priest there read the *Molitva Sfântului Vasile* (the prayer of Saint Basil), which seems to be the common prayer in the Romanian language area.

[18] Its newest edition was published in 2007. The exorcist prayer (*Moleben za besnovatykh*) is in the third chapter of the second volume of the service book. The first edition of the book was published in 1646. In the Russian Orthodox religious practice, the *otchitka* denomination is commonly used; they rarely call the ritual *exorcism*. The priests who do not have the episcopal blessing for practising exorcism can read simple healing prayers over the afflicted.

would worsen their condition. In the Peter and Paul Church or in the monastery, the pilgrims have to confess their sins as they arrive. Usually, it is suggested that they attend more than one exorcism session, which entails high costs as regards travel and accommodation. It can occur that a person stays for months. There are several hotels in the city, the ones related to the Church being mentioned above. It is possible to eat on the premises of the monastery (for many pilgrims, even a free food service is available), but one can find plenty of restaurants in the vicinity of the monastery. In exchange for a donation, certain guests have the opportunity to stay in one of the guestrooms of the parish Peter and Paul. Elite guests[19] may have a private exorcism in a specially designated hall in the house next to the Peter and Paul church. Social inequalities are not entirely dissolved either at the place of worship or during the exorcism, at least not in the communication between the personnel and the pilgrims. This obviously only happens in the communication between the pilgrims and the saint and God.

The Gate Church of John the Baptist, where Father Herman performs his mass exorcisms, is located at the main entrance of the monastery, above the arched gate decorated with murals. The church is small; it barely has the capacity to take in the crowd gathered for the ceremony (approximately three hundred people on each occasion), and usually, the narthex of the church is also filled with people. Father Herman performs the ritual almost every day; or more than once a day if one includes the private exorcisms. On Mondays and on important holidays, there are no exorcisms.[20] When Father Herman travels home to his native town, where he also performs exorcisms in one of the local churches (wherever they allow it), the exorcisms in the Lavra are suspended. Since the pilgrims pass information among themselves and there is also the possibility to call the monastery before travelling there, they usually manage to coordinate their needs with possible opportunities.

The exorcisms in the Gate Church of John the Baptist have been going on since the early nineties. Pilgrims from all around Russia come here to hear the sermon and the exorcist prayer of Father Herman, and to find out whether their troubles are caused by demons. We cannot consider the few hundred people who usually participate in the ritual as diabolically

[19] When I asked who was considered an "elite guest" I got the following answer: ministers, bankers, generals, famous actresses, singers. I even met a poet and singer who had been coming back regularly for years. She is an enthusiastic supporter of the Peter and Paul church to this day.

[20] It is important to notice that this is a report on exorcisms about ten years ago in the Lavra. As Father Herman is ageing, exorcisms are less frequent nowadays.

possessed. For many of them, the ritual serves divination functions, providing an explanation and a remedy that are easier to accept for the afflicted and the family than the explanation provided by official biomedicine. In a similar fashion to what happened at medieval places of worship and holy graves, while the priest reads out the exorcist prayer, it is observed whether the signs of possession and the presence of the Devil or demons within the man would manifest on contact with the cross (see Brown 1981). The signs of diabolical possession are classic symptoms, such as body seizures, bizarre and involuntary movements, extraordinary strength, aggressive gestures and voice, unnatural sounds (for instance a male voice in women or children), cursing, swearing, not tolerating sacred objects, sacred texts and bell ringing.

At the time of my fieldwork, Father Herman was nearly 70 years old. Many people think that his appearances recall the holy fathers of ancient times; his face resembles that of icons.[21] He is a tall, straight-backed man with a stern look and a lean figure. His ascetic lifestyle, his self-sacrificing, tireless, persistent service and his authoritative, respect-commanding presence all make a deep impression on the people seeking his help. His spiritual powers are estimated to be tremendous, and the fact that God has blessed him with the ability to exorcise is attributed to his pure way of life. Father Herman is a high-ranking monk (archimandrite[22]) who took his vow as a youth after having completed his studies at the Moscow Theological Academy and stayed here at the monastery. Today, he no longer lives within the walls of the monastery; his current residence is close to the Lavra in a guesthouse next to the Peter and Paul church. He is the *nastoiatel*[23] of the Peter and Paul church. It is he who supervises the

---

[21] Among his followers there are some who keep the portrait of Father Herman in their room with the icons.

[22] Archimandrite (cf. Greek *arkhimandritis*) is an honorary title that nowadays is no longer exclusively given to *hegumens* leading the community. It is one of the highest ranks a monk can obtain; directly above him in the ecclesiastical hierarchy is the bishop. The title is given to individuals who excel in spiritual or organisational activities. Father Herman was given this rank as a sign of appreciation for his activities carried out over the course of his life.

[23] The *nastoiat'el'* fulfils a leading function in the parish (Russian: *prikhod*); he coordinates the order of the rituals, the people serving at the church and the dealings of parish life. In Sergiev Posad, it is common to have five to seven priests in the service of a parish; in addition there is usually a deacon and a few helpers assisting the ritual. Often these assistant positions (*altarnik, ponomar*) are filled by people having had religious education. The priests of village churches are also called *nastoiat'el'*, but they serve alone and usually once a day at weekends. In

finances and decides how to spend the surplus. At the time of my fieldwork, he was the supervisor of six priests, one deacon, several men assisting rituals and a group of nuns, as well as a few lay residents and employees of the monastery.

Over the past two decades, he has been charged with the renovation of two churches in the city which administratively belong to the Lavra. By 2007 the renovation of the second (Peter and Paul) church was already completed and, here as well, he had established a well-conceived system of institutions around it (school, guesthouse, refectory—*trapeza*—for the employees and the priests of the parish, and a refectory for special guests); and adult courses, the lecturers of which were teachers from the Academy complemented by some well-educated priests from Sergiev Posad.[24]

Father Herman is worshipped as a saint by his closest followers. Some of the thousands of people turning to him for help stay forever in the city, and a few stay at the parish which provides them with a home and an employment. This, evidently, means a quasi-monkhood or a quasi-"nunness" (for lack of a better word); and many of them dress and live accordingly. But every employee is characterised by a strict Orthodox dress code and behaviour, which means wearing dark coloured clothes that cover all parts of the body, and a headscarf. The people who reside here have to maintain a strict attendance at masses, must keep fasting, and are expected to demonstrate modest behaviour. From a local perspective, the lay people and nuns or quasi-nuns working here form a very unique community which we could describe as traditional and visionary. The members of the group have often experienced miracles; many among them have had visions about Father Herman before they even knew him. Their acquaintance, on the other hand, has truly marked their lives.

Similar to what Giovanni Levi described in his microhistorical analysis, the family relations of the exorcists and the power relations at home play an important role in how the exorcist's career evolves (see Levi 2001). Father Herman comes from the Kuban region and to this day has

many cases, it is a male relative, often a son who helps out at the altar; and I have also seen, over the course of my fieldwork, a priest who had no assistance at all.

[24] The money gathered at the Church of John the Baptist contributes to the income of the Lavra. Therefore, it is crucial for the Peter and Paul church to attract pilgrims who confess there, who participate in the *soborovanie* ("the holy unction") and those who take part in personal exorcism all give donations to the parish. Father Herman not only successfully executed the restoration of the churches, but has built several buildings in Sergiev Posad that provide a home to the ventures within the parish, as well as to the employees, helpers and various guests.

close ties to his family and native land. He travels home on a regular basis. Relatives both close and distant, as well as local pilgrims, often visit Sergiev Posad. Some residents and employees are originally from Father Herman's hometown. For them, even the pilgrimage to the holy site is a great experience; others take the chance of staying and working here as a great opportunity. There are people who bring their families and send their kids to the local religious school, hoping that the education they will receive there will serve as armour against the problems of the age. The people on the inside who have been serving there for years are aware of a minor discord and a competition for the imagined or real favours of Father Herman. He and his prayers are capable of miracles because he lives the life of a saint—say those who live close to him. If something good happens to them, they interpret it as the result of God hearing the prayer Father Herman had said for them. They live in this environment; their main tasks are to assist the guests, to make sure they are catered for (according to their social status and the size of their donation), to assist the priest during the exorcism and to ensure the smoothness of the ritual performed in different locations for different persons.

Based on my observations, the exorcisms performed in the Gate Church of John the Baptist go as follows: before Father Herman arrives, an elderly nun (*inokinia*) reads prayers (from three o'clock in the afternoon); this is followed by Father Herman's one-and-a-half-hour sermon (from four to half past five in the afternoon) the text of which has been unchanged for years. This sermon is a type of catechesis containing the fundamental tenets of the Orthodox faith; furthermore, it contains basic information about demons and the ways in which one can defend oneself against them. The sermon is followed by the reading of the exorcist prayer. During the prayer, Father Herman burns incense and then sprinkles everyone profusely with holy water. After that, every participant is sacramentally anointed.[25] Finally, Father Herman leaves the church, and the younger priest assisting the ritual stands at the exit to hold the crucifix.

[25] The holy unction occurs more often within the Orthodox Church than in the Catholic Church. In our case, it is applied with healing purposes as a part of the *soborovanie* ritual, which is a prayer recited over afflicted people by a group of seven priests coming from different churches (in the Russian Orthodox Church). It is common for the afflicted to confess beforehand. It is important to mention that in the Peter and Paul Church, they hold *soborovanie* on a regular basis where the participants are more or less the same pilgrims who are present at the exorcism in the Lavra—evidently there is a very slim chance of everyone being granted this sanctimony during their stay in Sergiev Posad. It is important, however, that the two rituals complete one another, and thereby the chance of healing is multiplied.

While everyone kisses the crucifix as they leave, the young priest improvises a supplementary sermon to the crowd.

The crowd starts to gather at the Gate Church around two o'clock in the afternoon. Slowly, the people fill up the church and the narthex. The late arrivals stop at the entrance. The people in the crowd have very diverse social backgrounds: every adult age group is represented, but apparently there are more women than men and just a few children. Those suffering are usually accompanied by a relative, and children come with their parents. Based on their clothes, the crowd consists mostly of poor people, but occasionally we see "New Russians" (*novye russkie*[26]) appearing among them; and in the narthex and at the entrance, a few members of the press usually show up. It is easy to distinguish the helpers: there are only a few of them, they have a determined, authoritarian presence, and they are always active and punctual, making sure that the ritual goes smoothly, preparing all the accessories and ensuring silence in the crowd. There is a hierarchy among both the male and the female helpers, as is usually the case within the Church. Without a doubt, the highest authority among them is that of the elderly nun who has been serving Father Herman for almost two decades (basically an *inokinia* who had not taken her vow).[27] Besides reading prayers, she also participates in keeping order; she makes sure that there is a path in the crowd for the entrance of Father Herman. She does all this with an authoritative attitude, similar to her attitude as a relentless host in the guesthouse: no one can refuse either food or beverage at her place.[28] Besides the elderly nun, there is another old lady who collects the *zapiski* (notes with the names of the troubled people), the candles and the money that they hand forward in the crowd. She lights the candles and cleans the candleholders. The crowd becomes so thick that it is impossible to move, let alone to move forward, unless all move in synch with their neighbours. (Interestingly, there is always room for Father Herman to get to the altar at the beginning and

---

[26] On the *novye russkie* (the New Russians) see Humphrey 2002, 175-201.

[27] The old lady had been healed of cancer by praying at the relics of Saint Sergius (personal communication). Subsequently, Father Kirill, one of the elders (*startsy*) mentioned in the introduction, gave his blessing to her to help father Herman and to stay in Sergiev Posad. She left her family in a neighbouring *oblast'* and has been living here and helping out ever since. Meanwhile, she tries to provide for her family as well.

[28] The old lady is the guardian of morality around Father Herman. She makes sure to reprimand the longing looks of younger women bustling around Father Herman. Her close acquaintances told me that sometimes she anoints the eyelids of women who throw inappropriate glances at him.

during the ritual, and to move around in the crowd in any direction when it is the turn of the chrism.) A man (not a member of the clergy, just a simple employee and helper from the Peter and Paul church) scans and observes the crowd, supervises the behaviour of the people present, orders silence and peaceful behaviour and makes sure everyone wears the cross; he also emphasises that people have to fast and confess before coming here. Meanwhile, he repeatedly warns non-Orthodox people to leave because here they only accept Orthodox Christians. A young priest comes in with Father Herman, holding at his back an abundance of *zapiski* gathered at the Peter and Paul church by the people arriving at the exorcism. His task is to assist Father Herman during the ceremony, to lift the buckets containing holy water and to hold the sacramental oil. After Father Herman leaves, he is the one to hold the crucifix at the exit; profiting from the silence, he adds his thoughts to Father Herman's sermon, confirms the anti-witchcraft discourse, the antipathy against Muslims and Buddhists, and so forth. This person remains the same for a lengthy period of time, although over the course of Father Herman's activities, several have fulfilled this function. The number of helpers present at the exorcism is basically low—four or five people altogether.

I have noticed the authoritative and pronouncedly aggressive tone of the (ecclesiastic and worldly) helpers since the beginning. Father Herman is no exception in this regard. I was not the only one to notice it; journalists also make regular remarks about it, adding quickly that this is understandable, as is his grim personality, since he has been assigned a very difficult service: he is fighting the enemy of humanity, Satan, the dark forces. They usually stress that Father Herman is exhausted by the service ("it is as if he carried heavy stones all day long"); but the people living in his direct environment know that before the exorcism in the Lavra, he deals with selected guests next to the Peter and Paul church, in a more personal environment: first he talks with them; then he eats a meal with them; subsequently, if there is need, he performs exorcism on some of the guests. Naturally, he is also present at the morning liturgy, thus he serves all day long.

It is important to explain certain aspects of this. Russians, in general, tolerate such a type of aggressive and authoritative treatment much better than would be the case in the cultural environment I am used to. This is also manifested in their child-raising customs. They set very clear boundaries during child-raising, and these boundaries are respected and enforced by any community, even beyond the family (even the community of people travelling together in a minibus, the *marshrutka*). The way the crowd cooperates with the helpers to maintain order before the exorcism is rooted in this same mentality. Everybody considers it their duty to call to order any person "misbehaving" next to them. Or, in Orthodox circles, they believe that sects (meaning the believers of Protestant denominations, both historical and neo-Protestants), followers of Eastern Churches, yoga practitioners, believers in different magical and mystical doctrines, energy healers, people with supernatural skills (*ekstrasensy*) are all in the wrong and are all damned unless they become converted. Father Herman does not tolerate any other religion at his ceremony, which he emphasises at the beginning of his sermon. I witnessed as he sent a Baptist woman with her children out of the church (he had known them from before). Evidently, any Orthodox Christian person having participated in some sort of sinful activity, but feeling remorse for it and having confessed it, can come to the exorcism, which can thus help them to start a new life. In other Orthodox churches, the "right of entry" is usually not so strict. In most cases, keeping to the dress code is more or less enough to enter the monastery (in many places women in trousers can borrow skirts; or if that is not an option, necessity teaches women to ingeniously improvise a skirt using a scarf over their trousers). Women cannot attend Father Herman's ceremony without wearing a scarf and a long skirt either. The same rule applies to the Peter and Paul church; moreover, wearing these items of clothing is required over the entire territory of the parish.[29] Dressing decently and covering the body is usually compulsory in Orthodox churches.[30] Men have to wear long-sleeved shirts, long trousers and their head has to be uncovered.

In what follows, I will describe the ritual. The elderly *inokinia* arrives at three in the afternoon; she goes to the altar and starts reading the prayers kneeling down. The church is so crowded by this time that you can barely move. The people listen to the prayers in silence; meanwhile, the newly arrived people pass forward their *zapiska*, candles and greater or lesser amounts of donation (at the time of my fieldwork, this meant an amount of around 100, 500, 1000 roubles, lesser amounts being more frequent; I passed along the money on several occasions, which allowed me to note the amounts). On one occasion, someone refused to pass on the money; I presume it was out of fear of contact with the possessed.

---

[29] I was also made aware of this at the very first occasion.

[30] This expectation requires serious efforts in today's Russia, since the trend is the exact opposite. Interestingly, in Orthodox circles, it is a permanent topic to comment on the terribly distasteful clothing of tourists, while the non-observant religious locals are much less discrete. One of the popular topics is the western old lady who visited the monastery wearing shorts—which is nonsense because for years, the guards at the entrance would not have let her enter in these clothes.

The inner space of the church is divided with a cordon. The space before the altar, where the helper lady lights the candles and the elderly nun reads the prayers and where later, Father Herman would speak and sprinkle the holy water, is essentially closed off from most people. This is obviously necessary because of the huge crowd. Some people, based on prior coordination, kneel there throughout, that is, a duration of approximately three and a half hours. Coming earlier and positioning oneself closer to the separated area and also to the altar entails privileges: they will stand closer to Father Herman and thus will have more opportunities to touch the crucifix and his robes; they will also receive more of the holy water.

At around four o'clock, Father Herman arrives. His arrival is signalled by a low murmur. He is accompanied by a young priest, as I have previously mentioned. He goes inside the altar and puts on his ritual vestments.[31] Then he comes out and opens the windows wide (even in the winter), turns on the lights and finally stops at the pulpit (*kliros*) placed on the right of the altar and starts his sermon, which is one of the key elements of the ceremony; it plays an educational, socialising and guiding role. The teaching it contains is particularly important because when it comes to religious education, the population has been neglected for generations: it is quite rare for them to learn the fundamentals of Orthodox faith within the family. (And those who have a religious education usually do not go to exorcisms. They have learned how to live a balanced religious life, which does not include such extreme temptations and diabolical possession.[32])

The text of the sermon has been unchanged for years. It has also been published and translated into several other languages (German, Italian, English) (see Arkhimandrite Herman 2006). The published text has two introductions; one of them is a quotation from the diary of archbishop Nikon (*arkhiepiskop Nikon Rozhdestvenskii*) from 1910. The passage draws a parallel between the pre-revolution era and the post-perestroika period. Similarities can be found in the relationship between the Church and the intelligentsia, as well as in the impact of secularisation. Archbishop Nikon considers it a key issue whether someone accepts the existence of dark forces and demons. If yes, there is a chance to reconvert to the Orthodox faith.

This is followed by the foreword of Father Herman, which briefly determines the nature of the problems that people bring with them. People possessed by impure, evil spirits (demons) come in streams from all over

[31] He already wears a simple inner cassock at his arrival.

[32] These results come from interviews with members of the clergy or students from the Lavra.

Russia. It is a separate group of illnesses, which medicine defines as mental disorders; in the medical practice of many centuries of the Russian Orthodox Church, however, they are considered to be bewitchment and diabolical possession. "Under diabolical possession [*besnovanie*] we mean much more serious damage: in these cases, we say that the Devil has entered the person's heart" (Archimandrite Herman 2006, 5). The Orthodox priests read a special prayer in the church, which is a legacy of the holy fathers of the fourth century; they strengthen the afflicted with holy water and anoint them with holy oil (chrism), and then bless them with the holy crucifix. Meanwhile, the devils manifest themselves; they have a non-human voice: they caw and grunt, scream, cry, hit and shake the possessed, forcing them to perform bizarre body movements. Sometimes they bring the afflicted from other cities, tied to a pole. Father Herman claims that injuries, wounds, illnesses and sorrow are cast upon us by demons. Demons trick us, tempt us to sin, ambush us. If someone lives by the Ten Commandments, the divine blessing protects them, for they are surrounded by a protective shield that the evil spirits can see. But if someone is baptised and lives a sinful life, the protective shield dissolves around them; the demons rejoice over taking hold of the human. This is how illnesses begin; he quotes the teachings of Saint John Chrysostom *(Sviatoi Ioann Zlatoust: Slovo o zlykh dukhah).*

The first part of the sermon emphasises the participation-related requirements: only Orthodox believers are allowed to participate, they must be wearing a cross on their neck,[33] be after confession, purged and with the desire of a new life in their souls. He encourages the believers to confess and repent their sins and to convert. During the Soviet era, several generations had grown up without God, in atheism, as he says. Due to this, people have sinned a lot, often unconsciously. It is important that they confess all of their sins. He encourages everyone to write a list of all the sins of their childhood, adulthood and married life; even if it adds up to a hundred pages; then to go to the church and confess everything in order to obtain absolution. After that, abiding by the Ten Commandments, they should make every effort not to repeat the same sin again and to live the purest life possible.

A great number of pilgrims come from Northern and Siberian areas scarcely covered by the Church, from towns without a church or a priest,

---

[33] If somebody arrives without a cross, it is possible to buy one at the entrance. If it turns out at the beginning that someone did not bring a cross, Father Herman sends that person out. These people usually come back afterwards and fight their way back to their original places. I see some similarity between the place occupied during the exorcism and queuing in socialist times.

in order to find out the cause of their illness. Often, they suspect bewitchment. Father Herman tells the people to search for the source of all troubles within us. We only suffer for our sins; demons can only prevail over sinners. The helpless, suffering pilgrim starts to think about the causes of the illness, repents and asks for help. The faithless still blame others: they say their suffering is caused by the bewitchment of a witch. Yet witches are nothing compared to the power of Jesus Christ (Arkhimandrit Herman 2006, 10).

The people present usually listen to Father Herman's sermon in silence, hanging on his words. Only rarely are disturbing noises heard (as the participants change, so the behaviour varies; but silence and peace, occasionally interrupted by cries and sighs is more common than a huge noise).

Father Herman discusses the Ten Commandments in a specific order, emphasising everything from the eternal moral laws that respond to the problems of our days: prohibition of fornication, respecting the seventh day, going to church, keeping the commandment of celebrating holydays and resting. Morals have declined; half of marriages end in divorce, says Father Herman (even more, according to statistics). The importance of family has diminished. People should not divorce; they should endure. When the churches are empty, many go shopping to malls or stay at home and watch low moral shows on the television. The television, besides teaching sins, has a negative effect on work capability and emits harmful radiation. The children will have sleeping problems and will be exposed to jeopardy. Respecting the commandment seems easy; yet, nowadays very few go to the house of God at the end of the week.

Finally, Father Herman gives advice on how to protect ourselves against demons and evil spirits. The ancient Orthodox faith gives blessing and offers redemption for those who live by its rules. Saying the Lord's Prayer and the Jesus Prayer protects the person and scares off demons (Arkhimandrit Herman 2006, 27). Furthermore, they have a protective effect if we regularly sprinkle the house and the garden with holy water and smoke incense. The earthly remains of saints, sacred icons and holy oils have similar effects. The crucifix wards off the evil spirits. One must make the sign of the cross over everything that one buys on the market or in the store. Nowadays, a great variety of products are produced and distributed by godless, heretic and superstitious people. For an even better result, it is advisable to sprinkle with holy water everything we buy.

If someone's stomach, hand, feet or head suddenly gets sick, one must immediately make the sign of the cross over the sick body part repeatedly: not in the air but directly on the body. And one has to say the Lord's

Prayer more frequently. Coding (*kodirovanie*, the coding of the alcoholics), which is increasingly popular in today's Russia, is forbidden by the Orthodox Church. Coding is the conscious, deliberate settling of demons into the human body for a limited period with the consent of the sick by means of black and white magic. There exists a therapy to introduce substances into the bodies of alcoholics that cause immediate death if they consume alcohol. This aggression against human nature is reprehensible from the perspective of the Church (Arkhimandrit Herman 2006, 29). There is a possibility to order prayers against alcoholism; to take home three litres of holy water for drinking and to bathe in it every morning. Wine is also an indispensable beverage in ecclesiastical life; but it is important to consume it with moderation (only red wine, only on holidays and no more than one glass). Christian believers should not drink strong spirits, succedaneum, homemade brandy or cologne.

Father Herman's teaching can be summarised in two important thoughts: on the one hand, we are all prisoners and victims, consequences of our age and the godlessness we experience; on the other hand, we should not delude ourselves into thinking that our problems are caused by witches; they are sent by the Almighty because of our sins so that we have a chance to step on the path of redemption. Illness is an instrument in God's hand, which he uses to guide us onto his path. Demons are instruments of moral education.

The actual exorcism starts around half past five, after the one-and-a-half-hour sermon. Father Herman reads the exorcist prayer and smokes incense (in the usual manner: walking around, swinging the incense). In addition to the exorcist prayer, he also says an interactive prayer together with the afflicted into which everybody can include their own name and that of their relative and ask God's support in helping their recovery. It was only during the prayer that the crowd became somewhat noisy; for instance, a young woman groaned and wailed in the crowd. A university student, who came to the exorcism because of her drug addiction was kneeling in the entrance and was weeping loudly and painfully with tears streaming down her face. She was a blond, long-haired, young, modern urban woman in her twenties who, based on her clothes, was not the "church going" type. Other than this, even though there were many tormented, sickly faces in the crowd, people with visible problems were rarely seen. There was only one middle-aged businessman-like person whose head was shaking and visibly this bothered him a great deal; this was probably the reason he was there. I was told by journalists and my acquaintances that they had all witnessed more sensational exorcisms.

After the prayer, Father Herman sprinkles the crowd abundantly with holy water. There are buckets filled with holy water prepared in the centre of the church; from there, he splashes the water with a special instrument three times in every direction. He splashes so much water that the people are completely soaked; the water is even streaming down the murals. The people hold their heads up and face him as they wait for the water, as they do when receiving blessing, kneeling reverently. Here I must mention that during the ceremony, already from the start of the prayers, the crowd had to kneel. As soon as the water poured down on them, there was a ripple effect in the crowd as the people shook from the cold water suddenly hitting them. There was no room; I was suffering from forced immobility, stuck in the crowd. And judging by the words of the people around me, I was not the only one. Participation was an exhausting experience, both physically and mentally; not even because of the illness and the demons but rather due to the discomfort and the roughness.[34] Today, in the Russian Orthodox Church, experiencing physical pain during the ceremony is usually a sign of the demons' attack, which the observant believer has to endure and remain standing through the ceremony, even if it is long. The rough tone is addressed to the unclean people possessed by demons, who deserve this because of their sins. Their repeated participation proves that this treatment does not disappoint them.

After the splashing of the holy water, when the chrism comes with the holy oil,[35] everyone stands up. Father Herman traverses the crowd in several directions; there is always someone breaking the crowd and making way for him. Everyone is trying to "reach" with their foreheads and push forward trying to stick out from the crowd. They even address the priest: "*Bat'ushka,*[36] *suda*" [Father, over here!]; and they tell each other "*Bat'ushka pomogaet!*" [Bat'ushka helps us (or: is helping us)!]. Most people draw a cross into their hands with the holy oil from their foreheads; some draw the sign of the cross on the backs of their neck, over their hearts, on their necks, and on the sick body parts. They observe and imitate each other. The women and the men zealously anoint themselves with the oil. They attribute healing effects to the holy oil. The anointment serves also to seal off the orifices (ears and mouth) so that the demons cannot move around freely.

Following the anointment, Father Herman touches the people standing near him with the crucifix, the book and his stole who thus are in a

[34] These are personal impressions. Evidently, it might differ considerably how each person experiences the same event.

[35] The anointing of the sick is one of the sacraments of the Orthodox Church, cf. Greek *evkhelaion*, Ware 1997, 296–7.

[36] It is an informal and common way to address priests in Russia.

privileged situation. As he passes through the crowd, many try to touch his robes. At the end of the ceremony, Father Herman leaves, after which people slowly start to flow out of the church. At the exit, in front of the window and at the stairs, stands the other, younger priest who has only been assisting in the ceremony. He sprinkles the people once more on their way out; he holds out the crucifix for them to kiss. No one leaves without doing so. Meanwhile, he speaks enthusiastically, as if he had been waiting to finally be given the floor. His main topic was bewitchment [*porcha*] and its potentiality. In cases of illness, when the doctors are out of options, then it is indeed a case of bewitchment. He disparaged the specialists of magic called *ektrasensy* (cf. Lindquist 2006) claiming to have supernatural powers, and the witches, as did Father Herman; and he reiterated that these specialists send the demons upon the people, because they collaborate with them. The speech continues until the church is completely empty. The crowd scatters; most of them leave the monastery, go out for dinner then go to their accommodation. The subsequent day, most of them are already at the church early in the morning; they participate in every ceremony until the afternoon comes with a new exorcism.

Exorcism and Studying Eastern Christianity

Studies examining the history of Russia and the Russian Orthodox Church have proven that the issue of diabolical possession and the practice of exorcism have been present in the history of Russian Orthodoxy. We know from the historical monograph by Scott Kenworthy on the Trinity-Sergius Lavra that the monks who had been living here in the past centuries also believed in diabolical possession and there have also been exorcisms (Kenworthy 2010). In her book about *klikushestvo*[37], Christine Worobec explains that in the nineteenth century, while official medicine gained ground and the interpretation of the phenomenon was gradually medicalised and it became more and more frequent in the secular sphere to label the *klikushi* as hysteric women, the Church remained more tolerant and more understanding towards them and provided help for them through exorcisms (Worobec 2001). In view of Father Herman's figure and social role, it is important to highlight the parallel between him and Ioann Kronstadtskii (1829–1908). Worobec discussed in graphic terms the church ceremonies of Father Ioann Kronstadtskii, as well as the cathartic experience of mass confessions that he introduced, which turned the entire congregation into a roaring crowd of possessed people (Worobec 2001,

[37] The term means: "possession caused by a bewitchment of witches".

61–63). The exorcist reputation of Father Ioann Kronstadtskii (he was one of the exorcists of national importance of his age) proves the significance of miracles and of diabolical possession in pre-revolutionary Russia.

Galina Lindquist notes in her book about magic and healing written on the basis of her fieldwork in Moscow, that in modern Russia, the phenomenon of *klikushestvo* is not that common as it used to be when it had risen to epidemic proportions, but diabolical possession continues to occur to this day (Lindquist 2006). There are quite a few priests within the Russian Orthodox Church known for their ability to exorcise. They usually live in monasteries where they perform group exorcisms on a regular basis. We can only find a few general remarks concerning Orthodox Christian exorcisms in Lindquist's book (big crowd, pushing, dramatic, often dreadful rituals considered dangerous to the participants); but she describes in detail the healing of a possessed woman performed by a magician (*ektrasens*) from Moscow. Here we have a partly different terminology and a completely different healing method compared to ecclesiastic exorcism (Lindquist 2006, 66–9). Her analysis parallels the analysis of religious healing by Csordas (Csordas 1997); she even refers to his results. She notices that exorcisms are crowded, dramatic and often dreadful services, considered to be dangerous for the participants.

Historians and anthropologists have studied diabolical possession and exorcism in various cultures of the world. Several collections of studies have been published in several languages on this topic providing a representative selection of past years' research (Crapanzano and Garrison 1977; Levack 1992; Mageo and Howard 1996). Janice Boddy's overview of possession-related research, published in 1994, stresses that recent studies go beyond the issue of instrumentality and highlight the complex social significance of the phenomenon of possession with emphasis on the connection between contemporary social problems and moral issues (Boddy 1994).

In Hungarian, it was Éva Pócs who wrote a thorough overview of the phenomenon and related research of diabolical possession focusing on Europe and on Christianity (Pócs 2001). She explained that exorcism is more than simply chasing Satan who possessed the human body: it is a cleansing ritual in a wider sense, which is closely related to ecclesiastical benediction. Pócs mentions here that exorcism is also performed during the ritual of baptism (Pócs 2001, 187). This was also corroborated by several priests from Sergiev Posad who could relate their dreadful experiences concerning possessed infants. It is important to note in relation to my study that Father Herman's exorcisms were also beneficial rituals in a wider sense, which were able to help a wide variety of troubles, not only the possessed, but theoretically anyone.

Below, I will highlight four further studies which discuss similar topics in other Eastern Christian Churches. We learn from the monograph by Charles Stewart that on the island of Naxos where he conducted his research, exorcisms are rare; in the monastery of Phyl near Athens, exorcisms are performed regularly once a week (Stewart 1991). Here we also have mass exorcisms, with the participation of around three hundred people. One part of them are the afflicted, the others accompany them. It is usual to give the name of the afflicted and monetary donations when arriving at the monastery. The sermon is once again a key element of the ritual; contrary to the exorcist prayer, it is recited in a language that the people understand. (Father Herman reads the exorcist prayer in Old Church Slavonic, but he also preaches in Russian.) During the sermon in the Greek monastery, the priests discuss topics similar to the ones experienced in Sergiev Posad: they emphasise the healing power of religion and condemn those who seek the help of witches. Stewart published the prayer they recite and described the exorcism included in the baptism ceremony in detail; however, the book does not reveal the opinion of the pilgrims and the locals, nor that of the clergy about diabolical possession and exorcism.

Jill Dubisch undertook her fieldwork on a Greek island as well, near a place of worship (Dubisch 1995). In terms of our topic, an important part of her book is the description of a pilgrim who took a vow: a woman in her twenties is working her way up on her knees to the mountaintop where the pilgrimage church was located. On the way, she fights demonic forces that hold her back and cause her a headache. When she finally gets to the top she is relieved. The woman rids herself of the demons, not by the church ritual, but by a local vernacular ritual: she takes a vow and keeps it through great hardships. The people in the street are sympathetic with the sufferer; they encourage her and follow her struggle for hours, which is the complete opposite of how people distance themselves from the possessed in Sergiev Posad.

Gabriel Troc studied the exorcisms in a small village of the Transylvanian Western Carpathians called Poşaga and gives some sort of thick description of them (Troc 1998–1999). Troc is a local and knew the reactions and interpretations of the villagers well. The exorcisms in Poşaga were parallels of the Sergiev Posad exorcisms in many respects; they only attract a few people and were performed twice a week and were soon completely discontinued. The priest got into the crossfire of envy and accusations and was shortly transferred. Certain elements of the Poşaga exorcism are similar to the ceremonies of Sergiev Posad: the reception and the audition of the pilgrims at the parish; the presence of helpers; the settling of people in hope of recovery; the diversity of the illnesses and the troubles they treat; and the national reputation. In my opinion, in the case of women who have been participating in exorcisms for a long time, it is not just a simulation of being possessed, as Gabriel Troc ironically suggests, but an intense empathy. Financial gain, investments in building church property and in creating communities are also important here. The exorcism was performed in the village church, although in the vicinity of the village there is a monastery with a sacred fountain next to it.[38] The exorcism started in the evening and stretched into the night. The crowd often waited hours for the arrival of the priest. The sermon of Father Ioan included several topics also discussed by Father Herman (such as neglecting prayer and fasting; the dangers of sects, television and smoking; explaining illnesses, divorce and moral aberration). Although Father Ioan belongs to a much younger generation than Father Herman, he also preaches asceticism. During the exorcism, the priest read the prayers of Saint Basil the Great *(Sf. Vasile cel Mare)* and of Saint John Chrysostom *(Sf. Ioan Gură de Aur)* and he sprinkled the crowd with holy water around midnight.

Vlad Naumescu carried out his research in Ukraine in the Greek Catholic Church, not the Orthodox community. His study is about a group of monks who left the Church and about the exorcisms they perform in a monastery in Kolodiivka established by them (Naumescu 2008 and 2010). The author knew the exorcist monks well; and when describing their opinion and internal development, he also explored the context of the phenomenon. In a similar way to the places we have discussed above, here the social need for exorcism was also great; a significant difference, however, was that the entire monastery was specialised in exorcism. The monks followed Orthodox tradition in their exorcisms and in trying to lead an ascetic eremitical lifestyle. The charismatic personality of Father Planchak, the founder and leader of the community, plays an important role in the promotion of exorcisms. Since they had left the Church, it is not the Church who decides who has the right to exorcise. The monks can experiment with their capabilities, which, according to their views, are already given via germs to every Christian man since their baptism. The exorcisms in Kolodiivka go on from spring until late autumn on every last Tuesday of the month. On these days, many pilgrims arrive at the monastery and usually stay from morning until late night. The exorcist

[38] The Orthodox church in Poşaga burned down during the stay of Father Ioan, which was considered by many as an act of Evil.

prayers start around six in the afternoon; confessions are taken by several priests in the garden of the monastery from the morning onwards. The sacred anointment takes place before the exorcism. The study reveals little about the pilgrims and their points of view, but this was evidently not the main objective of the article.

The above-mentioned works clearly confirm that exorcism is still a contemporary practice in Eastern Christianity. We can discover numerous similarities between Father Herman's exorcisms and the ceremonies observed in Greek and Romanian Orthodox Churches, as well as with the exorcisms performed by the formerly Greek Catholic Ukrainian monks; these not only integrate well into Russian historical tradition, but also fit into a wider Eastern Christian tradition.

Conclusion

We know of two types of religious and moral explanations of illnesses. The first explanation states that the cause of the illness lies in the sinful nature of the human being and the illness is God's punishment. The other explanation claims that the malevolence of our fellow humans is accountable for the illness. The typical example of the latter is witchcraft accusation. Orthodox religion does not deny the power of witches; it does consider it, however, limited. Our faith in God and leading a true Christian life are sufficient for getting rid of the witches' powers. The Orthodox Church and Father Herman both believe that illness is a consequence of a sinful life; and they ask the people to confess their sins, instead of blaming witches for their troubles. They offer handholds and invite people to take the path of personal perfection.

It would be difficult to exhaustively answer the question of why exorcism is so appealing to such a wide audience in today's Russia. Why do people believe in the Devil? Why did religious explanations of troubles become so popular after so many decades of atheist campaign? The answers to these questions could only be delivered after further research. I have experienced over the course of my fieldwork that even those who only rarely think about demons consider their influence a real danger and are afraid of being possessed. By extending the above-mentioned questions, we get the fundamental question of modern (and not just Russian) research of religion: how is it possible that nowadays the role of religiosity is increasing worldwide rather than declining? This question is particularly relevant in former socialist countries. One thing is certain based on current research findings: the Soviet system has by no means eradicated Orthodox religiosity; like a subterranean brook, it surfaced and lives its renaissance in today's Russia. The matter of the continuity of tradition is another fundamental issue often discussed within the Church and in scholarly studies, and it is also important from the perspective of exorcisms. What seems a novelty in Father Herman's exorcisms is the mass nature of the ceremonies. This is a new tendency that can also be discovered in other contemporary Orthodox congregations.

The majority of people participating in exorcisms are not deeply religious and are not practising believers (*nevotserkovlennye*). For many, participation in the exorcism and learning about the Devil and about religion, in general, is an experience that motivates their later conversion. The individual life stories often relate several phases of the conversion process; many reach Orthodoxy through various religious movements and through religious experiences gained in other churches. Becoming converted is often coupled with the story of an illness or some other crisis and suffering. In Russia, an entire spectrum of healers is available and people usually try them, which is also how they discover exorcisms. The activities, beliefs and new religious views of these charismatic healers have a great impact on thousands of the population. The activities of Father Herman should also be analysed in this context.

Over the past two and a half decades, numerous disconcerting factors have influenced Russian society. New kinds of fears have arisen, new kinds of skills have had to be learned. Many could not handle the change-induced stress; they fell ill or became addicted to alcohol or drugs. Religious life provided help; religious communities offered a sense of belonging and support for many in this transitional—or as Inna Naletova called it—liminal era (Naletova 2007, based on Turner). The pilgrimages became appealing; the number of pilgrims increased, as did the exorcisms as well. There is a great need for spiritual leaders and miracles in Russia today. The hopeful believers pray to the saints and the living saints. Immediately after the perestroika, the elders (*startsy*) and the monks promoting asceticism had a strong appeal as spiritual fathers. Over the past decade and a half, some sort of change could be observed: the believers often selected a new spiritual father, usually a simple, married priest (a member of the white clergy). In the long run, it would be worth observing the career of the people coming from the "entourage" of Father Herman, as well as the fate of those who are healed by exorcisms. Furthermore, the following hypothesis should also be verified: Father Herman's impact is exclusive to those who come from a non-ecclesiastical environment.

Observing the exorcism suggests that for many, the presence of a leading character of an unquestionable authority is vital. All this tells a lot about the mass psychology of the post-Soviet man. If socialist systems were lacking in consumer products, and acquiring products was often associated with long journeys, waiting in line, big crowds and the experience of strong frustration and hard-to-reach rewards; today there is a shift in the quest for goods, from material to the spiritual: thousands of people take a journey, wait in line for spiritual and mental goods; they expect solace and recovery from the relics of saints, miracle-working icons and fountains or precisely from Father Herman. As participation in the liturgy and its apparent passivity represent an inner happening, contemplation and prayer, it is just as impossible here to get better without making the inner journey. Exorcism is just the beginning; a type of initiation on the path to recovery. If someone is determined to change, they must get rid of their sinful behaviours in the long run and then they will heal. The sermon offers advice, the ritual provides help, but without human determination, will and perseverance, success is impossible.

It would be great to clearly understand why there is a need today for exorcisms within the Catholic Church, why exorcisms are so important within Orthodoxy, and why the Devil and exorcism are such fundamental experiences in neo-Protestant religions. What are the common factors typical for the people of our time that trigger this interest and what personal and social problems do exorcists solve? We know that nowadays, in neo-Protestant religiosity, the concept of Evil, exorcism, healing and miraculous healing in general play a very important role in terms of group cohesion and enforcing faith (Wanner 2007). Within Orthodoxy, the person of the exorcist illustrates that asceticism and leading a wholesome life gives them power over the Evil haunting the world. One can get rid of the Evil and the troubles, be it illness or any other, through the mercy and the blessing of God (which, by promoting the doctrines and morals diametrically opposing its worldly equivalents, fills them with the hope of redemption). The efforts made for redemption's sake, however, are subject to personal freedom and decision.

Bibliography

Arkhimandrit Herman, Chesnokov. 2006. *Propoved' pered chinom izgnania zlyh duhov iz cheloveka* [Sermon before the exorcism of evil spirits].

Boddy, Janice. 1994. "Spirit Possession Revisited: Beyond Instrumentality." *Annual Review of Anthropology* 23 (1): 407–34.

Brown, Peter. 1981. *The Cult of Saints. Its Rise and Function in Latin Christianity.* London: SCM Press Ltd.

Crapanzano, Vincent, and Vivian Garrison. 1977. *Case Studies in Spirit*

Possession. New York, London, Sidney, and Toronto: John Wiley & Sons.

Csordas, Thomas. 1997. *The Sacred Self. A Cultural Phenomenology of Charismatic Healing*. Berkeley: University of California Press.

Dubisch, Jill. 1995. *In a Different Place. Pilgrimage, Gender and Politics at a Greek Island Shrine.* Princeton, N.J.: Princeton University Press.

Humphrey, Caroline. 2002. *The unmaking of Soviet life: everyday economies after socialism*. Ithaca & London: Cornell University Press.

Kenworthy, Scott. [2010a]. *The heart of Russia. Trinity-Sergius, monasticism, and society after 1825.* Oxford, and Washington D.C.: Oxford University Press, and Woodrow Wilson Center.

—. 2012. "The Revival of Monastic Life in the Trinity-Sergius Lavra after World War II." In *State secularism and lived religion in Soviet Russia and Ukraine*, edited by Catherine Wanner, 117–58. Conference papers. Washington, D.C.: Woodrow Wilson Center Press; New York: Oxford University Press.

Komáromi, Tünde et al. 2010. "'Spreading Grace' in Post-Soviet Russia." *Anthropology Today* 26 (1): 16–21.

Kormina, Jeanne. 2013. "Canonizing Soviet Pasts in Contemporary Russia: The Case of Saint Matrona of Moscow." In *A Companion to the Anthropology of Religion*, edited by Janice Boddy, and Michael Lambek, 409–24. Hoboken, N.J.: John Wiley and Sons.

Kormina, Jeanne, and Sergei Shtyrkov. 2007. "Letters of Believers as Advertising: The 'National Reception Room' of St. Xenia of Petersburg." *Antropologicheskii Forum* 9: 154–84.

Levack, Brian P. 1992. *Possession and Exorcism.* New York, and London: Garland Publishing, Inc.

Levi, Giovanni. 1988. *Inheriting Power: the Story of an Exorcist.* Translated by Lydia G. Cochrane. Chicago: University of Chicago Press [*L'eredità immateriale. Carriera di un esorcista nel Piemonte del seicento.* Torino: Einaudi, 1985.]

Lindquist, Galina. 2006. *Conjuring Hope. Magic and Healing in Contemporary Russia.* New York, and Oxford: Berghahn Books.

Mageo, Jeannette Marie, and Alan Howard. 1996. *Spirits in Culture, History and Mind.* New York, and London: Routledge.

Mitrokhin, Nikolay. 2004. *Russkaia Pravoslavnaia Tserkov'. Sovremennoe sostoianie i aktual'nye problemy*. Moskva: Novoe literaturnoe obozrenie.

Naletova, Inna. 2007. *Orthodoxy beyond the Walls of the Church: A Sociological Inquiry into Orthodox Religious Experience in Contemporary Russian Society.* Boston: Boston University, Graduate

School of Arts and Sciences.

Naumescu, Vlad. 2008. *Modes of Religiosity in Eastern Christianity: religious processes and social change in Ukraine*. Berlin: LIT Verlag.

—. 2010. "A Monastic Splinter Group and its Imagistic Practice of Exorcism." In *Eastern Christians in Anthropological Perspective*, edited by Chris Hann, and Hermann Goltz, 155–76. Berkeley, Los Angeles, and London: The University of California Press. (The Anthropology of Christianity 9.)

Pócs, Éva. 2001. "Démoni megszállottság és ördögűzés a közép-kelet-európai népi hiedelemrendszerekben [Demonic possession and exorcism in the popular belief systems of East-Central Europe]." In *Demonológia és boszorkányság Európában* [Demonology and witchcraft in Europe], edited by Éva Pócs, 137–98. Budapest: L'Harmattan, and PTE Néprajz Tanszék. (Studia Ethnologica Hungarica 1.)

Rodion, Sviaschennik. 2005. *Liudi i demony, Obrazy iskushenia sovremennogo cheloveka padshimi duhami* [People and demons. Temptations of contemporary people by fallen souls]. Kiev: Obschestvo liubitelei pravoslavnoi literatury, Izdatelstvo imeni sviatitelia L'va, papy Rimskogo.

Stewart, Charles. 1991. *Demons and the Devil. Moral Imagination in Modern Greek Culture.* Princeton, N.J.: Princeton University Press.

Tarabukina, Arina V. 2000. *Fol'klor i kultura pritserkovnogo kruga* [Folklore and culture of the temple milieu]. Candidate Diss., Rossiiskii gosudarstvennyi pedagogicheskii universitet im. A. I. Gertsena. http://www.ruthenia.ru/folktee/CYBERSTOL/books/Tarabukina/vstuplenie.html. Accessed: 10.03.2016.

Trebnik. 2007. *Trebnik mitropolita Petra Mogily* [The service book of Metropolitan Petr Mogil]. Kharkov: Folio.

Troc, Gabriel. 1998–1999. "Exorcism şi vindecare în Biserica Ortodoxă." [Exorcism and healing in the Orthodox Church]. *Caietele Tranziţiei* 2–3: 130–5.

Turner, Victor, and Edith Turner. 1978. *Image and Pilgrimage in Christian Culture.* Oxford: Basil Blackwell.

Wanner, Catherine. 2007. *Communities of the Converted. Ukrainians and Global Evangelism*. Ithaca, and London: Cornell University Press.

Ware, Timothy. 1997. *The Orthodox Church*. Harmondsworth: Penguin Books. [1963.]

Worobec, Christine. 2001. *Possessed: Women, Witches, and Demons in Imperial Russia*. DeKalb, Illinois: Northern Illinois University Press.

3. PUNISHING AND HEALING SAINTS, MIRACULOUS HEALINGS

MYTHICAL BEINGS PUNISHING THE BREAKING OF TABOOS ON SPINNING

MIRJAM MENCEJ

In many places in Europe, as well as outside of it, e.g. in Asia, there are legends told about figures, usually of female gender, who, according to folk belief, watch over spinning, punish lazy spinsters, make sure that no spinning is done on days when spinning is forbidden and so forth. Many legends tell of the visits of these beings, and how they punish spinsters who violate spinning taboos or fail to finish their spinning on time etc. They are also frequently described as being equipped with flax and spinning tools while in the act of spinning.

Thus, in Slovenia, Austria and Germany we find Perchta/Pehtra/ Perhta/Pehtra baba/Pehtrna/Pirta/Pehta/Percht/Berchta/Zlata baba, in Germany Frau Holle or Holda, Stampe/Stempe/Stempa, and in Switzerland Frau Saelde in the role of the "Spinnstubenfrau". The most prominent Slovenian researcher in these traditions, Niko Kuret, points out the similarities with beings which in Slovenia we also know by other names, such as Kvatrnica, Torka or Torklja. The Italians know a similar being named Befana, the French have Tante Airie, and we also find them with several different names in Central Asia, from Iran through Tajikistan to the basin of the lower Syr Darya and Amu Darya rivers etc. (Kuret 1997; 1989, II: 458). There are also various other beings with whom we could equate them to a certain extent, for instance the French Heckelgauclere, the Swiss Sträggele and Chrungele, the German Herke, the Slovenian/ Czech/Slovakian Lucy and others.

Let us, therefore, first look at beings within the European territory who watch over spinning and the observance of spinning taboos, the time of their appearance and the punishments that they were believed to inflict in order to enforce prohibitions against spinning. Then I shall look at the reasons for their appearance in precisely defined time periods and argue for the symbolic meaning of (taboos on) spinning.

Female figures watching over spinning

In 1858, Slovenian researcher Peter Hicinger wrote about Zlata baba (the Golden Hag), who, according to tradition, rages about the sky with the Wild Hunt during the nights *around the New Year*, and in 1859, Davorin Terstenjak wrote that Vehtra (Pehtra) baba was known from Tržič, across the Kamnik highlands, to Pohorje, that she was known as the queen of the "white wives" and that she was also called Zlata baba. During the winter she made "baba's mash" (baba's groats—an expression for sleet) and liked to spin. She blinded or buried a hatchet between the shoulder blades of anyone who treated her badly, and one year later returned their sight or pulled out the hatchet; she also slit open the belly of anyone who failed to observe the fast (Kuret 1989, II: 457). At dusk she was supposed to walk along the mountain ridges holding a golden pail[1] or *vehtra* (doormat) in her hand (Kuret 1989, II: 457; Kelemina 1997, 93, no. 57). She would kill women in Karner Vellach (Koroška Bela) who were still spinning on *Ember Friday before Christmas* if, by midnight, they did not spin twelve coils which she would throw through the window; however, there are no records pointing to her also overseeing the injunction against spinning during the Twelve Days of Christmas or at least on 5 January (her feast day), although in some places in Slovenia the custom of Pehtra's hunt or Pehtra's rounds used to be observed on that day (Schmidt J., "Perchtenglaube bei den Slovenen." *Zeitschrift für Volkskunde* 1, 1889, 418, cited in Rumpf 1976, 217; Kuret 1989, II: 460–8).

In Germany, Berchta or Bertha appeared as a wild woman who took the distaff away from those who had not spun all of their flax by the *last day of the year* (Saintyves 1987, 89). In the mountains around the Chiemsee, Berchta slit open the bellies of girls who had not spun everything by *New Year's Eve* and filled them with curlers. In the Tyrol, Percht watched over spinning wheels during the Twelve Days of Christmas, especially on her feast day, *5 January*—she destroyed the spindles of spinsters who had not finished their work by Christmas Day. In Tiers (South Tyrol), the girls had to spin all of the flax before the beginning of the *twelve nights*, or Berchta would unravel the remainder. In South Tyrol, Frauberta cooked and boiled washerwomen who spun during the *twelve nights* (Rumpf 1976, 215). In Orlagau, during the nights before *Epiphany,* she hunted through the spinning rooms for women who were

[1] In foreign translations she appears with "a golden spindle in her hand" (cf. Schmidt 1889, 414; cited also in Rumpf 1976, 218; Kilbourne Matossian 1973, 333: with a spindle and a tub of water), but the Slovenian word *ročka* means pail or jug, not "spindle".

spinning, to whom she would give a huge amount of flax which they would then have to spin in a very short time. If they failed in this, she would pull the flax off the distaffs, and tangle and defile it (Rumpf 1976, 216). In Saalfeld they said that Bergda would defile any distaff not cleared by the spinster by the *last day of the year* (Grimm 2012 [1888], 4: 1797, no. 512). "Much flax is placed by girls near the Hörselberg upon their distaff *at Christmastime* when Frau Holle starts her round, for she promises 'a good year for every thread'. But the flax must be spun by *Epiphany*, for on her return she threatens 'a bad year for every thread'" (Motz 1984, 154). In Ostfranken, Donndorf and Bad Steben, Berta defiled the distaffs of lazy spinsters, who should have spun everything by December 6 (Rumpf 1976, 219). In Franconia, Frau Holle defiled the flax of careless spinsters with her excrement (the distaff had to be cleared by *Christmas Eve*); Perchta could decide whether those who did not complete their tasks would have bad luck spinning for the entire following year. She could also slit open the bellies of such spinsters and fill them with waste and filth. This punishment was usually directed at those who had spun at the spindle at forbidden times (Motz 1984, 154 and 164, note 52).

In Slovenia there was also the figure of *Torka (also Torklja, Tvorka, Štorka, Turklja, Torek* etc.), whose synonymy with Pehtra baba, according to Slovenian researcher Niko Kuret, cannot be overlooked. Torka is the "guardian of Slovenian spinning", and in the Christian tradition also watches over the sanctification of the Ember Days (cf. Kropej 2008a, 331; Kuret 1997, 73). She most often prohibited spinning (in some places also baking, threshing and washing) on a *Tuesday*—from which some people derive her name (Sl.: *torek* "Tuesday").[2] According to beliefs from Pohorje, Torklja appeared on Tuesdays at eleven o'clock at night if people were spinning, baking or doing anything they shouldn't be and killed them, chewed them down to their bones, or tore them to shreds. A legend from Pohorje says that "If they were grinding or spinning after eleven, she came through the closed door, supposedly in the form of a huge woman, terrifically strong, and they had to stop; if they didn't, she destroyed everything. And if you were spinning, you never got up again!" (Gričnik 1995, 260). In Kamna Gorica and around Železniki people were threatened with legends of Torklja, who killed women who baked or laundered on

[2] Slovenian etymologist France Bezlaj holds that this is just a folk etymology. In his opinion the word came from India: "The ancient Indian spinning deity Tarku also has traces in Germanic languages (Herbig IF XXVI, 377–8) and could have come by some unknown paths to the Slovenes as well, although the Indian *tarku* ('spinning wheel') phonetically corresponds to the [Slovenian] word *trak* ('ribbon/band/strip')." (Bezlaj 1951, 351).

Tuesdays. No spinster was allowed to leave any thread on the wheel overnight, or Torka would come and spin all night, although not actually spinning anything; apparently, on one occasion a farmhand watched her, as a result of which she tore him to shreds. In the Notranjska region there was a rule that you were not allowed to spin on Tuesdays; any woman who broke the rule would be boiled alive by Torka (Kuret 1989, II: 459–60). According to a belief from Martinji Vrh, Torka is a monster who lives in the attic, behind the chimney or behind the stove, killing women who spun, sewed hems or boiled laundry on Tuesdays. One story tells of a disobedient girl who went to the attic to fetch a bundle of flax for spinning. From the attic you could hear: "I'm gnawing, I'm gnawing!" and in the morning her sister found her chewed-on bones lying in a pile (Kelemina 1997, 219, no. 199, I.). A woman who forgot the taboo against spinning on Tuesday was saved when her neighbours reminded her how to get rid of Torka—she should scream that all of the hills are on fire and her children as well. Torklja would then tell her that she should feel lucky that she screamed like that because otherwise, she would have boiled both her and all her flax in a cauldron (Zemon near Ilirska Bistrica) (Kelemina 1997, 219, no. 200). In some places Torka also came on *Fridays* and *Saturdays*. In the Ormož area in Slovenian Styria, "Torklja" pulled the meat from the bones of women who spun too long into the night on a Saturday. She also ripped all of the meat off the bones of mothers-in-law who spun and forced their daughters-in-law to spin on a Saturday night, so that all that remained were bones (Kelemina 1997, 219, no. 199, II.).

Spinning was especially forbidden on *Ember Thursday* or *Ember Nights* in general. In the Kamnik area people said that you shouldn't spin on Ember Thursday, or Torka would come (Cevc 1999, 93). In Gorenjska they said that Torka would come to spin in the evening if a spinster left thread on the wheel on Ember Thursday; sometimes they said that she spun the wheel in the form of a dog's leg in order to trample all of the flax. Several legends tell of how, if the taboo was not respected, the spinning wheel would begin to rattle at the stroke of eleven, and two farmhands would see Torka, a huge woman, who had started spinning at the wheel—when she noticed them, she tore them both to shreds. Another legend tells of spinsters in the Komenda area who intentionally left thread on the wheels and the distaffs on Ember night, because they didn't believe in Torka. Torka began to spin immediately, until she was chased off by neighbours with holy water, but the spinning materials and flax were destroyed (Kelemina 1997, 216–8, no. 198).

Since Torka is most often associated with Ember Days, she is also sometimes known as the *Kvatrnica* or *Kvatrna* (also *Kvatarnca, Kvatrna baba, Kvatrnječ etc.*) [Slo. kvatre "Ember Days t.n."] (Kuret 1997, 73; Novak 1987, 282). It was by this name that she punished women who spun during *Ember Weeks*, especially on *Ember Friday and Saturday*, by gnawing the meat from their bones or boiling them together with their skeins. In some places people would not spin on Ember Saturday because "otherwise the Kvatarnca would come" (Dolenc 1977, 182; see also p. 193–5: variants of legends about the taboo against spinning on Ember Days—M. Stanonik). In Rožak, the Kvatrna baba took particular care to ensure that work on Ember Days, especially the Winter Embers, was halted on time. A legend about a peasant woman who wanted to steam a large amount of flax on the Ember Friday before Christmas tells of how an unknown woman appeared all of a sudden and offered to help her. When the peasant woman went to borrow a tub from her neighbour, the neighbour warned her that the other woman was undoubtedly a Kvatrnica. The peasant woman remained with her neighbour, and around midnight, the Kvatrnica knocked on the door and told the peasant woman that if she went home she would boil her skeins with her on top (Kelemina 1997, 95, no. 60). A similar presentation of the cruel punishment meted out by Kvatr(ni)cas is shown in the following narrative, which was recorded by my students during the fieldwork we conducted in 2000 in Gorjane (in the Kozjansko district in eastern Slovenia):

> And there were also a lot of Kvatrcas on Ember Saturdays and Sundays… they went to a woman's house on Ember Saturday, and the woman put out a platter, and there was meat and such things hanging from the rafters and she wanted to serve them. But the woman did not come down and they all thought, what's this? Her neighbours asked her what was going on, and they heard: "I'm gnawing, I'm gnawing". It seemed strange to them. And they got the same answer six times. And then nothing but bones fell down. That was the punishment for working on Ember Saturday.[3]

In southern Germany (from Chamaven to Ostfalen), it was Herke who was responsible for watching over spinning rooms (Timm 2003, 194). Among the demonic beings associated with watching over spinning is also the Swiss Chlungere (Chlungeli, Chlungeri, Chlungere, Chunkle), whose name is frequently associated with *spinnen* (Ger.: "to spin") (Zürich and Solothurn cantons). She is described as having humps on her chest and back, a vulture's beak and long fingernails. She moved about during the *last nights of the old year*, punished lazy spinsters, sat like a nightmare on

[3] Inf. 35; recorded by Matena Bassin, Anja Kušar and Nina Rolc; Archives of the Department of Ethnology and Cultural Anthropology, Faculty of Arts, University of Ljubljana.

people's chests while they were sleeping, and strangled or flogged them. In the Canton of Zürich there was also a custom on "Chrungeli-Nacht" (23 or 30 December) that masked village youths break into the houses, accept food and play tricks on the spinsters, e.g. throw ash-covered spindles at each other, tangle the spinsters' tow—just like the legends say (Hoffmann-Kreyer 1940, 80).

Tante Airie is known on both sides of the border between France[4] and francophone Switzerland (Timm 2003, 98; Gennep 1999, 2429–33; Hoffmann-Kreyer 1940, 80). Researchers frequently connect her with the Italian Befane (Epiphanie) and the German Frau Holle (similarities include her cavern, working as a baker, rewarding the good, punishing the bad) or Berchte (punishing careless spinsters). Her activities included spinning with her distaff (Rocken) and a spindle, frequenting spinning rooms, and rewarding the best spinsters with gold and good husbands, while at *Carnival* she tangled up flax that had yet to be spun by lazy spinsters, and in a rage could even burn down houses (Timm 2003, 98); Gennep 1999, 2431). She was a role model for spinsters because she never put down her distaff, and she punished lazy young spinsters by tangling their flax. In the Montbéliard commune it was said that spinning wheels had to be completely cleared by *Christmas Day*, or Tante Airie would soil them with her urine and their work would be destroyed (Gennep 1999, 2741–2). In Saulnet, Tante Airie was exchanged for the Trotte-vieilles. These were fairies (*fées*) in the form of women with horns with which they used to grab naughty children and throw them into the stream in front of the door; however, they also rewarded good children (Gennep 1999, 2432–3).

In France and Switzerland, the Chaussevieille was a similarly horrific spectre for lazy spinsters over the period of the Twelve Days (Hoffmann-Kreyer 1940, 80; Gennep 1999, 2433). In the Alpes vaudoises, stories were told about the Tschausse-villha, who was supposed to be an old witch who harassed people in every possible way, especially during the *last days of the year*. In the Pays d'Enhaut, spinsters who spun at night were particularly warned that they would have to finish their work by *Christmas Eve*, otherwise the Tsaôthavîdhe would come during the year and tangle up the flax so that it could never be untangled (Saintyves 1987, 89). According to French legends, Berthe la Fileuse was considered to be a fairy protectress of spinsters—some folklorists associated her with Perchta. Every year at midnight, in the week between Christmas Day and New Year's Day, she appeared in the houses and brought misfortune to

[4] According to van Gennep, in spite of the record from 1891 he cannot find any evidence for this being in the three French provinces mentioned.

any house with disobedient children, tangling the flax or hemp not yet spun (Gennep 1999, 2437). In Fislis, Haut-Rhin, they used to say that women who spun too long on *Christmas Eve* fell under the power of Heckelgauclere, who would put twelve skeins in front of their window after midnight, which they would then have to spin on the same night (Gennep 1999, 2741).

In Switzerland, even the Wild Hunt sometimes played the role of punishing lazy spinsters (Hoffmann-Kreyer 1940, 79). Odin (Wodan), who from the 14th and 15th centuries onwards was considered the leader of the Wild Hunt, also sometimes had the same function of enforcing taboos against spinning: in Ivendorf (20 km northeast of Lübeck-Mitte) they said that Wodan's horse would trample the flax if it wasn't spun by *Christmas Day* (cf. Lecouteux 1997, 28–9). In present-day Holstein they still warn people about the taboo against spinning and leaving flax on the distaff during the *Twelve Days*, lest Wode (Wodan) should ride over (trample) it ("der Wode jage da durch") (Timm 2003, 187).

In Switzerland it was said that if a spinster failed to spin e.g. 10 bobbins *by the Wednesday before Christmas Day* (Weichnachtsfronfasten), Streggele would take away the flax (Motz 1984, 154). In legends from the Zug and Lucerne cantons, Strägele or Sträggele carried off any girl who didn't want to do her spinning (in a variant from Lucerne on the *third Sunday of Advent*)—all they found were torn braids of hair or, in another variant from Lucerne, the remains of a corpse. In Zürich Sträggele or Strunze came on the *Wednesday before Christmas Day* to get girls who didn't do enough spinning (Rumpf 1976, 225). In Lucerne the witch Sträggele harassed girls who didn't finish their work by *Ember Week* (Saintyves 1987, 89).

Peasants in Brittany say that on the night before St. Andrew's Day (30 Nov.), a very old fairy would come to see whether people were still spinning, and if she saw them spinning she would warn them that the following day was the holiday of St. Andrew (Sébillot 1981, 148).

According to Scottish belief, the Gyre-carlin is a mighty giantess reminiscent of Frau Perchta, with a disgusting visage, a long nose and supernatural abilities, who wounded the heels of her victims with an iron pike. Like Perchta, she carried off flax that had not been spun *by the end of the year* (Smith 2004, 176–7). In John o' Groats she was active from *Candlemas* to *Fastern's E'en (Shrove Tuesday)*, disturbing and frightening the whole family with her own spinning if the spinning wheel had not been put out of action and sained (blessed) at night (Smith 2004, 177). In Fife, superstitious females were anxious to spin off all the flax that was on their racks on the *last night of the year*; being persuaded that if they left any unspun, the Gyre-carlin, or as they also pronounce the word, the Gy-carlin, would carry it off before morning (*Jamieson's Scottish Dictionary*, 2nd ed., 1840, 496, School of Scottish Studies Archives, University of Edinburgh; Briggs 1976, 213).

In Sorbian belief, after eleven o'clock at night during the *Twelve Days,* the Spinnstubenfrau appears in the form of a Murawa (also Morawa, formerly Mora [i.e. "nightmare"]), spits on the unspun flax and sits on (haunts) the spinster like a nightmare (Timm 2003, 103).

The Unjats in the villages of Eastern Slovakia were not permitted to spin on *St. Sava's Day* (5/18 December)—they believed that a female demonic being called Sava would scold people who violated the taboo: Sava would bring a spindle into the house in a sieve and demand that the woman of the house would spin all the thread in a single night (Valencova 2009, 325). Like the above-mentioned demonic being, the taboo against spinning is also supported by Lucy(s), who was usually associated with beings such as Pehtra, Kvatrnica, Torka etc., and appears primarily in the Czech lands, Moravia, in parts of Hungary and Croatia, and in north-eastern Slovenia (Kuret 1997, 82; Kuret 1989, II: 245; Pócs 1999, 125). St. Lucy is the patron saint of spinsters in northern Croatia, more rarely in central Croatia and even more rarely along the Adriatic coast and in some places in Bosnia and Vojvodina. In some of these places there was also a belief that spinning was forbidden on *St. Lucy's Day*, 13 December. In some places in Croatia and also in Slovenia the main reason for prohibiting spinning (as well as sewing and knitting) on St. Lucy's Day was the fear of losing one's sight (Gavazzi 1988, 119; Kuret 1989, II: 251; Belaj 2006, 261). According to belief, in western Slovakia St. Lucy travelled about on her feast day, using a spindle to smite and pour charcoal on the heads of anyone who spun, causing them to have a headache; in other places she threw an entire basket of spindles into the house and demanded that they spun all of its contents in a single night, otherwise she would tear the spinster to shreds (Slovakia, Ukraine, Zakarpatska Region) (Valencova 2009, 325). In some places in south-eastern Austria, Perchta's counterpart Lutzel or Luzia performed similar gastrotomic activities to those of Perchta: she opened the heads of lazy people and filled them with refuse, or lacerated people's knees or heels and filled the wounds with salt (Smith 2004, 176).

Punishments for violations of taboos

Various explanations for the punishments for violations of this taboo meted out by these beings are actually nearly impossible to distinguish from each other: explanations that emphasise that these beings destroyed flax that was *not spun by a certain day* in fact implicate another frequent explanation, that *spinning had to be finished by a certain day, since from then on spinning would be forbidden for some time*, otherwise the being would punish the spinster—in both cases we can therefore state that such beings, in essence, enforced the prohibition against spinning during a certain period of time. And there is a third explanation that cannot be completely distinguished from these two: the punishment of *lazy spinsters*, who can be understood as those who (due to their laziness) did not finish their work on time.

Punishments for transgressions connected in one way or another with spinning encompassed on one hand the destruction, soiling, tangling etc. of the flax, the destruction of spinning tools or the setting of impossible tasks connected with flax: Perchta/Berchta/Holle/Holda etc. sometimes destroyed or took away distaffs, destroyed flax, soiled distaffs or made spinsters spin a huge amount of flax in a very short amount of time. Tsaôthavîdhe and Berthe la Fileuse punished spinsters by tangling the flax, as did Tante Arie, who also soiled it with urine. Heckelgaucklere, Sava and Lucy demanded that spinsters who had not finished their work on time or who spun at forbidden times should spin a huge amount of flax in a single night. Wodan rode over unspun flax, the Gyre-carlin took it away, and Murawa spat on it.

On the other hand, these beings could inflict various injuries on spinsters (and more rarely mere observers) and even cause their death: they slit open people's bellies, pulled out their intestines, filled them with waste, refuse etc., blinded them, gnawed them to the bone, killed them, steamed them, boiled them, strangled them and so on. In the stories, the Kvatrnica gnawed spinsters to the bone or parboiled them, Torka boiled them alive, gnawed them to the bone or licked the meat off their bones, tore them to shreds, and threw them to the ground so that they never rose again. She also tore to shreds those people who witnessed her spinning. Perchta/Berchta/Holle/Holda etc. steamed, boiled or simply killed spinsters who failed to observe the injunction against spinning, failed to complete their spinning on time or were lazy, or sliced open their bellies and filled them with waste and filth. Chlungere punished lazy spinsters—although exactly how, we don't know, nor do we know how the Wild Hunt punished spinsters. Sträggele carries off or harasses lazy spinsters or those who fail to finish their work; Murawa could sit on a spinster's chest; Lucy obviously robbed them of their sight, threatened to tear them to pieces, smashed in their heads, or gave them headaches; Sava and the old fée in France scolded or admonished them.

Many of these punishments were not as illogical as they appear at first sight. Smith holds that the punishments are analogous to the offences: "What the fictions under consideration convey is that if you spin or perform related tasks on a holiday, you can expect a penalty to match. Boil skeins, and you will be boiled alive. Spin, and your guts will be spun out of your belly" (Smith 2004, 174). But it seems that such direct parallels between the actions and the punishments are not always clear. Perchta, in a similar way to the prohibition on spinning, also punished people for other prohibited behaviour: when they did not observe the fast or did not eat certain foods, when they offended her, laughed at her, behaved badly towards her or stared at her, she also punished naughty or lazy children. As with lazy spinsters, she tore out the guts of naughty or lazy children and people who did not observe the fast, and filled them with straw, rocks and refuse.[5] People who saw her coming or who behaved badly towards her were punished with blindness, the same punishment that Lucy administered with regard to the spinning taboo. She administered punishments in the same way in cases both of failure to observe the prohibition against spinning and to observe the fast: she cut open people's bellies with a spindle. As Smith also points out, these methods of punishment are not exclusively connected with Perchta (Smith 2004, 176–7).

The punishments meted out by these beings, especially to spinsters and in particular unusual bodily injuries such as the gnawing of spinsters to the bone or pulling out their guts, undoubtedly deserve special treatment owing to their possible initiation roles, with which some researchers find parallels in shamanism, e.g. in the initiation dreams of Australian shamans (Josef Hanika, after Smith 2004, 169). Similarly, according to some, Perchta's act of carrying off children into the wild is reminiscent of the puberty initiation rites in "primitive" communities (cf. Motz 1984, 160).

---

[5] Smith in fact believes that at the outset, Perchta's task seems to have been the supervision of feasting and fasting: "Initially Perchta was the enforcer of communal taboos, hunting down those who spun on holidays or who failed to partake sufficiently in collective feasting (a propitious act designed to ensure future plenty). However, with the growing involvement of peasant women in the market economy (particularly for textiles), Perchta's role changed to the punisher of the lazy" (Smith 2004, 178). Gastrotomy was originally meant to discourage undue abstinence or its opposite (Smith 2004, 176).

Prohibitions of spinning in the annual cycle

In European beliefs we find other mythical beings and saints who prohibited spinning on specific *days of the week*[6] (some of the beings that watched over spinning in the annual cycle were sometimes also guardians of individual days of the week, as we have seen in the case of Torka), or just *at night*. These latter (e.g. fées, lutins, revenants in France, mora, kikimora, Paraskeva Piatnitsa in Russia etc.) did not necessarily threaten people with punishments, but people believed that they spun at night, when everyone in the house was asleep, so the injunction against spinning was certainly enforced through the belief in their presence near spinning wheels or spindles (cf. Sébillot 1981, 142–3; cf. Krinichnaia 1995, 5–6).

However, in this paper, I will focus solely on beings who enforced prohibitions against spinning in the *annual cycle of holidays* and whose main function was therefore above all to enforce prohibitions against spinning on certain days or in certain periods during the annual cycle. I will concentrate on the chronological context within which these beings appeared and in one way or another punished the failure to observe prohibitions against spinning. Whenever a time is given, we can conclude that the majority of these beings that we find throughout Europe appeared in the dead of winter, i.e. the time from the Winter Embers/Christmas/New Year's Day, to Epiphany. Erika Timm notes that none of these beings (Perchta, Holle, Stampe etc.) appeared regularly over the course of the year, but emerged with increased frequency during these twelve days, in the middle of winter or on certain days over the course of the Twelve Days (Timm 2003, 249). Pehtra/ Holle/ Bergda/ Berchta or Bertha appeared above all on the nights between 25 December and 6 January: on Christmas Day, on the last day of the old year, around New Year's Day, and also 5 January (on her feast day) or before Epiphany (6 January); Heckelgauclere on Christmas Day, Murawa during the Twelve Days, Tante Airie on Christmas Day, Tschausse-villha or Chlungere on Christmas Day and on the last days of the old year, Berthe la Fileuse in the week between Christmas Day and New Year's Day, Strággele on the Wednesday before Advent or the third Sunday of Advent and during Ember Week, the Gyre-carlin on the last night of the old year and Wodan at Christmas or during the Twelve Days. Torka and/or Kvatrnica, who appeared overwhelmingly

[6] E.g. The east-Slavic St. Paraskeva Piatnitsa, female figures Wednesday, Sunday (personification of the Assumption), in Central Asia Bibi Seshambe (Woman Tuesday), Bibi Chorshambe ("Woman Wednesday"), among the Turks Pershambe-Kary ("Woman Thursday") (Krinichnaia 1995, 8), Romanian Marţi Nopate ("Tuesday Night") and Vineri-Noapte ("Friday Night") (Kuret 1997, 73) etc.

during Advent Ember Week (Thursday, Friday, Tuesday, Saturday; sometimes also every Tuesday, Friday or Saturday night), also appeared during the Twelve Days, and the same occasionally holds for Pehtra, Lucy on her feast day (13 December), and Sava on the feast day of St. Sava (5/18 December). Slovenian researcher Niko Kuret thus uses the single name "Midwinter Woman" (*Sredozimka*) for Indo-European or Eurasian beings who appeared in Europe and Asia in the middle of winter under various names[7] and who, according to popular belief, were the protectors of customs and morals (especially the patrons of spinning and guardians of prohibitions against spinning) and at the same time the guides of souls (especially children's) (Kuret 1997, 66–9). Only rarely do we find them on other days of the year: Tante Airie could appear at Carnival (as well as Christmas), the old *fée* before St. Andrew's Day, and the Gyre-carlin could appear in the period from Candlemas to Shrove Tuesday.

We can therefore see that these beings, as a rule, enforced taboos against spinning in the very same period when we find the most widespread prohibitions against spinning in Europe in general, even when they are not supported by the appearance of and inflicting of punishments by mythical beings. The prohibition against spinning occurs on several days in the year,[8] but if we ignore individual, and expressly local saints on whose feast days spinning was forbidden for one reason or another, one of the periods during which taboos on spinning were most widespread throughout Europe was the *Christmas period*, as has also been established by van Gennep (Gennep 1999, 2740). The injunction could apply only to Christmas, for the period from Christmas to New Year, from Christmas (in Germany even from the winter solstice, 21 December) to Epiphany or even from Christmas to Candlemas (2 Feb.). Thus, spinning was forbidden at Christmas in Switzerland, France, Belgium, and Scotland; from Christmas to New Year in Scotland and Denmark, on New Year's Day in Switzerland and France, and in certain places in Scotland from Christmas to Candlemas. During the twelve nights, i.e. the period from Christmas to Epiphany, spinning was forbidden in France and among Slavs in general, from St. Thomas' Day (21 Dec.) to Epiphany in Germany, and only on Epiphany or the day after in France and England (cf. Mencej 2009a).

[7] Characters similar to Frau Holle and the Russian Baba Iaga are also found in Central Asia—Tajikistan, Afghanistan, in the area of the lower course of the Syr Darya and Amu Darya rivers (Robert Blechsteiner, Perchtengestalten in Mittelasien, Archiv für Völkerkunde 8, Wien 1953: 58; cited in Kuret 1997, 68–9).
[8] For a detailed review of European holidays on which the taboo against spinning is in effect, see Mencej 2009a.

The cycle of twelve nights between Christmas and Epiphany, in spite of the name the "twelve nights" or "Twelve Days", can actually last for varying lengths of time, as van Gennep points out: in France, for instance, it begins on St. Catharine's Day (25 Nov.) and lasts until Epiphany (6 January); sometimes it lasts from St. Andrew's Day (30 Nov.) until Epiphany or from St. Lucy's Day (13 December) to Epiphany; from Christmas to New Year, from Christmas to Epiphany or even from Christmas to Candlemas (Gennep 1999, 2308–9). So, we shouldn't be surprised to find taboos on spinning on other holidays during this period in the widest sense. The taboo on spinning was fairly widespread on *St. Lucy's Day*, especially among Catholic Slavs (Slovenia, Croatia, Slovakia), in Sweden and in Germany, often supported by a threat of Lucy(s). We find a taboo on spinning during the *Advent Ember Week* in Slovenia, Switzerland and Romania. Spinning was forbidden in some places among Slavs on *St. Catharine's Day* (in Croatia, Slovenia, Ukraine, Slovakia), which is just before Advent. We also find injunctions against spinning on *St. Andrew's Day* in France (supported by the threat of an old *fée*) and Slovakia, on *St. Nicholas' Day* in Slovenia and Slovakia and on *St. Barbara's Day* in Croatia and Slovakia.

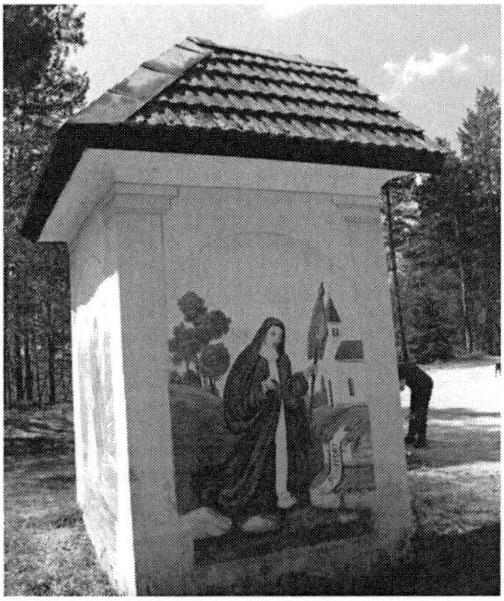

Saint Jedrt (Saint Gertrude), mural on the wall of the chapel next to the village of Ožbolt nad Zmincem (Slovenia), 2006. Photo by Nena Židov.

Liminal periods

This period can undoubtedly be understood as a *turning point in the year*. It probably does not need to be made explicit that the Twelve Days in the narrow sense, i.e. the period from Christmas to Epiphany, is understood everywhere as a time of the intrusion of the other world: it is a time in which the world is open (*mundus patet*), which is manifested in numerous beliefs or legends about the Wild Hunt, witches, various demonic beings, the souls of the dead (which wander about our world during this time); it is a time of magic and soothsaying etc. The ancient custom near the turning point of the year—the winter solstice, i.e. the pagan holiday of the "birthday of the unconquered sun" (*Dies Natalis Solis Invicti*) on 25 December, has been obscured to a great extent by the celebration in western Christendom of the birth of Christ. The rituals, beliefs and customs which accompanied the former "New Year" holiday were transferred to various holidays: those which were related to the coming of the dead were transferred for the most part to All Souls Day, costumed processions to St. Nicholas' Day and St. Lucy's Day, magical practices to St. Andrew's Day, which falls at the end of the ecclesiastical year (when costumed processions are also held), and to St. Thomas' Day and New Year's Eve.

In fact, apparitions and masked people appear throughout Advent, indicating a belief in ancestors who return to this world. Fortune telling is also popular throughout this period (Kuret 1989, II: 129–31, 212–3 and 261). On *St. Barbara's Day*, 4 December, in Slovenia and in Croatia in the area of Slavonski Brod we find processions of *polažarji*,[9] the successors of pre-Christian costume processions in the role of the souls of the dead (Kuret 1989, II: 218; Gavazzi 1988, 117). Since the twelfth century, the Christian custom of winter processions with demons on *St. Nicholas' Day*, 6 December, has obscured the tradition of the old costumed processions characteristic of Indo-Europeans, which represented the departed and other daemons who brought blessings for the New Year, later changed into demons and fiends in Christianity; St. Nicholas joined them only after the twelfth century (Kuret 1989, II: 210, 222–4 and 226). The feast day of *St. Lucy*, 13 December, was the shortest day of the year according to the old Julian calendar and thus also a turning point in the year since, in its time, St. Lucy's Day was the day of the winter solstice, and according to the

---

[9] Belaj also mentions *čarojičari*, who appear during the period before Christmas (when St. Barbara's Day also occurs), and which are known primarily among the Orthodox population (western Bosnia and the area of Vojna granica) (Belaj 2007, 191).

ancient tradition, also the end of the old and the beginning of the new year: on that day the world was open to the incursions of otherworldly beings, animals were able to talk, girls believed that they would dream about their future husbands (Feilhauer 2000, 249; Kuret 1989, II: 244 and 250). On this day processions of masked "Lucys" were held in certain places in Slovenia, Croatia, Czech lands and Moravia, and in parts of Hungary (Kuret 1989, II: 244–7). *St. Thomas' Day*, on which the taboo on spinning begins in Germany, is celebrated before the actual shortest day and longest night of the year. It is on this day, according to the belief of Slovenes living in Rož (Rosental in Austria), that witches have the most power, the world is open, and fortune telling can be conducted. After the change to the calendar in 1582, St. Thomas took over some of Lucy's duties, and he was also assigned some of the duties of *St. Andrew*, who had been considered the primary winter saint in the folk tradition (Kuret 1989, II: 259–60). Although the taboo against spinning in Slovenia on *St. Sebastian's* Day, 20 January, is expressly local, according to some beliefs this day marks the end of winter, similarly to *St. Vincent's Day*, which marks the middle of winter, or, as Kuret puts it, the "eagerly awaited spring", when, according to belief, birds chose their mates. *St. Agnes' Day*, on 21 January, when spinning was likewise forbidden in some places in Slovenia, was connected with spinning as St. Agnes was the protectress of sheep, and people brought tufts of wool to church on her feast day (Schauber, Schindler 1995, 33). As on St. Sebastian's Day, on St. Agnes' Day the servants were relocated and these days therefore represented a kind of turning point in the year, a line of demarcation in the hiring of the workforce (Kuret 1989, II: 517–21).

The *Ember Weeks*[10] similarly represented major breaks in the cyclical flow of the year, especially the Advent Ember Week, when spinning was particularly strictly forbidden.[11] The celebration of the Ember Weeks obscured the former pagan rituals in honour of the sanctity of agriculture, during which deceased ancestors were honoured in Rome, something also confirmed by various customs during the Christian Ember Weeks—in Slovenia one had to pray for the deceased during these weeks, milk was

[10] At first the Embers were seasonal fasts and were not held on prescribed days—they were held in March, June, September and December (the reason for this is the impermanent dates of the agricultural holidays, which were set according to the weather and the climate zones). The present Ember times were determined only by Pope Gregory VII (1020–85) (Kuret 1989, II: 168–9).

[11] The Church never ordered a taboo on spinning on Ember nights; this taboo obviously comes from a pre-Christian tradition which was preserved after Christianisation (Kuret 1989, II: 168–9).

given to the poor so that they would also pray for the departed and so forth. The Ember nights were generally ruled by ghosts, witches and other malevolent beings. Children born during Ember Weeks became *vedomci*, humans with the power of metamorphosis and the ability to communicate with the other world (Kelemina 1997, 92; Kuret 1989, 168–72; Šešo 2007, 257–8). According to Slovenian (Stara Fužina, Gorenjska region) beliefs, on these days *vedomci* would fly, those who spun on Ember Thursdays were "all witches", and it was during this time that the Friulian *benandanti* fought their battles (Novak 1987, 282; Ginzburg 1992, 109).

On the other hand, a great number of these ancient rituals at the end of the old and the beginning of the New Year were transferred to the celebration of *Carnival*—a time when we also meet Perchta and Tante Airie, and some places in Scotland the Gyre-carlin, from Candlemas until Shrove Tuesday. Therefore, it is not surprising that the second period during which a strict taboo on spinning was most widespread in Europe, as has also already been established by van Gennep, was Carnival (Gennep 1999, 2740). The end of Shrovetide or the Carnival funeral represented the end of winter and beginning of spring (Kuret 1989, II: 39). Soothsaying was also characteristic of this time, and the most characteristic event was the arrival of masked individuals representing deceased ancestors.[12]

Some of the other holidays when spinning was likewise forbidden also represent a turning point in the annual cycle, the end of the old and beginning of the New Year or the beginning of a new half/quarter of the year. For instance, *Saint Brighid's Day*, the Christianised Imbolc (1 February) of the Celtic calendar, one of the four turning points in the Celtic calendar, is a day when the use of spinning wheels or spindles is strictly forbidden (Torma 2002; Danaher 1972, 13–4). In Bulgaria no spinning is done on *St. Triphun's Day* (also 1 February), which represents the first possible beginning of spring; in other European traditions the dividing line between the two halves is often represented by *Candlemas*, 2 February, when spinning is forbidden in Scotland. This is a day which usually marks the beginning of spring or the middle of winter. In the Pyrenees, Candlemas is not paid as much attention as elsewhere in Europe, but all the more attention is paid to *St. Agatha's Day*, which they celebrate three days later (5 February), but whose day according to Violet Alford was once 2 February. Neither spinning nor washing may be done on this

[12] Of course, Carnival, which arrives with the end of winter and the beginning of spring, has a strong connotation of fertility: Frazer already interpreted Carnival as a holiday which ensures the growth of the crops, and although Burke believes that the people did not understand it this way, he does state that fertility is a very important concept for the understanding of Carnival (Burke 1994, 191).

day (Alford 1937, 68–9). In wassailing on St Agatha's Day in the Pyrenees, the shepherds reserve part of the gifts they gather for the dead and so we can conclude that in the Pyrenees, St. Agatha's Day was also associated with beliefs about the coming of the dead. St. Agatha's Day falls during Carnival, and she is also the patron saint of the harvest, especially of fruit trees[13] (in Bigorre) (Alford 1937, 97–8; Alford 1937, 107). After the appearance of Christianity, we know that the ancient beliefs and customs surrounding the New Year were also transferred to *Easter* (in addition to Christmas Day and New Year, Epiphany and Carnival), so it is no wonder that at that time we also encounter typical New Year's customs such as driving out witches and evil forces by making noises, explosions etc., putting out the old and lighting the new fire, and magical practices to drive out evildoers in the coming year—and in some places, also a taboo on spinning (Sweden, Polesian Brest, perhaps Greece, Belgium, Slovakia) (Kuret 1989, I: 181, 185, 188 and 213). *St. Martin's Day*, 11 November, can also be understood as a turning point as it divides the year into halves of winter and summer. On this day the turning of all wheels is forbidden in Ireland, as well as spindles and spinning wheels, and spinning is also forbidden in Denmark and among the southern Slavs. According to numerous interpretations, this day is an important turning point in the year, especially for Indo-European stockbreeders, which can be seen from the Celtic calendar. According to Miles, St. Martin's Day is the closest possible approximation of the day of the old celebration of the beginning of winter in November, the day when snow began to fall in central Europe and the pastures were closed to livestock (Miles 1976, 172 and 202). Miles believed that these days were joined by the celebration of the New Year from the German division of the year, which according to this calendar began on 11 November (Miles 1976, 172–3; Mencej 2001, 192–6 and 204–6; 2005). We also frequently encounter taboos on spinning during the *wolf holidays*,[14] which in the Balkans (Serbia, Macedonia, Bulgaria) are usually celebrated around St.

[13] According to various interpretations she supplanted the goddess of agricultural fertility, Demeter (Ceres), who was venerated under her Greek nickname Agatha (*agade*, "good") and later the Latin Bona Dea (good goddess) by Greeks throughout Sicily and particularly in the city of Catania (cf. Kuret 1989, II: 542).

[14] However, the taboo on spinning, although here also appearing at the turning point between summer and winter, is nevertheless most often just a part of a wider taboo on any kind of work with wool, which symbolically takes the place of sheep, and working with livestock in general, so that the wolves wouldn't "see", since in this way, the people want to prevent the wolves from slaughtering the livestock during the winter.

Martin's (Mrata's) Day, and more rarely around St. Michael's Day, as well as St. Andrew's Day, St. Dimitri's Day and St. Sava's Day. As I have demonstrated elsewhere, in the folk calendar the wolf holidays represent a strong line of demarcation between the summer and winter halves of the year (Mencej 2001; 2005; 2009b). We find a similar situation of the autumn dividing line between summer and winter in Estonia and in other agrarian peoples of northern Europe who mark the end of the year with the harvest (which usually falls around St. Michael's Day, 29 September) and the transition to the winter work cycle, which begins with the celebration of St. Andrew's Day, 30 November (when an old *fée* forbids spinning in France). Within this period, particularly significant roles are played by St. Martin's Day on 11 November, which is the symbolic initiator to a successful new agrarian year, and St. Catharine's Day, 25 November, and the end of the year approximately coincides with All Saints Day. On the whole, the turn of the agricultural year in Estonia more or less coincided with All Souls' Day, the traditional rites of which included the worship of deceased ancestors, the keeping of silence, but also the interdiction on spinning and other kinds of housework. The souls of deceased ancestors are invited for a meal on this day (Hiiemäe 1995, 16–20).[15]

To summarise: all holidays in which we encounter a taboo on spinning in European rituals of the annual cycle therefore have the characteristic of a turning point in the year, a dividing line between the old and the new year, winter and spring, between one part of the year and another, a rupture which also always implies the intrusion of the other world—the appearance of the souls of the dead, represented as masked people, witches, demonic or supernatural beings. The intrusion of the other world is also clearly represented in numerous beliefs or legends about supernatural beings, such as Perchta/Holda/Holle, Tante Airie, Torka, Heckelgaucklere, Sträggele, and Gy(re)-carlin, who on certain holidays would check to see whether anyone might be spinning, and any spinster so caught would be punished by having their flax destroyed, or some other punishment would be meted out. Often these were not only a matter of belief and legend, but also constituted rituals—masked people who represented those beings, breaking into houses, frightening or giving gifts

[15] This type of division of the year would be recognised in Galicia in the celebration of the chestnut festival (Magosto), when the youths eat chestnuts at the beginning of winter, 1 November, and during Carnival. As Mandianes-Castro demonstrates, there is a symbolic association between chestnuts and the dead, which indicates that the chestnut festival is an "inverse Carnival": during Carnival the dead visit the living, while during the Magosto festival, the living visit the dead (Mandianes-Castro 2004, 101).

to children, making their rounds and so on (e.g. Lucy, Perchta, Chrungele). We can probably apply the same explanation to the injunctions on spinning during the night: night is the time of demons and supernatural beings and therefore also the time of the intrusion of the other world (cf. Smith 2004, 173; Mencej 2008b). Besides, some of the days of the week when spinning was forbidden also bore a connotation of the turning/liminal day of the week and/or intrusion of the other world:[16] Thursday was once a Sabbath-like day of rest and according to Romanian belief was the day which the souls of the dead and the fairies chose as a day when they entered into contact with the living, Sunday was later proclaimed a day of rest, Saturday evening was already the beginning of Sunday[17] etc. (Bächtold-Stäubli and Hoffmann-Krayer 1987, 1: 572–3; and 2: 333; Smith 2004, 170; Timotin 2009, 193). However, it is still not clear why it was *spinning* that was forbidden in these periods.

Circular movement

In another paper (Mencej 2008a), I have argued that according to legend, folk belief, folk poems, ancient sources and philosophical treatises, there is a firmly established notion in the European world view about the passage between the two worlds through circular movement—be it in the form of a whirlwind, whirlpool, mill, spindle or spinning wheel. When one wishes to communicate with the other world, this can also be evoked on purpose, through various magic techniques or various forms of circular movement, such as rolling, circumambulation, turning around, whirling, spinning round, walking around and so forth.

Here I would like to argue that one important, if not the most important, reason for spinning being forbidden at certain times of the annual (or life) cycle is precisely the fact that spinning always involves *circular movement*: of a spinning wheel, a spindle or of the thread itself. Therefore, it is no surprise that during periods when spinning was forbidden, often it was not merely spinning that was forbidden, but the turning of *any kind* of wheel.[18]

---

[16] However, folk beliefs about the quality of the days of the week vary considerably from country to country, according to different criteria (Tolstaja 1995, 31–3).

[17] According to folk beliefs, the beginning of a new day was after dusk of the previous day.

[18] For instance, in Slovenia on St. Nicholas' Day, 6 December, there is a *taboo on turning mills* at the same time as the taboo on spinning; on St. Catharine's Day, 25 November, *all wheels* must be still; in Germany on 21 December, St. Thomas'

The idea of passing from one world to the other through circular movement while spinning is clearly evident from the actions or descriptions of goddesses or mythical beings who are entrusted with the passage of people's souls from birth to death and vice versa. In Plato's famous Vision of Er the *Moirae* (Clotho, Lachesis and Atropos, the Greek Goddesses of Fate), for instance, by sitting around the *Spindle of Necessity*, Ananke, the central axis of the universe, "through which all the orbits turned"[19] and guiding its revolutions, allow the souls of the people-to-be-born into their new incarnation on Earth.[20] We could therefore understand the spinning motion of the spindle, turned by the Moirae, as a channel through which a passage of souls from the other world into this one was made possible.

In the Moirae concepts such as death, fate, birth, and spinning are interwoven: for Homer the expression *moira* is an abstract concept of fate, and *Moira* is a chthonic goddess who brings death, understood as an aspect of man's fate. In Hesiod these three goddesses have individual names—Clotho, Lachesis and Atropos[21]—and are no longer connected only with the death of men, but with man's fate in general. In literary sources, the Moirae are clearly connected with spinning processes (Cottica 2004, 185–6).[22]

In Indo-European mythology and the mythology of the Near East in general, we encounter many mythical creatures or goddesses that are associated with spinning on the one hand, and with the domain of fertility/birth and death on the other (Krinichnaia 1995, 7–8; Toporov 2002, 47–9; Kilbourne Matossian 1973, 329–30; Cottica 2004). But this association of spinning with fertility (and therefore also with death) seems logical: "In the ancient religious sphere, spinning was a powerful

---

Day, *all wheels* (*machines with wheels*) must stop. In Ireland we find a taboo on spinning together with a taboo on turning *any kind of wheel* (mills, carts, bicycles) on 1 February, St. Brighid's Day, and 11 November, St. Martin's Day. In Denmark *nothing* is *allowed to turn around* (in a circle) between Christmas and New Year. In Sweden *no wheel is allowed to turn around* on St. Lucy's day. The wheels must *all* be packed away during Shrovetide in the Ansbach region of Germany (cf. Mencej 2009a).

[19] Politeia X, 616b–617d.

[20] Politeia X, 620d–620e; see also 617d–620e; (http://humanitieslab.stanford.edu/PhilosophicalStages/1642).

[21] Hesiod, Theogony 211–20 (http://www.sacred-texts.com/cla/hesiod/theogony.htm).

[22] However, as Cottica states, spinning symbolism was not originally included in the concept of the Moirae; they absorbed it or appropriated it from older goddesses of fate known in Minoan and Mycenaean mythology (Cottica 2004, 185–6).

metaphor of fertility and of the ability to give birth, ensuring the continuity of human gender" (Cottica 2004, 185). For instance, Istustaya and Papaya, the Hittite goddesses of destiny, are described in documentary sources "while spinning the life of the King" while in others they are mentioned in conjunction with other Hurritic and Hittite goddesses whose influence extends to the domestic sphere and to the moment of birth (Cottica 2004, 186).

The *Parcae* in Roman representations were three women spinning one's destiny, but when they are assimilated with the Latin goddess *Dea Parca*, who is traditionally associated with birth, and the goddess Fata Scribunda, the spindle attribute usually disappears, being replaced by a book or a globe (Cottica 2004, 191). The *Nornir,* the feminine beings who represent the notions of fate in Norse mythology and are in charge of birth and death also have a widespread connotation of being spinsters or weavers.[23] The pantheon of Prince Vladimir, mentioned in a chronicle from 980 AD, mentions the (only female) goddess *Mokosh*, who was supposed to have been directly connected with spinning. Toporov has demonstrated a possible linguistic connection between the word "mokos" and the meaning "spinning". A Russian proverb says: "Don't leave your tows [lying around], otherwise Mokosh will spin them" (Krinichnaia 1995, 7–8; Toporov 2002, 47). Mythological stories also tell of how, when everyone is asleep, you can hear spindles turning—it is the sound of Mokosh spinning wool (Krinichnaia 1995, 7–8). In ancient Russia (in the north), Mokosh was conceptualised as a woman with a large head who spun at night. She has exaggerated sexual traits (large breasts, long, loose hair), and stories (the Russian Slovo) denigrating Paganism emphasise the theme of her debauchery; this reminder of her debauchery has been preserved to the present day in the appellative *mokos'ja* (in the dialect of Podmoskovje), which means a woman who behaves immorally. But Mokosh is also the protectress of women in labour and the overseer of childbirth, and also appears as a mother (Toporov 2002, 49). In later folklore she is associated with rain, wetness, water, ground, darkness, night, odd numbers, sheep's wool, yarn, and spinning (Toporov 2002, 48; Kilbourne Matossian 1973, 329). The Slovenian legend of Mokoshka (from Trg Šent Florjan in Ložnica), if she is to be related to Mokosh, similarly confirms an association between Mokoshka and children: it suggests that she is particularly fond of carrying off children, especially

---

[23] However, Karen Bek-Pedersen argues that in spite of this widespread popular opinion, one would search in vain for an absolutely clear and unequivocal representation of spinning or weaving *Nornir* anywhere in Old Norse mythological texts (Bek-Pedersen 2007a; 2007b; cf. also Simek 2000, 237).

those that are not being raised well by their parents, an activity also attributed to Perchta (Kelemina 1997, 220, no. 201, I.).

Christianity, of course, for the most part assimilated the pagan gods into its doctrine by changing them into saints or demons: one of these saints is the Russian *Paraskeva Piatnitsa*,[24] who obviously succeeded Mokosh. Tows, spun sheep's wool and even cloth were thrown into her wells (Toporov 2002, 48). Since the distaff was reminiscent of the description of Piatnitsa (often portrayed as tall and thin with loose hair), Russian peasant women sometimes referred to distaffs as *piatnitsy*. At first, she was the patron saint of spinning, weaving and housework (Krinichnaia 1995, 8). They also offered her the first sheaf of flax. In this connection, they forbade doing such work on "women's days" during the week, i.e. on Wednesday and especially on Friday. They believed that women who spun on Friday or holidays were invisibly stabbing Paraskeva Petka (also St. Barbara or the Virgin Mary) with their spindles, or that Piatnitsa walked about the world stabbed by the spindles of lazy spinsters. Another variant of the motivation for the prohibitions was the fear that they would soil the eyes of deceased relatives with a mote (of flax) (Kilbourne Matossian 1973, 330).[25] Piatnitsa had many functions, but she especially fostered marriage and fertility, spinning and weaving (Kilbourne Matossian 1973, 330).

We find a similar set of conceptualisations in images and beliefs in Slovenia associated with *Saint Jedrt* (Gertrudis, Gertrude), whose feast day is 17 March: she is depicted with a stick crawling with mice, and sometimes holds a distaff in her hand while mice gnaw on the thread. This is a day when the spinning must be finished and the spinning wheels must be still. According to the interpretations of some researchers, she drove off a pagan feminine deity who took over people's souls after death; these were portrayed as mice and were seen as the souls of the dead who refused to leave the earthly plane. From this, stems the belief in some places that St. Jedrt is the protectress of the souls of the dead on the first night after death (Kuret 1989, I: 106–7).

The question is whether the mythical beings that watch over spinning can also be understood as the successors of former feminine deities of spinning and often of fertility (i.e. birth and death). Although Smith holds that Perchta and other similar beings are merely personifications of the

---

[24] Both names mean Friday, the fifth day of the week (same as Petka).

[25] I would like to thank Aleksei Iudin for sending me information on Piatnica (email 13 Dec. 2007).

feast days or fast days,[26] many researchers have connected them with older pagan goddesses (Smith 2004, 169–70). Jakob Grimm connected Holda/Holle e.g. with the maternal goddesses like Nerthus and Isis, who paid special attention to flax and spinning, similarly also Frigg; with respect to spinning tools also with Artemis[27] (Diana), Leto, Athene, Amphitrite and the Nereids, who hold a spindle or a distaff in their hands. Also, frequently mentioned in association with these beings are goddesses such as Hecate, Selena, Freya (often equated with Frigg, the fertility goddess who also functioned as the leader of the dead), Astarte, Atargatis/Dea Syria (Hittite superior goddess), Minerva, the Germanic goddess Tanfana/Tamfana, the Germanic Mistress of Wild Things (the force of nature which is both life-giving and life-taking), the Irish St. Brighid etc. (Grimm 2012 [1888], I: 270; Motz 1984, 161–3; Kuret 1989, II: 458; Ellis Davidson 1993, 116–7; Pócs 1999, 125–6; Timm 2003, 212, 255; Smith 2004, 168–9). Éva Pócs claims that the line of seers, usually women (who had particularly Germanic and Celtic historical roots, but existed in village communities of several European peoples between the Middle Ages and the Modern Age, as we know from the witch trials in the Alpine regions) who were taken and inaugurated into the soul troops around Christmas time, and who kept regular contact with the dead through their doubles, "lived on in the cult of Artemis and Diana up to the Middle Ages, in close relationship with the shaping of the belief system of the witches in the early Middle Ages". Other chthonic figures who appeared as the leaders of the march of the dead and as the guardians and initiator spirits of seeing women included Hecate, the Austrian and south German Perchta, Holda, the Swiss Frau Saelde, the Slovenian Pehtra baba, Freya and Lucia or Lucy. She also emphasises their role with respect to spinning and other feminine occupations, and their attributes of distaff and spindle. This female line corresponds to Ginzburg's female type of magicians (*benandanti*) who were initiated during the procession of the dead visiting humans and who were mostly concerned with healing, seeing the dead, and seeing treasure, and whose origin he finds in the Scythian fertility goddess of the dead with snake attributes ("snake goddess") (Pócs 1999, 124–6; cf. also Ginzburg 1992, 89–152).

---

[26] He argues that the origin of the word Perchta and Befana is a "feast of Epiphany" in the sense of the "Manifestation of Christ" which, later on being no longer understood, was reinterpreted to "Eve/Night of Perht", "Day of Percht"; the majority of other similar beings may also be seen as personifications of feast or fast days.

[27] Called the "Lady of the Golden Spindle" (Iliad 20, 70); cf. Motz 1984, 161; the protectress of small children, and the overseer of childbirth (Graves 1987, 76–7).

Whether Perchta etc. or Midwinter Woman in general follow directly from the line of all of these goddesses or not (which is not the subject of the present discussion), the fact is that the beings who oversaw spinning or whose traditions connected them with spinning also often possessed aspects that were both associated with *fertility* and were at the same time *chthonic*—they are often, although not always, associated with birth, with the souls of (newborn) children and also the souls of the dead. For instance, Perchta, as Timm finds, is shown above all in three interconnected roles: as the bearer of children, as the kidnapper of children and as the protectress of children's souls (Timm 2003, 259). Women who immersed themselves in Frau Holle's well were given the gift of fertility, Berchta shared a cave in the Tyrol with unborn children, and anyone who wanted a child had to pay her a visit; besides, the tradition frequently depicts her surrounded by a crowd of children who had died before baptism (Motz 1984, 155). According to the beliefs, Percht lived with small children in a cave near Lucerne (variant: cared for unborn children on a hillside in Wasserkufen). Anyone who wanted a child could take one from there. In Entlebuch, Switzerland, they said that small children came from Seltenbach (the stream of Mrs Selten—a variant of Perchta, who was called Frau Zälti there), while in Transylvania, that Frau Holle cared for unborn children in caves, mountains and wells. It was said that the Frau-Holen-Teich pond in Meissner made women who lay in her well healthy and fertile, and that the newborn came from her well, and that she brought them out. In Silesia, the Spillaholle (from Ger.: *Spindel-Holle*) brought children, whom she dragged into the well because of their laziness, to parents who were unable to have children (Timm 2003, 260). We find Perchta (Percht, Berchta, Holda, Holle, Stampe, Pehtra) surrounded by a crowd of unbaptised deceased children throughout her entire region (Timm 2003, 262–3; cf. also Kretzenbacher 1941, 86, who writes of Bercht as "Seelenführerin"; Kuret 1989, II: 458; 1997, 66; Kropej 2008b, 182). Certainly, the fundamental trait of Midwinter Woman was that she was a leader of souls, especially the souls of children (Kuret 1997, 66–7). Pehtra's fertility aspects in the Slovenian tradition can also be seen in the song sung by herders to call her as she walked along the ridges with a golden pail in her hand: "Vehtra baba, deža daj, Lanu ti dam debel kučaj". ("Vehtra baba, give us rain, I give you flax, a thick bunch") or "Vehtra baba, daj pšenice, Moji kravički travice". ("Vehtra baba, give us wheat, And grass for my cows") (Kelemina 1997, 93–4, no. 57, Gorenjska region; Kuret 1997, 67; Kilbourne Matossian 1973, 333).

Pehtra's association with children can also be explained by her occasional punishment of lazy or naughty children and more rarely of rewarding good ones: in Heidermoos/Inntal in Upper Austria she carried off naughty children, in Lauthenthal she threatened to carry off naughty and lazy children (Rumpf 1976, 219). Particularly in Alpine regions, Perchta meted out punishment by cutting open the bellies of naughty children and filling them with straw and rocks (Motz 1984, 154). According to southern German and Austrian beliefs, Perchta walked about during the twelve nights and rewarded those who followed the rules, punishing the negligent, greedy, lazy and curious; disobedient children and even adults were in danger of her slicing open their bellies, removing the contents, including the intestines, and filling them with refuse (Smith 2004, 168). We encounter the same conceptualisation in Slovenia (in a legend from Mežakla, which possibly indicates former rituals): Pehtra was said to come into the valley before the Epiphany, reward good children and kill naughty ones with fire tongs and pull out their intestines with them (Kuret 1989, II: 461). According to belief, in the Slovenian Carinthia and Goriško regions she walked about during Carnival and particularly at Epiphany, frightening children: "Perhta baba, hodi zdaj,/ kjer otrok se najde kaj,/ bucne vampič z vilami,/ tih' k' so zlo nasiteni ('Perhta baba, walks now,/ where there are children to be found,/ pokes their bellies with pitchforks,/ of those who are overstuffed')" (This could otherwise be understood as her overseeing the fast, cf. Smith 2004). In Bovec, she had a hatchet and walked about on the day after Epiphany frightening children; in Trenta, the "Perte" (a variant of Pehtras) distributed good and bad things at Epiphany (Kelemina 1997, 94, no. 58). In Rož (Rosental), among Slovenes in Austrian Carinthia, Pehtra came into the house, gave out gifts, usually dried apple slices, and threatened naughty children (Kuret 1989, II: 465). In lower Styria they said that on Christmas Day children disappeared from houses that were not well-cleaned—this was the work of the Pudelmutter, which is another name for Percht. In Upper Styria, Perchta carried naughty children away with her on Christmas Day. According to a legend in the Tyrol, Stampe sees a beautiful child and takes him into a cave. Germans in Moravian Kuhländchen said that Spillalutsche (= Spindel-Luzie, "Spindle Lucy") killed children who lagged behind and took them off with her. In Niederwald in Silesia, she took lazy children to her home, Spillalutschenstein. In Dillingen (Saar) they said that Frau Holle received her name because she "takes away" (Ger.: "holen") children. In Meissner, Holle liked to lure children to her pond; she made the good ones happy and foisted the bad children upon others—and here the circle is thus complete, as Timm observes. In Hausberg in Harz, children not only came from Frau Holle's well, but parents also threatened the children that they were going to put them back in it. The Silesian Spillaholle also took lazy children away before giving them to other parents (Timm 2003, 261–2). Similarly, the Trotte-vieilles kidnapped naughty children and threw them into a stream in front of the door, while they gave gifts to good children, and, according to belief, the Wild Hunt in Switzerland sometimes carried off disobedient children too (Gennep 1999, 2432–3; Hoffmann-Kreyer 1940, 79).

Why is it that these goddesses, saints and mythical beings are so often connected with spinning on the one hand and with birth and/or death on the other?[28] If we leave the symbolic meaning of a thread behind,[29] we see that if circular movement is a movement characteristic of a liminal space between the worlds and is at the same time an indicator of a passage from this to the other world (and vice versa) where the souls of the people-to-be-born abide, the connection between spinning (the turning of a spinning wheel or a spindle) on the one hand and birth and death on the other hand seems only natural. The turning so often applied to goddesses of birth and destiny usually refers to the technique of spinning,[30] which requires some sort of *turning* of a thread (Belmont 1971, 176–7; West 2007, 383).[31]

---

[28] West argues that a close semantic connection between turning and eventuating is perhaps relevant to the image of the goddesses' spindle that spins round because it twists the loose wool into a firm thread. A pervasive image of spinning for the fixing of human destinies might be understood as suited to symbolise the conversion of loose, incoherent possibilities into something definite, that, like a human life, grows continuously longer but sooner or later is cut off (West 2007, 383, 385).

[29] Spinning is an especially appropriate attribute of goddesses responsible for birth and death, since there is also a strong symbolic connection between thread and body tissue. The allegorical image of the "mother-as-a-distaff" together with that of the "child-as-the-flax-on-a-spindle" shape the metaphorical representation of "life-span" as "flax-spun" (Badalanova Geller 2004: 231). In the symbolism of Western civilisation to spin and weave means to create body tissue. The spinning goddesses therefore spin because their activity has magic power: in this way they spin the body tissue of a newborn child, they wind a band around a baby—but the winding sheet is also wrapped around the corpse in a spiral, like thread around a spindle, which should, according to Matossian, explain the association of the Goddess of life and death with spinning and weaving (Kilbourne Matossian 1924: 331; cf. also Cottica 2004, 200). The Hittite word for a spindle even derives from the verb "to live" (Cottica 2004, 200).

[30] Belmont argues that the turning movement of these goddesses is primarily connected with their task of the turning of a child in the mother's womb to the head down position before its birth.

[31] The word for a spindle or a spindle-whorl actually derives from the same verbal root *uert- in various languages (Old Church Slavonic *vrěteno*, Middle High German *wirtel*, Welsh *gwerthyd*).

Through turning the circular motion of a thread, a spindle or a spinning wheel, these goddesses are therefore able to communicate between the worlds, to enter the other world and draw the souls that are to be born into a new existence in the world of the living (and vice versa).

Conclusion

But to return to our original question: Why, then, was spinning forbidden precisely during the periods or on the holidays which we mentioned at the beginning? Why was circular movement, i.e. spinning, not allowed on the days/periods when the door between the world of the living and the world of the dead was open? Now, if it was possible to draw the souls of the newborn babies from the other world through circular movement (spinning), it could just as well be possible to draw dangerous demons, i.e. death itself from the other world. If the spinning, circular movement of the spinning wheel or spindle was a way to enter the other world, then we can understand the taboo on spinning as a preventive measure against drawing death to this world during the time when the door to the other world was open.

This is especially so if we understand the annual cycle as a two-phase temporal cycle, where "each year includes a double action where spin in one direction is succeeded by spin in the other" (Lyle 1990, 65), with time therefore going forwards and backwards, thus circling or spiralling there and back to the starting point, whereby backwards movement has a connotation of being the time of death (Lyle 1990, 62–5 and 94–5). In this model "[...] a ritually marked period of time (is) analogically related to backward movement, which is, in the Indo-European case, connected with death and reverse movement" (Lyle 2008, 15). If we apply this model to the year, then the period of reversal and death would most typically be found between Christmas and the Epiphany (25 December to 6 January). Just as spinning was therefore forbidden at times of death in the life cycle, since "death, which is already the reversal of the direction of the corpse,[32] forbids any other reversals in the time when the body still lies at home" (Belmont 1971, 179; cf. also Mencej 2009a) it was also forbidden in the "reversed" periods in the annual (as well as daily) cycle. The circular

[32] While death is associated with reverse movement, life is associated with forward movement. The notion about birth being connected with forward movement and death being connected with reverse movement at the level of the human life cycle corresponds well with Emily Lyle's hypothesis of a two-phase annual cycle.

motion of the thread/wheel/spindle[33] in the periods of reversal thus becomes the movement that brings death and infertility to our world.*

References

Alford, Violet. 1937. *Pyrenean Festivals, Calendar Customs, Music & Magic, Drama & Dance*. London: Chatto and Windus.

Badalanova Geller, Florentina. 2004. "The Spinning Mary: Towards the Iconology of the Annunciation." *Cosmos* 20: 211–60.

Bächtold-Stäubli, Hanns, and Eduard Hoffmann-Krayer, Hrsg. 1987 [1927–41]. *Handwörterbuch der deutschen Aberglaubens* 9. Berlin, and New York: Walter de Gruyter.

Bek-Pedersen, Karen 2007a. "Are the spinning Nornir just a Yarn?" *Viking and Medieval Scandinavia* 3: 1–10.

—. 2007b. "Nornir in Old Norse Mythology." PhD Diss., manuscript, University of Edinburgh.

Belaj, Marijana. 2006. "Sveci zaštitnici u hrvatskoj pučkoj pobožnosti [Patron saints in Croation folk religion]." PhD Diss., manuscript, Filozofski fakultet Sveučilišta u Zagrebu.

Belaj, Vitomir. 2007. *Hod kroz godinu: pokušaj rekonstrukcije prahrvatskoga mitskoga svjetonazora* [Walking through the Year: An Attempt of the Reconstruction of Ancient Croatian Mythical World view]. Zagreb: Golden marketing—Tehnička knjiga.

Belmont, Nicole. 1971. *Les signes de la naissaince. Études des représentations symboliques associés aux naissances singulières.* Paris: Librarie Plon.

Bezlaj, France. 1951. "Nekaj besedi o slovenski mitologiji v zadnjih desetih letih [A few words in Slovenian mythology in the last ten years]." *Slovenski etnograf* 3–4: 342–53.

Briggs, Katharine. 1976. *An Encyclopedia of Fairies*. New York: Pantheon Books.

Burke, Peter. 1994. *Popular Culture in Early Modern Europe*. Cambridge: Cambridge Scholar Press.

Cevc, Tone. 1999. "Pripovedno izročilo iz Kamniškega kota [Folk narratives from Kamnik region]." *Traditiones* 28 (1): 89–100.

[33] I would like to thank Karen Bek-Pedersen and Freda Bayne for clarifying a few facts of spinning to me.

*I would like to thank the Humboldt foundation for their financial support during my research stay at the University of Mannheim in 2008, where I collected most of the literature for the present paper and where the paper started to take shape.

Cottica, Daniela. 2004. "The Symbolism of Spinning in Classical Art and Society." *Cosmos* 20: 185–210.

Danaher, Kevin. 1972. *The Year in Ireland. Irish Calendar Customs*. Minneapolis, Minn.: Mercier Press.

Dolenc, Janez. 1977. "Pripovedno izročilo v severnem poljanskem narečju [Folk narratives in northern Poljane dialect]." *Traditiones* 4 (1975): 175–96.

Ellis Davidson, Hilda. 1993. *The Lost Beliefs of Northern Europe*. London and New York: Routledge.

Feilhauer, Angelika. 2000. *Feste feiern in Deutschland. Ein Führer zu alten und neuen Volksfesten und Bräuchen.* Zürich: Sanssouci.

Gavazzi, Milovan. 1988. *Godina dana hrvatskih narodnih običaja* [Croatian annual folk customs]. Zagreb: Kulturno-prosvjetni sabor Hrvatske.

Gennep, Arnold van. 1999. *Le folklore français* 3. Paris: Robert Laffont.

Ginzburg, Carlo. 1992. *Ecstasies. Deciphering the Witches' Sabbath*. London: Penguin Books.

Gričnik, Anton. 1995. *Noč ima svojo moč, Bog pa še večjo: Pohorje pripoveduje* [Night has its power, but God's is even bigger: Pohorje narrates]. Ljubljana: Kmečki glas.

Grimm, Jacob. 2012. *Teutonic Mythology.* Reprint. Cambridge: Cambridge University Press. [London: George Bell & Sons, 1888.]

Hiiemäe, Mall. 1995. *The Estonian Folk Calendar, Estonian Customs and Traditions*. Tallinn: Perioodika.

Hoffmann-Krayer, Eduard. 1940. *Feste und Bräuche des Schweizervolkes*. Zürich: Atlantis.

Kelemina, Jakob. 1997. *Bajke in pripovedke slovenskega ljudstva. Z mitološkim uvodom* [Belief Legends and Narratives of Slovenian People. With a Mythological Introduction]. Bilje: Studio Ro.

Kilbourne Matossian, Mary. 1973. "In the Beginning, God Was a Woman." *Journal of Social History* 6 (3): 325–43.

Kretzenbacher, Leopold. 1941. *Germanische Mythen in der epischen Volksdichtung der Slowenen.* Graz: Steirische Verlaganstalt.

Krinichnaia, N. A. 1995. *Nit' zhizni. Reministsentsii obrazov bozhestv sud'by v mifologii i fol'klore, obriadakh i verovaniiakh* [The thread of life. Reminiscences of the images of fates in mythology, customs, and beliefs]. Petrozavodsk: Izdatel'stvo petrzavodskogo universiteta.

Kropej, Monika. 2008a. *Od ajda do zlatoroga. Slovenska bajeslovna bitja* [From "Ajd" to "Zlatorog". Slovenian mythological beings]. Celovec: Mohorjeva družba.

—. 2008b: "Slovene Midwinter Deities and Personifications of Days in the Yearly, Work, and Life Cycles." In *Space and time in Europe: East and West, Past and Present*, edited by Mirjam Mencej, 181–98 Ljubljana: Oddelek za etnologijo in kulturno antropologijo. (Zupaničeva knjižnica 25.)

Kuret, Niko. 1975. "Die Zwölften und das Wilde Heer in den Ost-Alpen." *Alpes Orientales* VII: 80–9.

—. 1989. *Praznično leto Slovencev* I–II. [Annual cycle of Slovenian holidays]. Ljubljana: Družina.

—. 1997. *Opuscula selecta. Poglavja iz ljudske kulture* [Chapters from folk culture]. Ljubljana: SAZU.

Lecouteux, Claude. 1997. "Chasse sauvage/Armée furieuse. Quelques reflexions." In *Le mythe de la chasse sauvage dans L'Europe médiévale*, edited by Philippe Walter, 13–32. Paris: Editions Champion.

Lyle, Emily. 1990. *Archaic Cosmos: Polarity, Space and Time*. Edinburgh: Polygon.

—. 2008. "The Indo-European Ritual Year as a Two-Phase Cycle, Including a Period of Reversal." In *Space and Time in Europe: East and West, Past and Present*, edited by Mirjam Mencej, 147–52. Ljubljana: Oddelek za etnologijo in kulturno etnologijo.

Mandianes-Castro, Manolo. 2004. "Le Magosto: fête des châtaignes et des morts en Galice." In *Fêtes et rites agraires en Europe. Métamorphoses?*, edited by Bonnet Jocelyne, and Sébastien Fournier, 101–12 Montpellier: L'Harmattan.

Mencej, Mirjam. 2001. *Gospodar volkov v slovanski mitologiji* [The master of the wolves in Slavic folklore]. Ljubljana: Oddelek za etnologijo in kulturno antropologijo. (Zupaničeva knjižnica 6.)

—. 2005. "The Slavic Summer/Winter Opposition in the Pastoral Year and the Christian and pre-Christian Figures Identifiable as the Master of the Wolves." *Cosmos* 21 (1): 79–111.

—. 2008a. "Walking in circles." In *Space and time in Europe: East and West, Past and Present*, edited by Mirjam Mencej, 35–66. Ljubljana: Oddelek za etnologijo in kulturno antropologijo. (Zupaničeva knjižnica 25.)

—. 2008b "The Night is Yours, the Day is Mine! Functions of Stories of Night-Time Encounters with Witches in Eastern Slovenia." *Estudos de Literatura Oral* 13/14, (2007/2008): 189–206.

—. 2009a. "Spinning Taboos in Europe." *Social and Spiritual Aspects of Material Culture*, 135–58. Skopje: Odjelenje za etnologiju.

—. 2009b: "Wolf Holidays Among Southern Slavs in the Balkans." *Acta Ethnographica Hungarica* 54: 337–58.

Miles, Clement A. 1976. *Christmas Customs and Traditions. Their History and Significance*. New York: Dover.

Motz, Lotte. 1984. "The Winter Goddess: Percht, Holda, and Related Figures." *Folklore* 95 (2): 151–66.

Novak, Anka. 1987. "Iz duhovne kulture Bohinjcev [From the spiritual culture of the Bohinj people]." *Traditiones* 16: 279–87.

Pócs, Éva. 1999. *Between the Living and the Dead*. Budapest: Central European University Press.

Rumpf, Marianne. 1976. "Spinnstubefrauen, Kinderschreckgestalten und Frau Perchta." *Fabula* 3–4: 215–42.

Saintyves, Pierre. 1987. *Les contes de Perrault et les récits parallèles (leur origins); On marge de la légends dorée, Songes, miracles et survivances; les reliques et les images légendaires.* Paris: Robert Lafont.

Sébillot, Paul. 1981. *Légende et curiosités des métiers*. Marseille: Laffitte.

Simek, Rudolf. 2000 [1984]. *Dictionary of Northern Mythology*. Cambridge: D. S. Brewer.

Smith, John. B. 2004. "Perchta the Belly-Slitter and her Kin: a View of some Traditional Threatening Figures, Threats and Punishments." *Folklore* 115: 167–86.

Šešo, Luka 2007: "Vjerovanja u bića koja se pretvaraju u životinje [Beliefs in beings transforming into animals]." In *Kulturni bestijarij* [Cultural bestiarium], edited by Marjanić Suzana, and Antonija Zaradija Kiš, 253–86. Zagreb: Institut za etnologiju i folkloristiku, Hrvatska sveučilišna naklada.

Timm, Erika. 2003. *Frau Holle, Frau Percht und verwandte Gestalten*. Stuttgart: S. Hirzel.

Timotin, Emanuela. 2009. "Irodia, Doamna Zânelor. Notes sur les fées roumaines et leur cohorte fantastique." In *Les entre-mondes. Les vivants, les morts*, edited by Karin Ueltschi, and Myriam White-Le Goff, 179–94. Paris: Klincksieck.

Tolstaja, Svetlana. M. 1995. "Mythologie et axiologie du Temps dans la culture populaire slave." *La revue russe* 8: 27–42.

Torma, Thomas. 2002. Imbolc, Candlemas, and the Feast of St. Brigit. *Cosmos* 18: 77–85.

Toporov, Vladimir N. 2002. *Predzgodovina književnosti pri Slovanih. Poskus rekonstrukcije (Uvod v preučevanje zgodovine slovanskih književnosti)* [Prehistory of Slavic literature. An attempt at reconstruction]. Ljubljana: Oddelek za etnologijo in kulturno antropologijo. (Zupaničeva knjižnica 9.)

Valencova, Marina M. 2001. “Vreteno [Spindle].” In *Slovenska mitologija* [Slavic Mythology], edited by Svetlana M. Tolstaja, and Ljubinko Radenković, 102–3. Belgrade: Zepter Book World.

—. 2009. “Priadenie [Spinning].” In *Slovar slavianskyh drevnostei* 4. [Dictionary of Slavic antiquities], edited by Svetlana Tolstaia et al., 321–8. Moskva: Mezhdunarodnye otnoshenia.

West, Martin L. 2007. *Indo-European Poetry and Myth*. Oxford: Oxford University Press.

DIVINE HEALERS IN ROMANIAN MANUSCRIPT CHARMS (17TH–19TH CENTURIES)

EMANUELA TIMOTIN

This paper deals with a recently edited corpus of Romanian curative or protective magical texts preserved in manuscripts dating from the seventeenth to the nineteenth century (Timotin 2010 and 2015) and focuses on several holy figures invested with healing attributes.[1]

The investigation will take place in three stages. Firstly, it will explore whether charms assign one or several therapeutic functions to a certain divine healer. Secondly, it will study hagiographical details in order to discover whether a saint's healing role proceeds from specific motifs of his *Vita* or from innovative reinterpretations. Finally, it will try to establish whether a saint is invested with curative functions in manuscript charms only or whether he is assigned the same abilities in other sources, such as in the contemporary literature or the oral tradition.

1. A charm written in 1833, preserved in the Romanian Academy Library in Bucharest in MS 3479 (fol. 69^r), grants St. Cyprian with the power to protect those who suffer from evil spells.[2] The text is conceived as a prayer to the new moon and illustrates a charm-type which enjoyed a wide popularity in Romanian magical literature: it is preserved in ten manuscripts, written between the last quarter of the eighteenth century and the middle of the nineteenth century. In a highly reshuffled form, it is passed on both in numerous chapbooks published between 1867 and 1931, and in the oral tradition, as attested by several charms against evil spells

[1] For St John the Baptist and for St Sisinnios as healers of fever in Romanian manuscript charms, see Timotin 2009a, 368–71.

[2] The manuscript is described in Ştrempel 1987, 143–4. The text is edited in Timotin 2010, 334 and 2015, 252–4.

recorded in north-eastern Romania in the second half of the twentieth century.[3]

St. Cyprian, who lived in Antioch during the reign of the emperor Decius and whose feast day is celebrated on 2 October, is referred to in the very title of the charm:

> Carte de fapt a Iencului ciubotar cu soţul său Safta, cu agiutoriul sfântului mucenic Chiprien, ce au biruit pre Eliman vrăjitorul, cel plin de toată răutatea.
> ("Booklet against evil spells of the shoemaker Iancu and of his wife Safta, with the help of the holy martyr Cyprian who defeated Elymas, the very mean sorcerer".)

Despite this mention, the saint plays no part whatsoever in the development of the magical text, which assigns the therapeutic function exclusively to the new moon, as do other charms illustrating this charm-type.

This evocation reflects the scribe's efforts to provide the users of the charms, the shoemaker and his wife, with the supplementary protection of a saint renowned for his power against sorcerers. Cyprian is considered to be the most appropriate to fulfil this task because, according to his hagiography, he himself had been a powerful sorcerer before his conversion to Christianity. His past before conversion makes Cyprian the perfect celestial protector against evil spells, and in order to reinforce his abilities, the charm also recalls his triumph over the sorcerer Elymas. The detail is, however, apocryphal, since at no point in his life did Elymas confront Cyprian. His fame as a sorcerer, however, is greater, for he opposed a highly important Christian figure, the Apostle Paul (Acts 13, 4–12) who, like Cyprian, fought against Christians before adopting Christianity.

The figure of St. Cyprian seems to be specific to this charm: the saint does not appear in other Romanian charms from the manuscript or oral tradition, neither does he belong to the group of saints venerated in the popular tradition. The devotion granted to him is always due to the influence of the Christian cult. Thus, it appears that his mention in the charm against evil spells reflects the scribe's attempt to slightly Christianise the prayer to the new moon.

The scribe was undoubtedly familiar with the saint's hagiography, as his signature at the end of the copied texts reveals that he was a priest. His

---

[3] For the three components of the transmission of this charm-type, see Timotin 2009b.

education must have allowed him to identify another reason for designating Cyprian as a protector against evil spells. The Romanian name of the magical disease the prayer to the new moon was supposed to heal is *fapt*, a word inherited from the Latin *factum*, participle of the verb *facere*.[4] The word first appears in Romanian, with the meaning "evil spells", at the end of the seventeenth century in the translation of the *Lives of the Saints*, specifically in St. Cyprian's *Life*. It is therefore likely that the scribe attached the saint's figure to the prayer to the moon because he connected the "evil spells" (*fapt*) referred to in the hagiographical text to those evoked in the charm. This ingenious addition was also innovative because the priest did not mention the saint's real opponent, the governor of Antioch who had ordered St. Cyprian's martyrdom, referring instead to the famous sorcerer Elymas.

2. Another occasional presence in the Romanian charms is St. Nicetas, who appears in a "Charm against ghosts" (*Pentru strigoi descântec*) written in 1777 and currently preserved in the Romanian Academy Library in Bucharest in MS 2183 (fol. 161^{v}).[5] Unlike the prayer to the moon, the charm-type against ghosts seems to be illustrated exclusively by this lone version.

Unlike St. Cyprian, who played no active role in the development of the magical scenario, St. Nicetas, who was martyred in 372 and whose feast day is celebrated on 15 September, occupies a key position. He is described as the only character able to defend those attacked by ghosts, and the charm stresses the warrior attributes which allow him to fulfil this task: he is holding a sword of fire and a whip.

> Cruce pre ceriu, cruce pre pământ, cruce în cest loc unde mă culc. Easte cruce, easte şi cetate cu ferestri de pietri nestemate şi şade sfântul măcinic Nichita cu sabie de foc şi cu cnut în mână şi păzeaşte de la miiază de noapte până la cântători şi de la cântători până în vărsat de zori, ca un stan de piatră denaintea uşii.
> ("Cross onto the sky, cross onto the earth, cross onto this place where I am sleeping. There is a cross, there is a fortress with windows of precious stones and there sits the holy martyr Nicetas holding a sword of fire and a whip and he guards it [= the fortress] from midnight to the cock's crow and from the cock's crow till dawn, staying as a rock in front of the door.")

---

[4] For the use of this word in popular medical terminology, see mainly Şăineanu 1999, 316–8; Bălteanu 2000, 158–60.

[5] For this manuscript, see Ştrempel 1978–1992, II. 205; the charm against ghosts was not identified in the description of the codex.

The text provides several details about the ghosts: they are malevolent nocturnal beings, acting between midnight and dawn, and they disturb people's sleep.[6] The strong invocation of the cross, placed at the beginning of the charm ("Cross onto the sky, cross onto the earth, cross onto this place where I am sleeping"), represents the fragment of a prayer.[7] This invocation, along with the description of St. Nicetas as a protector against ghosts, suggests that the malefic beings were assimilated into the devil.

This assimilation must have been the main reason for St. Nicetas' presence in the magical text. Thus, although the saint's evocation as a protector against ghosts seems specific to this charm and has no equivalent in other Romanian magical texts, written or oral, Nicetas has always been famous as an opponent of the devil. This reputation is probably based both on the extrapolation of the signification of his name—"victorious"—and on some events recorded in his *Vita*: he fought against Athanaric's pagan troops and he remained faithful to the Nicene Creed. The saint's main features are also emphasised in the iconography. Medieval Orthodox representations portray him as a military saint, and in a sixteenth-century Russian icon, he is seated on a throne and holds a demon, which crawls at his feet, by its neck (Réau 1958, 974–5; especially Walter 2003). Such representations are likely to have influenced Romanian folklore, too, since several traditional legends collected in the second half of the nineteenth century praise Nicetas as a warrior saint and recall that he holds the devil by its hair.[8]

Thus, though St. Nicetas' presence in Romanian charms is occasional, since evidenced so far in only one magical text, it tallies with other testimonies, iconographical or literary, which assign him the power to defeat devilish actions. Hence the charm against ghosts becomes an important document in his Eastern European cult.

3. While Saints Cyprian and Nicetas are invested with specific roles, the Saints Cosmas and Damian are multifunctional healers. They are evoked in eighteenth-century manuscript charms which present various magical

---

[6] For a comprehensive description of the Romanian beliefs concerning the ghosts, see Taloş 2002, s.v. *revenants*, *sorcières*.

[7] A similar prayer appears in the incipit of a charm against snakebite, recorded in 1971; for this text, see Ciubotaru 2005, 505–6.

[8] Fochi 1976, 306. For the attributes with which Saint Nicetas is currently invested in the Romanian popular tradition, see Taloş 2002, s.v. *Nikita, saint*.

scenarios and are meant to cure snakebite,[9] wolf-bite[10] or feverish diseases.[11]

The two saints never take part in the plot. They are referred to exclusively at the beginning of the magical texts, following the pattern of the prayer to the new moon against evil spells, the curative effects of which had been strengthened by the evocation of St. Cyprian. The same phenomenon is largely present in the charms of the oral tradition. Scholars have therefore emphasised that such writings are the only ones to pay constant attention to the two holy figures, who are sporadically referred to in sayings as well (Bogrea 1971a, 124).

The saints are constantly evoked in charms (even though they play no active role in them), because they are traditionally worshipped with great honour, especially on their feast days, the first day of July and the first day of September.[12] Popular veneration grants them two nicknames. The first, "the silverless doctors" (*doctorii fără arginţi*, *doctorii fără bani*, *doctorii fără parale*), is a translation from the Greek *anargyroi* and stems from their hagiography according to which they accepted no payment for their services. The second is more general: "God's healers" (*vracii Domnului*) (see Taloş 2002, s.v. *Cosmandin*; Muşlea and Bîrlea 1970, 404).

In charms, the saints' names were included in two versed rhythmic fragments, forming a pair with *amin, amin* ("amen, amen"). These metrical constraints explain the many and even risible deformations to which Cosmas' and Damian's names were submitted, but these distortions also prove that the users of the magical words were unaware of the two *anargyroi*'s attributes.

In these versified structures, Damian's name is often modified:

Amin! Amin!
Cosmă, Dămin" (Pamfile 1997, 105).

---

[9] The texts are preserved in the Romanian Academy Library in Bucharest in MS. 1320 (fol. 21^{r}) and 4743 (fols. 184^{r-v}). For a description of the manuscripts, see Ştrempel and Moisil and Stoianovici 1967, 547; Ştrempel1978–92, IV. 291–2; and Ştrempel 1978–92, IV. 107. The texts are edited in Timotin 2010, 277 and 278.

[10] The charm, preserved in the Romanian Academy Library in Bucharest in MS. 1320 (fol. 21^{r}), is edited in Timotin 2010, 291.

[11] The charm is preserved in the Romanian Academy Library in Bucharest in MS 4903 (fols. 23^{v}–24^{r}); for the description of the manuscript, see Ştrempel1978–92, IV. 152); the text is edited in Timotin 2010, 314.

[12] For their celebration on 1 July, see Pamfile 1997. 105; for their feast on 1 November, see Muşlea and Bîrlea 1970, 404. For the protective virtues attributed to the two saints in South-Eastern Europe, see Candrea 1999, 228.

Amin! Amin!
Cosma, *Damnin*! (ibidem)[13]

The popular etymology is also partly responsible for its miscomprehension and, consequently, for its complete disappearance. Various examples prove that it was understood as a compound name formed from the preposition *de* (< lat. *de*) and the word *amen*. The oldest such mention appears in the eighteenth-century charm against feverish diseases:

Amin. *Cozma di amin*
("Amen, *Cosmas of amen* ") (MS. 4903, fol. 23^{v}).

Similar deformations are frequent in the charms of the oral tradition:

Amin, amin, *Cozma de-amin*
("Amen, amen, *Cosma of amen*")[14]

In other cases, under the influence of the Romanian *amin*, Damian's name is replaced by short structures formed from the preposition *de* ("of") and a name ending in (*-in*), which is deprived of any meaning in the context:

Amin, amin/ Cosmă *de vin*
("Amen, amen, *Cosma of wine*") (Rosetti 1975, 111).

Sometimes, the disappearance of Damian's name goes together with the reshuffling of Cosmas' name:

Doamne ajută-mi, *Cuzman*!
["Lord, help me, *Cuzman"*];

Amin, Amin, / *Cosman* de amin
("Amen, amen, *Cosman* of amen") (Bogrea 1971b, 136).

The two saints' names may also merge into a single one, *Cosmandin* or *Cozmanin*:

Amin, amin,
Cozmanin
[Amen, amen, *Cozmanin*][15]

---

13 For other similar examples, see Bogrea 1971a, 125.
14 See the numerous examples inventoried in Bogrea 1971a, 125; Moraru 1993, 41.

As Vasile Bogrea argues, such elaborations must have been influenced both by the similar designation of Constantine, the first Christian emperor, and by a lexical pattern specific to oral culture, in which the names of two patron saints or supernatural beings are combined to create the denomination of a feast day, as in the popular feasts of *Antanasii* or *Todorusalii* (see Bogrea 1971a, 125). A charm recorded in 1971 sheds new light on the unfortunate fate of the saints' names: while Damian is read as a compound, as in the interpretative pattern described above, Cosmas' name has become a meaningless common noun, as seen in its connection to the undetermined article:

> Amin, amin
> *C-un Cozman de in*
> [Amen, amen, *with a Cozman of wine/linen*] Ciubotaru 2005, 314).[16]

Such examples show that the famous holy doctors Cosmas and Damian are constantly called upon in Romanian charms. However, their role in healing the patient is never described and they are referred to only at the beginning of magical texts, often under corrupted denominations. Such mentions prove that, because of their fame as "silverless doctors", the evocation of the saints has gradually become a passkey, automatically added to charms in order to increase their therapeutic power. Although the two important Christian healers were endowed with the ability to cure various diseases, their multifunctional roles obliterated any interest in their hagiography. This situation is not specific to Romanian charms. One can find similar mentions of the two saints in French charms, which either evoke them in the final part

> En l'honneur de Dieu
> et de la Vierge Marie,
> Saint Cosme et saint Damien.
> Amen (Camus 1990, 75).

or introduce them using an innovative chronology in which Cosmas and Damian are contemporaries of Christ and heal Christ himself:

---

[15] For examples with Cosmandin, see Bogrea 1971a, 125. For the use of Cozmanin, see Ciubotaru 2005, 426.

[16] The Romanian word *in* can be interpreted both as "linen", and as a dialectological form of the word *vin* "wine".

Que Dieu te guérisse de cette pointe
Comme saint Côme et saint Damien
Ont guéri notre Seigneur Jésus-Christ
Lorsqu'ils l'ont descendu de l'arbre de la croix;

En l'honneur...
De saint Côme et saint Damien,
Qui ont guéri les plaies de Notre Seigneur Jésus-Christ
Sur le bois de la croix (Camus 1990, 76 and 92).

4. While the Saints Cosmas and Damian are called forth at the beginning of charms used to cure various diseases, the archangels are constantly referred to in the final part of a text against the evil eye. The writing resembles a prayer and circulated exclusively in the manuscript tradition during the period I am dealing with, specifically in nine codices written between the end of the eighteenth century and the beginning of the nineteenth century.[17]

The texts, which rely on a Greek model, [18]conceive the disease named the evil eye as the result of the malevolent, envious gaze of an unknown person who has looked in the patient's eyes and provoked the magical ailment. The patient assimilates the one who provoked the evil eye to the devil and begs God himself to turn His good and beneficent gaze upon him. In order to reinforce his plea, the patient recalls that God also saved the three young men whom the pagan king Nebuchadnezzar cast into the fiery furnace (*Daniel* 3). He then asks God to provide him with a strong guardian angel and concludes his supplication by invoking various saints, among whom only the Virgin and the archangels are always included.

The archangels' invocation at the end of the prayer, with no reference to the part they would play in the healing, might seem like a simple stereotype, functionally similar to the mention of Saints Cosmas and Damian at the beginning of various curative charms. However, one who is familiar with the compositional motifs of prayers will note that archangels are constantly called upon either in prayers regarding their feast days, or in prayers based on the enumeration of the names of various saints, neither of which is the case in texts against the evil eye.

A closer examination reveals that the archangels' presence is intimately connected to the other textual motifs.

As mentioned above, the patient begins his supplication to God by recalling the episode regarding the three young men in the fiery furnace

---

[17] The texts were edited in Timotin 2010, 263–73 and 2015, 147–60.

[18] According to H. Leclerq, this writing belonged to the Greek unofficial *Euchologion*; for the Greek text, see Leclerq 1936, col. 1939.

(*Daniel* 3). By resorting to such an argument to strengthen the patient's persuasive plea, the Romanian texts and, implicitly, their Greek model, are not innovative. On the contrary, the three young men are a constant presence in charms against the evil eye: their Hebrew and Babylonian names appear in a Coptic amulet dating from the eleventh-twelfth century, which was meant to cure various ailments, including the evil eye,[19] and they are also mentioned in a twentieth-century Greek charm especially for fever, but also against the evil eye (Arnaud 1912, 520).

The fiery ordeal to which the king Nebuchadnezzar submitted the three young men was regarded as analogous to the torments of a sufferer from fever and the episode was constantly included in charms against feverish diseases.[20] However, its mention in texts meant to heal the evil eye could be equally comprehended as a "persuasive analogy" for relieving the pains of a patient subjected to a continuous, malevolent gaze (Tuerk 1999). The Old Testament narrative includes a detail that the texts against the evil eye never mention, but which establishes a strong relation between the three young men and the one suffering from the evil eye: the three men were not alone in the fiery furnace, but were mysteriously accompanied by a fourth figure resembling the Son of God (Daniel 3, 25). This character, an angel (Daniel 3, 28), represents the proof that God continuously watches over and guards his servants. Accordingly, the one suffering from the evil eye hopes that he will likewise attract the divine gaze and receive the support of a strong guardian angel. In fact, the request for such an angel, who will continuously watch over the human assigned to him by God, is textually formulated, because the angel's beneficent scrutiny is supposed to make any evil look disappear.

The evocation of the archangels at once reflects the patient's fervent desire to attract the divine gaze and creates a subtle analogy between the divine beings and the sufferer. Seated close to the divine throne, the archangels continuously watch the divine light and, according to the texts, they see the light,[21] they resemble the light[22] or they shine brightly.[23] The

---

[19] See the text and the commentary in Bosson 1998. The editor focuses on the presence of the three young men in texts meant to heal fever, a presence considered easily comprehensible, since the ordeal by fire to which they were submitted was considered analogous to the patient's sufferings.

[20] For bibliography, see Bosson 1998, 111.

[21] See Ms. 1507: "Doamne, Dumnezeul nostru,... păzeşte-l pre el de tot răul pentru rugăciunile Preacuratei Maicii sale..., şi *ale văzătorilor de lumină arhangheli* ('God, our Lord, protect him [the patient] from any evil, for the prayers of your Blessed Mother... and of the archangels who see the light')". (fols. 64^v–65^r). The same fragment appears in MS 4083 (fol. 24^v), 3451 (fol. 70^r), 5425 (fol. 14^v).

situation of the patient is thus similar in many respects to that of the celestial beings: they are all subject to a powerful influence (God/the one who casts the evil eye); this influence is transmitted immaterially (as light or as a look) and it always affects the body upon which it is directed, which either becomes bright or falls ill.[24] Thanks to this transformative contact with the divine brilliance, the archangels become ideal assistants for one subject to a malevolent gaze. Hence, they join God and guardian angels as some of the most effective healers of the evil eye.

In conclusion, the saints' presence in the Romanian manuscript charms is by no means a unitary phenomenon. The saints mentioned here never heal, if by healing one means the thorough description of acts which restore one's health. It seems, however, that their qualities as protectors or divine *analogoi* of the sufferers are enough to earn a frequent presence in charms. Endowed with one or more therapeutic functions, occasionally or repeatedly referred to in charms, these saints, by the mere evocation of their names, actualise their hagiography and invite us to discover the particular reasons for which they were called upon. Their therapeutic roles are based on specific details of their *Vita*, which are sometimes reinforced by further interpretations, which can be divided into three categories: first, those that rely on internal developments of the saint's cult (St. Nicetas); secondly, those that are strengthened by the scribes' creativity (St. Cyprian); and finally, interpretations meant to evoke a situation analogous to that of the sufferer in order to provide him with the desired healing (the archangels).

---

22 See Ms. 2040: "Doamne, Dumnezeul nostru, milostiveaşte-te spre zidirea ta şi pre robul tău de toată stricăciunea şi supărarea ce i s-au făcut din dăochiu izbăveaşte-l... pentru rugăciunile preablagoslovitei, slăvitei stăpânei noastre,… ale arhanghelilor celor în chipul luminii ('God, Our Lord, have pity on your creation and deliver your servant from any evil and grief caused by the evil eye…, for the prayers of our Blessed Lady and of the archangels who resemble the light')". (fol. 112v). A similar fragment appears in MS 1335 (3v).

23 MS. 3275: "Doamne, Dumnezeul nostru, milostiveşti-te spre sluga ta aceasta... şi-l păzeşte pre dânsul mai presus de toate răotăţile, pentru rugăciunile preablagoslovitei stăpânei noastre... şi luminătorilor arhangheli ('God, our Lord, have pity on this servant of yours and protect him from any evil, for the prayers of our Blessed Lady and of the archangels who emanate light')". (fol. 175r). A similar fragment appears in MS 3404 (fol. 8r).

24 The same analogy between a patient suffering from a malevolent gaze and a Christian figure surrounded by the divine light is present in a nineteenth-century Greek exorcism, meant to heal various diseases, including the evil eye. In this text, the patient no longer evokes the archangels for healing, but rather the Transfiguration of Christ; see Arnaud 1912, 520.

The saints presented in this analysis play either an active or a passive role in the magical scenario, and the beginning of the charm appears to be the most variable part of a magical text, allowing the addition of new characters, especially saints, to the main plot. Though such is the case both for the charm that mentions St. Cyprian, and for those that mention Saints Cosmas and Damian, the texts introduce them for different reasons. The former reveals the scribe's intention to slightly Christianise the charm, while the latter shows how the two illustrious healing saints' figures ended up completely effaced by their reputation and how the utilisation of their names turned into a stereotype.

References

Arnaud, Louis. 1912. "La *baskania* ou le mauvais œil chez les Grecs modernes." *Échos d'Orient* 15: 385–94, and 510–24.

Bălteanu, Valeriu. 2000. *Terminologia magică populară românească* [The Romanian popular magical terminology]. Bucureşti: Paideia.

Bogrea, Vasile. 1971a. "Sfinţii-medici în graiul şi folclorul românesc [The holy doctors in the Romanian language and folklore]." In *Pagini istorico-filologice* [Historical-philological Studies], 124–34. Cluj: Dacia. (Cu o prefaţă de acad. C. Daicoviciu, ediţie îngrijită, studiu introductiv şi indice de M. Borcilă şi I. Mării.) [1924–1926.]

—. 1971b. 'Post-scriptum la "Sfinţii-medici" [Postscript to "The holy doctors"].' In *Pagini istorico-filologice* [Historical-philological studies], 135–8. Cluj: Dacia. (Cu o prefaţă de acad. C. Daicoviciu, ediţie îngrijită, studiu introductiv şi indice de M. Borcilă şi I. Mării.) [1924–1926.]

Bosson, Natalie. 1998. "Animadversiones. Amulette-palimpseste magique du Musée du Louvre." *Orientalia* n. s. 67: 107–14.

Camus, Dominique. 1990. *Paroles magiques. Secrets de guérison*. Paris: Imago.

Candrea, Ioan-Aurel. 1999. *Folclorul medical român comparat. Privire generală. Medicina magică* [Medical Romanian folklore in comparative perspective. Overview. Magical medicine]. Iaşi: Polirom. (Studiu introductiv de Lucia Berdan.) [1944].

Ciubotaru, Silvia. 2005. *Folclorul medical din Moldova. Tipologie şi corpus de texte* [Medical folklore from Moldavia. Typology and corpus of texts]. Iaşi: Editura Universităţii "Alexandru Ioan Cuza."

Fochi, Adrian. 1976. *Datini şi eresuri populare de la sfârşitul secolului al XIX-lea: răspunsurile la chestionarele lui N. Densusianu* [Popular customs and beliefs at the end of the 19th century. The answers to N. Densusianu's questionnaires]. Bucureşti: Minerva.

Leclerq, Henri. 1936. "Œil (Le mauvais œil)." In *Dictionnaire d'archéologie chrétienne et de liturgie*, t. XII/2, by Fernand Cabrol, and Henri Leclercq, 1936–43. Paris: Letouzey et Ané.

Moraru, Sergiu, coord. 1993. *Folclor din Ţara fagilor* [Folklore from the Beech county]. Chişinău: Hyperion.

Muşlea, Ion, and Ovidiu Bîrlea. 1970. *Tipologia folclorului. Din răspunsurile la chestionarele lui B. P. Hasdeu* [Folklore typology based on answers given to Hasdeu's questionnaires]. Bucureşti: Minerva.

Pamfile, Tudor. 1997. *Sărbătorile la români. Studiu etnografic* [Romanian traditional holydays. Ethnographical study]. Bucureşti: Saeculum I.O. (Ediţie şi introducere de I. Datcu.) [1910–1914.]

Réau, Louis. 1958. *Iconographie de l'art chrétien* III. *Iconographie des saints*. Paris: PUF.

Rosetti, Alexandru. 1975. *Limba descântecelor româneşti* [The language of the Romanian charms]. Bucureşti: Minerva.

Şăineanu, Lazăr. 1999. *Încercare asupra semasiologiei limbei române. Studii istorice despre tranziţiunea sensurilor* [Essay on the semasiology of the Romanian language. Historical studies on the transformation of meanings]. Timişoara: Editura de Vest. (Cu o alocuţiune-prefaţă de B. P. Hasdeu, ediţie îngrijită, studiu introductiv şi indice de L. Vasiluţă.) [1887.]

Ştrempel, Gabriel, Florica Moisil, and L. Stoianovici. 1967. *Catalogul manuscriselor româneşti* IV [The Catalogue of the Romanian Manuscripts]. Bucureşti: Editura Academiei.

Ştrempel, Gabriel. 1978–1992. *Catalogul manuscriselor româneşti* I–IV [The catalogue of the Romanian manuscripts]. Bucureşti: Editura Ştiinţifică şi Enciclopedică.

Taloş, Ion. 2002. *Petit dictionnaire de mythologie populaire roumaine.* (Traduit par Anneliese et Claude Lecouteux). Grenoble: ELLUG and Université Stendhal.

Timotin, Emanuela. 2009a. "Queen of the Fairies and Biblical Queen. Notes on the Romanian Heodias." In *Folk Religion and Folk Belief in Central Eastern Europe,* edited by Éva Pócs, 363–76. (*Acta Ethnographica Hungarica* 54 [2]).

—. 2009b. "L'invocation à la lune dans les charmes roumains. Tradition manuscrite et tradition orale." In *Romania Orientalis–Romania Occidentalis. Volum omagial închinat Profesorului Ion Taloş*, edited by Ion Cuceu, and Alina Branda, 651–60. Cluj: Editura Fundaţiei pentru Studii Europene, and Editura Megas.

—. 2010. *Descântecele manuscrise româneşti (secolele al XVII-lea–al XIX-lea)* [The Romanian manuscript charms (17th–19th Centuries)]. Bucureşti: Editura Academiei Române. (Ediţie critică, studii lingvistice şi filologice.)

—. 2015. *Paroles protectrices, paroles guérisseuses. La tradition manuscrite des charmes roumains* (XVIIe–XIXe siècle). Paris: Presses Universitaires de Paris Sorbonne.

Tuerk, Jacquelyn. 1999. "An early Byzantine inscribed amulet and its narratives." *Byzantine and Modern Greek Studies* 23: 25–42.

Walter, Christopher. 2003. "St. Nicetas (Nikita) the Goth." In *The Warrior Saints in Byzantine Art and Tradition*, 231–3. Aldershot: Ashgate Publishing Ltd.

DREAM HEALING: THE NOCTURNAL WORLD OF HEALING AND BEWITCHMENT

ÉVA PÓCS

In this study, I discuss religious dreams, or more precisely certain "significant" or, according to a typical category from antiquity or the Middle Ages, "God-sent" dreams, regarding which a Hungarian informant from Bukovina of Sándor Bosnyák said: "Not every dream has a significance, only the special dreams. It is not a superstition, I'm telling you, a lot of things come true" (Bosnyák 1977, 197). Within the category of significant and religious dreams, I focus on the role of healing, while to complete the theme of healing dreams, I will also discuss dreams related to bewitchments.

There are three foundations to my analysis: 1) Research among Eastern Hungarian groups in Csík (Ciuc) and Gyimes (Ghimeș) in Romania,[1] in the framework of which I examined the roles played by dreams in contemporary societies. As a wider geographical and historical context and cultural historical background, I have used the material of other studies of mine, as well as more distant examples in this present study from collections from other present-day communities, thus underlining the universal nature of the phenomenon of dream medicine. 2) The rich material on nocturnal visions and on dreams of the judicial records of Hungarian witch trials. This partially extinct world is very informative to the present research on dream healing. 3) Similarly, the parallel to our

[1] We carried out research in Csíkkarcfalva and Csíkjenőfalva (Cîrța and Ineu, Hargita county, Romania) between 1996 and 1998 with students in ethnography of the University of Pécs; in Gyimesközéplok (Lunca de Jos, Harghita county, Romania) and in Gyimesbükk (Ghimeș-Făget, Băcau county, Romania) we have been involved in ongoing research since 2002 with the participation of university and doctoral students. In this present study, besides my own collections, I have used the data of my former students and colleagues, for which I would like to express my gratitude now.

present-day ethnographical research has presented itself in the abundant ancient and medieval material on *incubation* (healing dreams solicited ritually at sacred places). The extensive volume of research relating to incubation is due to the large volume of preserved written sources. Nevertheless, as we will see, the popular forms of it, not documented in written sources, are also quite abundant and diverse; they are also less associated with the saints and divinities of the official Church, and they include the dead and various creatures of the spirit world of folk beliefs.

The research on cultural history and religious history in the past century addressing categories of dreams, and anthropological studies on present-day communities, show evidence that besides the well-known "individual" dream categories, such as the nightmare, the wishful fantasy etc., every society has dreams defined by local cultural patterns (for more on this, see for instance: Dodds 1951, 103; Stewart 1997; Burke 1997). This is confirmed by my own research in Csík (Ciuc) and Gyimes (Ghimeş) with one specification: the categories are only separated for the sake of research. One of the most important lessons of the examined dream material is the constantly intertwined nature of the individual satisfaction of "dream needs" and of the culturally determined dreams. Essentially, every dream has both features, although the ritually solicited (incubation) dreams are somewhat more culturally determined than spontaneous dreams.

The conjunction of the two categories and the effect of cultural patterns on the narratives of individual dreams would be an interesting research topic, but one which would require a more complex analysis of texts and contexts of dream narratives than the present study. (As also emphasised by Charles Stewart 1997.) Similar studies were last conducted by Lehel Peti; he analysed the effect of cultural patterns on narratives in his new study on the dreams of the Csángó (Peti 2012, 163–208). My research material, however, is too thin to be suitable for an analysis of the regularities of dream narratives; therefore, in what follows, I will not distinguish between the categories of "dream experience" and "dream narrative". Medieval and ancient data also rarely allow any conclusions, although researchers have occasionally attempted to examine them from this perspective. Dodds, for instance, by analysing the healing miracles of an incubation sanctuary in Epidaurus, was able to establish an otherwise obvious regularity that with a proportionate distance in time from the moment of awakening, the dream narrative becomes increasingly "culturally determined". He analyses in this context a narrative similar to the *Gunthram Legend,*[2] conveying the duality of the narration of someone observing the dreamer from the outside and of commenting on the dream experience directly: while the outsider observer sees the snake licking the feet of the patient, the patient dreams of a handsome boy who bandages his feet (Dodds 1951, 114).

Anthropologists of the second half of the past century have raised the question: what is the reason for certain societies considering dreams important (socially acknowledged) while others do not? (See for instance Tedlock 1987; Stewart 2004, 77–81). My article is about significant dreams in societies where they are considered important. There might be other difference-inducing factors in societies as regards "important dreams" and "unimportant dreams": since the theories of Freud and Jung, some answers are also offered by psychology, although more from the perspective of the individual than from that of society. It may, nevertheless, be stated that dreams are important in societies where sacred communication is also "important": that is, in deeply and generally religious societies. Peter Burke established that in medieval and early modern societies of Europe, and in the case of certain tribal societies, dream usually referred to religion, which is not true in the case of modern America (Burke 1997, 41–2). This is true, since in societies where the impact of religion is smaller, the role of dreams as supernatural communication is equally small—thus, dreams cannot be as "important" as they are for instance in the societies of Csík or Gyimes, where religiosity, although with great individual differences, seemed to be universally intensive during the time of my study.

The majority of the people in these communities believed in the reality of the other world possibly experienced in dreams, in the reality of the deities—Christian or not—, or the spirit creatures and the dead appearing in dreams, and in the importance of otherworldly messages manifesting in dreams. The normative role of the other world of the dream plays an important role in their everyday life (as Peter Burke also underlined in his description of these societies, where dreams are considered as a chance to gain an insight into the other world, a visual representation of the other world; that is, a sacred/supernatural way of communication: Burke 1997, 27). This might be the case in several communities of Modern Age Europe, as our data on parallels suggest. In these communities we experience the presence of the category of the "imagistic mode of religiosity" proposed by Harvey Whitehouse (Whitehouse 2004); it is about the importance of religious experience, of the emotional attitudes

[2] For the analysis of the Gunthram Legend, see Lixfeld 1972.

within religion, of compassion, of direct experience, of striving to have an "encounter", which all manifest most easily in dreams, visions and in the phenomena of *unio mystica.*[3] Certain types of dream and spontaneous visions mean the possibility of directly communicating with the creatures of religion, and in this regard, they are important additions to complement the official liturgy and communal rituals.[4]

In my study, I thus treat dreams as a kind of sacred communication.[5] For the sake of simplicity, I will universally refer to them as "dreams". From a psychological perspective, dreams and visions are far from being the same thing, but I will not distinguish between them in this study, since in many cases it is not even clear which one it is; from our point of view, the experiences of the two may be of equal value.[6] The dreams analysed below are about an alternative existence considered to be a reality (a Christian or non-Christian other world, deities, and spirit worlds), which has relations in many regards with the communities of this world's societies. I agree with Vilmos Keszeg, who wrote that "in a community which considers dreams and visions as revelations, a way of sacred communication, dreams play a practical role: they are the credible representations of the past or the future, they confirm a religious ideology, a social and moral system of values…" (Keszeg, Peti, and Pócs 2009, 32–3).

In the communities that I study, certain religious dreams are distinguished: they are considered as true and significant dreams, perhaps not universally by the entire community, but by certain "dream-sensitive" members who

---

[3] Here I have to mention the research of Lehel Peti, who discussed these aspects of the imagistic mode of religiosity in relation to the religiosity of the Csángó from Moldova, who are geographically close to our field of research; see Peti (2008). József Gagyi has also studied certain aspects of the social role of dreams and visions close to the regions of our research, in Csík (Ciuc) and Udvarhely (Odorheiu): see for instance Gagyi 1998. Both studies have provided important lessons in our research.

[4] As many have established in relation to religious dreams, see e.g. Le Goff 1992, 200. Eric Dodds studied the "irrationality" of ancient Greeks when he wrote that dreams offer a possibility to meet distant people, gods, the dead and to have personal contact with a god: Dodds 1951, 102–7.

[5] Ágnes Hesz was the first to study dreams of the dead as sacred communication in Gyimes: Hesz 2005.

[6] On the vision forms of sacred communication, and on the categorisation of dreams and visions in summary, see Pócs 1998; Keszeg, Peti, and Pócs 2009: *Előszó*; cf. the work overviewing religious visions by Benz, in which he discussed the issues of separating, or the inseparability of categories of dream vision, ecstatic vision, etc.: Benz 1969, 108–14.

experience/live their religiosity more deeply and approach religious creatures with stronger emotions. For them, such dreams have a normative function. Among these, the healing dreams occupy an important place.

I will discuss three large categories of these dreams: 1) healing saints and deities; 2) spontaneous and ritually solicited dreams of the dead who heal in dreams; 3) the dream world of witchcraft (malefactor and healer witches appearing in dreams, spirit creatures who can identify bewitchment).

Healing deities, saints

The spontaneous and ritually solicited healing dreams basically all belong to the wider category of "dream divination", if we interpret "divination" in the original sense of the word as a divine revelation referring to hidden things. In the case of dreams, including divine healing or divine revelation, the essential point is the communication with those appearing in the dream: to acquire information from saints.[7] In the healing dreams, it is the protective/defensive function of religion that is dominant, while in divination dreams, it is its normative role, but the content, form and function of the two types of dreams can often be identical or interwoven.

Spontaneous forms

My research material indicates that the "spontaneous" appearance of healing saints and deities in dreams appears to be a common phenomenon. In these dreams, religion primarily has a protective function, and plays an important role in the religiosity of certain people. We could mention numerous narratives from Csík (Ciuc) and Gyimes (Ghimeș) about dream encounters with the consoling, aiding Virgin Mary, Christ or saints: Jesus consoles the patient in his dream, predicts the outcome of their illness, heals them in his dream, or at least provides some help or guidance to patients with regard to their recovery.[8] The saintly figures mostly "appear"

[7] Relating to this, see the categories of divination by Zuesse 1987. Ritually prepared dream divination is known everywhere in Europe (on this see, for instance, the overview by Ronald Grambo 1973) in order to have a problem solved by the deity appearing in the dream through their answering a question which has been asked (Dodds 1971, 217).

[8] Besides my own collections I have found dream narratives in the material collected by students in Csík (Ciuc), and, although not very dominantly, a few narratives appear in the collections of Anikó Salamon 1987, 174–8; and Zoltán Magyar 2003, 708–9; and in the study on Gyimesbükk (Ghimeş-Făget, Băcau county, Romania) by Mária Antal 2004.

to those seeking help in cases of unexpected disasters, conflict situations, illnesses, or fear of death experienced during nocturnal solitude:

> You know, what I am telling you and I'm not lying, I was so ill from typhoid fever […]. I was very ill, at my father's place. And then I got worse and I was unconscious, and once, when I regained my consciousness, there was a little candle, it was burning on the table, and then I saw Mary, she was not facing me, I saw her from behind, but she was so beautiful, and from the moment I saw her I got better day by day, and then I healed… (70-year-old woman, own collection, Gyimesközéplok [Lunca de Jos], Harghita county, Romania, 2005).

Narratives in which saints appear solely in the role of comforter are frequent. People narrate their encounter with the saints with deep enthusiasm and emotional charge:

> Well, I was so ill, I lay down, but I couldn't sleep, because I was suffering so badly. And my husband was away from home all day, only in the night, because he had things to do as well. And one night I saw Jesus Christ. As I was sitting in my bed, I tipped forward, and I saw him in my dream as the Lord Jesus came in through the window and stepped next to my bed. He was just like in the pictures. Don't cry, he said to me, woman, just ask me, because I will not leave you! When I woke up in the morning, he stepped away from my bed and left through the window. And from that morning on I started to feel better, I felt that I was relieved. And from that moment on I got better, I could get up and I could work… (Gyimesközéplok [Lunca de Jos], Harghita County, Romania, Magyar 2003, 708–9).

It is the dream replicas of earthly remedies that appear in the narratives with an ideal "good physician" at the centre who worries rather about the individual and not the illness. He heals, gives medicine, or recommends a treatment. The psychological effects of the kind behaviour of the saint, his comforting words, the laying on of hands, and caressing are just as important as rational methods. The curative laying on of hands is especially significant; touch as a "physical" healing method is in some way the reification of an emotionally charged attitude. The consequences of the touch of heavenly saints are often spectacularly real. Based on data from Tordatúr (Tureni, Cluj County, Romania) the healer saint in the dream appears as a man wearing a grey hat who puts his hand on the head of the patient suffering from headache and sends him to church to fetch healing water from behind the altar, saying, "…wash your head with water from that fountain, and your head will never ache again." The end of the narrative is as follows: "For a long time afterwards I felt the touch of his hand on the top of my head…" (Csőgör 1998, 212).

It is frequent that a patient receives advice on what ritual to perform to honour a particular saint or place of worship in order to be healed. In other cases, the dreams about saints relate to expiatory rituals performed on instructions received in dreams, for instance relating to fasting. According to texts from the Mezőség (Cluj County, Romania) published by Vilmos Keszeg, the relatives of a possessed patient prayed and fasted following advice received during a dream:

> And they started to fast, he said, the girl was in the hospital. They started to fast, but two other daughters were married. Thus, three families were fasting. They fasted and prayed for a long time, and the little girl was lying ill in the hospital, and she said she woke up in the night to someone grabbing and shaking her, "wake up" someone said, "and come down because you are healed". The girl looked back and saw that he was dressed in white and had yellow hair down to his shoulders, she said… (Keszeg 1999, 317).

Present-day data from more distant areas suggest a similar picture; we know of healing dreams with similar motifs from Greek, Lithuanian, Latvian and Bulgarian narratives: in a dream, the saint gives advice on healing methods and medication; the saint appears, consoling and caressing the patient; he/she gives instructions on rituals or other actions, as an expiatory offering for the sake of healing (for instance, placing a "weeping icon" on the patient, cleaning a statue of Jesus, lighting a candle in the chapel, and so forth) (Višinskait 2007–2008, 233). Dreams involving such instructions constitute a transition towards ritual forms: here the ritual is induced by the dream, while in the other case, it is the ritual that induces the dream: in any case, we can observe the close interdependence of two realities, earthly society and norm-setting supernatural beings.

In dream narratives, the archaic features of the relations with the alternative, nocturnal world appear. The otherworldly existence appearing in the universe of visions and dreams resembles "normal" life, the events of the two worlds are interpreted as identical, and the healing in the dream is just as valid in the daytime. There is a transition between the two; they are both interlaced by the continuity of the events, the network of cause and effect relations. [9] Traces of dream encounters persist in earthly

[9] Ágnes Hesz also wrote about this aspect of dreams in the community she studied in Gyimesközéplok: "In societies where some sort of reality value is attributed to dreams (as it is in Gyimes) the reality of dreaming and of being awake coexist,

existence as well; if someone is healed in a dream that person will stay healed in the daytime; a medicine received in a dream, for instance, will remain in the patient's possession in real life.

Ritual forms

The most general form of ritual can be defined as: going to a sacred place where a healing force somehow produces its effects, where a saint can appear or where he or she "lives". The efficiency of the sacred site is increased if it is visited at a sacred time, thus the "when" and "where" of saints' manifestations are of prime importance.

In practice the majority of researchers and public alike use the term "incubation" (*incubatio* in Latin, and *Tempelschlaf* in German) in the sense of "being healed while sleeping in the church by a deity appearing in a dream" (the word "incubation" literally means "sleeping inside"); more accurate definitions are, however, that of Burke who puts them in the wider category of divination dreams (receiving a predictive dream in which the dreamer is advised on what to do) (Burke 1997, 29); or that of Gollnick who, besides healing, underlines other objectives: "going to a sacred place in order to get an answer in a dream to a problem or to obtain healing for an illness" (Gollnick 1999, 32).

Incubation is typically a phenomenon of European culture, which having first been associated with a certain place, age and culture by researchers, was named accordingly, since entering the public knowledge as a phenomenon of classical antiquity related to Greek and Roman sanctuaries, especially those of Asclepius. Incubation was universal in antiquity, including the East (Mesopotamia, the Hittites, the Jews, Canaan and Egypt; Porter 1981, 198–202; Gurney 1981, 158–9; McAlpine 1987, 158–60).[10]

---

they overlap and interact with one another" (Hesz 2005, 355). The intertwining and merging of the waking and dream existences have been described with different emphases in several societies; see for instance O'Flaherty 1984; Tedlock 1987; Burke 1997.

[10] Ancient Greeks and Romans were "operating" hundreds of dream temples from the earliest of times until Constantine the Great. Before Christianity, in all ages, these temples were mostly associated with Asclepius, the Panhellenic god of medicine. His most important sanctuary was in Epidauros (both classical and late antique); another sanctuary was the great Asclepeion in Pergamon (the "rival" of the one in Epidauros). Excavations have confirmed the authenticity of Pausanias' account from the second century AD, who described the *miraculum*-protocols of six stelae, and reported on architectural solutions of the Asclepion and the Abaton:

Research shows that in certain cases there is a direct continuity of incubation practices at sanctuaries of antiquity and the Middle Ages. Castor and Polydeuces, for instance, as gods who healed during incubation, gave up their temple in Rome to Saints Cosmas and Damian, and in another place to Cyrus and John, who also functioned as saints who healed in dreams. I could cite numerous other examples: other temples of Cosmas and Damian also used for incubation; the sanctuaries of Saint Thecla and of Saint Martin in Anatolia; the sanctuary of the Virgin Mary (Panaghia in Greek) in Southern Italy, Sicily and in the Balkans; Saint Therapon replacing Isis in Northern Africa, and so forth (overview by Hamilton 1906; Meier 1985; Sigal 1985, 117–47; Csepregi 2003; Csepregi-Vardabasso 2008). Ildikó Csepregi-Vardabasso has published important data regarding Cosmas and Damian, Saint Thecla, Saint Theodor and other incubation saints; her analyses demonstrate several "shifts" from pagan to Christian saints from the perspective of the importance of certain sacred places, and of the continuity of a cult. She describes and confirms with data the paradigm of the relation between the sacred person and the sacred place in which "an originally sacred place invests the proprietor with miraculous powers", when the saint healing in dreams is practically "created" for that sacred place (Csepergi-Vardabasso 2008, 344–6).

As regards the matter of the continuity between Paganism and Christianity, various researchers have had different views. Adolf Franz believed, for instance, that the pagan practice disappeared in most places without passing on its place to Christian saints in the second and third century; moreover, the Christian custom of sleeping in sacred places did not exclusively have as its objective the healing dreams, and healing saints appeared in dreams in other locations as well, not only in sacred places (Franz 1909, II. 438–41, chapter *Heiligenkult und Krankenheilung*). These "anti-continuity" arguments of Franz basically support the idea to which I would like to draw attention in this study: there is no clear distinction between ritual and spontaneous forms, between divine creatures appearing in sacred and/or (any) other locations; there are many variable, transitional cases, and healing dreams do not fall into strict categories.

---

the restricted area designated exclusively for those who sleep inside the temple in order to heal (Herzog 1931; Kee 1983, 78–87; Meier 1985, 73–4; Cox Miller 1994, 106–112). The miracle description from Epidauros tells us about a series of various illnesses (obstetric problems, infertility, alien objects inside the body, sick internal organs, diseases of the womb, etc.) and votive objects offered in gratitude, including the toad (associated with the diseases of the womb). (Herzog 1931, 71–84).

The views of clerics and theologians on dreams constitute an important source on medieval incubation. Without having to enter into detailed discussion, I must mention that the categories of significant dreams and god-sent dreams (according to Augustine: "dreams inspired by God") in which God, a saint or an ancestor appears, have been continuously present in Europe since antiquity in the works of philosophers, physicians, writers and poets, and with the expansion of Christianity, of ecclesiastical authors (Dodds 1951, 107–9; Bitel 1991, 52). The early Middle Ages were characterised by a general sense of mistrust. Apart from Gregory the Great and some other exceptions, most authors grouped dreams under the scope of Evil, making a distinction between the "true" dreams and "false" dreams. Only a limited area remained for true dreams, sent by God with angels and saints: dream divination was the only divination method in the Middle Ages not strictly rejected by Christianity.[11] Naturally, the Church was not able to extend its supervision to every dream; as researchers studying dreams appearing in Germanic and Celtic literature might experience, Europe, from this perspective, between the eighth and twelfth centuries was not entirely Christian after all. As some examples from early Christianity show, the pagan and Christian, official, ecclesiastic and "popular" forms (for instance those relating to the healing dead) coexisted and mingled (on mixed, transitional and pagan-Christian forms see Dodds 1951, 110).

The medieval (then early modern) data on incubation follow the change in the nature of the sacred places, places of worship, following the process of evolution in time: "sleeping inside" [a church] and healing during a dream was equally possible at the graves of martyrs, and next to images at places of worship (for an overview of the processes and phases of development of Christian places of worship, see Brown 1993). In the case of dream healings, it was the miraculous power—and its realness within the dream—of the relics, images, statues, and of the sacred place itself that made the impact, similar to the "daytime" healing miracles among pilgrims.

Due to the fact that most of the data has not yet been processed, we cannot have a clear picture of the medieval dimensions of dream healing, although we can rightly assume that it was quite common. Pierre-André Sigal analyses in his overview of French medieval material 2050 healing miracles of 76 saints (and sacred places), of which 259 were cases of dream healing (see Sigal 1985. This statistic was also cited by Gábor

[11] On ancient and medieval dream theories and categories, see among others: Le Goff 1992, 193–231; Dodds 1951, 118; Bitel 1991, 46; Kruger 1992, 17; Cox Miller 1994, part I; Berchman 1998, 133.

Klaniczay 2008, 54–5, in his overview of published studies on cases of dream healing in other countries, in which he gives examples for healing narratives). Dreams could have been solicited through ascetic spiritual preparations (vigil, prayer, fasting), but spontaneously sleeping at the sanctuary also played a significant role; moreover, we even have data confirming healing taking place without actually "sleeping inside", but merely experienced near the sanctuary. The records of these miracles refer to the dreams of every social stratum; we also have numerous narratives of the dreams of peasants.

Most of the recorded medieval and early modern healing narratives are rather similar to the present-day narratives; moreover, both the medieval and the early modern ritual dreams are identical with healing dreams not ritually solicited: in such a dream the saint heals (with the laying on of hands, with an operation or by giving medicine), or gives instructions or recipes. As regards Hungarian historical data, our miracle records have not been subject to such a comprehensive analysis. Gábor Klaniczay quotes the data on dream healings occurring at the grave of Saint Elisabeth from her canonisation trial; according to his analysis, six of the hundred and 29 miracles at the grave were dream healings (Klaniczay 2008, 54). In the previously mentioned study of Ildikó Csepregi-Vardabasso, we can find a suggestive example regarding the legend of Saint Margaret (Csepregi-Vardabasso 2008, 342). Sándor Bálint's research reveals that the only Hungarian place of pilgrimage of Cosmas and Damian was in Stanfalva (Stanești) in Moldova, of which we are informed in the 1647 record noted by Marcus Bandinus: a pilgrim called János Kazan testified that he had been healed of a serious illness. When he was warned in his dream, he had himself taken to and offered himself to Saints Cosmas and Damian (Tomisa 2003, 221). On the basis of recently analysed baroque miracle records, Gábor Tüskés mentions the dreams encouraging pilgrimage to a place of worship as frequent phenomena. He reveals that in these dreams there are instructions on how to carry out a healing act (usually to place a sacred devotional image on the sick body part), or to drink water from a holy well. All this does not clearly show the number of incubation dreams and their contexts in which healing saints appear (Tüskés 1993, 122–3). With systematic research, one could probably find more cases than the amount of data made public.

Our rather scarce present-day data are mostly Orthodox-related, but from the medieval material, we might perhaps draw the conclusion that incubation continued to be an extensive phenomenon in early modern times, and presumably remains so even today. Our present-day data on incubation are primarily related to miracle-working images, or the dream apparition of Mary from images at a place of worship where patients make pilgrimages on the feast day of the saint. The data from my own collection refer to incubation cases from Csíksomlyó (Şumuleu, Harghita County, Romania) Mátraverebély (Heves County, Hungary) and Máriagyűd (Baranya County, Hungary). From these cases and also from other places we know of the "soliciting" dreams that beckon people to the place of worship. These dreams were fairly common in medieval Christianity: the patients dreamed about the monastery or the church where they had to go; the saint appearing in the dream did not heal but sent the patient to a sacred place, the patient's state often improving along the way, before arriving at the holy place (see examples of Wittmer-Butsch 1990, 203–9). For instance, the twelfth-century Canterbury incubation cases described among the miracles of Thomas Beckett also suggest that the majority of rural patients arrived at the place of worship by being "solicited". Still, in their home village they discussed their dreams, which the priest then helped them to interpret with the help of his dream-book (Finucane 1977, chapter 5). Strohmaier's study on the miracle cases at the place of worship in Lower Austria, St. Maria at Waldegg, confirm that the cases of dreams soliciting patients were more common in the seventeenth and eighteenth century than regular incubation dreams: the patients were advised by an angel or by the Virgin Mary to go to a certain place of worship (Strohmaier 1997, 262–3). It was equally possible that the saint did not even appear in these ritual dreams: the otherworldly and holy nature of the dreams is in focus, accentuated by the aura of the sacred place (Wittmer-Butsch 1990, 207).

Regarding modern age sources of soliciting dreams, I can establish, despite the meagreness of my database, that my thin data show great similarities with what we know from earlier centuries. I cite one Hungarian example: in the diary of István Orosz, a holy man from Jászberény, we find that once the Virgin Mary, appearing in the dream of a relative of the patient, invited a diabolically possessed patient to Mátraverebély, asking them to come to see the miracle-working icon at Pentecost, where, she promised, the patient would be healed (Bálint 1942, 95).

In Orthodox regions, besides the Virgin Mary other dream-healers also play an important role: these include Saint George, Saint Theodore and Saints Cosmas and Damian. They heal, or recommend medicine, as in the "spontaneous" cases mentioned above, and they often practise dream divination: they predict the outcome (life or death) of the illness, and sometimes they identify the source of bewitchment (see Lawson 1910, 302; Blum and Blum 1965, 213; 1970, 59). In Bulgarian monasteries it seems that incubation was an especially popular practice; in certain places they even have a separate incubation space. According to Albena Georgieva, in one of the Saint George monasteries they even sacrificed a lamb in honour of the saint as a ritual preparation for the incubation.[12]

The dead and the fairies—spontaneous and ritual forms

In Europe in the past, and in many present-day rural communities, dream divination as a form of communication with the dead is closely related to the important protective, defensive, advisory roles played by the ancestors and those family members who have died within the society of the living. These roles concerning the otherworldly life of the dead were not entirely eradicated by Christian doctrines; on the contrary, to some extent the teachings supported these roles. (On certain fundamental questions of communication with the dead in relation to Europe, see Lecouteux 1987; Schmitt 1998; in relation to early modern Hungarians, see Pócs 1997; on certain specific references to Gyimes regarding communication with the dead, see Hesz 2005). There are numerous pagan and/or Christian variations from medieval Europe describing incubation as a means of communication with the dead (for instance sleeping on the grave or in the cemetery, during which one could acquire information, knowledge, initiation, healing and poetic inspiration from the dead either appearing or being solicited ritually—"resurrected"—in the dream). The rituals relating to divination by the dead were associated with the dates of the midwinter visitation period of the dead, the Christian Christmas and New Year celebrations. We have no room to present the rich Celtic (Irish, Welsh) and Germanic material referring to other methods of "incubation with the dead".[13] Let us mention a few concrete data to illustrate the similarities between the incubation practices of times and places distant from one another. According to thirteenth-century data from Yorkshire, someone went to a hill, lay down and said: "I'm thirsty", upon which an elegantly dressed person appearing on the spot handed him a cup. It contained an unknown delicious nectar and after drinking it all his thirst and weakness disappeared (from the work of Gervasius of Tilbury entitled *Otia Imperialia*: Menefee 1985, 5–6). Or in another healing narrative, the dead

---

[12] The kind, oral communication of Albena Georgieva; see her article—also dealing with incubation healing in Bulgaria—in this volume.

[13] I only mention a few works from the abundant literature dealing with the topic: Meisner 1917, 100–3; Kelchner 1935, 33–66; Chadwick 1968, 39–45; Davidson 1981, 118–36.

taught a mute person to speak with a piece of gold, telling him where it was hidden (Davidson 1981, 138).

Lay people and professionals (seers, cunning folk) were all able to see dreams in such a manner. Nordic literature mentions a method called *útiseta* ("sitting out"), which was part of more complex rituals, even called shamanistic by certain researchers. One example: Seidl described how people in Iceland and the Faroe Islands sat on graves at Christmas night and participated in the funerary mass in their dreams, during which they could acquire all sorts of information, including healing-related instructions (Seidl 1968, 419). Beyond the incubation forms, communication during the earthly visit of the dead is the most important common characteristic of the otherwise rather diverse European techniques for connecting with the dead. (On the communication during the periods of the earthly visit/stay of the dead see, for instance, Schmitt 1998, 173–8; Pócs 1999, 29–31).

Communication with the dead continued in several places even in early modern Europe and is still alive in the form of archaic views that are not so much in harmony with Christian doctrines and of rituals seeking contact with the dead ("seeing the dead", conjuring the dead). As regards present-day Hungarians, communication includes divination, asking for advice, and healing; the dead can also play normative roles similar to that of the saints, and can have protective functions as well. The dream apparition of the healing dead is less frequent than that of the beings helping their families. These dreams attribute a role to dead ancestors similar to that of the healing saints. For instance, we can learn about a dead person in the role of a medical advisor in a narrative from Gyimesbükk (Ghimeş-Făget, Băcau county, Romania).

> A man was very ill at his neighbour's. They took him everywhere, but they did not find the cause of his illness. One night he saw a deceased friend of his in his dream, who told him to stop going to the doctor and to seek recovery in home medicine, in herbal teas. He told him in his dream what kind of herbs he should collect and to prepare a bath from it… (Antal 2004, 166).

Regarding the ritually induced dream healing, the dreams and visions of the dead usually occur at the "sacred place" of the dead: graves and cemeteries. (For the cemetery as a sacred place close to the church in the Middle Ages, see Schmitt 1998, 182–4). The role of the aura of this sacred place, however, is similar to the role they play in Christian incubation. Peter Burke also noted this: he discussed that sleeping in a cemetery in early modern times (or sleeping with a Bible under the pillow) is equivalent to (Christian) incubation; the reason for this, according to him, is that cemeteries and churches were close, or next to one another (Burke 1997, 30). Several folklore collections indicate that in East-Central European folklore, at the celebrations related to the dead one can meet the dead appearing among the living in a spontaneously or ritually induced trance or dream (see for instance Róheim 1920; Seidl 1968, 419; Pócs 2002. All this is partially related to the methods of necromancy (conjuring up the dead) practised by those performing elite magic in the Middle Ages, and by the "clerical underground" (term by Kieckhefer), which I will not discuss in detail; see briefly in Kieckhefer 1994, 372–4). There were only slight differences between the Eastern and Western territories of Christianity, at most in terms of the timetable, in accordance with the different systems of the memorial days of the dead (on the two systems, see Ranke 1951).

Our most detailed and most varied descriptions of incubation healing related to the dead are from Finland. The *wise man* (*tietäjä*) described in the study of Matt Salo works in the period associated with the dead: in the night, at midnight, at Easter, on Saint John's day in the cemetery or at Christmas in the church, since it is then that the dead also make an appearance there. As a rule, what we have here is the incubation of the healer, or the patient, or—in most cases—both, as if it was an incubation dream guided by a helper. One variant: the patient relates his or her grievances to the healer, who then sleeps on it and in the morning establishes a diagnosis and a cure. In other cases, the healer consults the dead in the cemetery; he either awakens them with the known European techniques of necromancy in the circle he draws around himself, or simply sleeps there and dreams with them, and tells the patient in the morning what the matter is, and so forth (see Salo 1974).

We also have to mention here the Balkan rituals performed to conjure fairies and to heal the fairy illnesses caused by ambivalent fairies, which are very similar to the previously mentioned Finnish methods of communicating with the dead. These illnesses (locomotory disorders, epilepsy, muteness, blindness, etc.) usually afflict those who violate the taboos of fairies. Given that the character of the Balkan fairy world is very much related to the dead, the relationship between the Bulgarian, Serbian or Greek "fairy sorcerers" and the fairies can be considered as local variants of the communication with the dead. Healing takes place at "fairy locations" (where the illness has come upon the person due to the violation of a taboo) at "fairy times" occurring at specific periods (one week, month, year, etc. after the start of the illness). The patient and the healer settle down at the ritually created sacred place (for example, a circle drawn around them), the healer sleeps there with the patient and after having performed a sacrifice to the fairies he conjures them up, and they heal the patient in an incubation dream. (On the Balkan fairy world and on this method of communication, see Pócs 1989; 2009; 2017.)

It would be going too far and would require a more extensive study to discuss the rituals associated with the memorial celebrations of the dead in the Eastern Balkans, because dream healing is only an incidental part of these complex and multifunctional rituals, be it in the form of collective, organised rituals (such as the Bulgarian, Serbian and Romanian *rusalia* rituals) or communication between professional seers and the dead at celebrations associated with the latter (or in certain cases with fairies) (see for instance: Arnaudov 1920). Nonetheless, let us mention a typically Romanian example: in a village called Volenia, a sorceress falls into a trance on the occasions of the great feasts, she predicts the destiny of the people coming to her, she speaks with the dead, and based on these conversations, she orders medicine for the sick person (Puchner 1987, 267). We know of another incubation ritual in relation to the Bulgarian *rusalka* (which, according to Marinov, was once practised in several parts of Bulgaria). In this case, too, we are dealing with the locations and the traditional times of the fairies (which coincide with the times of the dead). During the week of Pentecost, the *rusalka senica* ("the week of the *rusalka*"; one of the habitual periods when the *rusalki* appear among the people), the afflicted go to sleep in meadows where the dittany *(rossen—Dictamnus Fraxinella Pers., D. Albus L.)* blossoms in quantities at this season (this flower has some kind of a mythical relationship with the *rusalki*). Before going to sleep they place offerings and gifts (milk, honey, sweet bread) for the *rusalki* on a tablecloth spread on the grass. The healthy companions of the patients, who are awake and observe the events from the sidelines, see that around midnight, when the patients are asleep, a whirlwind approaches accompanied by a buzzing, laughing, whispering noise, and this whirlwind carries sand, leaves, and dry twigs, etc., onto the tablecloth. All this is considered by the outside observers of the patients' dream as the manifestation of the *rusalki*. The objects "left by the *rusalki*" are taken home the following day and used for incense by the patients. Some repeat the ritual until they are healed (see Marinov 1914, 470–5; Kazarow 1933). Mihail Arnaudov describes several other similar cases in his monumental study on *rusalia* (Arnaudov 1920, 208–15).

This is a quite special form of breaching the borders between the dream world and the real world, which takes place between the realistic vision of the outsider observer and the dream vision of the patient. Regarding the objects taken from the scene, the locations marked by the visit of fairies have a similar radiative effect as the effect experienced at Christian places of worship.

These ritual systems founded upon the cyclical nature of the world of the dead are completed by certain symbolic techniques; in early modern times this was the field to which most of the European traditions of communicating with the dead were linked. These do not necessarily imply real relations experienced during a dream (or trance), but they do imitate the establishment of relationships through symbolic rituals. Such rituals artificially create the other world by drawing a circle, or a crossroads, or by walking around the house or the grave, peeking into the other world through a mirror or a crystal ball, or by looking through the water or sitting on a *Luca* chair (a chair fabricated on December 13, Saint Lucy's Day), and so forth. They also include numerous ancient techniques, used even in antiquity and earlier, and applied by early modern, learned *ritual magic*, which create an interesting amalgam with popular techniques. We encounter such rituals all across Europe. They are varied and tenacious, and until the twentieth century they were very popular at least as legends. (A rich source material on the subject can be found in Róheim 1920; Meyer to Bernd 1952, chapter 15: *Exkurs, Der Årgang*; Mykytiuk 1979, 15–16 and 92–93; Menefee 1985). We do not talk about them in detail because they are rarely related to healing and dream healing (they are mostly about divination connected to death and love, marriage, occasionally the outcome of illnesses, or information gathering from the other world: "seeing the dead", seeing treasures, etc.).

Dreams related to witchcraft

Hungarian witch trials provide rich material on the nocturnal world of witchcraft, which has preserved few traces in today's dream experiences and narratives. It is consequently obvious that the demon and spirit world of the witch and her enemies, which were manifested in dreams and visions, played a more important role in early modern times than today (see Pócs 1999, chapters 3–6; Klaniczay 2008). In this demonic nocturnal world, every actor of the given community's witchcraft affairs could have appeared in the alternative existence portrayed by the dreams: the malefactor witch, the "counter witch" or healer, and the individual who identified the bewitchment and the person who perpetrated the bewitchment (another witch or a third party). (On the social institution of witchcraft beliefs, their social roles and the distribution of these roles in the community, see Klaniczay 1990b; Pócs 1995). Thus, witchcraft beliefs, as the system coordinating how to cope with the disasters striking rural communities have, or more correctly had, a nocturnal/supernatural dimension regarding both bewitchment and healing. The foundation of this dimension is the supernatural aspect of the witch and her ability to appear as a nocturnal demon: one can communicate with a witch in her demon form even during a dream, whether she appears as the bewitcher or the healer. Moreover, this ability of European witches is connected to their *mora* nature originating from their relations with *mora* creatures.

The demon called the *mora* in several Slavic languages[14] is a specific triple creature: besides being the demon that attacks humans, it can simultaneously be a man and his alter ego (its "free soul"), which can appear as their own "guardian spirit" or "helper spirit". The earthly other world of the *mora* creatures is the nocturnal aspect of human settlements, an alternative nocturnal existence when European witch figures possessing *mora* characteristics turned into nocturnal demons, or as the Hungarians called them: "night walkers" (*éjjeljárók*), or "night women" (*éjasszonyok*). (On the *mora* relations of the witch and on the European "nocturnal witch", see overview by Pócs 1999, chapter 3). The *mora* creatures and the witches through their second self, their nocturnal alter ego, are at home in the "other" world as well (which, of course, is far from being identical to the Christian other world, rather being an earthly alternative existence). This alternative world can be experienced not only by themselves, but also by common mortals in their visions and dreams, filled precisely with these demonic creatures, who both appear as attackers and as guardians and helpers of people.

In recent ethnographical collections all this can only be found in fragmented beliefs; nonetheless, the early modern witch trial records reflect a lively nocturnal world, in which frequently repeating motifs are the dream apparition of the maleficent witch and of her adversaries fending off and eliminating the consequences of bewitchment.

Bewitchers and healers

A great variety of the attacks by witches as nocturnal demons are known from the protocols of our witch trials: this is no coincidence, as what drove persecutions were the bewitchment accusations against the witches based on the *maleficium* cases narrated by the witnesses. We could mention hundreds of cases of demonic attacks during dreams narrated at the trials; nonetheless, let us settle for one single example to get the taste of it (and to

[14] Germanic *mahr, mara;* English night*mare,* French cauche*mar*; their approximative Hungarian equivalent is *lidérc*.

introduce our central topic, the healing cases),[15] from the records of a witch trial in Hódmezővásárhely from 1750. The witch as a nocturnal demon does not always appear as herself, but often "takes the image" of someone else. This is illustrated by the following *maleficium*-narrative:

> She heard that Maria Linka was a suspicious person but she had nothing on her; but the witness was tortured by the image of her [Maria's] husband during the night; the witness gave two cups of wine to the husband of Maria Linka, he asked for a third one, and when she refused, he left seeming half-hearted, and that night she was tortured by someone in his image (Schram 1970, I. 285, trial of Mrs Mihály Horváthné Mária Linka, Hódmezővásárhely, 1750).

With regard to modern ethnographic data, I have encountered this demonic dream world during my fieldwork only a few times. From my data collected in Gyimesközéplok (Lunca de Jos, Harghita county, Romania) concerning the witch who attacks in dreams, let me mention the narrative of a man in his fifties, who was reported by a militiaman from the village and subsequently appeared in his dream as a "witch", beating and torturing him and exhorting him not to tell of him to anyone. Sándor Bosnyák writes about a case narrated by his informant from Hadikfalva (Dornești, Bukovina), in which a witch attempted to haunt the narrator during his dream, but remembering that he was able to grab her with his left hand, he was thus able to neutralise the witch (Bosnyák 1977, 219).

In the *maleficium* narratives of the trials the witch also appears as a dream healer. These cases are similar to the dream apparition of saints: they give medicine and/or advice on the use of medicine, or even heal the patient. Here is an example from a 1715 trial from Kassa (Košice):

> …the evil ones visited him in his dream and asked him: good man, where does it hurt and with what do you bandage your foot? […] In the shape of shadows, the evil ones went to him the second night as well, and advised him in his dream to wash his foot in sweet milk and it would heal (Bessenyei 1997, 39).

Or:

> …one night the witness saw a vision in which Mrs András Oláh went to her bed and told her: "show me your head so that I can let your blood, and you'll be healed". And she did cut the vein by her blind eye, and when she woke she touched the place of the incision but she couldn't feel anything

[15] On the attacks of the demonic witch we find abundant data material in the publications of trial protocols mentioned below.

> and it didn't leave a mark (Schram 1970, I. 285, trial of Mrs Mihály Horváth née Mária Linka, Hódmezővásárhely, 1750).

A healer in a 1717 trial from Dunaföldvár sent the patient to a sacred well in her dream (a "soliciting" incubation dream):

> …that night she saw Mrs János Pap in her dream, she put the pig-pail on her head saying: "take this pail to the sacred well in Gyapád, soak your head in it and you will heal" (Schram 1970, II. 468–9, trial of Mrs István Péntek).

The witnesses emphasise the kindness and leniency of the healer appearing in the dream. Meanwhile, another frequent phenomenon involves a less positive, rather ambivalent witch figure who, though healing in line with her role, accompanies this with a harsh attitude:

> …that night Mrs Benedek Réz from Gáva, in her own image, went to the witness's husband and said: "Get up you dog", the husband of the witness sat up at these words, and she brought him icy water in a tub, saying: "drink this, you dog, and you will heal", so he drank it, and after that he was healed from all his illnesses (Schram 1970, II. 315, trial of Mrs Benedek Réz née Anna Pásztor, Gáva, Szabolcs county, 1727).

Another accused dragged her patient violently by force to the stream:

> In the night, Mrs Pintér came accompanied by another, she called her to go to the stream to wash herself and to heal. As she didn't want to go, they pulled and dragged her towards the door… (Schram 1982, 206–7, trial of Mrs Péter Pintér née Anna Sebők, Horpács, Nógrád county, 1692).

How do these witch healers appear in the dreams of the sick persons, which usually feature saints in similar roles? In witchcraft affairs the bewitchers and healers are more or less identical: the bewitchment can only be repaired by the witch herself. In the case of the above-mentioned Mrs Benedek Réz this was explicitly stated: she was the one who had bewitched him, and even the real-life conflict resulting in the bewitchment is mentioned: "It was obviously Mrs Benedek Réz who had bewitched him, only because he couldn't help her with the threshing…" (Schram 1970, II. 315). The role of the witch within the community is ambivalent. It depends on the actual situation whether a healer with supernatural powers is playing the role of the bewitcher or the healer in the given witchcraft case. Numerous real healers were put on trial as witches whose appearance as nocturnal demons was only in a dream, or in the imagination; meanwhile, they played a very important role as actual healers in the rural social network of witchcraft. The foundation for the beliefs in which the witch appears as a dream healer (similar to their role as a malefactor demon) lies in their *mora* nature: their human/demon metamorphosis and their familiarity with the other world (see Pócs 1999, chapter 7, and Pócs 2017).

Elements of reality and dream are intertwined in the dreams related to witchcraft, mutually presupposing one another. Parallel to the daytime accusations, cases of bewitchment and their elimination can be seen as a closely related series of nocturnal events, in which any actors can appear in their dream spirit form (even the dreamer "taken" by the demons to the other existence). Dream healings are otherworldly reflections of real-life witchcraft affairs, or in other cases complements and continuations of them. In the *maleficium* narratives the earthly-otherworldly and daytime-night-time scenes are optionally alternating; a change of level between the two worlds is frequent even within one case. In a trial record from Szentes, a healer witch appearing in a dream tried to repair her own case of bewitchment:

> …that night Kata Kántor came into the room through the little hole in my window and stood by my head, and she asked: "what is this fat and grease for?" I replied: "they massage me with it so that I heal". Kata Kántor said: "It is useless for you." In the morning she went to her in *propria* ***persona*** and asked similar questions, but her reply was: you will never get better with that, but you need a bath, I will prepare it for you and you will heal." She prepared me a bath two times for five coppers and then I got better… (Schram 1970, I. 238–9, trial of Mrs Mihály Tóth née Katalin Kántor, Szentes, 1732).

It is marked in this text that the night-time dream healing and its daytime real-life sequence are intertwined and further complicated; the relieving solution eventually comes in the daytime reality. In 1736, a dreamer from Abaúj-Torna county woke her husband to tell him that in her dream the accused witch had advised her to prepare a bath from wheat and oat, which she left on the porch. They searched for it in vain, it was no longer there, but her husband brought new bath water instead, which they prepared accordingly:

> …as they cooked the wheat and the oats and bandaged the witness's foot with it, it was as if they had cut the pain in her foot… (Schram 1970, I. 17–8, trial of Mrs István Beke, Jablonca, Abaúj-Torna county, 1736).

This witch first appeared in the dream of another bewitched person and proposed that she bandaged herself: "Bandage your chest with burdock leaves and you will heal…", after which, she came to see the patient in the morning in her real guise and asked about her state, telling her that it was she who had visited her in her dream and advising her to prepare a burdock bandage; she also reproached her for not having followed her advice, and so forth (Schram 1970, I. 18, ibid).

Objects and signs from "the other side", the other transitional elements between the two worlds characteristic of healing dreams also appear here. From the data mentioned above, for instance, we find that the witch also gave a milk bucket along with the dream recipe, for which they had looked in the morning, though in vain.

Spirit battles

We have abundant data from seventeenth- and eighteenth-century witch trials concerning the nocturnal battles of people attacked by demons or their healers with hostile demons. The spirit battles against demons bringing bewitchment and illness to humans usually appear in the dreams and visions of the persons eliminating and healing the bewitchment, who pick up the fight by virtue of their supernatural skills; in rare cases, it is narrated by a third person, a witness from the dream. In the dream scenes of witch trials, the battles between the bewitcher and the healer, and those between the helper spirits are related to the *mora* nature of the witch, to her nocturnal metamorphosis and to the characteristic *mora* helper spirits. The latter might as well appear as the guardians of their own (human) selves as the helper of others (their own relatives). The adversaries are mostly the demonic alter egos of the witch. (For more on the spirit battles, see Pócs 2017.) The examples are narratives of dreams and visions experienced by the narrators themselves. The following is from the 1693 trial of Mrs Ignác Villás:

> …the devils who had made the binding, come upon me during the night […] during the second night they came upon me twice, but I fought them once again, so that I had to lie in bed because of it…

> …oh during the night they wanted to kill Mrs István Kis, they were five, but I was her defender, they all bewitched my hand, I can barely lift it, they destroyed it so bad… (Komáromy 1910, 151 and 154).

The battle is often the symbolic reflection of the real social conflicts of real-life witchcraft, or is complementary to an alternative existence, and the "success" of the battle favourably influences the resolution of real-life conflicts as well as the situation of the bewitched person.[16] In the case of the latter, it is about the rivalry between two healers; in another part of the trial text we find: "I can heal her if she is not greater than me" (Komáromy 1910, 153). In a 1693 witch trial from Debrecen a healer *táltos* woman complained as follows: "I was almost killed with my daughter by the witches for having healed you…" (Komáromy 1910, 166). The guardian spirit of the victim is often interestingly a family member:

> The witness had a lodger named Sára […]. She said: "Oh, my lady, they fought a battle with Mrs Bartha last night, there were many here, but the most powerful of them all was the young daughter of Mrs Bartha, who took the sword in her mouth and fought terribly. I was lying in my bed and watching. Mrs Bartha said: don't be afraid, Sára, no one will hurt you." She heard this from her lodger named Sára. The witness also heard Mrs Bartha say herself that when they came to fight her, if it hadn't been for her daughter, they would have killed her (Bessenyei 1997, 390, trial of the *táltos,* Mrs András Bartha, Debrecen, 1725).

The nocturnal helper of this *táltos* woman was her own daughter. In a 1629 witch trial from Kolozsvár it is the nocturnal alter ego of a father who appears in this role: Kata, the daughter of Mrs Gáspár Kis, complained about a witch attacking her regularly in the night in the image of a woman; she tortured and beat her, then (in her vision) she woke her father and called to him, showing him the "apparition": "…here it is, my father. My father fought her, I couldn't say a word, I was silent until dawn" (Komáromy 1910, 95–6).

In the data of witch trials and in present-day ethnographic data, similar battles appear in the dreams, trance experiences or imagination of other healers, seers and cunning folk. Apparently, they run parallel in the dream world to the real rivalry between bewitchers and healers, or two sorcerers or two healers, parallel to the "earthly" battles for the life or death of the patient. As the data from Sárrétudvari on Ilona Madar demonstrate, for instance, the "witch identifier" and the bewitcher do battle to heal: "They battle […], the one who is more powerful will beat the other to the

[16] In two books of Carlo Ginzburg, published a couple of decades ago, one on the witches' Sabbath, the other on its mythical precedents (Ginzburg 1966; 2003 [1989]) these battles are exceptionally highlighted and several types are merged under the common cover name of "European shamanism". Hungarian researchers (Gábor Klaniczay and myself) have also discussed certain types of these spirit battles: Klaniczay 1990a; Pócs 1991–2. It is, nonetheless, an incorrect generalisation to compare or confuse these mediators with Eurasian shamans. For more, see Pócs 2017.

ground..." and: "they fought a battle with each other, the one who bewitched, and the one who wanted to heal [the patient]…" (Collection of Ilona Madar; *Archive of Hungarian Folk Belief*). Confirmed by data from the collections of Homoródalmás (Mereşti, Harghita county) by József Gagyi, healing "is fighting a battle in which the spirits of one person are fighting the spirits of another" (Collection of Gagyi József, in *Archive of Hungarian Folk Belief*). There is a sort of neighbourly animosity based on the opposition of "own versus stranger" in these spirit battles, which makes it even more obvious that there are certain real-life rivalries reflected in the battles between sorcerers and healers.

Identifiers of bewitchment

My experience gained from Csík (Ciuc) and Gyimes (Ghimeş) shows that when it comes to the identification of bewitchment in the dream world of witchcraft, the Christian and non-Christian spirit worlds (Virgin Mary, saints, the dead) also appear in the role of the identifier alongside the demonic metamorphoses of the witch.

In the "daytime" social systems of witchcraft, the identification of the bewitcher plays an important role, even if they think they know for certain that it is a case of bewitchment and they also suspect the identity of the bewitcher. Some kind of bewitchment-identifying spirit creature also appears in the dream world of the malefactor and healing witches: dreams identifying bewitchment also belong to the wide category of divination dreams, in which real-life secrets are revealed without the limitations of time and space.

We can again observe the complementary role of reality and dream: the exploratory saint in the dream helps to decipher a real-life bewitchment. T.V., a woman from Gyimesközéplok (Lunca de Jos, Harghita county, Romania), received the solution to a family conflict from a celestial comforter: she heard in a common family story a voice revealing the identity of the bewitcher, which she interpreted as a celestial sign. Based on data from Csíkjenőfalva (Ineu, Harghita county, Romania), this would appear to be a guardian angel, who identifies the bewitchment in the dream of the bewitched person and sends the person to see the priest to be healed (in accordance with the local system of witchcraft, in which Orthodox priests and friars also join the social and ideological context of witchcraft, besides healing, they contributed with divination and ordeal procedures giving a curse sermon, striking down the guilty, thus revealing their identity. See for instance: Pócs 2004, Komáromi 2010). On the other hand, the story follows the pattern of one type of incubation dream, which "solicits" the dreamer to visit a sacred place:

> My sister told me, my younger sister from Szenttamás, that she saw in her dream: "Go somewhere and pay for a sermon because you had been bewitched…[17] They told me openly. A guardian angel appeared. So go and have someone pray for you." So she went several times to Hévíz, where there are Romanian priests, not to have bewitching sermons, but to have decent sermons. And they recited the gospels over her head, and she felt relieved, as if something heavy had been lifted from her (75-year-old woman, own collection, Csíkjenőfalva, 1998).

According to similar Bulgarian data, the incubation saint sends the bewitched patient to a priest in order to lift the bewitchment, or to reciprocate it (with a curse sermon).[18]

To summarise the different aspects of bewitchment and healing dreams we can say that this supernatural sphere of witchcraft is in close relationship with the realistic systems of witchcraft based on neighbourly and family conflicts. It provided "otherworldly" examples, norms and sanctions to the resolution of the related tensions and problems of everyday life.

Epilogue

In conclusion, let us underline certain specificities of the diverse manifestations of the dream world outlined above. The common features and similar phenomena of these rituals and beliefs are conspicuous in both elite and popular, Christian and non-Christian forms, in every era of European culture. These similarities, spanning over great distances in time and space, and regardless of their eventual historical continuity, can be associated with the general, universal specificities of communication between the human and the supernatural world, and with the common psychological factors of dreams and dreaming.

Another component of these common features is the similar role of healing dreams (in a wider sense: all divination dreams) in individual religiosity. These dreams might be important, always and everywhere, as the manifestations of the imagistic mode of religiosity in accomplishing the emotive function of sacred communication. As opposed to prayer and meditation, these direct encounters offer the experience of reality filled

[17] In Hungarian *megcsináltattak* ["you have been made"].

[18] According to the kind, oral communication by Albena Georgieva (Sofia).

with emotion; as opposed to praying to or touching an image, the "real" touch in the dreams stimulating the senses gains ground. Moreover, in another aspect, as borne out by our examples, the compensatory and normative, practical role of this type of religious dream is equally important. (Research about religious dreams has emphasised this aspect on several occasions; studies by Hungarian researchers I ought to mention as examples: Tüskés and Knapp 1998, and Gábor Barna 1998). The practical role is emphasised by the ritually solicited dreams, which are legitimised and made part of public knowledge through incubation rituals known by the entire community and traditionally practised by many at specific times, (and vice versa: the legitimising and normative roles of incubation dreams are surely important for practising the rituals).

Regarding the dreams related to witchcraft, these represent a rural community in which the normative role of the archaic supernatural world of witchcraft beliefs was still very decisive. Similar to the healing dreams of saints, these dreams might also have had a compensatory, and at the same time, normative and legitimising function (on another level of their archaic world view) in the life of contemporary rural communities.

Certain common features of Christian and non-Christian incubation dreams are manifested in the universal specificities of the bonds to a sacred place. In this regard, we can observe a sort of archaic (and essentially non-Christian) "materialisation" of the supernatural world. Sacredness manifests in places where the supernatural has some kind of concrete material aspect: it is present in the earthly remains and relics of saints, in the bones and ashes of the dead whose souls have gone to the other world. The image of the saint was supposed to represent (or supplement) this same realistic, material existence, just as bringing home objects from a sacred place also extends the "material" radius of the sacred place.

The concrete material existence of the supernatural, its materialisation (according to Laura Stark-Arola's terms: *mystical sacredness* versus *tangible sacredness*) appears in the dreams as well, whether the mythical creature be Christian or non-Christian. (Stark-Arola 1998, 85; she discussed the "geography" of sacred communication while studying the religious life of Karelia). We just have to think of the identical reality of dream and real life, of the reality of otherworldly encounters, touches and physical marks "brought" from the other world. This type of material relation between the living and the world of spirits, demons and God can also be considered as identical and universal specificities of Christian and non-Christian forms.

The dream narratives under examination are also representations of archaic concepts of spirit and of the other world, which have allowed the simultaneous apparition of humans, the dead, demons and saints in the other world of dreams in their physical presence and as spirit creatures. (See briefly on these issues in Pócs 1999, chapter 2. On the simultaneously various concepts of the other world, see Hesz 2008). This is not a marked shift from this world to the other, between human and body, ghost and spirit; we can speak rather about simultaneous, parallel existence and continuous transition, the "alternation" of several possibilities. Thus, otherworldly healing incidents could become the carriers of sacredness and simultaneously the very realistic, barely spirit doubles of earthly healing.

References

Antal, Mária. 2004. *A gyimesvölgyi csángó magyarok hitvilága* [The beliefs of the Csángó Hungarians of Gyimesvölgy]. Budapest: General Press.

Arnaudov, Mihail. 1920. "*Kukeri i rusalii. Vgradena nevesta. Studii varhu bălgarskite obredi i legendi.* Studii vărhu bălgarskite obredy i legendi [*Kukeri* and *rusalii.* The built-in bride. Studies on Bulgarian rites and legends]." *Sbornik za narodni umotverenniia i narodopis XXXIV.*

Barna, Gábor. 1998. "Az álmok szerepe Orosz István életében [The role of dreams in the life of István Orosz]." In *Eksztázis, álom, látomás. Vallásetnológiai fogalmak tudományközi megközelítésben* [Ecstasy, dream, vision. Religious ethnological concepts in an interdisciplinary approach], edited by Éva Pócs, 340–50. Budapest, and Pécs: Balassi, and University Press. (Tanulmányok a transzcendensről I.)

Bálint, Sándor. 1942. *Egy magyar szentember. Orosz István önéletrajza* [A Hungarian holy man. Autobiography of István Orosz]. Budapest: Franklin Társulat.

Benz, Ernst. 1969. *Die Vision. Erfahrungsformen und Bilderwelt.* Stuttgart: Ersnt Klett.

Berchman, Robert M. 1998. "Arcana Mundi: Magic and Divination in the De Somniis of Philo of Alexandria." In *Mediators of the Divine. Horizons of Prophecy, Divination, Dreams and Theurgy in Mediterranean Antiquity*, edited by Robert M. Berchman, 115–54. Atlanta, Ga.: Scholars Press.

Bessenyei, József, ed. 1997. *A magyarországi boszorkányság forrásai* I. [Sources of Hungarian witchcraft]. Budapest: Balassi.

Bitel, Lisa M. 1991. "In Visu Noctis: Dreams in European Hagiography and Histories, 450–900." *History of Religions* 31: 39–67.

Blum, Richard, and Eva Blum. 1965. *Health and Healing in Rural Greece.* Stanford: Stanford University Press.

—. 1970. *The Dangerous Hour. The Lore of Crisis and Mystery in Rural Greece.* London: Chatto and Windus.

Bosnyák, Sándor. 1977. *A bukovinai magyarok hitvilága* I. *(Világkép, mitikus alakok, jeles napok, álomfejtés)* [The beliefs of the Hungarians of Bukovina (World concept, mythical figures, marked days and dream interpretation)]. Budapest: MTA Néprajzi Kutatócsoport. (Folklór Archívum 6.)

Brown, Peter. 1993. *A szentkultusz kialakulása és szerepe a latin kereszténységben.* Budapest: Atlantisz. [*The Cult of the Saints. Its Rise and Function in Latin Christianity.* Chicago: University of Chicago Press, 1980.]

Burke, Peter. 1997. "The Cultural History of Dreams." In *Varieties of Cultural History*, 23–42. Ithaca, and New York: Cornell University Press.

Chadwick, Nora. 1968. "Dreams in Early European Literature." In *Celtic Studies. Essays in Memory of Angus Matheson 1912–1962*, edited by James Carney, and David Greene, 33–50. London: Routledge & Kegan Paul.

Cox Miller, Patricia. 1994. *Dreams in the Late Antiquity. Studies in the Imagination of a Culture.* Princeton, N.J.: Princeton University Press.

Csepregi, Ildikó. 2003. "Gyógyító álom—gyógyító nevetés [Healing Dream—Healing Laughter]." *Ókor* 3: 38–46.

Csepregi-Vardabasso, Ildikó. 2008. "A szent és a szent hely. A csodatevő erő földrajza [The holy man and the holy place: The geography of thaumaturgic power]." In *Démonok, látók, szentek. Vallásetnológiai fogalmak tudományközi megközelítésben* [Demons, seers, saints. Religious ethnological concepts in an interdisciplinary approach], edited by Éva Pócs, 342–51. Budapest: Balassi. (Tanulmányok a transzcendesről VI.)

Csőgör, Enikő. 1998. *Tordatúr hiedelemvilága* [Beliefs of Tordatúr]. Kolozsvár: Kriterion.

Davidson, Hilda Ellis. 1981. "The Germanic World." In *Divination and Oracles*, edited by Michael Loewe, and Carmen Blacker, 115–41. London: George Allen & Unwin.

Dodds, Eric Robertson. 1951. *The Greeks and the Irrational.* Berkeley, Los Angeles and London: University of California Press.

—. 1971. "Supernormal Phenomena in Classical Antiquity." *Proceedings of the Society for Psychical Research* 55. Part 203, March, 1971.

Finucane, Ronald C. 1977. *Miracles and Pilgrims. Popular Beliefs in Medieval England.* London, Melbourne, and Toronto: J. M. Dent and Sons Ltd.

Franz, Adolph. 1909. *Die kirchlichen Benedictionen im Mittelalter* I–II. Freiburg im Breisgau: Herder.

Gagyi, József. 1998. *Jelek égen és földön. Hiedelem és helyi társadalom a Székelyföldön* [Signs in the sky and on earth. Belief and local society in Székler land]. Csíkszereda: Pro-Print.

Ginzburg, Carlo. 1966. *I Benandanti. Stregoneria e culti agrari tra Cinquecento e Seicento.* Torino: Einaudi.

—. 1989. *Storia notturna. Una decifrazione del sabba.* Torino: Einaudi.

Gollnick, James. 1999. *The Religious Dreamworld of Apuleius' Metamorphoses. Recovering a Forgotten Hermeneutic.* Waterloo and Ontario: Wilfrid Laurier University Press.

Grambo, Ronald. 1973. "Sleep as a means of ecstasy and divination." *Acta Ethnographica Hungarica* 22: 417–41.

Gurney, Oliver R. 1981. "Babylonians and Hittites." In *Divination and Oracles*, edited by Michael Loewe, and Carmen Blacker, 142–73. London: George Allen and Unwin.

Hamilton, Mary. 1906. *Incubation or the Cure of Disease in Pagan Temples and Christian Churches.* St. Andrews and London: W. C. Henderson & Son, and Simpkin, Marshall, Hamilton, Kent & Co.

Herzog, Rudolf. 1931. *Die Wunderheilungen von Epidauros. Ein Beitrag zur Geschichte der Medizin und der Religion.* Leipzig: Dieterich. (Philologus, Supplementband XXII, Heft III.)

Hesz, Ágnes. 2005. "Álom halottakkal, mint élők és holtak közti kommunikáció [Dreams about the dead: Communication between the living and the dead]." *Ethnographia* 116: 349–63.

—. 2008. "Néphit vagy helyi vallás: lélek- és túlvilágképzetek Hidegségen [Folk belief or local religion: Concepts of the soul and of the other world in Hidegség]." In *"Vannak csodák, csak észre kell venni." Helyi vallás, néphit és vallásos folklór Gyimesben* 1. ["Miracles exist, if only you notice them..." Local religion, folk belief and religious folklore in Gyimes], edited by Éva Pócs, 15–75. Budapest, and Pécs: L'Harmattan, and PTE Néprajz Tanszék. (Studia Ethnologica Hungarica VIII.)

Kazarow, Gawril I. 1933. "Krankeninkubation in Bulgarien." *Archiv für Religionswissenschaft* XXXIV: 362–3.

Kee, Howard Clark. 1983. *Miracle in the Early Christian World. A Study in Sociohistorical Method.* New Haven, and London: Yale University Press.

Kelchner, Georgia Dunham. 1935. *Dreams in Old Norse Literature.* Cambridge: Cambridge University Press.

Keszeg Vilmos. 1999. *Mezőségi hiedelmek* [Beliefs of Mezőség]. Marosvásárhely: Mentor.

Keszeg, Vilmos, Lehel Peti, and Éva Pócs, eds. 2009. *Álmok és látomások a 20–21. századból* I. [Dreams and visions in the twentieth and twenty-first centuries]. Budapest: L'Harmattan. (Fontes Ethnologiae Hungaricae VI.)

Kieckhefer, Richard. 1994. "The Holy and the Unholy: Sainthood, Witchcraft, and Magic in Late Medieval Europe." *The Journal of Medieval and Renaissance Studies* 24: 355–85.

Klaniczay, Gábor. 1990a. "Shamanistic Elements in Central European Witchcraft." In Gábor Klaniczay: *The Uses of Supernatural Power: the Transformation of Popular Religion in Medieval and Early Modern Europe,* 129–50. Cambridge: Polity Press.

—. 1990b. "Hungary: The Accusations and the Universe of Popular Magic." In *Early Modern European Witchcraft. Centres and Peripheries,* edited by Bengt Ankarloo, and Gustav Hennignsen, 219–55. Oxford: Clarendon Press.

—. 2008. "Learned Systems and Popular Narratives of Vision and Bewitchment." In *Witchcraft Mythologies and Persecutions*, edited by Gábor Klaniczay, and Éva Pócs, 50–82. Budapest and New York: CEU Press. (Demons, Spirits, Witches 3.)

Komáromi, Tünde. 2010. "Crossing Boundaries in Times of Personal Crisis. Seeking Help from Orthodox Clergy in Transylvania." In *Religion and Boundaries: Studies from the Balkans, Eastern Europe and Turkey,* edited by Galia Valtchinova, 155–66. Istanbul: The Isis Press.

Komáromy, Andor. 1910. *Magyarországi boszorkányperek oklevéltára* [Source-book of Hungarian witch trials]. Budapest: Magyar Tudományos Akadémia.

Kruger, Steven F. 1992. *Dreaming in the Middle Ages*. Cambridge: Cambridge University Press.

Lawson, John Cuthbert. 1910. *Modern Greek Folklore and Ancient Greek Religion. A Study of Survivals.* Cambridge: Cambridge University Press.

Lecouteux, Claude. 1987. *Geschichte der Gespenster und Wiedergänger im Mittelalter*. Köln, and Wien: Böhlau.

Le Goff, Jacques. 1992. *The Medieval Imagination.* Translated by Arthur Goldhammer. Chicago, and London: The University of Chicago Press. [L'Imaginaire médiéval. Essais. Paris: Gallimard, 1985].

Lixfeld, Hannjost. 1972. "Die Guntramsage (AT 1645 A) Volkserzählung vom Alter Ego in Tiergestalt und ihre schamanistische Herkunft." *Fabula* 13: 60–107.

Magyar, Zoltán. 2003. *A csángók mondavilága. Gyimesi csángó népmondák* [Folk legends of the Csángó Hungarians in the Gyimes area]. Budapest: Balassi.

Marinov, Dimităr. 1914. "Narodna viara i religiozni narodni obichaii [Folk belief and folk customs]." *Sbornik za narodni umotvoreniia i narodopis* XVIII.

McAlpine, Thomas H. 1987. "Sleep, Divine & Human, in the Old Testament." *Journal for the Study of the Old Testament*, Supplement 38.

Meier, Carl A. 1985. *Der Traum als Medizin. Antike Inkubation und Moderne Psychoterapie.* Zürich: Daimon Verlag.

Meisner, Rudolf. 1917. "Ganga till fréttar." *Zeitschrift des Vereins für Volkskunde* 14: 1–13, 97–105.

Menefee, Samuel Pyeatt. 1985. "Circling as an Entrance to the other world." *Folklore* 96, 3–20.

Meyer to Bernd, Heinz. 1952. "Das zweite Gesicht im Volksglauben und in Volkssagen." Dissertation, Göttingen. Manuscript.

Mykytiuk, Bohdan Georg. 1979. *Die Ukrainischen Andreasbräuche und verwandtes Brauchtum.* Wiesbaden: Harrasowitz.

O'Flaherty, Wendy Doniger. 1984. *Dreams, Illusions and Other Realities.* Chicago: The University of Chicago Press.

Ogden, Daniel. 1999. "Binding Spells: Curse Tablets and Voodoo Dolls in the Greek and Roman Worlds." In *Witchcraft and Magic in Europe. Ancient Greece and Rome*, edited by Valerie Flint, Richard Golden, Georg Luck, and Daniel Ogden, 1–90. London: The Athlone Press.

Peti, Lehel. 2012. *A moldvai csángók népi vallásosságának imagisztikus rítusai.* [Imagistic rites of vernacular religion of the Csángó in Moldova]. Kolozsvár: Nemzeti Kisebbségkutató Intézet.

Pócs, Éva. 1989. *Fairies and Witches at the Boundary of South-Eastern and Central Europe.* Helsinki: Academia Scientiarum Fennica. (Folklore Fellows' Communications 243.)

—. 1991–2. "The Popular Foundations of the Witches' Sabbath and the Devil's Pact in Central and South-eastern Europe". Acta Ethnographica 37: 305–70.

—. 1995. "Maleficium-narratívok—konfliktusok—boszorkánytípusok. Sopron vármegye 1529–1768 [Maleficium narratives—conflicts—witch-types: Sopron county 1529–1768]." *Népi kultúra—népi társadalom* XVIII: 9–66.

—. 1999. *Between the Living and the Dead. A Perspective on Witches and Seers in the Early Modern Age.* Budapest: Central European University Press.

—. 1998. "Transz és látomás Európa népi kultúráiban [Trance and vision in the folk cultures of Europe]." In *Eksztázis, álom, látomás. Vallásetnológiai fogalmak tudományközi megközelítésben* [Ecstasy, dream, vision. Religious ethnological concepts in an interdisciplinary approach], edited by Éva Pócs, 7–57. Budapest, and Pécs: Balassi, and University Press. (Tanulmányok a transzcendensről I.)

—. 2002. "Tér és idő a néphitben [Space and time in folk belief]." In *Magyar néphit Közép- és Kelet-Európa határán* [Hungarian folk belief at the boundary of Central and Eastern Europe], 9–39. Budapest: L'Harmattan. (Válogatott tanulmányok I.)

—. 2004. "Curse, Maleficium, Divination: Witchcraft on the Borderline of Religion and Magic". In Willem de Blécourt—Owen Davies (eds.): *Beyond the Witch Trials 2. Popular Magic in Modern Europe,* edited by Owen Davies, 174–190. Manchester University Press.

—. 2009. "*Tündéres* and the Order of St. Ilona or, Did the Hungarians Have Fairy Magicians?" In *Folk Religion and Folk Belief in Central Eastern Europe*, edited by Éva Pócs, 379–396. *Acta Etnographica Hungarica* 54/2.

—. 2017. "Fairies: Small Gods, Small Demons. Remnants of an Archaic Fairy Cult in Central and South-Eastern Europe". In *Fairies, Demons, and Nature Spirits: Small Gods at the Margins of Christendom*, edited by Michael Ostling, 255–76. Houndmills, Palgrave Macmillans. (Palgrave Historical Studies in Witchcraft and Magic).

Porter, J. Roy. 1981. "Ancient Israel." In *Divination and Oracles*, edited by Michael Loewe, and Carmen Blacker, 191–214. London: George Allen and Unwin.

Puchner, Walter. 1987. "Zum Nachleben des Rosalienfestes auf der Balkanhalbinsel." *Südost-Forschungen* 46: 197–278.

Puhvel, Martin. 1989. *The Crossroads in Folklore and Myth*. New York, Bern, Frankfurt am Main, and Paris: Peter Lang.

Ranke, Kurt. 1951. *Indogermanische Totenvereherung* I. *Der dreißigste und vierzigste Tag im Totenkult der Indogermanen*. Helsinki: Academia Scientiarum Fennica. (Folklore Fellows' Communications 140.)

Róheim, Géza. 1920. "Lucaszék." In *Adalékok a magyar néphithez* II. [Data on Hungarian folk belief II.], 29–227. Budapest: Hornyánszky Viktor.

Salamon, Anikó. 1975. "Gyimesi mondák [Legends from Gyimes]." In *Mai népi hiedelmek* [Contemporary popular beliefs], 65–156. Budapest: ELTE. (Az ELTE Ókori Történeti Tanszékeinek Kiadványai 10.)

—. 1987. *Gyimesi csángó mondák, ráolvasások, imák* [Csángó legends, incantations, prayers from Gyimes]. Budapest: Helikon.

Salo, Matt T. 1974. "The Structure of Finnish Shamanic Therapy." Dissertation, State University of New York at Bingham. Manuscript.

Schmitt, Jean-Claude. 1998. *Ghosts in the Middle Ages. The Living and the Dead in Medieval Society.* Chicago: University of Chicago Press. [*Les revenants. Les vivants et les morts dans la société médiévale.* Paris: Gallimard, 1994.]

Schram, Ferenc. 1970. *Magyarországi boszorkányperek 1529–1768.* I–II. [Hungarian witch trials 1529–1768.] Budapest: Akadémiai.

—. 1982. *Magyarországi boszorkányperek 1529–1768.* III. [Hungarian witch trials 1529–1768.]. Budapest: Akadémiai.

Seidl, Franz. 1968. "Das Kreisstehen. (Ein Beitrag zum Wahrsagebrauchtum um die Jahreswende)." In *Festschrift für Otto Höfler zum 65. Geburtstag* II., edited by Helmut Birkhan and Otto Gschwantler, 411–22. Wien: Notring.

Sigal, Pierre-André. 1985. *L'homme et le miracle dans la France médiévale (XIe–XIIe siècle).* Paris: Les Éditions du Cerf.

Stark-Arola, Laura. 1998. "Sacred Centers and Preconceived Journeys: Insights into the Cultural Construction of Religious Experience in Orthodox Karelia." *Acta Ethnographica Hungarica* 43: 81–107.

Stewart, Charles. 1997. "Anxiety, Experience and the Limits of Social Constructionism in Modern Greek Dream Narratives." *American Ethnologist* 24 (4): 877–94.

l-Bodrog "Introduction: Dreaming as an Object of Anthropological Analysis." *Dreaming* 14 (2–3): 75–82.

Strohmaier, Johann. 1997. "Die Mirakelaufzeichnungen des Wallfahrtsortes Maria Landegg/NÖ." Doctoral diss., Universität Wien. Manuscript.

Stroumsa, Guy G. 1999. "Dreams and Visions in Early Christian Discourse." In *Dream Cultures. Explorations in the Comparative History of Dreaming*, edited by David Schulman, and Guy G. Stroumsa, 189–212. New York, and Oxford: Oxford University Press.

Tedlock, Barbara. 1987. “Dreaming and Dream Research.” In *Dreaming. Anthropological and Pyschological Interpretations*, edited by Barbara Tedlock, 1–31. Cambridge: Cambridge University Press.

Todorova-Pirgova, Iveta. 2008. “Witches and Priests in the Bulgarian Village: Past and Present.” In *Witchcraft Mythologies and Persecutions*, edited by Gábor Klaniczay, and Éva Pócs, 283–94. Budapest, and New York: CEU Press. (Demons, Spirits, Witches 3.)

Tomisa, Ilona. 2003. “Az örökkévalóság igézetében. A középkori szenttisztelet nyomai Hárompatakon [Under the spell of eternity. Traces of medieval worship of saints in Hárompatak].” In *Hárompatak. Egy ismeretlen néprajzi kistáj Erdély és Moldva határán* [Hárompatak. An unknown ethnographic small region at the borders of Transylvania and Moldova], edited by Ilona Tomisa, 211–25. Budapest: MTA Néprajzi Kutatóintézete.

Tüskés, Gábor. 1993. *Búcsújárás a barokk kori Magyarországon a mirákulumirodalom tükrében* [Pilgrimages in baroque Hungary in the mirror of the miracle literature]. Budapest: Akadémiai.

Tüskés, Gábor and Éva Knapp. 1998. “Egy dunántúli parasztasszony álomelbeszélései [Dream narratives of a Transdanubian peasant woman].” In *Eksztázis, álom, látomás. Vallásetnológiai fogalmak tudományközi megközelítésben* [Ecstasy, dream, vision. Religious ethnological concepts in an interdisciplinary approach], edited by Éva Pócs, 366–79. Budapest, and Pécs: Balassi, and University Press. (Tanulmányok a transzcendensről I.)

Višinskait, Asta. 2007–2008. “Narratives on Dream’s Effect on People in Lithuanian and Latvian Oral Folklore.” *Estudos de Literatura Oral* 13–14: 231–8. (Universidade do Algarve, Portugal.)

Whitehouse, Harvey. 2004. *Modes of Religiosity: A Cognitive Theory of Religious Transmission*. Walnut Creek: Altamira Press.

Wittmer-Butsch, Maria Elisabeth. 1990. *Zur Bedeutung von Schlaf und Traum im Mittelalter*. Krems: Gesellschaft zur Erforschung der materiellen Kultur des Mittelalters. (Medium Aevum Quotidianum, Sonderband I.)

Zuesse, Evan M. 1987. “Divination.” In *Encyclopedy of Religion* 4, edited by Mircea Eliade, 375–82. New York: Macmillan.

MIRACULOUS HEALING AT SACRED PLACES: PROCEDURES AND NARRATIVES

ALBENA GEORGIEVA

In our contemporary world, miraculous healing is marginalised; it is considered irrational and superstitious. Still, people continue to practise it and to believe in its effectiveness and, as field investigations prove, to this day it is quite established and active. One mostly seeks divine assistance when in sore need and as a last resort—when all other possible means of solving one's problems and medical remedies or other conventional healing techniques have failed.[1] In most cases, the precise problem that creates some kind of tension and impels the individual to address the supernatural is a temporary or longer-term separation from society. An intractable illness, difficulties in the family or at work, or stress-induced mental problems are the most typical reasons for a personality imbalance or isolation and alienation from the social milieu. And so, one undertakes a pilgrimage to try to manage one's threatened psychic and physical balance and wholeness, in the hope of becoming socially integrated and of feeling once more within the limits of *normality* (Georgieva 2008).

Healing Procedures

Folk tradition has established specific healing procedures at sacred places, some of which are fairly old and universal while others are rather rare and bound to a particular space and its cultural background.

The first step a pilgrim makes on their way to salvation is by undertaking a *journey* to a shrine. The departure from the habitual everyday activities which maintain life, but, paradoxically enough, deflect attention from the most important existential problems, is actually a departure from routine and monotonous living; it is a preparation for a sojourn on *another* level and for experiencing some *other* order. As Peter

[1] As Galia Valtchinova has formulated: "… divine agency is sought especially in social and political contexts where human agencies fail (or are nearly failing) to produce the intended effects" (Valtchinova 2009, 210).

Brown puts it, pilgrimage is a "therapy of distance" (Brown 1982, 87). The journey itself has an ancient archetypal symbolism and is one of the images representing psychological *individuation*—the process of personal growth and maturing. In myths and in fairy tales, the hero sets off on a journey, driven by an initial shortage or loss, which can be compensated for only with the help of something very special and difficult to find—"life-giving water", "golden apples" and the like. The fetching of the magic object is in fact the establishing of contact with the inner centre of the personality, the centre which gives strength and stability when dealing with obstacles and which makes life rational and wholesome (Franz 1978, 170). It is precisely the search for answers to one's problems—of the quest for one's own *life-giving water*—which leads the pilgrim to set off for the holy place. The journey presupposes effort and acquires the symbolic meaning of spiritual purification and concentration in passing from the *lower* to the *higher* levels of existence and perception (Baeva 2001, 139); in a way, it is a preparation for some specific and extraordinary experience.

Once at the sacred place, the pilgrim should exhibit his/her respect towards the divine power—for the saint who is the *master* of the shrine. Taking part in the ritual practices is necessary in order to become involved and to declare one's participation in the pilgrim community; submitting an offering—a *sacrifice*: money, candles or other objects—is the way to gain divine favour and to show one's humility and homage. Prayer is important: the pilgrim formulates in it his/her expectations and explicates his/her faith and willingness to change. Taking part in the religious ritual, submitting an offering and praying, are not healing procedures in themselves, but they are an important condition for achieving success, because they influence the pilgrim's mood and inner attitude.

One widespread healing procedure that is considered miraculous and quite effective is to *sleep overnight* at the holy place. It is mostly practised on the eve of the patron saint's day, because of the belief that then the divine power's presence is most sensible, but it can be just as effective on any other night as well. Those sleeping overnight in a monastery are expectant of a *miraculous dream* which should indicate how to overcome one's inner conflict or how to find a way out of one's difficult situation. As a healing method, induced dreaming—*incubation*—has been used since antiquity and persists in Christianity (Le Goff 1998, 321 and 333–4). It is based on the idea that dreams as a whole, and in ritual conditions in particular, are messages from the supernatural and the divine. They are not subject to the will and the desires of the dreamer and sometimes even oppose his conscious intentions: they *happen* to him and his role is only to understand their meaning. So, going to the sacred place and getting involved in its specific atmosphere due to the saint's *praesentia* (after Peter Brown), the pilgrim may expect a *special* dream with a healing or prophetical meaning.

Dreaming is furthermore a proven and effective way to enter into contact with the unconscious and to access its hidden contents: when the conscious is sleeping, the unconscious is activated and makes an effort to enter into a creative and healthy relationship with the conscious—to prompt true answers, to warn against risks, to correct fallacious and uselessly maintained views, to prevent bad deeds or evil intentions. The dream messages come from the individual's inner centre, which remains in the depths of the unconscious even when the personality is relatively wholly developed. This centre has therefore no other possibility to influence the conscious side of the psyche, except for trying to get in touch with it through the archaic language of images and symbols. Unless *deciphered*, this language is devoid of reason: it cannot be logically interpreted and does not communicate simple, consistent ratiocinations (Jung 1978, 33 and 37).

People dream all the time, but as a rule do not pay attention to dreams because in everyday life their thoughts are engaged in "more important" things. But when a conflict between the conscious and the unconscious occurs and the dreams become disturbing and nightmarish it is no longer possible simply to ignore or forget them. It then becomes important to pay attention to one's dreams and to try to find out what they are trying to convey through their strange images—what they *reveal*, what they *advise*…and if in moments of trouble or tension dreams overwhelm the conscious in order to protect or warn it, they acquire a greater significance when one has devoted time to comprehending and remembering them, or when one has undertaken a pilgrimage in order to open one's consciousness to them and to all the experience on the border between dreams and reality—between the unconscious and the conscious. For that reason, many stories are told at sacred places about vivid and remarkable dreams which have a healing or prophetic significance—after all, this is one of the very goals of the pilgrimage.

The most striking example in my field research is the case of Mariana Strugova from the village of Garmen in the Gotse Delchev region (South-Western Bulgaria). She went through considerable stress as a child and as a result became a sleepwalker, going around the house at night or even outside in the yard, doing things she could not recall when awake. This behaviour persisted even after her marriage, until one Saturday her mother and mother-in-law decided to take her to the Hadjidimovo monastery of St. George in the same region. While sleeping there overnight she dreamed that she had to pass close to a deep precipice, walking down a narrow path beside a cliff. When she seemed about to fall, a woman in black reached out a hand and drew her to safety. Mariana thereupon recovered and was no longer somnambulant.[2]

Another instructive example is that of Liubomira Iusekchieva, a Muslim from the village of Pletena who experienced a similar *miraculous* transformation while sleeping overnight in the same monastery. She was a schoolgirl in the tenth grade when on the first day of Kurban Bayram, she fainted on the way to school and lost the power of speech. In the hospital, she was told that all her tests were normal, but she was still unable to speak. Her grandmother took her to the Hadjidimovo monastery, where in the morning she recovered her speech and asked for food and water.[3]

Another widespread healing procedure is that of *washing* with the curative water of a holy spring (ayazmo). Washing, and especially bathing, were not everyday practices in the past and had a rather symbolic and ritualistic role rather than the daily and sanitary significance they have today. As the eminent ethnographer Dimitar Marinov testifies, Bulgarian peasants and even the bourgeoisie at the end of the nineteenth and in the first half of the twentieth centuries were not very prone to regularly bathing themselves. They bathed in the rivers only "for reasons of health" on St. George's Day (6 May), on St. John's Day (Midsummer—24 June) and during the Goreshtnitsi (Dog-Days—15, 16, 17 July), and also bathed with herbal water when ill (Marinov 1914, 489). With regard to this, we should keep in mind that in the Bulgarian villages until the middle of the twentieth century, and in many places until even later, there was no drainage and running water in the houses, which proves that in the past, the significance of washing and bathing was magical—preventive or healing—rather than hygienic.

Water is another well-known medium for establishing contact with the divine, and every source of water—lake, river, spring or well in mythology and in folk tradition—signifies the border between the human and supernatural worlds. This border is considered haunted—in the past by a monster and in our days by a saint who governs the water's properties and who—if conciliated—may become a mediator and an intercessor in one's struggle against the disease. Washing and bathing is a symbolic act of

[2] Mariana Assenova Strugova, born in 1962 in Garmen, higher education, accountant; recorded by Albena Georgieva and Ognian Enev on 06.05.2004 (St. George's Day) in the village of Garmen, Gotse Delchev region.

[3] Liubomira Iskrenova Iusekchieva, born in 1975 in Gotse Delchev, secondary education, a worker; recorded by Albena Georgieva and Snezhana Bakalova on 11.07.2002 in the village of Pletena, Satovcha parish.

purification—physical, as well as psychic—from the *infection*, which is the disease, and also from the *evil forces* which have caused it. People believe that after this purifying procedure, in most cases repeated three times for better effect, the disease and its cause are washed away with the water or remain in the thread or the garment which was part of the patient's clothing and which they afterwards hang on a tree or a bush near the spring. This thread or piece of clothing is the symbolic substitute of the patient and is his/her offering to the supernatural power haunting the water. After washing it is recommended that the patient should drink from the holy water over a certain number of days—generally—and the grounds for this practice are again symbolic and not so much connected with the water's real healing properties as with its magical power—it should purify the patient from *within*, expelling the implanted evil force.

In some sacred places the specific healing procedure of *squeezing* is practised. It is carried out in peculiar natural formations—a fissure in a rock (as at the Rila monastery, the best-known monastery in Bulgaria) or in the intertwined branches or—better—roots of a big tree (as is the case at today's very popular Krastova gora [Cross Mount] in the Rhodope Mountains). Squeezing through a magic place or object has an ancient origin and is a rather old tradition in Bulgarian folk healing practices. According to one belief, in ritual circumstances some specially prepared objects or natural forms acquire magical power and become a means of purification and for contacting the supernatural world—for passing through it, after which people and animals become resistant and immune to diseases. Such a ritual is carried out most often when epidemics break out. People are protected by squeezing through a *magic* shirt prepared from the wool of a black ram, when the whole process from shearing to spinning, weaving and sewing is completed over one night (from sunset to sunrise). A similar magical power to stop an epidemic can be acquired by a narrow gorge between rocks or between banks, when a *life-giving* fire (again ritually lit) is made near it and people and animals pass through it, thereby becoming resistant to the disease (Marinov 1914, 559–61).

Passing through a natural cleft or a gorge located in the vicinity of the sacred place is considered a particular trial and means of renewal. Like the mouth of a cave, it is attributed the symbolic role of an entrance to the magic supernatural reality, in which inner psychic resources and unconscious impulses are activated and in which the experience of a transformation is possible and expected. To successfully squeeze through the fissure is considered a kind of verification, signalling righteousness and purification from sin, and so it gives the patient inner strength and security.

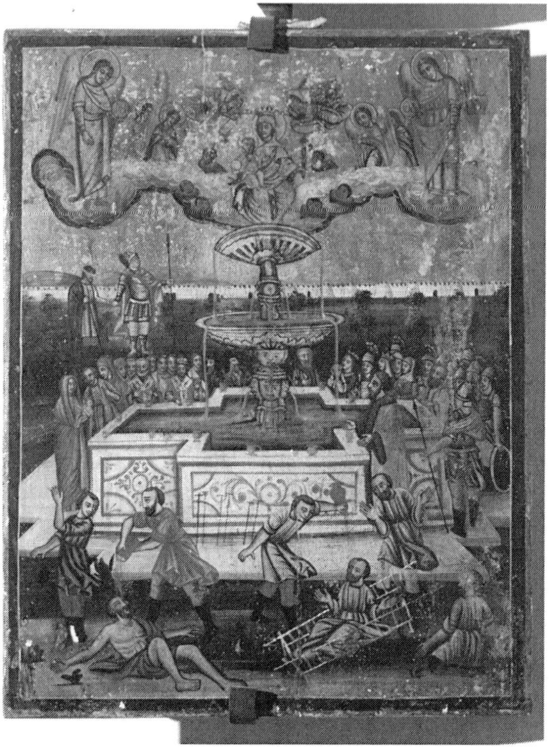

The Virgin Zoodochos Pighi (also called *The Virgin Life-Giving Source* or *The Virgin Spring of Life*) – icon from the Art Gallery in Burgas, Bulgaria. Photo Archive of the Institute of Art Studies at the Bulgarian Academy of Sciences. Courtesy of D.Sc. Ivanka Gergova, Corr. Member of BAS.

Another traditional "health-giving" practice is the ritualistic unlocking of the church door. As described by Vihra Baeva, the worshipper should be the first to arrive at the church on the day in question and while unlocking the door should not take the key out of the keyhole. They should then drop some money for the church through the door and should enter with the right foot first (Baeva 2008, 197–9). The practice is a symbolic opening of one's path and ensures not only health, but also good luck and success.

The common method for healing insanity in the folk tradition is *binding* the patient to a tree in the church for several days—three or forty. The observations of Galina Valtchinova indicate that psychic disorder is mostly expressed in losing one's social identity or in diverting from it, while the healing procedure aims to establish functional balance between the sound and curative natural object (the tree) and its cultural counterpart—the insane human body (Valtchinova 2005, 14). The church is targeted as a place for contacting the divine and God, and its architecture on a smaller scale represents the idea of the world's order. The church's role as a medium between the worlds makes it suitable as a divine agency and for miraculous healing, and its structural duplication of the world's order confirms its aptness for one's inner *arrangement* and *harmonisation*, for re-establishing one's strongholds in life, temporarily lost due to stress or a disease. This is the primary reason for expecting that when occupying the sacred place, the insane person will restore their social identity; that is, their *normality*.

Binding the patient to a tree, however, besides its practical aspect—to prevent possible violence and aggression on the part of the subject—has an additional symbolism. In psychology, as in mythology, the tree is an image of life and growth, an image of the gradual and persistent development of one's life's potential, in the way the tree's potential insensibly grows from its seed, fulfilling its definite pattern. For that reason, the tree or its stylisation—a pole, a column, etc.—is introduced as the axis mundi connecting heaven and earth, in fact connecting the *upper* world of consciousness, of birds and of bright creatures and deities, and the *lower* world of the unconscious—of daemons and dark forces. In depth psychology, the tree is also another image of individuation—the process of growth and maturing, the process of gradual unfolding and harmonisation of one's psychic characteristics (Franz 1978, 161). Binding the insane to a tree in a churchyard, therefore, is the patient's symbolic binding to the world's axis, which ensures connection and coordination between the different mental levels, or which, more precisely, presents the hierarchy and the *subordination* between these levels—the *subordination* which should be present in the individual's psyche, but which is misbalanced in the patient's. The proximity to and the physical contact with the axis, representing the world's centre and order, should contribute to the patient's reconciliation to this order and to the main norms and strongholds they have deviated from; it should mark the path of their growth and maturing and of the overcoming of their temporary social isolation.

Besides the common, by and large recurring healing procedures discussed above, there are some other rather rare rituals which may be encountered at particular sacred sites. One good example is, to my knowledge, unique to Bulgaria, and involves the making of special belts from a thread wrapped three times around a church, as a charm against childlessness. This is practised at The Church of the Dormition of Mary, known as *Mary the Golden Apple* in Gorni Voden (once a separate village, now a quarter of Asenovgrad, Plovdiv region—South-Western Bulgaria: see Baeva 2000a). Some of the practices of the general ritual complex could also be considered rare, for example, the "re-buying" of the sacrificial lamb as a symbolic offering at the Hadjidimovo monastery of St. George, which we have already encountered, where a desired sum of money is paid in order to take one of the lambs already offered by some other people to the monastery, and to bow with it in front of the icon of St. George.

No matter what local peculiarities there may be in the detail, everywhere in the past pilgrimage has been associated with *feasting*—festive meals, dances and general merriment rounding off the ritual activities. This was certainly the practice in the past, because over the years the church has opposed the noisy funfair and the peddlers, the passionate dances and the drinking of alcohol, considering them inappropriate and contradictory to the decency and the quiet expected of a sacred place. Today, this kind of celebration is frequently set apart from the church and the monastery, and is carried out on the central square if it is the settlement's fete day. In the past, however, the merriment with eating, drinking, singing and dancing happened in close proximity to, although *outside* the shrine; it was an organic part of the cult itself. The feast was a way of representing the community's ideal of well-being accomplished *here* on Earth: the abundant meals and the collectively shared emotions through singing and dancing symbolise life's wholeness and the people's unity and solidarity; it gives way to the joy of life and a sense of involvement in one's own social role and group; after all, it is a way of going beyond, although only for a while, everyday shortfalls and of sojourning in a harmonious and consistent world, where everyone may give free vent to their emotions and ambitions.

The miraculous healing is somehow the overcoming of the patient's temporal social isolation, resulting from disease or stress, and at the same time their reacquired harmonious incorporation into an appropriate social group. So the festive merriment affirming that incorporation and symbolically signifying it turns out to be not only an organic part of pilgrimage itself, but also a *healing procedure* in its own right. Since antiquity, music and dance have been an essential element of those ecstatic curative rites that have spread all over the world and are, in this sense, universal, and are defined by some authors as shamanism (Eliade 1996, 18). Most rituals with dance and music are characterised by inspiration and exhilaration which, introduced by the musicians and dancers, is experienced as freedom and spiritual power, as completeness and a fulfilment of desires. By participating in the common rhythm of music and dance, or merely becoming intoxicated by alcohol, thereby releasing some of the usual inhibitions, the individual feels naturally involved and exuberant. And, if seeking support in a solution to some difficult problem or in coping with a disease or stress, this exuberance may serve as a catalyst in accelerating inner transformation and in experiencing enlightenment and liberation from the imposed alienation and loneliness. It is precisely because the festive merriment can also act as a bridge to overcoming one's social isolation, and to this effect can cause *miraculous healing*, that in the past feasting was considered inseparable from the sacred and the religious. As Petko Ivanov has generalised, in contrast with Christianity, folklore's leading element is not God or the saints, but the celebration itself (Ivanov 1992, 276).

Narratives

Oral narratives inevitably accompany the healing procedures and play a decisive, constructive role in making a place sacred: they act as repositories for most of the memory and information about magic objects, healings or other miracles, and thus provide the necessary motivation for pilgrimage. Here, attention will be drawn to the process of narration and its functions in establishing, maintaining and spreading local religious culture.

To begin with, narratives *establish the sacred nature of a place*. In the territory accepted by the community as its *own,* and thus domesticated, oral stories outline those significant points on which contact with the divine is considered possible and which are marked by cultic activity and offerings. Usually, these are the places symbolically representing the process of winning over the inhabited world from nature and of defending the collective *own* identity—human, national, religious. Stories which are quite popular today involve discovering a miracle-working icon, a curative spring or a monastery treasure, or about building a monastery or a chapel, and about the miracles of one saint or another. These stories are communicated as a sign of agency and of supernatural presence in the human world, as a manifestation of divine patronage and intercession with God. The very building of the shrine and the cult practices and offerings are a *payment* for this patronage: they are the people's way of showing respect and gratitude.

The narratives about various chapels and monasteries and their retelling in direct communication are still the main channel for *structuring and maintaining knowledge* about the sacred. Various forms of media are also involved in that process—TV and radio broadcasts, books, magazines and special issues. This, however, does not change the situation in its essence—that the principal means for affirming existing knowledge is the pilgrimage itself. The gathering together of people who then share narratives among themselves is the real proof that the shrine truly is important and that there is a community which identifies with it and maintains it.

What are the exact dimensions of the knowledge transmitted in narratives? Oral stories explain the origin of the shrine and its building as a result of a miraculous sign; they also render all the emblematic cases when miracles happened, proving the effectiveness of this shrine. Narration, therefore, *outlines the local sacred history* from its beginning up to the present and including the significant moments in its progress. An instructive example in my fieldwork is the story of the Chapel of *St. Nedelia* (*St. Kyriaky*) near the village of Garmen in the Gotse Delchev region. It begins with a miraculous dream, in which St. Nedelia appears first before the protagonist Lina, and then her husband Stoian, insisting that they go and dig out an icon with her image, buried in a place indicated by her, where a monastery had existed in the past and where they should now restore it. Stoian refuses on the grounds of their poverty, but his body becomes paralysed and he is compelled to give his consent. They find the icon and another miraculous dream tells them to go with the icon around the neighbouring villages in order to collect money and materials to erect a chapel. The chapel is built and time passes by, and a most striking case is remembered when a paralysed boy starts walking after having slept overnight in the shrine, rather explicitly convincing listeners of the healing power of the place (Georgieva 2000).

As is obvious from the example, the events in the narratives reveal not only the *history*, but also *the symbolic significance* of the sacred place and its importance as a place of contact with the divine. Someone has been in contact with or has had something happen in the presence of a supernatural being; another has been healed or has experienced another miracle. The narratives reveal a possible outlet to *heaven*, the perception of which is somehow scattered in everyday activities, but the affiliation to which is essential for human life and provides it with indispensable strongholds and basic values.

This leads us to another important function of narration—*to motivate the cult practices* which are performed at the shrine. Narratives explain the origin of the cult in question and the meaning of the actions performed, especially if they are specific and unique, as is the case with the above-mentioned making of special belts against childlessness at *Mary the Golden Apple* church in Gorni Voden. But stories explain some more trivial practices as well, such as washing, bathing and drinking water from the holy springs, sleeping overnight at miracle-working shrines, squeezing through trees and caves, etc. The narrative's objective in this case is not only to reveal the symbolic significance of the actions, but also to prove their undoubted practical effectiveness: someone in the past—a relative, a friend, a neighbour—has been healed when washing with the curative water, or has begun to walk again after sleeping overnight at the shrine; a family has acquired a child as a result of the magic belt, etc.

In this sense, the narrative situation is also *a form of education*: the story introduces the shrine's history and symbolism, it reveals the meaning of the performed actions and formulates their expected effect, and thus it is persuasive and involves newcomers in the practices. To some extent, the narrative *initiates* newcomers—young people and children as well as those coming from other places. Usually, the story is accompanied by a demonstration of appropriate behaviour or by a willingness to show the particular objects involved. At the same time, the narrative incites the adoption of definite concepts, it admonishes and gives examples to follow. Sometimes the narrative situation even offers a chance for the *re-education* of particular interlocutors, winning them over to religious faith, persuading them of the effectiveness of a behaviour consistent with Christian norms, and above all in making them rethink their own experience and find a clear significance in some events which had remained confusing or unacceptable until that moment. To a certain degree, storytelling may develop into *a kind of sermon*, when the narrator enters into the role of the priest and, giving concrete examples, preaches about the advantages of faith as a world view and as a guide to behaviour in life. Such is usually the case with a number of charismatic leaders in the community who tell instructive stories, give answers to the questions and reassurances to the hesitations of the participants, and strengthen their faith with their own positive example of steady and natural belief (see Baeva 2000b).

The most important role of narration in the local religious culture is its capacity for *creating a community*. On the way to the shrine, one can learn about its history from a guide or a brochure; one can maybe even go there on purpose having already heard or read about it. One's real incorporation into the place, however, starts when someone decides to *relate* information about it to them. Narration is a situation: it presupposes time and attention for the plot to unfold and its significance to be comprehended; it presupposes the availability of someone who *knows* and is willing to talk about it; it presupposes that there are listeners willing to learn and to give their time. The narrative situation is a departure from the day's routine; it requires concentration on the story and its message, and at a sacred place, this almost inevitably involves concentration on religious faith and on its significance in human life.

The listener may not be so deeply interested in the topic; he or she may lack time and so may be in a hurry to "slip out" from the situation and to withdraw. But if one is attracted by the story, and especially if they have come to the shrine looking for help or some other benefit, one is going to listen carefully and participate with questions, commentary or one's own stories. In turn, this may attract new listeners or new narrators from the people gathered around or from those just passing by. And thus, the situation may develop into experiencing a real and moving communication, when the participants come to know each other, sharing their pains and problems, sharing also their hope to be able to cope with these problems, because *someone has already received help, has been cured, has started to believe...* This situation is especially characteristic of occasions involving sleeping overnight on the eve of the patron saint's day: some of the pilgrims start singing religious songs, others talk and exchange narratives, among which the predominant ones are miracle stories, and the very narration acquires the significance of a ritual, giving hope and affirming God's grace and power (Baeva 2008, 195).

The narrative situation *creates order* in the world—stories, especially when claimed to be *true*, *prove* the validity of the adopted norms and beliefs, the effectiveness of religious behaviour and of true faith. They suggest definite concepts and a point of view from which the painful and inexplicable problems fit the pattern of already existing precedents, transforming them from being unique into something paradigmatic and repeated. In the completed wholeness of the narrative, everything that happens is interpreted as corresponding to the unwritten principles of life, in a way regular, even *natural*: *a silly accident* turns into *a trial*, a *penalty*, *a warning*, *a reward*. Events acquire inner logic and purposefulness and from being chaotic and unaccountable, transform into something meaningful and bound with human destiny and behaviour, subject to human rationalisation and influence. The world depicted in the narratives reveals it as ordered: it is possible to assimilate and understand it; it is adaptable to control and change.

In sharing stories, the participants realise that all of them are equally dependent on fate and chance, yet at the same time equal in their potential to assume responsibility and cause a turning point or at least a change in their own destiny, thus finding the solution to their problems and achieving healing and enlightenment. The equality attained by narration amplifies still further the situation's effect: people unite their efforts in coping with difficulties and show affiliation to the spiritual values confessed by the community. The shared narrative repertoire constructs for them *a common identity* closely connected with local religious symbols and specific ritual practices. In this way, the sacred becomes their distinctive mark—*an emblem* of their *own* territory, but also *an emblem* of all who visit the shrine and who consider it their own stronghold and path to salvation.

The possibility for sharing, for achieving equality with others and for affiliation at the sacred place sometimes manages to overcome the individual's communication and socialisation difficulties and is experienced as a salutary healing effect, as an unexpected ability to cope with one's problems and as a miraculous achievement of long and painfully sought solutions to them. This accounts for the *therapeutic effect* of the pilgrimage centre. Partly, such an effect is due to the very involvement and presence in the established community of equal and wholesome individuals (*communitas* after Victor Turner) due to the participation in performed vigils, services, prayers and other ritual actions. Nonetheless, this effect is due to the deep experience and the rethinking of what is heard and shared in narratives. Stories provide examples and offer a point of view and life values which may stimulate the re-evaluation of one's own background, and which may lead to strong emotions and to a psychic transformation. This in turn may lead to salvation: to taking control of a crisis at once physical, yet much more mental. Placed in the meaningful wholeness of the narrative, events acquire existential significance and symbolism; they may have a releasing effect and may help the individual overcome the obstacles which seem external, yet which in most cases are erected unconsciously by that individual on their journey to other people and to complete development.

The support received at the sacred place and the release from inner psychic barriers (in psychology denoted as *frustration*) is the condition for one's incorporation into or return to one's appropriate group and social milieu and for the further realisation of one's potential in life. One's *salvation* or *healing* frequently becomes the turning point in one's world view and way of living; it becomes a strong motivation for one's *faith* and in turn is transformed into a *narrative*. Rendered in the first person or by the witnesses of the event, this narrative closes the circle and enters the narrative process as the serial proof of the shrine's *miracle-working power* (see also Baeva 1997, 65).

Narratives therefore, and especially narration as a process and a situation, are an important constructive part of the local religious culture; they are the dynamic and constantly actualised connecting unit between the elements of its structure. Narratives render the history and the symbolic meaning of the place and thus establish and maintain its significance as *sacred*; they attract and persuade people to join in ritual activities; they instruct the participants and involve them in other people's fates; they also act as a stimulant towards change and inner transformation, experienced as a miracle and in turn converted into a story. This mechanism of transmission, folklore in its essence and tested over the course of years, is fundamental to every local religious culture. It is intensified in periods of crisis, but its operation and scope may also be expanded through skilful management on the part of those in authority—priests or informal leaders. It may be used as well for imposing or for affirming the local community's prestige beyond its territory; sometimes it may even be involved in political campaigns. In any case, however, this process answers existential needs—the need for identity and the need to cope with one's deficiencies in life. This makes it quite vital and still resistant to change even in our contemporary era of globalisation.

Appendix A

Healed at Hadzhidimovo Monastery "St. George"

Mariana Strugova:[4] Well, I'm very pleased exactly on this day[5] to retell you an absolutely, absolutely true incident, and personally, it happened personally with me. I was less than ten years old, almost in my tenth year as a child, when with a cousin of mine we passed through our village, more precisely in Zagrade neighbourhood. We passed by a house, where in front of the house there is a gully, as a matter of fact, a big gutter full of water. And we unruly little children, my cousin, as we passed by, the woman from the same house was washing outside in that gutter her little children's clothes. And he only lightly pushed the clothes with his foot and they fell in the water. And there was much water in that gutter and the water carried them away. Well, then this woman got out and started persistently chasing us—all day long we tried to run away. But he was not from Garmen, he was from Ognianovo,[6] and every day he came here so that we could play together. And towards the evening, I had already forgotten about the incident, what had happened— all day long we ran and hid from that woman, and as I was playing out in the street, she came, took hold of me by the back and said: "Let me now, she said, let me tell you what the matter is about!" She took hold of me and from there—to the gutter, and my head in the water. I became blue, already about to… I am drowning: I got blue and was wet all over. Outside on the bench there were old women, they shouted at her, they didn't dare stop her, she was so enraged, so angry, that she was almost about to do the worst. The old women shouted at her: "Don't, you are going to drown the child!" She continued.

It was the same season as now, in May, and my father and mother came back on a motorcycle, then there were no cars, my father drove a motorcycle, may he rest in peace, he drove a motorcycle. They came from the field, they had been hoeing tobacco. And in the centre of the neighbourhood, in Zagrade under the plane-tree, some women stopped him and told him: "Asen, hurry", they said, "your child is at the gutter,

[4] Mariana Assenova Strugova, born in 1962 in Garmen, higher education, accountant, from 2005 working in the municipality; recorded by Albena Georgieva and Ognian Enev on 6 May 2004 (St. George's Day) in the village of Garmen, Gotse Delchev region.

[5] As pointed out below, the interview takes place during a big Christian holiday—St. George's Day.

[6] Ognianovo is a village near Garmen.

they said, and they are soaking her there in the water, they said, her head is in the water!" He threw the motorcycle aside, and went straight to me. The moment he saw her, he nearly killed her! He just took hold of her, squeezed her, raised her up… And a man: "Don't", he said, "don't get into trouble", he said, "because of… You better", he said, "refer to the authorities, he said, but you are going to get in trouble!" And he let her go.

From then on, after that incident, I came under a deep stress and began getting up at night: I'd go around, even in the yard, while sleeping, not knowing what I do—I had disassembled a chandelier while sleeping! I wake up in the morning and see the whole chandelier on the floor; I cannot fit it together afterwards. This happens at night, when I am asleep, all the time I get up and go around. I thought that… My mother started taking me to witches to cast lead[7] for me, but it wouldn't work, I continued in the same way, I continued and did it at night. I thought things would change when I got married. But they continued.

Two or three months after I got married, my mother-in-law told my mother: "Come on", she said, "let us get up and go", she said, "what you have done up till now, you have done", she said, "but let us go", she said, "and sleep overnight in the St. George's monastery in Hadzhidimovo". And this was a real, I would say, a real holiday for me, because this was the end of it all.

We went one evening, it was on one Sunday eve, and I will never forget what happened to me during the night in this very monastery. We were lying down in front of the chapel; we had spread blankets on the floor. I had fallen asleep. My mother is on one side, my mother-in-law on the other, and we are on the floor. I will never forget my dream. Well, I dream of a deep precipice. At the precipice's high side is a hill and along that hill only a narrow path for passing. I have to pass from one side to the other along that narrow path, facing the hill and leaning on it and trying to get hold of it, but there is nothing; it is a rock and there is nothing to get hold of. And I go, but slowly, slowly and I am near to falling down the precipice, and the precipice is full of water. And I say to myself: "That's the end, I'm falling! That's the end of it all!" And only in a second do I see in front of me, on the opposite side where I should have already gone, I see a woman, all dressed in black, reaching out a hand to me and saying: "I am going to help you, just give me a hand!" I reached my hand out slowly, little by little, cautiously, my fingers touched hers, and she took hold of my hand and got me across that precipice! I remember this as a

[7] Casting lead is a well-known method in folk medicine for healing from fright and in Bulgaria is practised mainly by Muslim women.

dream; I dreamed it and I will never forget it. And my mother told me: "Only, she said, as you were lying on the floor, she said, you got up, sat down, turned, looked over all of the icons; for five minutes, she said, you were looking with wide open eyes at the altar and only in five minutes, she said, you laid down and woke no more, nor did you move". From then on, up to the very present day, everything was over with me, what I suffered; up to the present day I don't have those problems any more.

Appendix B

Her Speech Recovered after She Slept Overnight in Hadzhidimovo Monastery "St. George"

Liubomira Iuzekchieva:[8] I didn't dream anything, only in the morning I was already speaking, that was the best.
And you didn't speak, did you?
No, and the light disturbed me.
And why didn't you speak?
Well, I don't know. It was Bayram, I was a student in the eleventh class, we started from home on the first day of Bayram—it was Kurban Bayram,[9] we started for school. And near the school, next to it—I don't remember any more. In the hospital everyone told me everything was normal, but I couldn't speak.
Did you faint or something?
I fainted, I knew absolutely nothing. I have an uncle, older than my father; he took me to the imam in Gyovren,[10] first to him. He said that we should go there [to the Hadzhidimovo monastery—A. G.]. We came back and from here they took me to Hadzhidimovo. I only slept overnight and on the following day asked for water and began to speak. But that imam told me that I was at the monastery. I remember quite well, there was a grandfather there—Tryphon, a very old priest, and he even… I'm not sure if his wife is still alive, the year before last she was still alive. I went to her as well on that morning when they woke me up. And Father Tryphon said that it should be repeated three times. Right in front of the church he

[8] Liubomira Iskrenova Iusekchieva, born in 1975 in the town of Gotse Delchev, living in Pletena, secondary education, a worker; recorded by Albena Georgieva and Snezhana Bakalova on 11 July 2002 in the village of Pletena, Satovcha parish.
[9] The Muslim holiday Eid al-Adha. All the inhabitants of Pletena, Satovcha parish, including Liubomira Iuzekchieva, are Muslim Bulgarians (Pomaks).
[10] Giovren is a village in the same region.

ordered me to sleep in front of the icon of St. Petka,[11] not of the Virgin Mary, but of St. Petka, so that this trouble should not happen to me again.
And who told you that?
Father Tryphon.
And where is this icon situated? Do you remember the place? I have been in that monastery.
When you enter on this side in the corner.
On the left?
On the left in the corner; even above it there is some of that oil which they put and light.
An icon-lamp.
You put coins on its side, and next to it I think it was the Virgin Mary "Miremana"[12] as we call her, the Virgin Mary, next to it, it was. Then is the one of Jesus, there are gifts on its side, those who bring lambs, and then you take the lambs back over there. They bring offerings to St. George.
Did you bring some offering?
We brought an offering. He said: you may bring one, or not bring one. Otherwise we did put some money on St. Petka's icon in the morning.
And what kind of offering did you bring then, do you remember?
A lamb. There was a man outside whom you pay for the lamb. You bring it in front of the icon which you want—not to eat it. You take it alive. You pay for the lamb and take it, and the person who is sick, takes it. You take it, then if you want, you may call father priest, someone from the officials there, to chant for you or whatever you want. If not, you leave it and you start praying with your own words, as I did that time.
You pray privately to begin to speak and to recover after that ritual with the lamb?
Yes, exactly. After that there was a man behind us who took the lamb back. You do not kill it and there you give money or what you will.
And do you remember how you prayed, with what words?
Not in words, I just closed my eyes and prayed to myself, voicelessly, to myself.
Well, it means, as you recovered your speech, it means you believed that you would receive help? Did you believe that?
When we went from our village, there was a woman with me, Lydia, they took us together. I didn't know what she went for and I didn't care, for I was half a person. My grandmother was with me, the mother of my father,

---

[11] In Greek *Agia Paraskevi*.
[12] Obviously, she means the Muslim denomination *Mariam*.

she was with me. The first thing which, when I was awake in the morning, was that I was very thirsty. And only when I asked her, I told: "Will you give me some water, because I am very thirsty?"—And then she said: "Dear Allah, the child has asked for water!" Those were her first words. And she gave it to me right away, because they told every one of us to fill some water and to leave it somewhere nearby, holy water so to say. So, she did it, she gave me water. After a while I said: "Is there something to eat?" And then she was delighted and said: "Dear Allah, the child also wants to eat!" She started chanting for me. I don't know what she was chanting, for she chanted in Turkish. That was it. Father Tryphon came and advised me three times to go around the church where we were. The first time he told me to walk slowly, the second time—faster, and the third time he said I should run, but I could not run, although I wanted to go faster.

And what after that?

Then we came back here and I started recovering, I started to communicate normally.

And have you visited that monastery again?

Yes, I have.

Again on a holiday or…?

On holidays also, on St. George's Day, or when I pass nearby and go to the church, I may light a candle. I once visited a family in Hadzhidimovo and went up there,[13] I go there.

You don't make a cross when you light a candle, do you?

I do not cross myself. I light candles both for the dead and for the living, for everybody. Not only there, when I go in Blagoevgrad also, I have been to the Rila monastery, I go in, only I do not cross myself, I don't have an inclination. Simply I am of another faith.

Snezhana Bakalova: You will do it physically, no problem, but it is not from the heart.[14]

LI: That's right.

SB: It's the same with me.

LI: For a week I bore a cross from the monastery without a problem, they gave it to me from the monastery, and Father Tryphon told me: "you will bear it for one week". Then I took it off and I still preserve it, but nobody can touch it, that's it, nobody can see it, that's it—the way it was tied when he gave it to me, nobody can touch it.

And what else did he give you besides a cross?

---

[13] Hadzhidimovo monastery is situated high above the town.

[14] Snezhana Bakalova is from the same village, Pletena, and of course is also a Muslim.

Nothing, only a little cross, inside is the little icon which I bought, and a coin. He gave me the coin, taking it from the icon, somebody had put it there, and he took it and said: "This is for good luck, child, he said, and let the Lord be with you!" And tied it, "and you should bear it for one week", he said.
And what did he tie it in –paper?
No, I gave him my handkerchief.
And you still preserve it?
I have put it in a place where nobody can touch it, nor can see it, and I have not touched it since then. That is, this happened in 1990. I can tell you for sure. Liubomira Iusekchieva.

References

Baeva, Vihra. 1997. "Lichni razkazi za chudesa—mezhdu vsekidnevnoto i sacralnoto [Personal narratives of miracles—between everyday life and the sacred]." *Bălgarski folklor* 5–6: 59–71.

—. 2000a. "'Zlatnata iabalka' v Gorni Voden—izmereniiata na praznika ['The golden apple' in Gorni Voden—the dimensions of a holiday]." *Bălgarski folklor* 2: 26–36.

—. 2000b. "The Charismatic Figure in the Context of Popular Christianity—Two Possible Patterns." In *Bulgarian Studies at the Dawn of 21st Century: a Bulgarian–American Perspective*, edited by Anisava Miltenova, 138–46. Sofia: IK Gutenberg.

—. 2001. "Poklonnicheskoto patuvane—pogled otvatre [The pilgrimage—a look from inside]." In *Ritsari i mirotvortsi na Balkanite. Pohodi, preseleniia i poklonnichestvo* [Knights and peace-makers on the Balkans. Conquests, pilgrimage and migrations], edited by Snezhana Dimitrova, and Elena Tacheva, 136–42. Blagoevgrad: Mezhdunaroden balkanistichen seminar.

—. 2008. "Pravoslavniiat hram kato myasto za iztselenie v savremennostta [The orthodox shrine as a healing place in the present days]." In *Etnologiia na prostranstvoto* 1. [Ethnology of space], edited by Rosen Rosenov Malčev, 192–203. Sofia: ROD.

Brown, Peter. 1982. *The Cult of the Saints. Its Rise and Function in Latin Christianity*. Chicago: The University of Chicago Press.

Eliade, Mircea. 1996. *Shamanizmat i arhaichnite tehniki na ekstaza.* Translated by Todorka Mineva. Sofia: Lik Publishing House. [Le chamanisme et les techniques archaïques de l'extase. Paris, Payot, 1951.]

Franz, Marie-Louise von. 1978. "The Process of Individuation." In Jung, C. G. et al. *Man and His Symbols*, 157–254. London: Picador Pan Books Ltd. [1964]

Georgieva, Albena. 2008. "'Miraculous Healing' as a Process of Integration." In *Macedonian Folklore. Papers from the 16th International Symposium for Balkan Folklore: "The Folklore and the Common Cultural Values on the Balkans"* 65: 87–94.

Ivanov, Petko. 1992. "Folklorat i hristiianstvoto kato duhovni formi na zhivot [Folklore and Christianity as spiritual forms of living]." In *Obshtuvane s teksta. Sbornik s teoreticheski statii i eseta* [Communication with the text. A collection of theoretical articles and essays], edited by Angel Angelov, and Alexander Kiosev, 261–97. Sofia: Universitetsko Izdatelstvo "Sv. Kliment Ohridski."

Jung, Carl Gustav. 1978. "Approaching the Unconscious." In Jung, C. G. et. al. *Man and His Symbols*, 1–94. London: Picador Pan Books Ltd. [1964]

Le Goff, Jacques. 1998. *Vaobrazhaemiiat sviat na Srednovekovieto.* Translated into Bulgarian by Elka Rousseva. Sofia: Agata Publishing House. [L'Imaginaire médiéval. Essais. Paris: Gallimard, 1985]

Marinov, Dimităr. 1914. "*Narodna viara i religiozni narodni obichai* [Folk belief and religious folk customs]." *Sbornik za narodni umotvoreniia i narodopis* 28.

Valtchinova, Galina. 2005. "Svetetsat i traktovkata na ludostta v traditsionnata kultura [Christian saints and the treatment of "madness" in traditional Balkan orthodox cultures]." *Bălgarska etnologiia* 2: 5–17.

—. 2009. "Introduction: Ethno-Graphing 'Divine Intervention'." *History and Anthropology. Special Issue: Ethnographies of "Divine Interventions" in Europe* 20/3 (September): 203–18.

4. HEALING METHODS, MEDICAMENTS

AN ATTEMPT TO IDENTIFY HOMER'S "MOLY" AS MANDRAKE

NORA ZERGI

There is a miraculous and unidentified plant in Greek literature called the "moly". It makes its first appearance in Homer's *Odyssey*, and although it next surfaces only a few centuries later, in Theophrastus, after that it goes on to a great career in later medical-botanical literature. Identifying antique references to plants is always a great challenge, but the possibilities of such studies are often very limited. Many scholars have tried to pin down the *moly*, and the fact that heretofore about twenty different species have been suggested as a solution shows that something must be confused in the tradition. While I am convinced that the question ultimately cannot be settled beyond doubt, for pharmacodynamical reasons I would like to make a case for two plants out of all those 20.

Why two? To answer that, let me quote the passage in the *Odyssey* already referred to:

> So saying, Argeiphontes gave me the herb, drawing
> it from the ground, and showed me its nature. At the root it
> was black, but its flower was like milk. Moly the gods call it,
> and it is hard for mortal men to dig; but with the gods all
> things are possible (Odyssey, X. 304–6).

Here we learn the following about the plant: its flower is white, its root black, and "it is hard for mortal men to dig". In Sanskrit, *mūla*, from which *moly* is said to derive, means "root", suggesting that the culture naming the plant thus perceived its root to be distinctively important. If a plant is difficult to dig up due to its often-branching roots or the depth to which some of these go down, naming the plant after such a distinctive feature could easily be justified.

A related image often recurs in medieval medical-botanical manuscripts: Hermes is depicted with a plant in his hand, in the company of Homer, in some versions a doctor standing between them. The texts identify the plant as *herba immolum*, which clearly contains *moly*.

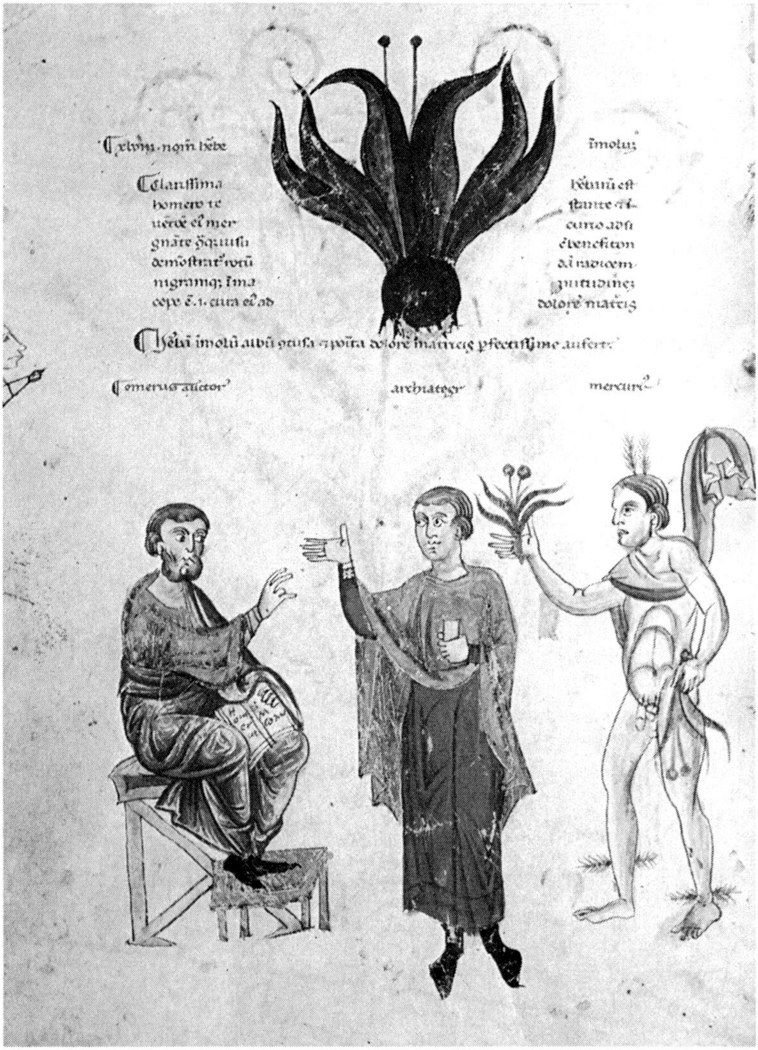

Homer, a doctor and Hermes with *moly* in his hand. "Medicina Antiqua", in *Codex Vindobonensis* 93, 61v. Österreichisches Nationalbibliothek. http://commons.wikimedia.org/wiki/File:Kraut_Moly_und_Allegorie.jpg, accessed: 16.04.2010.

Although these depictions have their own interesting elements, in this paper I will only concentrate on the plant, because some details might appear not to match. Its flower is not white—indeed it seems to be more a cluster of berries, and not a flower at all (disregard for a moment how one is biologically related to the other). We do not actually see the roots, so we do not know their colour or shape. If it was not Hermes and Homer in whose company the plant appears, we might not even think of the plant being the *moly*. And this leads to a further question: are Homer's *moly* and the medieval *herba immolum* the same plant?

To avoid long and boring excurses, the answer is no. The key to this "no" comes roughly midway between Homer and the Middle Ages, in the works of Dioscorides and Galen. Dioscorides' work, *De materia medica* dates from the first century AD, and includes the passage:

> Some call peganon agrion what in Cappadocia and in Asian Galatia is said to be moly.

Dioscorides is here writing about *peganon agrion*, but in the list of its other names he mentions that in Cappadocia they call the plant *moly*. He then goes on to write a separate passage about *moly*:

> moly—its leaves are similar to agrostis, … the flowers resembling leukoion, milky-coloured, … the root is small, bulb-like.

About two centuries later, we read the following in Galen:

> Moly. Some call it peganon agrion, others harmala, the Syrians besasa, while the Cappadocians moly, since its root is black and it has a milk-like flower.

Here it is apparent that for Galen the two plants *moly* and *peganon agrion* are identical. Since for centuries his writings constituted the Bible of medical learning, and since, in the descriptions, botanical details were not exactly prominent, due to this identification by the early Middle Ages *moly* and *peganon agrion* had merged irrevocably.

This plant we can much more easily identify in terms of modern taxonomy: the *moly* or *herba immolum* of the medieval codices is very probably the plant *Peganum harmala*. The shape and flower (or berries) of this plant show appropriate similarity to what we saw in Hermes' hand. *Peganum harmala L.* is known to be an antidepressant and an anxiolytic, but consumption of its seeds can also lead to psychedelic experiences. To this day, it is often used recreationally or as a part of religious rituals. In other words, it is a plant worthy of a god. It is even more suggestive that it is native to Asia Minor, has a white flower and a large lateral root system that would indeed make it "hard for mortal men to dig".

But one solid reason why I do not think we can claim to have solved the age-old riddle is the near millennium that elapsed between Homer and Dioscorides, during which no identification with *peganon* arose. Another reason is that the effects just outlined do not fit the Homeric story. Let us recap in a few words what happened before Circe turned Odysseus' companions into swine by a so-called *kykeon (κυκεών)*:

> She brought them in and made them sit on chairs and seats, and made for them a potion of cheese and barley meal and yellow honey with Pramnian wine; but in the food she mixed baneful drugs, that they might utterly forget their native land (Odyssey, X. 233–6).

It is here that I would like to propose a theory, bringing another magical substance, toxic honey into the picture. In Greek, it is referred to as *meli chloron* or meli *mainomenon*, and for its hallucinogenic properties it was popular among priests, priestesses, mages and all sorts of witches. Its active substance, grayanotoxin, can easily be identified, and the symptoms of poisoning can be relieved with atropine. This antidote, in turn, can be found in large quantities in the plants of the nightshade family (*Solanaceae*), including mandrake (*Mandragora officinalis L.*), deadly nightshade (*Atropa belladonna L.*) and jimsonweed (*Datura stramonium L.*).

Mandrake is a widely known and popular magical plant. Most people know the legends about it, including how difficult it is to dig up. Its flowers are white, its root brown and branching. If the *kykeon* mixed by Circe contained toxic honey, thus inducing confusion and delusions, this could have been treated with the atropine from the mandrake, the antidote to grayanotoxin. I do not wish to demythicise the story and tie down its references to measurable empirical reality: nevertheless, it is, I think, a remarkable reference—did the Homeric Greeks observe how the effects of these two well-known magical substances cancel each other out? Further research can possibly offer some answers, but my examination of the extensive corpus of antique and medieval medical texts about *moly* and mandrake has not yet unearthed any apparent awareness of a connection.

As I noted earlier, more than twenty different species have been put forward by scholars as more or less likely candidates for being the mysterious Homeric *moly*. My examination has not singled out any of them conclusively, but it is perhaps safe to say that the *moly* of the medieval lexicons (*herba immolum*) can be identified with *Peganum harmala* on the basis of most of its descriptions and most of its depictions as well. However, if in the Homeric story we keep in mind the effect of the magic plant, it seems more appropriate to identify the *moly* with the well-known mandrake.

Biologically uneducated lay people even today relate plants to each other (and use the same name to refer to them) based on the plants' external characteristics. This might help explain the merger of biologically different species in antique and medieval botany. If we want to untangle such identifications and mergers, we need to pay very close attention not only to the description of the plant, in the hope of learning sufficient details for exact taxonomical placement, but also to what the text says the plant does: in this way we can gain additional information that could possibly make our work easier.

References

Boisacq, Émile. 1938. *Dictionnaire étymologique de la langue grecque*. Heidelberg: C. Winter.

Dioscorides. 2008. *De materia medica*. Irvine: Thesaurus Linguae Graecae Digital Library.

Galen. 2008. *De simplicium medicamentorum*. Irvine: Thesaurus Linguae Graecae Digital Library.

Homer. 1995. *The Odyssey*. Translated by A. T. Murray. Cambridge: Harvard University Press.

Koca, I., and A. F. Koca. 2007. "Poisoning by mad honey: A brief review." *Food and Chemical Toxicology* 45: 1315–8.

Stirling, János. 1995–1997. *Lexicon nominum herbarum arborum fruticumque linguae latinae I-IV*. Budapest: Enciklopédia.

Sütlüpinar, N., A. Mat, and Y. Satganolu. 1993. "Poisoning by toxic honey in Turkey." *Archives of Toxicology* 67: 148–50.

TELESMA AND STOICHEION: MAGICAL STATUES IN BYZANTIUM

ANNA JUDIT TÓTH

I.

Statues and their extraordinary abilities were favourite themes in Byzantine folklore, the motif frequently occurring in Byzantine literature as well as in modern folklore. Although many elements of Greek folk beliefs are derived from ancient religion, this is an exceptional case, where we have reports on each step of the development and can gain an insight into the dynamics of survival. One of the first reports on magical statues comes from the chronicle of John Malalas. We can read the following description in Book 10 of this work:[1]

> There lived and flourished in the time of the reign of Domitian the most learned Apollonius of Tyana who travelled round making talismans everywhere in the cities and their territories. He went from Rome and came to Byzantion. On entering Byzoupolis, which is now felicitously known as Constantinople, he made many talismans there too at the request of the Byzantines, one for the storks, one for the river Lykos which runs

---

[1] The research leading to these results has received funding from the European Research Council under the European Union's Seventh Framework Programme (FP7/2007–2013) / ERC grant agreement № 324214. Malalas was a Greek chronicler of Syrian origin who lived in Antioch in the sixth century; he wrote the first extant world chronicle in which he discusses history since the creation of the world until the events of his age, that is, until the reign of Emperor Justinian I. Only the last four books of the lengthy eighteen book-long chronicle are considered to have a source value; in the previous books the chronicler basically gathered rationalised myths and anachronistic historic legends. Among them is a garland of stories in which he describes with a unique elaboration a magical technique practised with the help of statues. Modern edition of the chronicle: Thurn 2000. I reference the chapter numbers of this edition, while also giving the page references of the Bonn edition (Dindorf 1831). Source of the English translation: Jeffreys 1986.

> through the middle of the city, one for horses, as well as other miraculous things. Then Apollonius left Byzantion and made talismans in other cities. He came to Syria from Tyana and entered Antioch the Great. The Antiochene landowners asked him to make talismans there to satisfy their needs. He made one talisman against the north wind, putting this talisman at the east gate. Likewise, he made a talisman in the city against scorpions, so that they should not dare approach the region. He placed this talisman in the middle of the city, making a bronze scorpion and burying it and setting a small column over it—and the scorpions vanished from the entire neighbourhood of Antioch. He made many other things there. The citizens asked him to make a talisman against mosquitoes, so that the city of Antioch should not have them anymore. He did so, by telling them to celebrate in Antioch of Syria on the 7th Daisios-June the chariot-races known as Graste's, during the month of Daisios. But he set up the talisman at the new moon of the month Daisios, and told them that on the seventh day of the same month, the day of the chariot-races of Graste, they were all to carry on canes small busts of solid lead with the features of Ares and a shield of red leather hanging down on one side, and on the other a red dagger equally hanging, both tied up with a linen thread. He told them to chant as they paraded, saying, "No mosquitoes in the city!" and after the end of the chariot-races everyone was to put the talisman in his own house. And there was not a single mosquito to be seen in Antioch the Great (Malalas X.51, 263–5).

The word translated as talisman is *telesma* in the Greek text, which was used in the modern sense of the word in late antiquity and Byzantium, although it usually referred to large-scale statues in public spaces. Apollonius was considered to be the creator of the most famous *telesma*s in Byzantium, but we also hear of other sorcerers. According to Chapter XIII.52 in Malalas, Apollonius of Tyana renovated an earlier *telesma*: the citizens of Antioch led the sorcerer to a small porphyry column, erected in the time of Caesar by a certain Debborius, a philosopher and *telestes* (ibid., X.52, 266), in order to protect the city from earthquakes. The talisman was damaged by the "fire of Typhon", presumably by lightning, thus the city's notabilities were afraid it had lost its protective powers. At their demand, Apollonius erected a new talisman. According to X.9, the sorcerer Ablakon hid under the statue of Tiberius a chest in which he had placed a talisman, which was supposed to protect Antioch from floods. In Chapter XIII.3 we can read about a bronze statue of Poseidon, a talisman against earthquakes, discovered by the citizens during construction work, which they melted and transformed into the statue of Constantine. Although Malalas does not call it a *telesma*, we do however see justified mention here of the statue in Chapter VIII.21: during an epidemic, the philosopher Leius instructed the people of Antioch to carve a face which would end the epidemic into a cliff on the mountain.

Malalas is not the only one who writes about the activities of the talisman-making Apollonius of Tyana, although his description is the most detailed. From a historical point of view, the legend is not authentic; the life and deeds of Apollonius of Tyana, the Neo-Pythagorean philosopher who lived in the first century AD, is known from much earlier and better sources which ignore the talismans.[2] While numerous sources of the Byzantine era already mention the *telesma*, their tradition lived on in the times of the Arabs and the Turks. Several other sources prove that by the end of antiquity they had attempted to "charm" statues in practice as well.

The character of the ancient cities was determined by a great number of statues: effigies of gods and statesmen. This was also the case with Constantinople. Built by Constantine to be the capital of Christianity, he ensured that it would not be overshadowed by the splendour of the ancient Eastern metropolises, and so he had ancient monuments of Hellas transported in quantities to Constantinople. These statues, either depicting gods, or immortalising profane themes, were inherently related to the pagan past; however, they were not damaged even after pagan cults had been banned. As C. Mango revealed, statue demolition for religious reasons did not exist in Byzantium (Mango 1963, 58). On the contrary, we even find examples of an originally pagan statue reinterpreted and considered as a Christian monument.[3] Meanwhile, the advancement of

[2] Apollonius of Tyana was a well-known Neo-Pythagorean philosopher from the first century: for more about him, see: Dzielska (1986, 99) and Duliere (1970). Byzantine and Arabian folklore remember him mostly as a sorcerer; several sources testify to the talismans he allegedly made, e.g. Chronicon Paschale 467.; Ps-Iustinus: *Quaest et resp.* 24.; Cedrenus 346, 432; Hesychius 25; Nicetas Choniates 861. Since these are late sources, their authenticity is surely questionable (Dzielska 1986, 100–2).

[3] Example of Mango (1963): *Patria* II. 47: here they mention an equestrian statue which certain people think is of Joshua, others believe it is of Bellerophontes. We find a similar example in Malalas' story: IV.9. 78–9, in which Constantine the Great recognises Saint Michael in a statue near Byzantium associated by the local people with the Argonauts, and thus the artefact is dedicated to the archangel. We know of this statue from other sources that it depicts Attis; on the association of Attis with Saint Michael, see Mango 1984. The situation is similar in the West, in Rome, where the equestrian statue of Marcus Aurelius is also considered to be that of Constantine. It is a question whether it is always a matter of oblivion, or, by "administrative means", it was possible to attribute a statue to another person, or as a pagan temple such as the Pantheon, which due to its convenient layout could be

Christianity introduced basic aesthetic changes: the Christian churches, at least in the East, completely lacked statues; portrayal became essentially two dimensional, the statues related to idolatry were replaced by icons, while monumental sculpture played only a negligible role in Byzantine art. It is no wonder that from then on people were suspicious of statues. The sinister aura surrounding these sculptures was further enhanced by another circumstance: the populous metropolises of the Eastern Roman Empire weathered the storms of migration, which resulted in a population which already included Christian citizens living their everyday lives among the artefacts of a dead culture, thus it is not surprising that more and more superstitious beliefs were related to the statues of gods no longer worshipped and to those of forgotten warlords.

Some of these stories are about statues manifesting spontaneous vital signs; others claim it was with the intervention of a sorcerer that they acquired magical powers. Among the latter, the legends of Apollonius of Tyana form a well-defined cluster. The stork and the turtle of Constantinople are well known, and the existence of the statues of Antioch mentioned by Malalas is also confirmed by other sources. Obviously, no one wished to actually protect their homes against storks, turtles or horses; the sources for the legend were clearly some of the peculiar animal statues of the city of Byzantium, the function of which the urban folklore wished to explain. We know for certain that there was a Stork Street in Constantinople, which was named after three stone storks facing in three different directions which most probably were believed by the locals to work as talismans. The dangerousness of the storks was explained in their dropping venomous snakes into the wells, thus poisoning the water (Polites 1920, 52, Hesychius: *Patria Konstantinupoleos* 25). We also know that the statue of the turtle used to walk away during the night-time, and consume all the debris (Moffatt 1990, 107). The statue of the scorpion was buried by Apollonius, because objects with a magical purpose, such as voodoo dolls and curse tablets, were usually hidden, e.g. buried in graves. As will be seen from later examples, statues appearing from underground thus caused twice as big a fright.

Many similar stories are known from other authors. Zosimus (*floruit* 490–510) writes about a sorcerer called Nestorius who transformed the statue of Achilles at the Acropolis of Athens into a talisman against earthquakes (Zosimus IV.18). Olympiodorus of Thebes (*floruit* 412–425) claims that the city of Rhegium was protected by an "ἄγαλμα τετελεσμένον"

---

consecrated as a Christian church. On the Byzantine approach to statues, see Dawkins 1924, Guberti Bassett 1991 and 1996, Saradi 2000.

against the fire of Etna and against the barbarian troops attacking from the coast; in one foot of the statue would have been a "never sleeping fire", in the other "incorruptible water" (Dodds 1947, 65; Olympiodorus 261). He tells a similar story with an opposite meaning from the time of Constantine (Olympiodorus 268), when they found silver statues in Thrace, at a place which was looked upon by the locals as an ancient shrine. The statues faced north and wore barbaric clothes. Problems began with the finding and the digging up of the statues: a few days later the Goths broke into Thrace, then a little later so did the Huns, and then the Sarmatians, for since there were three statues, they could expect three enemies.

If we consider the above-mentioned features as the basic characteristics of a talisman, we have to add one more item to the list: the Palladium of Troy. According to the twelfth chapter of the fifth book of Malalas, the Palladium protecting Troy was also a kind of talisman. The aim of this mythical statuette was always to provide magical protection to the city it was currently kept in. According to the myth, the image was stolen from Troy by Odysseus and Diomedes. In historic times, numerous Greek cities claimed to have kept Athena's original *xoanon* within their walls. The Romans believed that it was Aeneas himself who saved the statue from the demolished city, or that he received it from Diomedes: in any case the statue was kept at the Temple of Vesta and was treated as the token of perpetuity of the city. The Byzantines unequivocally considered the statue to be a talisman, comparable to those made by Apollonius. Malalas and Cedrenus believed it to be the creation of a philosopher called Asius, and called it by the same names as the creations of the philosopher from Tyana: *telesma, stoicheion* and *zodion* (Malalas V.12, 108, the entry *Palladion* in the Suda encyclopedia and the analogous Cedrenus's text (I.229.) depend on this text). The ancient statue did not interest them for its Roman references, and from the sixth century on it was increasingly common to think that this *xoanon* ensured the magical protection of Constantinople as well. According to the authors (*Patria* II. 45; Mal. XIII.7. 320, Procopius *Bella* V. 15.14), Constantine the Great, when founding the capital, brought the Palladium from Rome and placed it in the Forum hidden under a column supporting his own statue.[4] This procedure had nothing to do with the respect the Romans paid the statuette; it was instead following the procedure of the magician of Antioch, who buried his talismans *under* statues and columns, underground.

---

[4] This is the statue of Constantine, which might have portrayed the emperor as Helius.

The assessment of magical statues was more hostile among contemporary ecclesiastical authors than laymen. It is not impossible that this hostility against statues in Byzantine art, and in the domain of Orthodoxy in general, was not only targeting avoidance of the sin of idolatry, but also stemmed from the fear of being exposed to the effects of the statues' magical powers; the clergy was well aware that "the believers" had an unquenchable desire for magic, so often chastised by the Church Fathers. Although we do know of cases where magic was used in front of icons, it is less common.[5] The fact itself that the talismans worked was never doubted, even by Christians. Justinus posed the question[6] of how God could have allowed the pagan talismans to continue to function. He reached the conclusion that it was obviously for their subservience and expedience, because when one of the statues demanded loudly that Apollonius should be respected as a god, he silenced it. According to other authors, these talismans had no power whatsoever in the Christian era, yet still the people tenaciously believed in them (Ioannes Chrysostomus 490, 886).

We also find a great number of magical statues from later ages. A great part of these sources are compilations based on earlier works, e.g. the chronicle of Malalas, but we have clear evidence that the belief in *telesma*s did not turn into lifeless antiquarian data. (The Malalas text is cited in the Chronicon Paschale (467), it was known by Tzetzes (Tzetzes: *Chiliades* II.60, 925); Cedrenus 346, 432; Nicetas Choniates 861; *Suda* sv.; Palladion; Zosimus 4.18). After the Dark Ages of the Arab-Byzantine wars and the Iconoclast movement, the older term used for magic statues was replaced by a new word: *stoicheion*. Authors knew and understood the word *telesma* as well, but they used it only when citing their source (Blum 1946, 317). From the middle byzantine period our most valuable sources, along with the chronicles and antiquarian works (e.g. the *Suda* lexicon),

[5] An example could be in the *Vita S. Andreae Sali* (Nicephorus Presbyter 776c–781b), where a woman allows the magician to do magic in front of her icons, which thus lose all their actual powers, basically their character of an icon.

[6] Ps-Iustinus Quaest. et resp. 24. This text can be dated to the end of the fourth century, so it is the earlier source of Apollonius' *telesma*s. According to Speyer (1974, 56) the texts portraying Apollonius in a positive light should be retraceable to pagan texts. I am not convinced of that. I find the opinion of M. Dzielska (1986, 99) more plausible; he says that the Church fathers had an ambivalent attitude towards the magician, even those who disapproved (for example: Isidorus of Pelusium 405b) could not deny admitting some of his positive features. Anastasius Sinaites (*Quaest. et Resp.* XXIV, 524) writes less understandingly about talismans.

are the representatives of the *Patria* genre,[7] which, as a broadly defined travelogue listing and describing the main sights of Constantinople, contain a remarkably large amount of data on magical statues. Among them we can find new types: statues that were possessed by demons. These statues often manifest vital signs completely spontaneously, without any magical manipulation. This was not characteristic of the Apollonius stories.

According to one story, when they removed the "Hellenic"—meaning pagan in contemporary vocabulary—statue of Phidalia from Constantinople, the region was shaken by an earthquake, which could only be appeased by a procession led by the emperor (*Parastaseis* 4; *Patria* II. 86). The command of precaution was not to remove any old statue, because it might cause trouble. In the Suda encyclopedia, the entry *kynegion* also warns that one must respect and be cautious of ancient statues, especially if they are pagan. According to the story in the Patria collection, the reader Theodorus and Himerius *chartularius* went to the Kynegion to peruse the ancient statues. While they were discussing the history of the place, one of the seemingly stable statues fell and struck Himerius dead. Theodorus, scared to death, fled to a church, and reported the incident. The relatives of the deceased, the representatives of the emperor and a certain "philosopher" called Ioannes arrived at the scene; interpreting the incident based on the documents of Demokritus, the latter established that the man had been killed by the statue, that is, the *zodion*. On the philosopher's advice, the emperor buried the statue (*Suda*, *kynegion* entry; *Patria* II. 27).[8]

In this story, magic plays a passive role: a spirit or some kind of negative energy possesses the statue, which causes unpleasantness to the people; the spirit has to be conciliated or exorcised. In other cases, the statues were used quite consciously for magical purposes. By means of sympathetic magic, just as a wax doll can replace the target person, a statue can also be identified with a person or even an entire population. In these stories, the magic is quite active indeed. The method was known by early Byzantine authors, but where the source of the magic was a pagan

---

[7] *Patria* was a late Antique and medieval genre, which described the sights and legends of one city. We know of the existence of several such works, however, only the ones relating to Constantinople remained in our age. On the literature of *Patria Konstantinupoleos,* see Dagron 1984; Cameron and Herrin 1984; Berger 1987; Berger 1988. Edition of the related texts: Preger 1901.

[8] Although it seems inconsistent with Democritus' materialist atom theory to refer to him as a professional magical authority, there is a serious tradition of presenting Democritus as a magician, cf. Vakaloudi 2000b, 125; Diogenes Laertius IX. 9.38.

sorcerer, Christians intervened unwillingly e.g. by finding buried statues. In the texts of the middle byzantine period, the situation changes. In the *Patria* we can read about Michael I Rhangabe, who had the arms of the Tyche statue (i.e. the statue of Fortuna) cut off in Constantinople, thus paralysing Destiny, in order to prevent it from giving power to the rebels of the circus factions, instead of the emperor (*Patria* II. 101).

In another story, the one who performed the magical ritual was the patriarch himself, John VII of Constantinople, or John Grammaticus, an iconoclast patriarch (834–843). Several chronicles have noted that once a great barbarian army led by three chieftains attacked Constantinople (Theophanes Continuatus 155; Cedrenus II. 145, 308; for more on this, see also Brehier 1904). The patriarch led his people to the hippodrome, where there was a three-headed statue. With proper incantations he magically "tied" the three barbarian chiefs to the heads of the statue, and ordered all three heads to be cut off. They successfully managed to get rid of two out of the three, and as a result, two chiefs died suddenly. Only the third chief managed to reach the capital with his dwindled army.[9]

Nicetas Choniates talks about the statues of two women in the Forum, known in the twelfth century as the Roman Woman and the Hungarian Woman. When the statue of the Roman Woman unexpectedly fell, Manuel I Comnenus immediately had the statue of the Hungarian Woman knocked down so that it would not become a bad omen for the Romans, i.e. the Byzantines (Theophanes Continuatus 196.) The crusaders breaking into Constantinople also demolished a great number of statues, not least for fear of magic. They found a buried statue in the hippodrome which seemed to be depicting a Bulgarian. They melted the statue, fearing that someone might use it against them (Nicetas Choniates 848).

The belief in the *telesma*s was not limited to Greek antiquity and Byzantium. The Arabs adopted the legendarium of Apollonius, calling him Balīnās, and they assigned to him the creation of even more talismans in the Middle Eastern and Central Eastern cities than had the Greeks (Dzielska 1986, 77 and 112). During the Arabian expansion and the Islamisation of the bigger Byzantine cities, they inevitably adopted and sustained the local beliefs related to these cities. The statues appear among

[9] Cedrenus tells analogical stories (II. 38.), but here the magician who protects the city from the Bulgarians is an "*astronomos*", i.e. an astrologist called Ioannes, and not a cleric. When they were fearing the attack of Tsar Simeon, the *astronomus* Ioannes went to see the emperor, and encouraged him to sever the head of a certain statue, because he had previously tied it to Simeon with magic (he uses the verb *stoicheioo*, which cannot be properly translated in this context), and thus beheading the statue would cause the death of the Bulgarian.

the Arabs, imbued with other functions, for instance, as guardians of treasures.[10] The term and idea of *telesma* became part of the Arab folklore and magic in the form of *tellestim*.[11] The "magic books" attributed to Apollonius were translated into Arabic and new ones were written.

The belief in *telesma*s appears in the West as well, although much more sporadically than in Byzantium. Our earliest data might suggest that belief in the urban *telesma* statues was common in the East and in the West. This is implied in the documents of Gregory of Tours (538–594), according to whom in old Paris the rituals of the old times kept fire hazards and snakes away: it transpires from an incident involving the cleaning of a bridge when bronze statues of the animal in question were removed, that it reappeared in the city after the removal of these statues (Gregory of Tours VIII. 3).

However, the great cities of antiquity, along with their statues, had disappeared in the West by the Middle Ages, and so the *telesma* beliefs had to be rediscovered during the High Middle Ages, partly through direct interaction with the Arabs and the Byzantines, and partly through the books on talisman magic translated from Arabic (a summary of Western talisman magic was made by Láng 2007, 62–82). In Italy the belief may have been continuous.[12] The third way of transferring this tradition

[10] We hardly find any examples for this function in Latin and Greek literature, while in Arabian folklore it is quite common and it can be traced back to Egypt in the age of the Pharaohs, thus this story-type was basically associated with the Nile region and possibly points out the land of origin of magical statues where the tradition of a belief in animated statues goes back thousands of years. The Arabian traditions claimed that the guardian of the pyramid of Chefren was a granite idol, with a spear in his hand and a snake lying on his head, so that if someone was approaching, it would precipitate itself upon and kill that person. The guardian of the pyramid of Cheops was a sitting idol holding a spear, with flashing eyes, who eliminated intruders with his voice—these descriptions were presumably inspired by statues of Pharaohs (Fodor 1971, 133). Another version claims that the spirit of the pyramid of Cheops was a naked, yellow, beardless young man with enormous canines, the one of Chefren was a beautiful naked woman, and the one of Menkaure was an old man with a basket and some incense in his hands (Fodor 1971, 134). The Arabian authors refer to the "Coptic writings" as the source of these stories, and the origin of the legends does indeed go back a very long time; the Sphinx was already considered to be the guardian of the cemetery of Giza in the times of the Pharaohs (Fodor 1971, 132).

[11] Garnett and Stuart-Glennie 1896, 390: the oriental *tellestim,* similar to its modern Greek counterparts, belongs to a building.

[12] We know of a number of stories in which popular imagery invested a building or statue of the city with apotropaic powers: the protection of Naples was ensured by Virgil himself; that of Florence was ensured by their Mars temple, and by the

happened purely *via* Christian authors: the Church Fathers of antiquity had known the *telesma* statues, which were not only important to the uneducated people, as the Neo-Platonist philosophers also firmly believed in them. This explains how animated statues could have occurred in the *Civitate Dei* of Augustine (VIII.23), and how Saint Thomas Aquinas had also known of them (*Contra Gentiles* 3.105).

In Greece, the idea of *stoicheion* lived on even after the Osmanic conquest. In Neo-Greek folklore, *stoicheion*, or as they pronounce it today, *stichio* means household patron spirit, according to Richard and Eva Blum (Blum and Blum 1970. footnote 1: "*stichi (from stoicheion spirit) refers to ghosts and to the protective house spirits*"). It is a common belief throughout the entire country. In Santorini, they had a custom of burying a rooster or some other animal in the foundation of the house, which thus became the household's "*stichio*" (Blum and Blum 1970, 303). According to Ch. Stewart "στοιχειόμενο" = "positively haunted" (Stewart 1991, 103). Each place has its own *stoicheion*: houses, bridges, trees, fountains, rivers. There is an interesting distinction which is a modern linguistic development: στοιχείο = element, στοιχειό = spirit (Stewart 1991, 267). This new type of *stoicheion* became common in the post-Byzantine era: nonetheless, there already exist unequivocal sources confirming its existence in Byzantium. In the fourteenth century, Joseph Bryennius mentions the belief in the Nereides and *stoicheions* controlling certain places among popular superstitions, and he also describes how people

astrological constellation during which the temple was built under the rule of Augustus. Certain venturous persons even felt like putting this magic into practice. Guido Bonatto, who also attempted to reconcile the Guelphs and the Ghibellines of his city with the help of astrology, wanted to make the city invincible by burying a statue of a horse made of metal or stone with magic powers (Burckhardt 1878, 270; Weinreich 1909, 165). While the legends concerning the passive and immobile Byzantine *telesma*s referred to existing statues, the mobile Egyptian and Arabian guardians of treasures fall into the realm of fables. Nonetheless, their parallels can be found in the West as well. According to a legend from the twelfth century, Virgil, who was considered to be a magician in the Middle Ages, built a palace in which they placed the symbolic statues of the peoples conquered by the Romans, holding a bell. If one of these peoples were organising an uprising, their statue rang the bell, and the bronze soldier standing atop of the palace raised his spear in the direction of that rebel territory (Fodor 1971, 138; Comparetti 1875, 259). Pope John XXII prohibited the enclosure of demons into images or other objects: Dodds 1947, 64.

offered sacrifices to the *stoicheion* of the house.[13] Leo Allatius uses the word in the same sense in the seventeenth century when he describes these spirits in his work *De quorundam Graecorum opinationibus* (Allatius 1645, cap. XXI). Between the two phases—the earlier, dangerous demon and the modern, benevolent guardian spirit—a transitional phase must have existed, traces of which can be found in the texts of Greek ballads. The motif of the walled-up wife is widespread in South East European folklore (Megas 1976; Oikonomides 1981): in the Greek versions, the builders offer a foundation sacrifice in order to accomplish the building of a bridge. In many cases, the advice was given by a dragon and/or the spirit of the river, the *stoicheion* (Megas 1976, 11, 74–77 identifies the dragon and the river-spirit), and the victim will be the *stoicheion* of the new bridge (Spyridakes 1962, 319–325; Megas 1976, 21–105; Garnett and Stuart-Glennie 1896, 70–73).[14]

II.

We can establish at least three phases in our sources: the word *telesma* was replaced by *stoicheion*, first in the meaning of magical statue, later in that of natural spirit. The words *stoicheion* and *telesma* appear to be synonyms at first sight, and different authors use them when describing the same story. Nonetheless, each individual author uses only the one of them. Moreover, until the sixth century only *telesma* was used, while later we primarily find the denomination *stoicheion*.[15] The semantic field of the word *stoicheion*, according to my observations, is unequivocally broader: it is used to denote any statue having a magical effect; the *telesma*, on the other hand, is indeed a talisman: it holds apotropaic powers, and it serves to fend off potential dangers that might occur in the future. The *telesma*

[13] Oeconomos 1930, 227 published the short text in its entirety. Blum (1947, 323) mentions an even earlier example from a 14th century manuscript of the poem Digenes Akritas.

[14] The motivation for the sacrifice is multiple in the texts. According to Lawson (1910, 262) and Oikonomides (1981, 53), the original aim of the ritual was to propitiate the spirits. Politis (1871, 138) claimed that the wife's transformation into a *stoicheion* was the original version. All of them make a common mistake in assuming that the foundation sacrifice was a rite known in Greek and Roman antiquity (Polites 1871, 138; Megas 1976, 13; Oikonomides 1981, 54; Tóth 2010). Every source on Greek human sacrifice seems to be fictional (Hughes 1991, 73–78), and even these myths and anecdotes lack any trace of foundation sacrifice.

[15] According to Dzielska, its earliest occurrence is dated in the middle of the seventh century (Dzielska 1986, 103; cf. Blum, C. 1946, 322).

stories are schematic, the magic of the *stoicheion* having a more complex character. Considering that both of them were based on the manipulation of statues, we have to pose the question whether they derived somehow from the statue cult in Greek religion. The answer is no. It is true that in ancient Greece, the god and its statue were not separated from one another; in the vase paintings, instead of its statue, they portrayed the god itself, while they did not expect the statues to prove their specialness by manifesting signs of life[16] (e.g. by weeping, moving, laughing or healing illnesses). Two major monographs, the books of Faraone and Tarn Steiner (Faraone 1992 and Tarn Steiner 2001), have recently been written on the statue–religion–magic relationship in Greek culture. Neither of them found new evidence of the consecration of cult statues or animated cult statues; their examples come from myth or Late Antique theurgy. The essential Greek cultic object was the altar, not the cult statue. Greek theology provided no explanation for the character of the connection between a god and his statue. The idea that a large public statue might possess magical powers is undoubtedly a Late Antique and Byzantine development. Nonetheless, magic dolls were already known to the Greeks. While harmful wax dolls could not have survived over thousands of years, 38 dolls made of durable material have been discovered (Ogden 1997, 24). They cannot be confused with toy dolls or other dolls of cultic function: they were often hidden in graves placed in a coffin-like lead or ceramic box; some had curses written on them, or the name of the person they were supposed to bewitch, their hands were tied behind them and often their body was twisted and their head and limbs contorted (Ogden 1997, 24; on the further use of wax dolls, see Faraone 1989; Faraone 1991). They were called *kolossos*, which is identical to our word colossus. Willamowitz recognised that *kolossos* referred to any statue portraying a person, regardless of the size, and it was not until the first century BC that it gained its present meaning (Willamowitz-Moellendorf 1927).[17] In certain cases, the data suggest that they were not used in malicious, legally and

---

[16] A substantial number of examples was assembled by Otto Weinreich 1909, 146. His examples are all from the Age of Emperors, and from Roman times; in Rome, contrary to the Greeks, the observation of holy objects had a great tradition, and their movements, as for instance in the case of the spears of Mars, were considered a bad omen.

[17] Willamowitz's opinion is generally accepted, although there are researchers who suppose that the term has always referred to larger-than-life statues, e.g. Dickie 1996, and who interpret the sources from this perspective—however, I find it completely unconceivable that anyone in antiquity had the means to have life-size wax statues made.

morally stigmatised magic rituals, but rather in public, social rituals (Faraone 1991, 180). In addition, although there are only sporadic data to confirm it, the idea of a statue serving as the double of a human body, and suitable for accommodating a soul, was also known (Ogden 1997, 104).[18]

Most of the occurrences, however, lead us to a level of religion which was not acknowledged by the state, and often even sanctioned under criminal law; this contradicts the fact suggested by the sources, namely that the Late Antique *telesmas*, and especially those attributed to Apollonius, were benign. Moreover, their establishment, according to the traditions, was not performed in secret, but publicly. Even the Christian authors, otherwise against magic, considered the function of these statues to be useful and harmless. This contradiction requires an explanation.

In the Roman imperial period, data multiplied surrounding an idea according to which the statue itself could come alive. This change is actually indicated by Lucian, when the Greek gods in his satire complain that in the Olympian hierarchy they were dragged behind the pure golden eastern gods.[19] Lucian, who was entirely sceptical in religious matters, describes in *Philopseudes* (18.ff) the peculiar beliefs of his peers and his friends.[20] There is a statue portraying the Corinthian general Pelichus in

[18] Erecting a statue has been long considered as a potential remedy for instances of haunting. Pausanias, the author of the travelogue of Hellas, writes about his homonym, the Spartan king Pausanias, whose spirit haunted a temple where his compatriots had starved him to death. The gods even set a plague on the city; the deliverance from these troubles was eventually achieved by erecting a statue of the king next to the temple (Plut. *Moralia* 560 e-f, Thucydides I.134. Pausanias III.17). According to another story—perhaps a legend—from the sixth century BC, the Crotonians attacked the city of Siris and killed the priest of Athena and also fifty youths who sought shelter at the altar. After this abomination, an epidemic devastated the city; finally, following the advice of the oracle of Delphi, they erected life-size statues of all fifty of the martyred boys (Justin. 20.2). There are several shared elements in the two stories: in both cases they had to appease victims of murder aggravated by sacrilege, such as the murder of asylum seekers in a sacred place. In these cases, the effigy of the victim was suitable for reconciling the spirit; in other cases, however, the effigy might serve as the location of demonic activity. Apollonius of Tyana performed an exorcism on a young man who was believed by his peers to be insane and drunk. Apollonius ordered the demon to signal its departure by knocking over a nearby statue (Philostratus: *Vita Apollonii* IV.20).

[19] Earlier the material of the god statue had not increased its cultic value, the most appreciated statues having been roughly-shaped *xoanons* of ancient origin.

[20] An important feature of Lucian's story is that the characters participating in the satirist's dialogue are not uneducated peasants or craftsmen, but intellectuals. It has

the house of the protagonist Eucrates. After the statue cured Eucrates from a bout of fever, he and his household honoured it with cultic respect, and the statue took regular walks during the night—a common characteristic of other magical statues as well. Incidentally, this statue never harmed anyone if they stayed out of his way, unlike another statue mentioned by Lucian, that of Hippocrates in the house of the physician Antigonus: this statue used to throw things around if he had not received the usual sacrifices he was due (Lucianus: Philopseudes 21). By contrast, the statue of Pelichus also took baths, and one could hear him dabbling in the night. This was not a cultic statue in the strict sense of the word, Pelichus not even being a real hero; in fact, in the dialogues the probability that the statue of the old man was indeed portraying the Corinthian war chief is barely mentioned: for them, the historical Pelichus was not interesting. Here we simply have a sculpture, originally meant as a mere decoration in a private home which, due to a "miracle", earned the cultic respect of the household. Similar stories are attested not only by satirical authors, but historians as well. The statue of a certain Neryllinus in Troas was paid similar cultic respect.[21] Several statues of athletes had also been attributed similar healing powers, such as those of the wrestler, Polydamas of Skotoussa (Pausanias VI.5) or the boxer, Theagenes of Thasus (Pausanias VI.11.2); both cured fever. According to Pausanias, they had several statues, all of which disposed of this power. There is even a story of vengeance associated with the statue of Theagenes in Thasus (Pausanias VI.11.6; Eusebios Praep. Ev. V.34.9ff; Dio Chrysostomus Or.31.96). After the death of Theagenes, a rival of the sportsman had been flogging the statue every night until the statue eventually fell on him and killed him. The family raised charges against the statue, which was thrown into the

---

been commonplace to attribute superstitious thinking to women and lower social classes, however, it is probably a prejudice. For the Byzantine and early modern periods see: Hartnup 2004, 4–7; for antiquity: Bonner 1931. Bonner (1932, 42) cites Alexander of Tralles, a physician, who complains that it was especially the rich patients who trusted more in magic than in medicine.

[21] Athenagoras (*Apologia* 26). Unfortunately, it was impossible to establish who this otherwise unknown Neryllinus was. From the context, Weinreich assumes that he was some kind of magician, like Alexandros of Abonuteichos and Peregrinus Proteus, both mentioned in the same place, and both protagonists of Lucian (Weinreich 1909, 141). The other possible identification would be M. Suillius Nerullinus, the consul of the 50th year, the proconsul of Asia around 67/70. In this case, the statue and its cult would be associated with the cult surrounding Roman officials exercised in the East. I do not believe that the two arguments would be mutually exclusive: the fact that Athenagoras mentions him along with two magicians might suggest that he too had ignored Neryllinus' original identity.

sea as a punishment. Following this, however, a famine came upon the people of Thasos, which lasted until they eventually took the advice of the oracle of Delphi and brought the statue back from the sea and put it back in its original place (a similar story survived of the pentathlonist, Euthyches according to Eusebius Praep. Ev. V. 34).

The most conclusive vital sign of the statue would be the ability to speak; we do not hear of such statues in Byzantium, since it would have required a conscious fraud, and the belief of superstitious people would not have been enough. In the Roman imperial period, on the other hand, we often hear of talking statues, such as the *telesma*, which demanded a god-cult for Apollonius; or the statue described by Eusebius, which encouraged the persecution of Christians (Eusebius HE. IX.2–3). As we see in another text by Lucian about the meeting of gods, the Olympians complain: "Soon every stone and altar will be an oracle if it is soaked in oil, enwreathed and there is an impostor around the corner" (Lucianus Deorum concilium 12). We actually have a statue, the head of a philosopher, probably that of Epicurus, into the mouth of which they carved a hole and, by introducing a metal tube, could make the statue talk from a distance (Poulsen 1945).

The earliest roots of the belief in *telesma* and *stoicheion* can be recognised in these anecdotal stories, but their direct antecedent can be found in the doctrines of a philosophical school. The origin of the term *telesma* is a verb, *telein*, the original meaning of which was "to initiate into mystery cults"), while its participle *tetelesmenon* was a frequent epithet of magic statues, *telestes* being its creator. These words were terms of Late Antique theurgy, a branch of Neoplatonic philosophy.

The word theurgy comes from *theos* (= god) and *ergon* (= work): the aim of the theurgist was knowledge of god, not through rational argumentation or meditation, but ritual-magical deed; theurgists sought to conjure the spirits and influence their activities. Here magic was practised with a religious purpose. This is the opposite of *goeteia*, an ancient term for "black magic", which uses the concepts and names of gods in a religion for its own dark purposes, trying to coerce the demons to serve these aims. At the same time, we cannot always draw a line between the two, as they have several things in common (Dodds 1947, 61). Iulianus, who lived at the time of Marcus Aurelius, was the first person to be called a *theurgus* (Dodds 1947, 55). He wrote the famous collection of "*Chaldean oracles*" and a lost book with the title *Telestike*,[22] which might

[22] For more on this, see Dodds 1947, who distinguished between two basic occurring forms of theurgy, the *techne telestike*, which operates with statues, and the divination and conjuration of spirits through means of human mediums.

have included elements of the rituals mentioned in Malalas' books. The sources make it probable that Iulianus was a professional wizard. His books and the *Chaldean Oracles* were rediscovered by the Neoplatonic philosopher, Porphyrius; theurgy and Neoplatonism are inseparable in the works of Iamblichus.

Telestike, or statue-magic, was a method of theurgy, as Proclus says: "Farther still, it would also be absurd that the telestic art should establish on the earth a place fit for the oracles and statues of the Gods, and through certain symbols should cause things generated from a partial and corruptible matter to become adapted to the participation of a deity; to be moved by him, and to predict future events… [but] we see that this is possible from telestic works." (Proclus *in Tim.* IV. 287.C). By means of certain *"symbolons"*, the science of the *telestes* can make the statues of gods, objects made of perishable material, suitable for taking a share in the god, to become mobile through him and tell the future (Proclus *in Tim.* III, 155). "The telestic art purifying it and putting certain letters and *symbolon*s around it animated the statue" (Proclus *Theol. Plat. I.28.70;* Dodds 1947, 61–5; cf. Proclus: *In Tim.* I.51.25; III.6.12; In Crat. 19.12). We find a clear description from the Byzantine era by Michael Psellus on how to make a statue with magical powers (Psellus ep.187): one had to place plants, stones and seals with magical properties inside the statue (cf. Iamblichus: *De mysteriis* 233.10; Augustinus: *De Civitate Dei* X.11; Proclus: *In Tim.* III.6.13). The effectiveness of the *symbolon*s is based on the doctrine of cosmic *sympatheia*, a mysterious web connecting the living and the lifeless parts of the universe. The *symbolon*s create hierarchical concatenations on a par with a traditional god or a planet. The ritual manipulation of the *symbolon*s affects the universe as well as the god himself. Since the *symbolon* "participates" in the essence of the god, it can be a commodity for the telestic statue of the same god.[23]

The doctrine of *sympatheia* and the methods applied by the *theurgos* can unequivocally be traced back to the second century BC, it probably being Bolus of Mendes (around 200 BC) who made the doctrine of *sympatheia* a determining part of magic (Kákosy 1984, 49). Nonetheless, theurgy is not tantamount to magic; the principle of sympatheia allowed Iamblichus and his followers to defend traditional religious rituals against criticism: ritual is not an empty, outward deed, it establishes real

According to Lewy (1978, 5), the word Theurgos without a name always refers to him, and the word *logion* (prophecy) to the text of the *Oracula Chaldaeica*.

[23] Proclus: *in Tim.* III.155.18. On the significance of the symbolons at Iamblichus, see Athanassiadi-Fowden 1981, 7. The role of *symbola* és *synthemata*: Iamblichus: *De mysteriis* I.11.15–21; II.11; IV.2; VII.4.5; the theurgic *unio mystica*: VI.5.7.

connection with the transcendent.[24] This approach to theurgy, maybe unwillingly, created something earlier unknown in Greek religion: the theology of the idol.[25]

The magic power of materials was principally ensured by their astrological symbolic value both in magic and theurgy, since every celestial body had a corresponding plant, gemstone, even vowel. (The seven Greek vowels were often used as magic spells, and it was associated with the five planets, and the Sun and the Moon. Dornseiff 1925, 82; Diels 1899, 44; Kákosy 1984, 136; Kákosy 1978, 271.) We even know of special scientific books, for instance the collection known by the title *Kyranides*, which categorised alphabetically the substances used in magic. Unfortunately, our sources do not discuss in further detail where the statue got its soul from; we can presume, however, mostly from the works of Proclus, that some god or *daimon* inhabited the statue. The earliest accounts of *telesma*s attributed to Apollonius emphasise the interactions based on the doctrine of *sympatheia*, and not the demonical elements; accordingly, Pseudo-Iustinus also described Apollonius as someone who knew the sympathetic relations of natural forces: the document of *Biblos Sophias* discussing talisman magic primarily focuses on the secret names of celestial bodies, months, and so forth.[26] Not once are demons mentioned in the extensive work of Malalas; he rather discussed secret names and special magic tools, thereby presenting magic as a sort of science which could be used for both good and bad purposes.

III.

The other two words, *zodion* and *stoicheion*, cannot be discussed independently of each other. The term *stoicheion*, mainly known in the sense of "element", has gone through a significant change of meaning in

---

[24] Iamblichus: *De mysteriis* II. 11. 96–97; III.20.149.

[25] Theurgists were the first to establish a ritual difference between common statues and "animated" cult statues. The entry *Heraiskos* in the Suda encyclopedia mentions a person called Heraiskos, who was believed to be able to distinguish between animate and inanimate god statues (Suda, s.v. Heraiskos).

[26] Although the Arabic "specialised literature" in this topic is better known, we also know some texts in Greek, which were entirely dedicated to the issue of how to produce talismans, e.g. *Biblos sophias, Apotelesmatika pragmateia*. The procedure was inherited from antiquity: according to a magical papyrus, for instance, one had to carve the inside of a statue of Apollo made from laurel wood, and place magic spells written on gold, silver or lead plates in it, and the statue would provide oracles (PGM I. III. 296).

the course of antiquity. In one phase of this transformation it gains an astronomical meaning, being used to denote the demons of so-called decans. The word *zodion*, literally meaning "little animal", can be exclusively interpreted in terms of astrology, and means zodiac sign (Malalas 5.12. p. 81; Suda s.v. Palladion; cf. Mango 1963, 63).[27] Both words indicate that the magical statues cannot be interpreted independently of astrology and astrolatry. Among the three terms, *stoicheion* is the one with the most complicated history, since it had been used to denote many different things over the course of time. There are numerous articles discussing the long and meandering history of the word, during which the original meaning of "row" was first transformed into a philosophical element, a principium, then to a letter, a celestial body, a demon and finally a statue (on the linguistic history of the word, see articles by Diels 1899; Dornseiff 1925; Dieterich 1925; Blum 1946, 315; Vollgraf 1949; Koller 1954; Burkert 1959). For this very reason it has long been disputed whether the word did indeed imply a magical connotation, or if it only meant statue, and erection of a statue. The issue is discussed by C. Blum's article, primarily illustrated with the case of Cedrenus. In certain sentences, the non-magical interpretation might indeed be possible; however, it does not come through in all cases, for instance when the subject of the verb is the River Lycus: here the binding is obviously not to be taken literally, but in a magical sense (Blum 1946, 316. He primarily argued with the articles of Diels 1899; Polites 1920, 51).

How could this word, originally meaning "element", have gone through such a change over the centuries? The word has two possible connotations which might be associated with magic. *Stoicheion* can mean letter, and the letters of the alphabet were of particular importance in ancient magic. Repeating the seven Greek vowels had a magic effect, and they occur on numerous Egyptian magical papyri as well. Many phenomena related to letter magic proved to be ineradicable despite all good efforts of the Church Fathers. The talisman against earthquakes mentioned by Malalas was placed in an underground chest, which makes it possible that it was actually a text containing magic spells.

Although we cannot entirely exclude this explanation, there is another, no less interesting and far-reaching interpretation of *stoicheion*. The term was used in astrological literature in the sense of "celestial body" (Mango 1963, 63; Blum 1946, 315). An apocryphal text from the third century AD bears the title, *The Testament of Solomon*. It is about King Solomon, and

---

[27] The word can either refer to a specific astrological constellation under which the talisman has to be made, or an astral demon.

most of the book is a catalogue of demons in which the king forces the demons one by one to confess their names, what constellation they belong to, and which angel could expel them. Some spirits live in specific celestial bodies, while others are only dangerous to people with a specific zodiac sign (McCown 1922). In Chapter 8.1 a demon appears, interwoven from seven souls who call themselves *stoicheion*: their names are Deception, Strife, Clotho, Jealousy, Error, Power and the Worst of All. The seven demons corresponded to the ensemble of the five planets, the Sun and the Moon. In Chapter 18.1 there is a demon made of 36 pieces who is also called *stoicheion*. These are the spirits of *decans*. Egyptian astrology divides each zodiac sign into three parts, *decans*, for they each covered ten degrees of the Ecliptic, which gave a total of 36. For all 36 *decans*, or 36 *decan* spirits, the Egyptians had a corresponding body part, and thus the spirits were primarily responsible for causing illness (Vakaloudi 2000a, 185: there was a particularly strong *sympatheia* between the human body parts and the 36 *decans*, cf. Orig. *conta Celsum* IV.150; Greenfield 1988, 237; Kákosy 1978, 241. The demons of the *decans* became gods, and no longer corresponded to actual stars. Kákosy 1978, 243–6: *decan* illustrations).

There is a meagre reference by Malalas suggesting that there might have been astrological aspects of making *telesma*s: the mosquito repellent talisman had to be set up at a new moon, but there are other sections that suggest that the astrological constellations at the time of the ritual had significant meaning. Psellus did not explain what ensured the magical powers of the objects placed inside a statue. We can assume, however, that it was their astrological symbolic value. The seven Greek vowels also corresponded to the seven astrological celestial bodies (Dornseiff 1925, 82f; Diels 1899, 44; Kákosy 1984, 136; Kákosy 1978, 271.ff; the latter gives examples in his book for the personal use as amulets of statues of decans and planets from Egypt to Agrippa von Nettesheim). The Christian John Malalas considers it necessary to mention this connection at the very beginning of his work, when discussing the Biblical book of Genesis (Malalas I.1). Taking all this into consideration, it seems logical that the original meanings of the word *stoicheion* were "celestial body" and "astral spirit" in an astronomical sense, before the later "magical statue" connotation developed.

The three names, merely by their etymology, provide explanations regarding the functioning of talismans and the magical mentality behind them; meanwhile, they raise new issues. The fact that the previously used term *telesma* was replaced with *stoicheion* in later chronicles, even if the original story was otherwise left unchanged, already suggests the existence of some kind of a living ritual, and not simply a dead, antiquarian cluster of information transmitted unaltered from one chronicler to the next; the word pair *telesma-stoicheion* must have played a role in everyday magical practices. But why did they change the expression denoting talismans if the ritual itself, the preparation of the object and its function remained the same? The ritual described by Malalas appears to be completely innocent and gentle, while in other texts we read about demons. Blum claims that the verb *stoicheioo* had always meant magical binding—did it only mean that originally, though, investing one object with magical powers, or had it already the sense of binding a demon to a statue as well? Blum, who mainly discusses talismans in his article, commits himself to the former argument, while Greenfield, in his extensive demonology, for instance, defends the primacy of the demons: and we do find demons called *stoicheion* before the examples of their being associated with statues (Blum 1946; Greenfield 1988, 190–195). Another question is how the statue came alive: was the object given an independent soul through a magical procedure? Or was it an already existing soul, a demon that they had bound to the statue? The sources allow both possibilities. In my opinion, the terms *telesma* and *stoicheion*, although appearing as equal synonyms in the texts from the middle byzantine period, were originally far from overlapping, and their sphere of application and origins could have been different.

The denomination of *telesma* itself refers to the performed ritual: the statue has been "initiated". The term *stoicheion*, however, appears first as the name of a demon before becoming a statue. The association of the two can be easily explained by the fact that some of those who performed magic with statues believed that their magic actually bound astral spirits to statues. However, the meaning of *stoicheion* as a bewitched statue first appears only in the seventh century, and as we will see from our sources discussing the demon inside the statue, it will turn out that it was not an astral demon after all. We can suppose that the semantic field of the word *stoicheion* had already been expanded earlier, and was used in the sense of demon in general, not just an astral demon. The explanation for this could be that the word *stoicheion*, before gaining its magical connotation, had gone through a Judeo-Christian filter. *Stoicheion* occurs several times in Paul's Epistles, clearly referring to the celestial body and the spiritual being behind it (II Cor. 6. 14–16, Gal. 4.8–9)[28] and denouncing worship of them. This idea is reiterated by the Church Fathers. Judeo-Christian

[28] Greenfield 1988, 191, note 578: "the majority of commentators this century have understood stoicheia in this context as denoting personally active spiritual beings, despite attempts by one or two to make them impersonal elements."

mentality had a tendency to identify pagan religions with astrolatry; the basis for this mentality must have been the actual experiences of the Jewish people living in the close vicinity of Babylonians, Chaldeans, and others. Stigmatisation of pagans with astrolatry persisted after antiquity. On the one hand, Malalas originated pagan religion in a euhemerist way, from the cult of ancient kings, while on the other, he traced it back to the worshipping of planets (Malalas I.1, I.8). Accordingly, every pagan god could be associated with astral spirits.

From a Christian point of view, the astral spirit and the statue associated to it are both demonical; from a pagan perspective it is not: the statue initiated by a *telestes* due to *sympatheia* relations does indeed gain its power from a "planet spirit"; there are no essential differences between the two, it is only the moral judgement that is different. This, over the course of time, transformed the statue-related magic of *stoicheion*s into such a dark phenomenon that the associated demon would no longer be a celestial spirit, but according to Byzantine sources it is a *biothanatos*. This type of magic can also be traced back to the Hellenistic age, although the magic stems from a less intellectual region than theurgy.

According to the aforementioned story in *Patria Konstantinupoleos*, two officials of the already Christian and Orthodox emperor were walking among the ruinous monuments of Constantinople, looking at statues, when a statue fell on one of them and crushed him to death (Suda sv. Kynegion, *Patria Const*. 35.28. = 162. cap. 27). The court philosopher from the palace who arrived at the scene drew the conclusion that the culprit was a *biothanatos*. Contrary to what it appears to be, the word does not mean "living dead", but the soul of someone who had died a violent death: the original form was *biaiothanatos* and it played an important role in ancient magic (Delatte 1932, 141; Ogden 2004, 149).

It is an existing phenomenon, regardless of culture, to think that those who die before their time cannot find peace in the grave. The spirits invoked to assist in ancient magic were the "*aoroi*", souls of those who had died prematurely: children, youths who passed before marriage, or of those who died a violent death (*biothanatos*, mostly spirits of executed victims or gladiators), and the "*ataphoi*", the unburied (Tertullianus: *De anima* 56). They would wander on Earth as a vengeful spirit (*alastores*) until their time, predestined by fate, was up (Apuleius: *Apologia* 129). This explains why battlefields were a favoured location for magical practices: the people who had perished there fell into all three categories, they died before their time, in arms, and did not have a proper funeral. (Pausanias writes about the battlefield at Marathon where they often saw ghosts of the fallen soldiers, which he explains by the Greeks not having provided a proper funeral for the dead of the enemy—something also confirmed by archaeological excavations. Pausanias I.32.3–4). On one occasion, Apollonius of Tyana exorcised the spirit of a soldier from a little boy's body (Philostratus: *Vita Apolloni* III.28. Further examples: Ogden 2004, 13–4). The idea proved to be long-lived, almost ineradicable, since the Church Fathers had to insist time and again that it was not the spirits of people with violent deaths who became demons, but those of evil people.[29] During both late antiquity and in Byzantium it was considered possible for a sorcerer to force such demons into a statue and thus gain control over them. This is the case for probably all the statues mentioned as *stoicheion*. This procedure is a much darker method than that of the *theurgos*, because it is dangerously close to certain forms of necromancy, a practice condemned both legally and by public opinion.

IV.

The terminology of the Byzantine "magic statues", as well as the meaning of the related terms, changed over the centuries, the benign talismans being replaced by more harmful and active forms of magic. The different terms and various theoretical conceptions behind the terms still came from the same age, both dating back to the early centuries AD, though the idea of "telestic" statues had already received its final form in late antiquity, in contrast with the magic of the *stoicheion*s, whose connection with statues cannot be older than the middle byzantine period.[30] It is not the aim of the present study to find an explanation for these changes—we can even posit the possibility that the change is illusory. The *stoicheion* statue is a late innovation; however, in Christian sources the idea of harmful, malignant statues can, on the whole, be traced back to antiquity (Dieterich 1925, 13 with the examples of Politis' *Paradoseis*, cf. Origenes: *Contra Celsum* VII.69). This tradition has always been dominant in Byzantium, although in the early centuries it coexisted with the tradition of benign, Neoplatonic talismans. Both survived the dark age of Byzantium, but in the Middle Ages there was no longer any reason to maintain the terminological and

---

[29] Ioannes Chrysostomus *De Lazaro hom.* PG 48. col. 983. Suda, sv. psychikos anthropos: ψυχαὶ τῶν βιοθανούντων οὐ κατὰ τὴν τῶν πολλῶν δόξαν γίνονται δαίμονες, ἀλλὰ τῶν ἁμαρτανόντων.

[30] The opinions (e.g. Mango 1963, 59) suggesting that the malign, demonic statues represent the older form are probably false. Greenfield (1988, 190–195) argues for the priority of the demon because we hear earlier of *stoicheion* demons than *stoicheion* statues, but this change is independent of telesma-stoicheion chronology. Cf. Dieterich (1925, 13)

conceptual distinction between the old, rivalling ideas: theurgy, magic and the Christian reflection of magic. The result was a new synthesis, which is abundantly attested both in Byzantine literary sources and Greek folklore.

References

Primary sources

Anastasius Sinaites. *Quaest. et resp.*

Anastasius Sinaites. 1865. "Questiones et responsiones." In *Patrologia Graeca* 89., edited by Jacques-Paul Migne, 327–826. Paris: Vrayet.

Apotelesmatika pragmateia.

"Apotelesmatika pragmateia." 1927. In *Anekdota Atheniensia I,* by Armand Delatte, 397–445. Paris, and Liége: Édouard Champion.

Apuleius: *Apologia.*

Apuleius. 1912. Apulei *Platonici Madaurensis Pro se magia liber (Apologia).* Edited by Rudolf Helm. Lipsiae: Teubner.

Athenagoras: *Apologia.*

Athenagoras. 1857. "Apologia." In *Patrologia Graeca* 6., edited by Jacques-Paul Migne, 890–973. Paris: Vrayet.

Augustinus: *De Civitate Dei.*

Augustinus. 1955. *De civitate Dei* I–II. Edited by B. Dombart, and A. Kalb. Turnhout: Brepols.

Biblos sophias.

"Biblos sophias kai syneseos apotelesmaton." 1908. In *Catalogus codicum astrologorum Graecorum* VII., edited by Franciscus Boll, 174–81. Bruxelles: Lamertin.

Cedrenus.

Cedrenus. 1838–1839. *Compendium Historiarum* I–II. Edited by Immanuel Becker. Bonnae: impensis Ed. Weberi.

Chronicon Paschale.

Anonymus 1860, "Chronicon Paschale." In *Patrologia Graeca* 92., edited by Jacques-Paul Migne, Paris: Vrayet.

Dio Chrysostomus: *Or.*

Dio Chrysostomus. 1940. *Discourses 31–36.* Cambridge: Harvard University Press. (Loeb Classical Library 358.)

Diogenes Laertius.

Diogenes Laertius. 1972. *Lives of Eminent Philosophers.* Edited by R.D. Hicks. Cambridge: Harvard University Press.

Eusebius: *Praep. Ev.*

Eusebius. 1857. "Praeparatio Evangelica." In *Patrologia Graeca* 21., edited by Jacques-Paul Migne, Paris: Vrayet.
Eusebius. *HE*.
Eusebius. 1857. "Historia Ecclesiastica." In *Patrologia Graeca* 20., edited by Jacques-Paul Migne, Paris: Vrayet.
Gregory of Tours.
Gregorius Turonensis. 1884. "Historia Francorum." In *Monumenta Germaniae* Historica, scriptorum rerum Merovingicarum, pars 1. edited by W. Arndt, and Br. Krusch. Hannoveriae: Impensis Bibliopoli Hahniani.
Heliodorus: *Aithiopika*.
Heliodorus. 1855. *Heliodori Aethiopicorum libri decem ab Immanuele Bekkero recogniti*. Lipsiae: Teubner.
Hesychius.
Hesychius. 1901. "Patria Constantinupoleos." In *Scriptores Originum Constantinopolitanarum* I., edited by Theodor Preger, 1–18. Lipsiae: Teubner.
Iamblichus: *De mysteriis*.
Iamblichos. 1966. *Les mystères d'Egypte*. Edited by Edouard Des Places. Paris: Les Belles Lettres.
Ioannes Chrysostomus.
Ioannes Chrysostomus. 1862. "Homiliae." In *Patrologia Graeca* 48., edited by Jacques-Paul Migne, Paris: Vrayet.
Isidorus of Pelusium.
Isidorus Pelusiota. 1864. "Epistolae." In *Patrologia Graeca* 78., edited by Jacques-Paul Migne. Paris: Vrayet.
Lucianus: *Philopseudes*.
Lucian. 1921. "Philopseudes." In *Works* III. Edited by A. M. Harmon. Cambridge, Mass., and London: Harvard UP, and William Heinemann Ltd.
Lucianus: *Deorum concilium*.
Lucian. 1921. "Deorum concilium." In *Works* III. Edited by A. M. Harmon. Cambridge, Mass., and London: Harvard UP, and William Heinemann Ltd.
Malalas.
Dindorf, Ludwig, ed. 1831. *Ioannis Malalae Chronographia ex recensione L. Dindorfii*. Bonnae: Impensis Ed. Weberi.
—. Thurn, Hans, ed. 2000. *Ioannis Malalae Chronographia.* Berlin: de Gruyter. (Corpus fontium historia Byzantinae XXXV.)
Nicephorus Presbyter.

Nicephorus Presbyter. 1863. "Vita S. Andreae Sali." In *Patrologia Graeca* 111, edited by Jacques-Paul Migne, 621–906. Paris: Vrayet.

Nicetas Choniates.

Nicetas Choniates. 1835. *Historia.* Edited by Immanuel Bekker. Bonnae: impensis Ed. Weberi.

Olympiodorus.

Photius. 1860. Bibliotheke. In *Patrologia Graeca* 103, edited by Jacques-Paul Migne, 256–80. Paris: Vrayet.

Origenes: *Contra Celsum.*

Origène. 1967–1976. *Contre Celse.* Introduction générale, tables et index par Marcel Borret. Paris: Les Editions du Cerf.

Parastaseis.

"Parastaseis syntomoi chronikai." 1907. In *Scriptores Originum Constantinopolitanarum* II., edited by Theodor Preger, 19–73. Lipsiae: Teubner.

Patria.

"Patria Konstantinupoleos." 1907. In *Scriptores Originum Constantinopolitanarum* II, edited by Theodor Preger, 135–289. Lipsiae: Teubner.

Pausanias.

Pausanias. 1903. *Graeciae Descriptio* I–III. Edited by Fr. Spiro. Leipzig: Teubner.

Philostratus: *Vita Apollonii.*

Philostratus. 1870. *Opera.* Vol.1. Edited by Carl Ludwig Kayser. Teuber Lipsiae.

PGM.

Karl Preisendanz. 1928–1931. *Papyri Graecae Magicae. Die griechischen Zauberpapyri* I–II. Leipzig: Teubner.

Proclus: *In Tim.*

Proclus. 1903–1906. *In Platonis Timaeum commentaria.* Edited by E. Diehl. Leipzig: Teubner.

Proclus: *In Crat.*

Proclus. 1908. In *Platonis Cratylum commentaria.* Edited by G. Pasquali. Leipzig: Teubner.

Proclus: *Theol. Plat.*

Proclus. 1968–1977. *Theologia Platonica—Théologie platonicienne* 6. Edited by H. D. Saffrey, and L. G. Westerlink. Paris: Les Belles Lettres.

Procopius: *Bella.*

Procopius. 1963. *Bella* I–II. Edited by Jacobus Haury. Lipsiae: Teubneri.

Ps-Iustinus: *Quaest. et. resp.*
Pseudo-Iustinus. 1857. "Quaestiones et responsiones ad orthodoxos." In *Patrologia Graeca* 6., edited by Jacques-Paul Migne, 1249–400. Paris: Vrayet.
Psellus.
Michael Psellus. 1876. *Epistolai*. In *Mesaionike Bibliotheke* V. Michel Psellou Historikoi logoi, epistolai. Edited by K. N. Sathas. Paris, and Venetia: Maisonneuve et C.
Suda.
Suidae Lexicon I–V vols. 1928–38. Edited by Ada Adler. Leipzig:Teubner.
Tertullianus: *De anima*.
Tertullianus. 1844. "De anima." In *Patrologia Graeca* 2, edited by Jacques-Paul Migne, 642–752. Paris: Vrayet.
Theophanes Continuatus.
Theophanes Continuatus. 1838. *Chronographia.* Edited by Immanuel Bekker. Bonnae: impensis Ed. Weber.
Thucydides.
Thucydides. 1942. *Historiae in two volumes*. Edited by Henry Stuart Jones. Oxford: Oxford University Press.
Zosimus.
Zosime. 1971. *Histoire Nouvelle* I–II. Edited by Francois Paschoud. Paris: Les Belles Lettres.

Secondary sources

Allatius, Leo. 1645. "De Graecorum hodie quorundam opinationibus." In *De templis Graecorum recentioribus ad Ioannem Morinum; De narthece ecclesiae veteris, ad Gasparem de Simeonibus; nec non de Graecorum hodie quorundam opinationibus, ad Paullum Zacchiam.* Coloniae Agrippinae: Apud Iodocum Kalcovium et socios.
Athanassiadi-Fowden, Polymnia. 1981. *Julian and Hellenism*. Oxford: Clarendon Press.
Berger, Albrecht. 1987. *Die Altstadt von Byzanz in der vorjustinianischen Zeit.* Bonn: Habelt. (Poikila Byzantina 6.)
—. 1988. *Untersuchungen zu den Patria Konstantinupoleos.* München: Byzantin–Neugriech. Seminar. d. Freien Univ. Berlin.
Blum, Claes. 1946. "The Meaning of στοιχεῖον and its Derivatives in the Byzantine Age. A Study in Byzantine Magic." *Eranos* 44: 316–25.
Blum, Richard, and Eva Blum. 1970. *Dangerous hour. The Lore of Crisis and Mystery in Rural Greece*. London: Chatto and Windus.

Bonner, Campbell. 1932. "Witchcraft in the Lecture Room of Libanius." *Transactions and Proceedings of the American Philologic Association* 63: 34–44.

Brehier, Louis. 1904. "Un patriarche sorcier à Constantinople." *Revue de l'Orient Chrétien* 9: 261–8.

Burckhardt, Jacob. 1878. *The Civilization of the Renaissance in Italy*. Vienna, and Oxford: Phaidon Press, and Oxford University Press.

Burkert, Walter. 1959. "Στοιχεῖον. Eine semasiologische Studie." *Philologus* 103: 167–97.

Cameron, Averil, and Judith Herrin, eds. 1984. *Constantinople in the Early Eighth Century. The Parastaseis Syntomoi Chronikai.* Leiden: Brill.

Comparetti, Domenico. 1875. *Virgil im Mittelalter*. Leipzig: Teubner.

Dagron, Gilbert. 1984. *Constantinople imaginaire. Études sur le recueil des Patria*. Paris: Presses de Univ. France.

Dawkins, R. M. 1924. "Ancient Statues in Medieval Constantinople." *Folklore. Transactions of the Folklore Society* 35 (3): 205–48.

Delatte, Armand. 1932. *La catoptromancie grecque et ses dérivés*. Liège: Vaillant-Carmanne.

Dickie, Matthew W. 1996. "What is a *Kolossos* and How Were *Kolossoi* Made in the Hellenistic Period?" *Greek Roman and Byzantine Studies* 37: 237–57.

Diels, Hermann. 1899. *Elementum. Eine Vorarbeit zum griechischen und lateinischen Thesaurus*. Leipzig: B.G. Teubner.

Dieterich, Karl. 1925. "Hellenistische Volksreligion und byzantinische-neugriechische Volksglaube." *ΑΓΓΕΛΟΣ Archiv für Neutestamentliche Zeitgeschichte und Kulturkunde* 1: 2–23.

Dindorf, Ludwig. 1831. *Ioannis Malalae Chronographia ex recensione L. Dindorfii*. Bonnae: Impensis Ed. Weberi.

Dodds, Eric R. 1947. "Theurgy and its Relationship to Neoplatonism." *Journal of Roman Studies* 37: 55–69.

Dornseiff, Franz. 1925. *Das Alphabet in Mystik und Magie*. Leipzig: Teubner.

Duliére, Walter L. 1970. "Protection permanente contre des animaux nuisibles assurée par Apollonius de Tyane dans Byzance et Antioche. Evolution de son mythe." *Byzantinische Zeitschrift* 63: 247–77.

Dzielska, Maria. 1986. *Apollonius of Tyana in Legend and History*. Roma: L'Erma di Bretschneider.

Faraone, Christopher A. 1989. "Clay Hardens and Wax Melts: Magical Role-Reversal in Virgil's Eighth Eclogue." *Classical Philology* 84: 294–300.

—. 1991. "Binding and Burying the Forces of Evil: The Defensive Use of 'Voodoo' Dolls in Ancient Greece." *Classical Antiquity* 10: 165–205.
—. 1992: *Talismans and Trojan Horses. Guardian Statues in Ancient Greek Myth and Ritual.* New York, and Oxford: Oxford University Press.
Fodor, Sándor. 1971. *Arab legendák a piramisokról* [Arabian legends of pyramids]. Budapest: Akadémiai.
Garnett, Lucy M. J., and J. S. Stuart-Glennie. 1896. *Greek Folk Poesy.* London: David Nutt.
Greenfield, Richard P. H. 1988. *Traditions of Belief in Late Byzantine Demonology.* Amsterdam: Hakkert.
Guberti Bassett, Sarah. 1991. "The antiquities in the Hippodrome of Constantinople." *Dumbarton Oak Papers* 45: 87–96.
Guberti Bassett, Sarah. 1996. "Historiae Custos: Sculpture and Tradition in the Baths of Zeuxippos." *American Journal of Archeology* 100: 491–506.
Hartnup, Karen. 2004. *"On the beliefs of the Greeks." Leo Allatios and popular orthodoxy*. Leiden: Brill.
Hughes, Dennis. 1991. *Human Sacrifice in Ancient Greece*. London NewYork: Routledge.
Jeffreys, Elisabeth et alii. 1986. *The Chronicle of John Malalas. (A translation by Elisabeth Jeffreys, Michael Jeffreys, Roger Scott).* Melbourne: Australian Assoc. for Byzantine Studies.
Kákosy, László. 1974. *Varázslás az ókori Egyiptomban* [Magic in Ancient Egypt]. Budapest: Akadémiai.
—. 1978. *Egyiptom és az antik csillaghit* [Egypt and the antique astrolatry]. Budapest: Akadémiai.
—. 1984. *Fény és káosz. A kopt gnosztikus kódexek* [Light and chaos. Coptic gnostic codices]. Budapest: Gondolat.
Koller, Hermann. 1954. "Stoicheion." *Glotta* 34: 161–74.
Láng, Benedek. 2007. *Mágia a középkorban* [Magic in the Middle Ages]. Budapest: Typotex.
Lewy, Hans. 1978. *Chaldaean Oracles and Theurgy. Mysticism, Magic and Platonism in the Later Roman Empire*. Paris: Études Augustiniennes.
Mango, Cyril. 1963. "Antique Statuary and the Byzantine Beholder." *Dumbarton Oak Papers* 17: 53–75.
—. 1984: "St. Michael and Attis." *Deltion tes Christianikes Archaiologikes Hetaireias* 12: 39–62.
Maspero, Gaston. 1893. "Le double et les statues prophétiques." *Études de mythologie et d'archéologie égyptiennes* 77–91.

McCown, Chester C. 1922. *The Testament of Solomon.* Leipzig: Hinrichs.

Megas, Georgios A. 1976. *Die Ballade von der Arta-Brücke*. Thessaloniki: Institute for Balkan Studies.

Moffatt, Ann. 1990. "A Recording of Public Buildings and Monuments." In *Studies in John Malalas*, edited by Elisabeth Jeffreys, Brian Croke, and Robert Scott, 87–109. Sidney: Australian Association for Byzantine Studies.

Oeconomos, Lysimaque. 1930. "L'état intellectuel et moral des Byzantins vers le milieu du XIVe siècle." *Études sur l'histoire et sur l'art de Byzance. Mélanges Charles Diehl*. 1: 225–33.

Ogden, Daniel. 1997. *The Crooked Kings of Ancient Greece*. London: Duckworth.

—. 2004. *Greek and Roman Necromancy*. Princeton: Princeton University Press.

Oikonomides, D. B. 1981. "He thysia eis oikodomemata." *Epetéris Hetaireias Byzantinón Spoudón* 45 (2): 43–132.

Polites, Nikolaos G. 1920. "Telesmata." *Laographia symmeikta* I: 48–57.

Poulsen, Frederik. 1945. "Talking, weeping and bleeding sculptures. A chapter of the history of religious fraud." *Acta Archaeologica* 16: 178–95.

Preger, Theodorus. 1901. *Scriptores Originum Constantinopolitarum*. Lipsiae: in aedibus Teubnerii.

Saradi, Helen. 2000. "Perceptions and literary interpretations of statues and the image of Constantinople." *Byzantiaka* 20: 37–77.

Speyer, Wolfgang. 1974. "Zum Bild des Apollonios von Tyana bei Heiden und Christen." *Jahrbuch für Antike und Christentum* 17: 47–63.

Spyridakes, G. K. 1962. *Hellenika Demotika Tragudia (Ekloge)* I. Athenai: Akadēmia Athēnōn.

Stewart, Charles. 1991. *Demons and the Devils*. Princeton, N.J.: Princeton University Press.

Tarn Steiner, Deborah. 2001. *Images in Mind: Statues in Archaic and Classical Greek Literature and Thought*. Princeton: Princeton University Press.

Tóth, Anna Judit. 2010. "Az artai híd balladája [The ballad of the Arta Bridge]." *Vallástudományi szemle* 6 (1): 72–83.

Vakaloudi, Anastasia D. 2000a. "Δεισιδαιμονια and the Role of the Apotropaic Magic Amulets in the Early Byzantine Empire." *Byzantion* 70: 182–210.

—. 2000b. "The magic arts of necromancy and ventriloquism as cited in the first Byzantine period sources." *Byzantiaka* 20: 119–35.

Vollgraf, Wilhelm. 1949. "Elementum." *Mnemosyne* 4.S.2: 89–115.

Weinreich, Otto. 1909. *Antike Heilungswunder*. Giessen: Töpelmann.
Willamowitz, Ulrich von. 1927. "Heilige Gesetze: Eine Urkunde aus Kyrene." *Sitzungsberichte der Preussischen Akademie der Wissenschaften* 19: 155–76.

PORK AS A WONDER DRUG, OR RELIGIOUS TABOO AS MAGICAL MEDICINE

ILDIKÓ CSEPREGI

Ritual healing is a broad concept, which renders the use of the term flexible and practical, as it covers a whole range of forms of magical and religious healing practices and often even some of the narrower range of official medicine, as well as combinations of these. Possibly this emulates the way in which the patients and healers of times gone by experienced the same complexity as a unified phenomenon. Here I shall be discussing a particular aspect, the use of religious taboo in a ubiquitous and elaborate form of ritual healing, in the practice of incubation. Incubation, that is, sleeping inside a place of worship was highly popular both in the colourful religious ritual in antiquity and in Medieval Christianity, continuing afterwards in Islam and at many of the cultic healing places of the Roman Catholic, Greek Catholic, Coptic and other churches throughout the early modern period right into the present day. (For a thorough introduction to the practice, both pagan and Christian, see Deubner 1900, Hamilton 1906, and for the most recent overview on the Greek material, see Ehrenheim 2015).

The practice of incubation continued practically undisturbed right through the changes in religious world views, retaining its function (healing and occasionally divination), its manner (intentionally sleeping at a sacred place), its milieu or medium (sleep, dreaming, encountering the healing agent in one's sleep, in a dream), the characteristics of the dream encounter (conversation, personal touch) as well as the structure of the narratives describing miraculous recoveries (formal analogies among incubation miracle accounts). In many places, even the shrine itself remained the same, only the figure of the local healer changed. This is how the cult of the popular incubation healers of antiquity came to be the terrain of the Christian physician saints. As religious world views changed, people whose faith differed from the religion of the shrine also tended to seek the assistance of popular cultic places and healers that were believed to be effective. This may partly have been due to the fact that the figure of the healer evolved into a form which worshippers might have expected to find in the previous healer. Even more frequently, however, it was the predicament produced by their disease that compelled people to try everything including visiting a cult place different from their own faith but believed far and wide to be effective. Situations of this kind can also turn recovery into a test of faith, while trust in the healer can act as the condition or the very means of recovery. The healing methods of Christian incubation saints, no matter whether we are talking about *living* saints or *relics*, were extremely similar to the repertoire of their ancient forerunners.[1]

The advice given in these dreams, which is sometimes supplemented by directions from the church staff, often involved some of the elements of contemporary medical science, sometimes including minor surgical interventions, recommending baths, abstinence from certain foods, or gymnastic exercises; they enlisted a broad range of herbs and drugs and also abounded in symbolic and magical means, the use of which was legitimised by the cult place or the figure of the holy healer. In what follows I would like to illustrate the use of pork as prescribed by incubation healers in dreams, a remedy embracing characteristics from the fields of magic and medicine as well as representing a test of faith-remedy when administered to patients for whom it counted as a religious taboo, based on both Greek and Christian examples.

Saints Cosmas and Damian were the most popular physician saints both of Byzantine and of later, medieval Latin Christianity. The emergence of their cult as healers may go back as far as the fifth century AD. It spread from the Syrian parts of Asia Minor through the entire Mediterranean, sometimes in the wake of the Greek physician-deity Asclepius or of other local healers. Written accounts of their miraculous cures date back as far as the sixth century and these went on to become transformed and expanded over the centuries. One of the miracles performed by these two saints is about a Jewish woman with breast cancer. (KDM 2). She goes to the shrine of Cosmas and Damian, sleeps inside it and in her dream is given advice to eat pork in order to be healed. She relates the dream to the servants or family members present with her at the church and resolves to postpone her decision about breaking the

---

[1] The most widely known are Saints Cosmas and Damian, Saint Thecla, Saints Cyrus and John and Saint Artemios; the lesser known include Saint Demeter, Saint Thérapon, Saint Febronia and Saint Dometius. For their miracle accounts in Greek and in modern translation see Festugière 1971; Fernandez Marcos 1975; Crisafulli and Nesbitt 1997; Dagron 1978; Gascoux 2006. References to their miracles are abbreviated as KDM, MT, MCJ and MA, their numbering is standard and retrievable in the above editions.

commandments of her faith. Cosmas and Damian appear to the woman, still hesitant, for a second and a third time in her dreams and repeat their instructions, emphasising that there is no other way in which she can recover. (A dream repeated three times is a very frequent feature in Christian incubation). The woman is suffering acute pain, so she finally bids her servants to bring her pork, but the latter are convinced that the presence of the saints is mere fantasy, while their commandment is a grave transgression against the law and the ancient customs, and so they try to dissuade their mistress. Eventually they obey, but when the woman is about to eat she notices that her husband is approaching her on one of his frequent visits to her in the church. Alarmed, she hides the meat under her dress. In the meantime, the Lord hears the prayers of the two saints and makes the woman's malady leap over from her body to the meat. When the husband departs, the woman feels prepared to eat the meat and discovers the miracle. The story ends with her conversion to Christianity and her baptism.

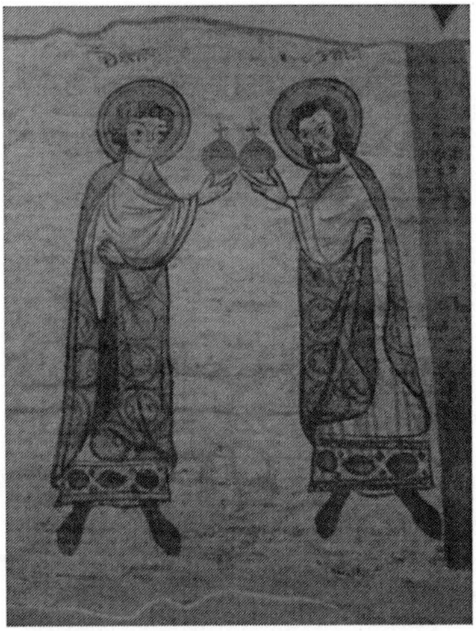

Fig. 1. Sts Cosmas and Damian.
Church fresco, Csaroda, Szatmár
County, Hungary, 15th century.
Photo by Gábor Klaniczay.

It is worth noting that in the story, conversion and confessing the Orthodox Christian faith are conditions for the attention of these saints in the sense that the mere willingness to convert is sufficient for regaining health. What are the contexts in which this miraculous cure lends itself to interpretation? Besides the presence of pork used to effectuate the cure, this story encompasses other important factors used in miraculous healing: first, the unclean substance, which is often used to attract the malady and carry it away; secondly, this transfer of the illness from the patient to the substance, which is in itself a curative method used in magic, but only one of the numerous instances when religious healing employs magical elements. Finally, if we examine the use of pork in magical-ritual healing, we find that it highlights another ever-present feature: the test of faith, and more precisely, a religious taboo advised as a remedy.

Pork in Greek ritual healing

By way of comparison, let me quote here an instance of healing from Asclepius where pork, a religious taboo for the patient, is recommended as a remedy. (This story survived in a 10th century Byzantine encyclopedia called the Suda under the entry Domninos, while its original source is Damasios, *Vita Isidori* fr. 218; in: Edelstein and Edelstein 1998, T 427).[2]

> ... The kind of life that [Domninos—5th century AD] lived was not sufficiently perfect for us to call him a true philosopher. Asclepius of Athens prescribed the same cure for Plutarch from Athens and Domninos from Syria, because the latter kept coughing blood, that was his disease, while Plutarch suffered from something different. The cure prescribed them to eat as much pork as they could. Plutarch, however, did not subscribe to this kind of remedy even though it did not go against the laws of his forebears. Instead, as soon as he woke up, he leaned on his elbow where he lay, looked up at the statue of Asclepius (as he happened to have slept in the hall of the shrine) and said, "My good Lord, what would you have prescribed for a Jew suffering from the same disease, surely you would not have advised him to eat as much pork as he could?" This is what he said, and Asclepius soon replied, through his statue and proposed a different type of cure in a kind and friendly voice.

However, the story does not end here. Domninos who, being a Syrian, also did not eat pork, decided not to take advantage of the deity's lenience but

[2] All the references with T refer to Edelstein's *Testimonies* and have been translated by Emma Edelstein.

to use the original cure of eating pork, even though for him it was religious taboo:

> Domninos credited the dream and even though it was against the law, meaning the ancient law of the Syrians, he did not follow Plutarch's example but ate pork both then and from that time onwards. It is rumoured that if he missed this for even one day the disease would return until he filled himself up with pork again.

Frazer points out the ambivalence of the Syrians' pork taboo. The fact that a pig could be neither eaten nor sacrificed points to its being a sacred animal, but at the same time, anyone who touched one became unclean. (Frazer 1890: Chapter LXIX).

In Lucian, Alexander the false prophet prescribed pork for a man with colic and although the text aims to mock the poetic capacities of Alexander, the remedy itself is remarkable in this religious-magical context:

> The man complained of colic, and Alexander, wishing to direct him to eat a pig's foot cooked with mallow, said: "Mallow with cumin digest in a sacred pipkin of piglets" (Μάλβακα χοιράων ἱερῇ κυμίνευε σιπύδῳ. Lucian 1925, 211).

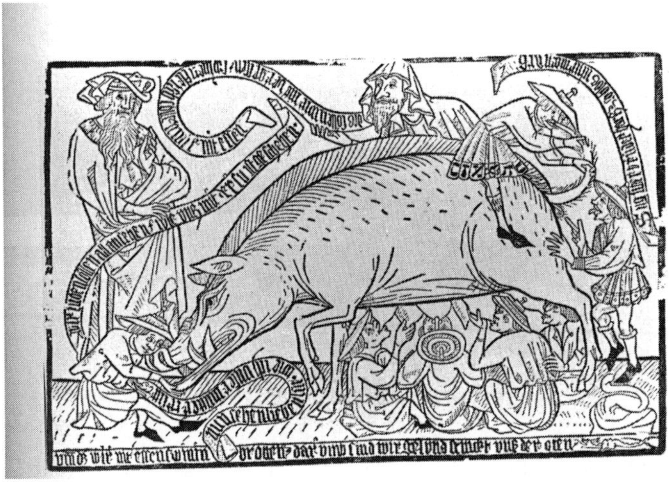

Fig. 2. The sow of the Jews (Judensau). German engraving from the 16th century. Adapted from Fabre-Vassas: "The Singular Beast", 1997, Fig. 10.

What scarce evidence exists makes it difficult to say whether pork or pig fat were in fact widely recommended in ancient miraculous healing. According to Ludwig Deubner, this may have been one of the popular cures in magical medicine, and his examples include a prescription which Aelius Aristides received in a dream. (Deubner's 1900, 48. 1 reference to: Aristides, Hieroi Logoi I. 43, cf. Behr 1981, 285). Deubner may be exaggerating the extent to which pork was used as medication, but he does offer an excellent interpretation of the way in which pigs were offered up and sacrificed in the cult of Asclepius. (The most famous pig in the context of Asclepius was the silver statue which Asclepius asked for as a fee from an incredulous patient he had cured, "as a memorial of her ignorance". Epidaurus, Iamata, Edelstein and Edelstein 1998, T 423.4; Deubner's other sources are Philostratos, Vita Apoll. I. 10; Herondas, IV 15. On pigs as offerings to other deities, see Deubner 1900, 40). Sacrificing piglets was very common in ancient Greece in general, because it was the cheapest meat and cheapest animal sacrifice and pigs were frequently depicted on votive tablets as well. (On the popularity of sacrificing pigs in general and in the cult of Ascelpius in particular, as well as for further references on the epigraphic evidence on pigs, see Ehrenheim 2015, 31-34).

One thing that is certain, however, is that pork does appear as magical medicine in the admonitions of a magical papyrus which encourages readers to eat grilled pork lungs. (πολλὰ πίνοντα καὶ μὴ μεθύειν· χοίρεον πνεύμονα ὀπτήσας φάγε. Wessely 1893, 25; cf. Deubner 1900, 48). The magical papyri also show pork in a completely different way as they command the person who receives the magical phrases not to eat pork to assure the efficacy of the conjuration: "And I adjure you, the one who receives this conjuration, not to eat pork, and every spirit and daimon, whatever sort it may be, will be subject to you." (PGM IV. 3007-86, A tested charm of Pibechis for those possessed by daimons; tr. W. C. Grese, in Betz 1986, 96).

Illness as miasma, healing as cleansing and repulsive remedies

In cases when the pork or the pig fat represented anything unclean or repulsive for the patient, its use can be seen as analogous to cures which entailed rubbing mud or some kind of faeces onto the body. In such cases the mechanism is in part a test of the patient's faith, but more importantly exploits the notion whereby disease, particularly any that involves symptoms visible on the skin, is some form of impurity or miasma. Ritual healing has the potential to wash this off—indeed, one of Apollo's bynames was "the Washer"[3]—while Asclepius often used to wash his patients in their sleep. Pausanias reports that there is a place by the river Samikon which was dedicated to the nymphs, daughters of Anigros. People who came here for healing would first promise some offering to the nymphs and then scrub their bodies clean in the river, afterwards swimming across the river, while the traces of illness would stay in the water. (Pausanias, Guide to Greece 5. 5. 11). On occasion, the Christian physician saints also used to apply ablutions; one instance is reported when Saint Artemios took out the inner organs of his patient, rinsed them out and put them back in their place. (MA 25). Another method for removing miasma is to place some similarly filthy and disgusting substance on the body which would then attract the impurity that caused or indicated disease. (Parker 1983; Mouliner 1952).

Saint Thecla also recommends dirt as a remedy, yet we find a far more illustrative example in the case of Elias the leper among the miracles of Cyrus and John (MT 18). The hagiographer writes that Elias bore stigmas on his skin as a sign of the sin he had committed, and neither his adherence to the laws of Moses, nor the science of Galen and Hippocrates could help him. The saints advised him to cover his entire body with camel dung which Elias promptly executed, exempting only his face, which indeed continued to bear the marks of his disease and of his incredulity and disgust. (MCJ 13). This cure can be associated with the methods of magical healers executing purging procedures while at the same time it serves as a test of faith in the healer.

Test of faith remedies

A far more remarkable result of prescribing pork is that it forced the sufferer to make a crucial choice about his or her faith and take the side of

[3] Plato 1921: *Cratylos* [405a] "Socrates: His name and nature are in harmony; you see he is a musical god. For in the first place, purification and purgations used in medicine and in soothsaying, and fumigations with medicinal and magic drugs, [405b] and the baths and sprinklings connected with that sort of thing all have the single function of making a man pure in body and soul, do they not? Hermogenes: Certainly. Socrates: But this is the god who purifies and washes away (ἀπαλοούων) and delivers (ἀπολύων) from such evils, is he not? Hermogenes Certainly. Socrates: With reference, then, to his acts of delivering and his washings, [405c] as being the physician of such diseases, he might properly be called Apoluon (ἀπαλούων, the washer) …

the saints' credo. In this respect, the previously mentioned case of the Jewish woman who decided to eat pork in the church of Cosmas and Damian is akin to the stories which tell that a pagan first needed to convert to obtain a cure, or when heretics needed to take the Eucharist in the Orthodox fashion. The host in these stories is used as if it were a pill, to be swallowed for the sake of the cure and on each and every occasion it appears only for patients for whom taking the Eucharist in the prescribed manner meant a religious taboo. (I have written in detail on this topic in Csepregi 2006). Taking the Eucharist in a dream or promising to take it once awake, in the way the saints defined as Orthodox, often along with reciting a particular creed, could be the pre-condition of further recovery or constitute the remedy in itself. And just as a miraculous remedy could be instantaneous and produce an immediate cure, taking it with a biased heart could lead to immediate disaster, as in the case of the pagan who pretended to be a Christian, who to confirm his disguise even took the Eucharist and was seized immediately by convulsions and died (MCJ 32).

Conditions like this, which serve to endorse the healer's exclusive authority, may be ritual acts which are in line with or which contradict the sufferer's faith, but they can also be blasphemous commandments which test their faith. (For instance, the advice given by Cosmas and Damian to the paralysed man according to which he should try to sleep with the mute woman lying right close to him. When the man finally gathers his strength and crawls over to the woman, she cries out and the paralysed man runs away; in other words, both are cured: KDM 24). In other cases, they are absurd instructions in stark contrast to any kind of medical practice. (In Saint Artemios' miracles, for instance, a butcher with a paralysed hand had to shave his fellow patient while another patient had to slap somebody on the face in the church, elsewhere the remedy suggested by the saint was to strike someone with a hammer).

A faith-related condition in connection with pork is also told among the miracles of Saints Cyrus and John (MCJ 54). The hagiographer embarks upon the account of the epileptic little boy Isidoros, "a pagan", with a laudation of the scholarly forebears of the patient: Dionysos had come from Damascus and was among the most honoured and aristocratic of men, coming from a family of long-standing glory—his ancestors had included the famous philosopher Nicolaus, teacher to Herod, son of Antony and Cleopatra. This Nicolaus gave life to twelve children who followed in line, excelling in philosophy, increasing the family's fame and glory. Dionysos' child Isidoros was attacked at the baths by a demon when still a child and doctors were called in vain, but his illness only grew worse. The father sent the son, together with his mother, to the church of

Cyrus and John. The saints appeared to the mother in her dream, proposing the following cure: the boy's body should be covered in pig fat from head to toe, "because they were also trying to cure the woman's soul", since the mother "was suffering from an error of the Greeks and was eating pork in relation to the death of Adonis". In the cult of Aphrodite, the taboo of touching pork was associated with the death of Adonis, the great love of the goddess. Adonis had been fatally injured by a wild boar, hence the loathing of that animal by the goddess and her followers. All of this is encapsulated in the Greek saying, "Offering Aphrodite a pig for sacrifice", meaning to give someone an improper or inappropriate gift. (The pig, however, is ambivalent in Aphrodite's cult, since we know that, while it was taboo, it was also Aphrodite's sacrificial animal at Argos and Cyprus where a special feast was dedicated to it (Hysteria). The same ambivalence is also reflected in Aesop's Fable No. 197. On the pig in medieval and early modern Europe, see Fabre-Vassas 1997).

The woman in the story had to surmount the difficulty of offending a religious taboo and rub her son's entire body with pig fat; this the demon could not stand and, as if stricken by some divine punishment, it instantly departed from the boy's body. What is more, the boy's physical illness went hand in hand with the mother's spiritual illness, and just as other heresies and incredulity are described elsewhere as the sickness of the soul, here too her pagan belief is set in medical terms, its symptom being her aversion to pork. And the cure is a double one: it rectified the mother's erroneous religious belief, and the son, so we read, gained protection against demons for the rest of his life.

In the next miracle from the same collection the cure proposed by the saints is again related to pigs, and in a very interesting context. As the story reveals, the cure was magical in a double sense. Here the pork is not actually related to the sufferer's illness so much as to the person causing the disease; secondly the curative magic also relies on other sources. What is more, besides the cure, the origin of the disease itself is also magical and the story itself happens with a famous physician (MCJ 55).

Theodoros was a physician, one well versed in the sciences and of great renown who, not knowing the cause of his own paralysis, tried to cure himself by all the means he usually applied to genuine paralysis not caused by magic. (It is important to note that the hagiographer acknowledges the effectiveness of medicine!) The doctor fled to the church where the saints prescribed him the following cure in his dream: he should buy a pair of pig's lungs, roast them over charcoal, baste them with wine and rub them into his ailing body parts. However, the saints' ambition was more than merely to cure Theodoros' illness—they also wanted to identify the cause. They therefore gave the following advice: Theodoros should send a servant to his house in Cyprus and dig the floor up under the doorstep of his bedchamber. As soon as this took place and the magical substance which had nearly proved lethal emerged (no further details revealed), Theodoros would know straight away who the author of the plot had been, "and that person was soon snatched away by death, avenging Theodoros with the approval of the martyrs. It was a Jew who, as such, cannot be held clear of such suspicion". (An example of the Jewish magus contemporary to the present text is the legend of Theophilos of Adana from the early seventh century: Bibliotheca Hagiographica Graeca 1319–1322).

The miracles of Cyrus and John are arranged into thematic units. The above two episodes appear in a group of miracles which feature strangers and foreigners, and both narratives share the trait whereby the disease is originally caused by magic and the remedy for which is pork, which represents a religious taboo. One scholar who analysed this miracle, Natalio Fernandez Marcos, sees the pig as a remedy which is a specific cure against magic perpetrated by a Jew. (Fernandez Marcos 1975, 196).

Some other reminiscences of ancient magic in Christian miracles

Pork and the related magical elements such as causing the disease to leap across to the meat in the miracle of Cosmas and Damian are not the only echoes of antiquity in early Byzantine healing miracles. There is another story among the miracles of Cosmas and Damien in which the saints encourage the protagonist to go into the hippodrome at midnight and bury three jugs of castor oil. When the person is caught lurking, he is taken to court on the charge of doing magic, where he can only prove his innocence if he is willing to drink the "magic potion" he buried at night—meaning the content of all three jugs. The resulting abdominal cramps do a great job of curing him of his disease and, more importantly, also blow away his fanatic attachment to horse racing. This type of magical healing was legitimised through and for Christianity. Let me analyse a very different case, that of the genuinely "pagan" gesture which has survived persistently. One such example is found in a story about Cyrus and John: a man fell into a curious state of trance after taking the Eucharist and began to make an odd slurping noise through his nostrils. According to the hagiographer, this habit is particularly appreciated by the pagan deities (for more on this magical practice, see Bonner 1942, 87). Tertullian also writes about this gesture and although its genuine meaning (which is obscene or is related to the magical activity of demons) stays hidden in the Christian texts, it cannot be concealed from these saints who promptly punish the perpetrator by blindness (Tertullian, Apologeticus XXIII. 5).

In another miracle of Cyrus and John we witness a case of a binding spell—a small doll, trussed around its arms and legs, is found and released, which gradually brings about a step-by-step recovery for the patient in his paralysed arms and legs (for such dolls and bound figurines used in Greek magic, see Gager 1992, 15; and Ogden 1999).

It is highly likely that healing gestures of antiquity survived vigorously in the notions of newly converted Christians, even after the original magical meaning faded. It is also easily imaginable that the chronicler of the episode, the hagiographer, knew of such cases and intertwined them with his narratives as examples meant to deter.

No matter how fictional or literary hagiography is as a source, and even though it is practically a mandatory element of the genre to feature some individuals who do not believe in miracles (believers of a different faith, sceptics, supporters of the medical approach), it is certainly possible that shrines were sought out even by people whose faith differed from the professed denomination of the shrine. Besides the "test of faith" element there is another important theological message related to the appearance of pork and, in that context, of Jews and other non-Christians in accounts of miracles. Presenting the true faith and the genuine healer who even overcomes the methods of magic and whose effectiveness in healing tempts followers of different creeds to commit to Orthodox Christianity offered an excellent opportunity for religious propaganda.

We must bear in mind, however, that these collections of accounts of miracles also used to provide entertainment literature during that time. As a result, it is an important characteristic that they aim to relate the most colourful and complex stories possible, including characters and situations which render the narrative itself more interesting but which are not necessarily a true representation of reality. I am thinking, for instance, of the role of physicians in healing miracles, who were usually subject to bitter polemics and mockery or were otherwise forced to acknowledge the effectiveness of magical healers. This in no way means that the church or the hagiographers in question actually opposed the representatives or means of scientific medicine—polemics was merely a requirement of the genre. A similarly "mandatory" element is to feature non-Christians in the miracles who import their related religious and social associations, like Jews import their taboo on pork.

It is interesting to observe the Janus-faced nature of healing rites employing magical elements when used in Christian corpuses. On the one hand, these are used by the saints, while on the other, they are often ridiculed or simply prove useless in contrast to the power of healing endowed by God. The episode of curing the noted physician and sophist Gesios, one of the non-fictional characters of the collection, can be read as a mockery of this kind. Gesios was an Alexandrian teacher, physician and philosopher, a figure held in high esteem by both the pagans and the Christians of his age. His sixteen-volume compendium of Galen was still in use as late as the tenth century. The saints prescribed him the following humiliating procedure for his backache: he had, in broad daylight, to go in circles round the yard of the church with a saddle on his back, a bell round his neck and a bit in his mouth, with all the people to behold him, shouting, "I am a stupid fool!", while the saints sarcastically asked whether Democritos or Heracleitos had ever prescribed such a cure. Here the saints aim to mock the way of life of the Alexandrian scholar and scientific medicine as such, but do this in a way which can also be read as a grotesque parody of both magical and medical practices.

References

Betz, Hans Dieter, ed. 1986. *The Greek Magical Papyri in translation*. Chicago: University of Chicago Press.

Bonner, Carl. 1942. "A Tarsian Peculiarity." *Harvard Theological Review* 35: 1–11.

Csepregi, Ildikó. 2006. "Mysteries for the Uninitiated. The Role and Symbolism of the Eucharist in Miraculous Dream Healing." In *The Eucharist in Theology and Philosophy: Issues of Doctrinal History in East and West from the Patristic Age to the Reformation*, edited by István Perczel, Réka Forrai, and György Geréby, 97–130. Leuven: Leuven University Press.

Crisafulli, Virgil S., Nesbitt, John W., and Haldon, John F. 1997. *The Miracles of St. Artemios. A Collection of Miracle Stories by an Anonymous Author of Seventh-Century Byzantium*. Leiden: E. J. Brill.

Dagron, Gilbert. 1978. *Vie et miracles de sainte Thècle: texte grec, traduction et commentaire*. Bruxelles: Société des Bollandistes.

Deubner, Ludwig. 1900. *De Incubatione capita quattuor*. Lipsiae: B.G. Teubner.

—. 1907: *St. Kosmas und Damian. Texte und Einleitung*. Leipzig: Teubner.

Edelstein, Emma, and Ludwig Edelstein. 1998. *Asclepius: a collection of the testimonies* I–II. Baltimore, and London: The Johns Hopkins University. [Baltimore: The Johns Hopkins Press, 1945.]

Ehrenheim, Hedvig von. 2015 *Greek Incubation Rituals in Classical and Hellenistic Times*. Liège: Kernos.

Fabre-Vassas, Caroline. 1997. *The Singular Beast: Jews, Christians and the Pig*. New York: Columbia University Press.

Fernandez Marcos, Natalio. 1975. *Los Thaumata de Sofronio. Contribucion al estudio de la incubatio cristiana*. Madrid: Instituto Antonio de Nebrija.

Festugière, A-J. 1971. *Sainte Thècle, Saints Côme et Damien, Saints Cyr et Jean (extraits), Saint Georges*. Paris: Edition A. et J. Picard.

Frazer, James George. 1890. *The Golden Bough. A Study in Comparative Religion*. London: Macmillan.

Gager, John G, ed. 1992. *Curse tablets and binding spells from the ancient world*. New York: Oxford University Press.

Gascou, Jean. 2006. *Sophrone de Jérusalem, Miracles des saints Cyr et Jean. BHG I 477-479*. Paris: de Boccard. (Études d'archéologie et d'histoire ancienne.)

Gil, Luis. 1969. *Therapeia. La medicina popular en el mundo clássico*. Madrid: Ediciones Guadarrama.

Hamilton, Mary. 1906. *Incubation. The Cure of Disease in Pagan Temples and Christian Churches*. London: W. C. Henderson.

Lucian. 1925. *Alexander the False Prophet*. Translated by A. M. Harmon. London: Heinemann. (Loeb Classical Library IV.)

Moulinier, Louis. 1952. *Le pur et l'impur dans la pensée des Grecs d'Homère a Aristote*. Paris: Librairie C. Klinksiech.

Ogden, Daniel. 1999. "Binding spells: Curse tablets and voodoo dolls in the Greek and Roman worlds." In *Witchcraft and Magic in Europe*, edited by Bengt Ankarloo, and Stuart Clarke, 1–90. Philadelphia: University of Pennsylvania Press.

Parker, Robert. 1983. *Miasma. Pollution and Purification in Early Greek Religion*. Oxford: The Clarendon Press.

Plato. 1921. *Plato in Twelve Volumes*, Vol. 12. Translated by Harold N. Fowler. Cambridge, MA and London: Harvard University Press and William Heinemann Ltd.

Wessely, Carl. 1893. *Neue Griechische Zauberpapyri*. Vienna: Tempsky.

SOLDIERS OF CHRIST ON EARTH AND IN HEAVENLY JERUSALEM. PSYCHOTRONICS: A CONTEMPORARY ESOTERIC HEALING SYSTEM

JUDIT KIS-HALAS

The metaphor of Heavenly Jerusalem contains rich meanings in Judeo-Christian eschatology, and plays an important role in the Christian history of salvation. In this study, nonetheless, I will discuss it as a basic symbol of *Psychotronics* or *spirit surgery*.[1] In my article I would like to point to the new meanings (mainly relating to the ideas of the New Age and Neo-Paganism) associated with the Judeo-Christian religious interpretations.

The main reference points of my analysis will be within Western esotericism, the relationship between New Age ideas and medicine or traditional "popular" healing methods, and alternative healing therapies in Hungary. Consequently, the methodology of this present analysis, even though the topic is closely related to the field of religious studies, essentially follows the approaches of comparative folkloristics, historical ethnography, and the ethnology of religion.

My conclusions are based on healing narratives in which visits to a specific otherworldly location—Heavenly Jerusalem—are referred to. The text corpus consists of three well-distinguishable source groups: 1) semi-structured interviews and personal narratives recorded during my fieldwork;[2] 2) lectures given at the spirit surgery training courses and

---

[1] In order to avoid word repetition, I use the two terms alternately, as synonyms. (J. K.-H.)

[2] I've been conducting fieldwork since the year 2000 among various healing and esoteric practitioners who are also experts of contemporary popular magic (aura seers, clairvoyants, seers of the dead, etc.) in the country town of Siklós and its vicinity in South-West Hungary. My data come partly from semi-structured interviews, and partly from informal conversations, cf. Kis-Halas 2009a, 513–4.

published in an internally disseminated publication, the *Szellemsebész Hírlevél* (Spirit surgeon Newsletter);[3] 3) relevant entries in online social forums and blogs.

These texts, created with different goals and in various ways, outline the roles played by the Heavenly Jerusalem metaphor in the central narrative of spirit surgery, and at the same time, allow us to consider some of the interpretations of the healers and their clientele.

By extending data collection to the online contexts, I follow the approach of my previous studies discussing New Age phenomena and alternative spiritualities in Hungary (Kis-Halas 2007; 2008; 2009a; 2009b; 2012b; 2014a; 2014b); that is, I consider the interactive forums of the Internet as typical manifestations of secondary orality. This concept was introduced by Walter J. Ong in his seminal study on "The Literate Orality of Popular Culture Today"; he also discusses it in detail in his book describing the paradigm shift of orality (Ong, 1971; 1982). These written texts possess the characteristics of live speech: they are in the present tense, they coordinate, and are dynamic and reflective; indeed, chat forums develop a communication model very close to live speech (Czeizer 1998). The semi-structured interviews, conversations and forum entries in cyber space have helped in providing an insight into the psychology of the various discourses about spirit surgery. In this case, we can consider these forums as specific, virtual fields of empirical methods of cultural studies, of an "ethnography of cyber space" (Csordás 1997). Naturally, the communication taking place in cyber space exists in virtual reality, no matter how closely it bears the traits of live speech; the identity of the participants is also virtual. We also have to accept that it can only provide indirect information on the social reality it represents.[4] Meanwhile, we cannot disregard that this virtual space, by its easier and faster interoperability, becomes more and more indispensable to the communication between religious (and other) communities, to the organisation and operation of religious life and to the exchange of the textual and visual manifestations of theories, experiences and ideas. The Internet can be the social scene of communication about religion, or "religion online" (Cowen and Hadden 2004, 120; Kis-Halas 2007; 2008; Hubbes 2013). The network-like organisation is not only useful in terms of information

[3] It will be referred to by the acronym *SzH* in this paper. (J. K.-H.)

[4] Gaidukov points out the discrepancy between the virtual world and reality in relation to the Rodnoverie movement, especially in terms of credibility. He sees that the people expressing themselves in cyber space might as well be "clones"; the sources of information are unverifiable and all this leads to misunderstandings and debates (see Gaidukov 2013, 327–8).

communication, but can also be a pattern for the organisation of virtual religious groups (Possamaï 2007, 162–3).

In the first part of this study, I will define the wider theoretical context of the methods of spirit surgery, assigning its place among New Age movements, Hungarian Neopagan ideologies and contemporary alternative healing systems. In accordance with Paul Heelas (1996) and Wouter Hanegraaff (2007) I prefer to call it a movement. After that, I will take into consideration the basic characteristics of Psychotronics: the conceptual framework, the practitioners and the healing methods. In a subchapter of the latter, I will discuss the healing processes projected to the transcendent sphere, in which Heavenly Jerusalem plays a central role.

Esotericism, Neo-Paganism, Medicine

Western Esotericism—New Age—alternative spiritualties

In current religious studies and in public discourse, a considerable slice of contemporary religious phenomena consists of forms of manifestation and trends described by the notions of New Age religion, New Age spirituality, and Neo-Paganism. Although delineating and defining the essence of certain movements and trends is quite difficult due to their heterogeneity and their diversity, nonetheless they can be well discerned by their phenomenological features, which also accentuate the differences among them.

Western esotericism constitutes a common theoretical cluster of references to many of these currents, described by Antoine Faivre with the following four criteria: 1) every component of the universe is in correspondence with one another: "they are a collection of signs/hieroglyphs waiting to be deciphered"; 2) nature is considered a living entity; 3) the relationships of the universe become decipherable and clear through some form of mediation (for instance symbols, rituals, meditation, spiritual mediators, etc.); and 4) the goal is to acquire experiences that lead to spiritual enlightenment (second birth, transmutation). Faivre proposes the alchemical term of transubstantiation/transmutation because, in this case, the transformation is substantial and irreversible (Faivre 1994, 10–5).

Faivre mentions two further characteristics, although he believes that their existence is optional, and that, therefore, they are not indispensable criteria of the definition of Western esotericism: syncretism (the concordance between different traditions) and the importance of transmitting knowledge (Faivre 1994, 14–5; 1998, 2). The same characteristics are also emphasised by Miguel Farias (2006, 105) and Sabina Magliocco (2015, 636–7).

In Western civilisations, New Age ideologies developed together with the counterculture movements of the 1960s from the "traditions" of Western esotericism described above (Hanegraaff 2007). Steve Bruce, exemplifying the cultic milieu of the New Age, underlines the holistic approach (the individual, the transcendent and the material world carry the same essence); extreme eclecticism (a medley of methods, isms, myths and symbols); and the central role of the individual (in the principle of the "divinity incorporated in the individual" and in the widely utilitarian approach acknowledging the individual as the highest authority) (Bruce 2000, 226–8; Kamarás 1999). George Chryssides sees the individual nature in the fact that for New Age followers, to "understand and interpret meaning in their lives is one of the most important goals that they want to reach with some sort of guidance from the outside" (Chryssides 2007, 14). Some Hungarian researchers, especially when comparing New Age movements with Christian mentality, in fact consider extreme individualism to be the most characteristic feature of these movements, and thus they do not interpret it as a religion, but rather as quasi-religious phenomena.[5] It is undeniable that, indeed, religious practices of New Age followers were not institutionalised under organised, ecclesiastic-style frameworks, but were rather conducted in a loosely organised manner: as Grace Davie describes it, "believing without belonging" (Davie 1990).[6]

It is also accentuated that in this milieu the individual behaves as a consumer: people create a spiritual package of their own, which they consider to be the most appropriate in the given situation. The metaphor of a spiritual supermarket is used by many researchers (Bruce 2000, 228; Kamarás 1999; Bowman and Sutcliffe 2000, 7); Wouter Hanegraaff calls

---

[5] By contrast, Christopher Partridge claims that the New Age and similar alternative spiritualities appear as "privatised" forms of religion in the process of "re-enchantment" in the secularised world (Partridge 2004). The official position of the Roman Catholic Church on New Age movements reveals a biased attitude, see *Jesus Christ the Bearer of New Life*; and *Jézus Krisztus, az élő víz hordozója.* Chryssides refuses to categorise the New Age within new religious movements. Moreover, he sees the essence of the New Age to lie in rejecting such a position, claiming that the answering of spiritual questions is the exclusive monopoly of religion (Chryssides 2007, 17).

[6] On the Hungarian reception of Davie's ideas, see Tomka 1996. Analysing data drawn on recent surveys on religious attitudes (religion vs. spirituality) of Finnish society, Kimmo Ketola observes that individualisation processes (spirituality) are strongly contested by experiential religions, see Ketola 2007. For more on the spirituality versus religion discourse, cf. Glendinning and Bruce 2006.

New Age religiosity the "spirituality of the market" (Hanegraaff 2007, 47). In Adam Possamaï's words, the followers "shop" according to their needs from the options offered by the cults (Possamaï 2007, 160).

Marion Bowman and Steven Sutcliffe define the strongly individual and consumer-type religious attitudes of secularised, industrial and post-industrial societies as being alternative spiritualities. They emphasise that this definition of spirituality is *emic* because it approaches the specific New Age religious milieu from the perspective of the followers. According to their interpretation, "spirituality is halfway between the 'official', widely institutionalised religion and the diverse lifestyles and subcultures of modernity"; between the saintly and the profane worlds. Thus, it becomes suitable for "being not only a pragmatic, but also a strategically efficient resource for a mobile individual searching for its place in the modern world" (Bowman and Sutcliffe 2000, 10). This attitude is well illustrated by the metaphor of a "quest", (Possamaï 2005, 31–2); the "seeker" is one of the most typical among the potential roles in New Age religiosity (Sutcliffe 2000, 20–3; 2004). Bowman and Sutcliffe, by using the "alternative" epithet, suggest the interpretation of these strategies as options. Meanwhile, they consider it completely inadequate to define spirituality, one of the characteristic attitudes of contemporary religiosity, as opposed to the all-time prominent cultural formations (Bowman and Sutcliffe 2000, 10–1).[7] If, according to Marion Bowman's model, we consider religiosity (from the perspective of the relation between the individual and religion) as "the dynamic interaction between beliefs, practices, attitudes, rational considerations, narratives; the experiences related to the practical efficiency of all these; and personal experiences", then alternative spiritualities may be known as contemporary forms of popular religion (Bowman 1992; Bowman and Sutcliffe 2000, 7; cf. also Knoblauch 2008; Kis-Halas 2007, 401; Draper and Barker 2011).

Neo-Paganism in Hungary

Before discussing the topic of contemporary alternative medicine, we have to briefly discuss the religious movements marked by the umbrella term

---

[7] Naturally, this attitude constituted the most fundamental point of reference at the establishment of certain trends and streams (such as Theosophy, and some alternative healing methods, etc.) in the process of self-determination and legitimacy. Some of the Hungarian Neopagan groups also define the determining elements of their identity as opposed to mainstream religiosity, according to Réka Szilárdi (2007, 108–9 and 112).

Neo-Paganism,[8] because these have played an important role—similar to that of the New Age—in the creation of the ideology of spirit surgery.

In the beginning (in the first half of the 1990s), the relationship between the New Age and Neo-Paganism had been considered differently by researchers of religion. At the time, there were basically two approaches: 1) Neo-Paganism is one of the New Age movements. Tania Luhrmann considers Neo-Paganism as a clearly discernible subculture (1991, 29–41); Wouter Hanegraaff sees it as a trend within the New Age (1996, 78–9); 2) Neo-Paganism is an individual religious system, which is also proven by its phenomenological features which differ from those of New Age movements, and the two systems only connect on certain points. Tamás Szilágyi and Réka Szilárdi, the authors of the pioneer study discussing Neopagan trends in detail, represent the latter point of view (2007). Today, most researchers lean towards the latter view. These different opinions underline that both systems are extremely heterogeneous, syncretic, and mostly variable, which has made their description from the perspective of the history of religion, theology and the science of religion very difficult. The current point of view is that Neo-Paganism is a religious movement, and even though it is completely distinguishable from New Age spiritualities, we cannot exclude the possibility of the two creating hybrid formations.

Neo-Paganism consorts with the spirituality represented by New Age movements in its presumption of universal connections, its interpretation of magic, its application of symbols as mediation methods and, furthermore, in its terms of religious and ethical tolerance. However, the sacralisation of the cosmos, including a respect for nature,[9] the revival of

---

[8] Other names for it: modern Paganism or contemporary Paganism (dissociation from the ancient interpretation). According to Michael Strmiska, "Paganism" without any prefix or epithet is also relevant because it focuses on the continuity between the religious practices of pre-Christian religions and contemporary followers (2005, 2). Ethno-Paganism and "a native faith movement" are mostly applied to movements of Eastern and Central Europe because these trends emphasise the ethnic character. The nomenclature is, thus, not uniform. The editors of the latest collection of studies, Aitamurto and Simpson, consciously employ a diverse terminology because it best expresses the diversity of Neopagan world views (2013, 5). Simpson and Filip describe the different "shades" of interpretation of Paganism through the analysis of Central and Eastern European Neopagan narratives and their terminology (2013).

[9] Chas Clifton (concerning the Wicca), goes as far as calling Neo-Paganism (and some other New Age trends) a nature religion (2006, 55–54) because, in accordance with Catherine Albanese who introduced the concept, they believe that in Neopagan cosmology, nature is in the centre of religious symbolisation: nature

pre-Christian cults and the identification with them, along with the emphasis on their historical continuity (remythologisation), the (not fully universal) neglect of hierarchic religious organisation, the belief systems based on duo- or polytheism, sexual tolerance and the promotion of gender equality (although not in every direction) are all characteristic of contemporary paganisms.

Tamás Szilágyi and Réka Szilárdi in describing contemporary Paganism in Hungary, wrote about a "Neopagan spiritual orientation", illustrating that in Hungary it is very difficult to talk about Neo-Paganism *par excellence*. The authors separate "purely" Neopagan movements from groups that are constituted of heterogeneous religious elements. While the former consequently follow certain "well-defined cults, traditions", the belief systems of the latter are rather characterised by religious eclecticism and syncretism (Szilágyi and Szilárdi 2007, 69–70). The possible (and very viable) symbiosis of the two types of religious systems is well illustrated by groups carrying the traits of the New Age and Neo-Paganism, such as the *Ősmagyar Táltos Egyház* (Ancient Hungarian Táltos Church) or the *Univerzum Egyháza* (Church of the Universe), which have strongly contributed to the shaping of the ideas appearing in healing methods of Psychotronics discussed in this study.

Health, energy, New Age

In his analysis of the traits of New Age religiosity, Wouter Hanegraaff underlines healing and personal growth as defining features. He points to the similarities between the alternative healing methods of the New Age and the attitude of traditional "popular" medicine. He not only considers the holistic approach (Hedges and Beckford 2000; Tighe and Butler 2007, 416–20) to be essential among them, but also emphasises that both systems place the illness under a symbolic, fundamentally religious and spiritual interpretive framework.[10] Unlike Western medicine, these interpretations do not simply consider illnesses as diseases, as biophysical facts, but as a physical and spiritual human experience. Thus, the physical and spiritual dimensions are also merged in the applied therapies (Hanegraaff 1996, 42–3). Medical anthropology distinguishes between two types of medical systems on the basis of the explanations of illnesses:

---

shapes and inspires "the establishment of religious beliefs, forms of behaviour and a set of values" (1991, 7).

[10] The use of medical metaphors for religious experience has a long tradition in many cultures and religions, cf. Sontag (1983); Lupton (1995); Barnes and Sered (2004).

the "personalistic", a medical system in which illnesses are caused by the intrusion of some kind of perceivable agent (supernatural creature, or a person with supernatural powers), and the "naturalistic", a medical system wherein the illness is considered to be an imbalance within the body or between the body and its environment (Foster 1976; Hanegraaff, 1996, 44–5).[11] Another important conclusion by Hanegraaff was that in the New Age approach (similar to traditional cultures), healing was fundamentally religious, because in both religion and medicine, it is the desire to have physical and spiritual health and cleanliness that is expressed; furthermore, the central figures and the symbols of religion may serve as the source of healing. In this sense, recovering from an illness and the process of healing can in fact be considered as radical forms of salvation (Hanegraaff 1996, 43–4).

Catherine Albanese, in her study revealing the analogies between quantum physics and New Age healing methods, also underlines the religious nature of healing: she calls New Age a "new healing religion". In relation to this, she also points out the terms playing a key role in the healing-related discourses of the New Age, such as (among others) the "healing energies of the universe", "harmonising", "chakras" and "vibration". Albanese also finds it remarkable that, according to the New Age approach, the healing of a human organism happens simultaneously at the level of the universe. Consequently, one's health can only be recovered if one's vibration is in harmony with the universe. Moreover, the opposite is also true: the imbalances in the universe can be settled by healing, "harmonising" the human organism in "correspondence" with the universe.[12]

In my opinion, the "energetic healing methods" of contemporary alternative medicine belong to the category Hanegraaff called "naturalistic" because illness is interpreted as the disruption of harmony between people and their environment. Their common denominator (as Albanese points out) is the energy providing the existential basis for all living creatures.

---

[11] Honko's classification, though it is somewhat overlapping with that of Foster's, is less applicable in our case. He distinguishes five explanations of illness: breach of taboo, soul loss, spirit possession, intrusion of an alien object in the body, presence of a worm or worms (1959, 23–37).

[12] Albanese takes the example of the work of Richard Greber, a physician committed to Theosophy, and in particular his *Vibrational Medicine* (1988); according to him, matter (and thus the human body) is nothing else but the sum of frozen photons of cosmic light; therefore, healing should start with the harmonisation of the energy level consisting of the most elemental particles, the electrons (1992, 75–7).

This energy is cosmic, often of divine origin, and every living being is able to incorporate it through certain orifices of the body called *chakras* and distribute it through the channels (*nadi*) which form a network in the body similar to blood vessels. Other views claim that living beings are able not only to absorb, but also to create their own energy called "life essence", which is produced in the *kuṇḍalinī*, the geometric centre of the human body.[13] The internal or external energies of a living creature are utilised according to their specific needs: we might say they are tailor-made and, what is more, that they create from this energy an "energy field" (Brennan 1988), the *aura*. The *aura* consists of several layers of different colours (seven, according to general belief), which correspond to certain body parts, internal organs, psychological characters, different zodiac signs, planets, elements, and so forth. It is not difficult to recognise here the Neoplatonic concept of associating "body" with "microcosm" and the "universe" with "macrocosm". The *aura* surrounds the body as a shell; its diameter is directly proportional to the energy needs and the state of physical-spiritual health of the living creature: the *aura* of a seriously ill person shrinks, while the aura of a healer with excess energy might extend to kilometres, or might even be infinite. Moreover, the *aura* is a two-sided projection screen: from the inside it carries the imprint of the living being's ever-changing physical and spiritual state, while it is simultaneously the illustration of external effects impacting the body. The *aura* is usually invisible because it consists of energy, of resonating particles, such as the previously mentioned quanta. Ordinary people with sensitive perception are also capable of perceiving this subtle resonance; moreover, "aura seers" are able to see it spontaneously with the naked eye without using any tools. Examining the *aura* is the basic diagnostic method of energy medicine. Specialists measure the vibration of the *aura* with dowsing, a divinatory method known since antiquity.[14] In any case,

---

[13] For the origins and symbolism of kuṇḍalinī, see Urban (2005). The term was first introduced in Western esoteric currents by Arthur Avalon (Sir John Woodroffe), whose book on Shaktic and Tantric yoga practice had soon achieved great popularity (Woodroffe 1950).

[14] In most cases, either a simple dowsing rod or a special device, called *sensibil* or *Moses' staff* is employed. The former is usually made of brass and is bent in an L shape. The shorter shaft must be held while measurements are made based on the movements of the longer shaft. The latter is an instrument made of wire bent in the form of a hand, which is held between the thumb and the index finger. As the practitioner makes combing movements along the patient's body, the occasional deflections indicate the state of the aura.

the energy field can be made visible to anyone with special devices, now popular at esoteric fairs in Hungary, too.

One of the principles of energy medicine is that all illnesses stem from the disruption of the capability of the patient to absorb and/or utilise energy. In certain cases there might be additional causes of illness characteristic of personalistic systems: the disruption of absorbing and distributing energy can be caused by supernatural creatures (such as revenants, evil spirits, demonic energy vampires) attacking the *aura* and the body, or by spending time with someone suffering energy deficiency (human energy vampire).[15] Energy healers (*bioenergetics specialists*), after having established a diagnosis on the basis of the *aura*'s examination, clear the energy-absorbing *chakras* and the energy-transporting channels; sometimes they restore the equilibrium of the energy imbalance by transmitting the appropriate amount of energy. Energy healers are thus able to absorb and transmit a greater amount of energy that is more efficient (of a higher frequency). This method incorporates "channelling", one of the most characteristic features of New Age religiosity, where the manifestations of the universe (energy, force, knowledge, etc.) become accessible to others by the mediation of a medium with special skills.[16] The possibility of acquiring the skills, and thus, to some extent, healing oneself is open to anybody who, after acquiring the appropriate knowledge, is initiated into one of the branches of energetic healing and becomes a "channel" himself or herself.[17]

Another important principle (also pointed out by Albanese) claims that, through the transmission of vitalising energy, all living beings are in

---

[15] Being an energy vampire is one of the most common explanations in the systems of energy medicine. For more on the subject in contemporary Russia, see DeNio Stephens 2004, 371–7. Drawing from my Hungarian data, I make a distinction between living and demonic energy vampires. While the first are human beings attributed with the ability of "sucking" one's life force, the second type is a supernatural demon, who may even possess humans, see Kis-Halas 2009b and 2012b. A healer from Győr (West Hungary) sees energy vampires as revenants dwelling in the patient's aura and devouring his health (S. Balázs 2004, 215).

[16] Hanegraaff mentions this among the important New Age trends: Hanegraaff 1996, 20. Hammer argues that in New Age ideology, channelling has not only become an effective tool in order to create "rhetoric legitimacy" besides science, but also an important source of wisdom and knowledge, see Hammer 2004, 55–6. So far, the most extensive overview on channelling has been provided by Michael Brown 1997. On the role of channelling in Theosophy see Hammer (ibid.); in UFO religion, see Grünschloß 2007; Flaherty 2011, 592–3; Östling 2016, 148.

[17] The essence of initiation into the *Reiki* healing method is exactly that, cf. Kis-Halas (2007: 404–407).

interaction with their environment: to a certain extent, they are capable of transmitting energy to or taking energy from it. The circulation of energy creates the harmony of the universe, thus maintaining health from the micro-level of the human being to the macro-level of the cosmos. This is the basis of the previously mentioned vibration medicine (Albanese 1992, 75–7). The energy flow between people is the cohesive strength of society. There are extremist theories claiming that the ultimate goal of human communication is not the exchange of information, but rather the exchange of energy.

Psychotronics: healing in hyperspace[18]

In what follows, I will discuss Psychotronics as a special method of energy medicine which is also a current religious medical system. The phenomenon is not unknown to Hungarian research in cultural and medical anthropology. László Kürti was the first to write about it in his study (2001) discussing the spiritual milieu in Hungary after the change of the political system in 1989, in which he unequivocally described Psychotronics as a form of Neoshamanism.[19] Imre Lázár introduced Psychotronics as a Neoshamanic healing method in order to describe the potential roles of alternative medicine in a postmodern society from the perspective of medical anthropology. In his study based on the experiences of several years of fieldwork, Lázár drew a detailed and valid picture of the methods applied by Hungarian neo-*táltos* healers (including Imre Kercselics, who also appears in this present study), and of spirit surgery.

---

[18] The concept of hyperspace appeared in science fiction as early as the 1940s, for example in Isaac Asimov's works. His Foundation series was translated to Hungarian in the early 1970s. As science fiction counts as one of the germinating sources of contemporary popular religious thought (in the cases of UFO and ET belief, for example), no wonder that the concept of hyperspace has been applied to the realm of the supernatural in our cases. For the role of science fiction in modern esoteric UFO and ET belief, cf. Grünschloß 2007; Flaherty 2011; Östling 2016, 419. Theoretical physics, however, has a great impact on Hungarian online discourses on *quantum healing*, as reflected by the frequent references to the book of American-Japanese physicist Michio Kaku, on the topic (1995).

[19] There have been very different interpretations of the notion of Neoshamanism. Some researchers and ethnologists of religion believe that it is part of the *revival* phenomenon, but only the revived practices of people once of shamanic faith, adapted to the contemporary social and religious environment, are included here. In a wider sense, however, it is one of the current attitudes of New Age religiosity: *spiritual path for personal empowerment,* see Adlam and Holyoak 2005, 531–2.

Lacking proper knowledge on the subject, the goal of my overview cannot be a philological analysis and scrutiny of the heterogeneous and syncretic belief system of spirit surgery. Nonetheless, wherever there is an opportunity, I will always discuss supposed ideological parallels, potential prefigurations, or even actual sources. In my analysis, I will apply an empirical approach, blending emic and etic points of view: I will describe the religious healing system from the perspective of the adherents, the followers and those who apply it; meanwhile, I will also give an interpretation of the phenomena in the objective scientific register (see Hanegraaff 1996, 4–6; Szilágyi and Szilárdi 2007, 10–11; Lázár 2006, 38). I primarily use as reference the doctrines and lectures of important healing personalities such as Vilmos Csontos Jr. and Imre Kercselics published in printed and electronic media, as well as the oral and written expressions of their disciples and of those who practise it. To this, I add the material of semi-structured interviews conducted during my fieldwork, as well as my own field notes.

Anomalous Terminologies

The medical system appears in the Hungarian esoteric discourse, and hence in the analysed texts as well, under various names. The most common terms are "Psychotronics" and "spirit surgery", which function as synonyms. We sometimes find the term "psychotronic surgery"; furthermore, online platforms occasionally refer to it as "spirit medicine", or "psychic surgery". To avoid misunderstandings, the teachers and practitioners of the method clearly distance themselves from the latter two methods.

It is worth briefly comparing the conceptual background and connotations of the various denominations in order to highlight the shades of differences and similarities between them. "Psychic surgery", which is widely known today, denotes the Reiki-like "surgical" method of Filipino healers.[20] During this procedure, the healer operates without opening up the patient's body, relying entirely upon his psychic ability. This is also the origin of the name: it is a medical procedure performed not on a physical, but on a psychic/spiritual level.

Spirit surgery, properly known as "active (less frequently: 'Atlantean') spirit surgery", is one of the energetic healing methods we refer to below. The healer treats the "energy field", that is, the *aura* of the patient by

[20] Reiki is one of the most popular branches of energy healing, cf. Brennan 1988; Albanese 1991 and 2000.

involving the personal spiritual assistant of the healer, called the "*raffaelite*" (some sort of angelic helper).[21] The intensity of the interventions aiming to restore the harmony of the energy system can be different, but they can also be surgical procedures performed in the transcendent sphere—hence the term spirit *surgery*.

The term *Psychotronics* was first employed by the French engineer, Fernand Clerc, to describe the behaviour of brain waves as a streaming entity, a new type of energy. Psychotronics, in the contemporary sense, defines itself as a branch of parapsychology: an interdisciplinary science which studies the energy pervading people and their environment, creating a connection between matter and spirit. This is the meaning of the concept in French, Russian, Czech, Polish, German and American esoteric discourses.[22]

Vilmos Csontos Jr., who is the person considered to have introduced the healing methods we shall discuss, also consistently uses the term "Psychotronics" in his teachings. In his definition "Psychotronics is basically a mixture of Greek and Latin words that mean to heal with a soul/spirit that is alive and moving" (Csontos, V. Jr. Interview 2009). It is interesting that Břetislav Kafka, whom Vilmos Csontos Jr. claimed to be the author who most inspired him, is also considered to be a significant precursor of Czech (formerly Czechoslovakian) psychotronic research.[23]

To my mind, it is as if the simultaneous use of the terms Psychotronics and spirit surgery illustrate the dual identity of this special healing method, both in the authoritarian and the lay register: "Psychotronics" alludes to international references while "spirit surgery" represents a more accentuated national aspect, which we will discuss later in detail. The choice of terminology, nonetheless, cannot be regarded as deliberate: the concepts are equivalent synonyms.

---

[21] The connection between the Archangel Raphael and healing appears in the book of Tobias in the Bible: Raphael gives advice to the young Tobias on how to heal the blindness of his father, Tobit, by using the powder of a fish's dried gall. See Tobias 11. 7–13.

[22] There are psychotronic associations operating in several countries, among the goals of which we usually find the recognition of parasciences, see for instance US Psychotronics.

[23] Kafka studied to become a sculptor; then he started to deal with hypnosis. He first published his thoughts in 1949 in his book entitled, "New Essentials of Experimental Psychology". Further information on his life and works can be found on the website named after him, see "Kafka, B.".

In what follows, I will outline the world view of Psychotronics as a religious system, because this provides the ideological background to healing.

Cosmogony, cosmology, divinities

It is primarily Vilmos Csontos Jr., the founder of spirit surgery, who elaborates thoughts on the creation of the universe in his works and teachings partially published in the previously mentioned journal. From the stories, we can outline a fundamentally syncretic creation narrative blending Judeo-Christian theist ideas with scientific knowledge and theories from nineteenth-century Western occultism: it is a supreme deity bearing various names (God, Creator, Maker) who created the universe out of himself by means of his own illumination. Besides God, other creator deities may appear, for instance Enlil, known from Sumerian mythology, or the head of the alleged ancient Hungarian pantheon, the Sun God.[24] In the name of universal ecumenism, and gods and goddesses of Hinduism, supreme creatures of "ancient Hungarian" beliefs and certain deities of ancient civilisations (Sumerians, Greeks) also figure among the divine beings. This heterogeneity and syncretism clearly indicate the fusion of New Age and Neopagan orientations present in Psychotronics.

Among the creatures belonging to the spirit world, it is primarily the members of the Christian pantheon (Jesus, the Holy Trinity, Virgin Mary) and the angels, especially Archangel Michael, who play an important role. Jesus's mediator-advocate role is accentuated, similarly to the Virgin Mary, who occasionally is presented in a national perspective (*Boldogasszony*).[25] I will discuss in detail the ideas related to the Holy Trinity in playing a significant role in the healing procedure in the section on healing methods.

---

[24] Enlil creates the souls, the Sun God creates the healers, see *SzH* VI/1: 3, and Kercselics 2009/1.

[25] As liturgical texts (homilies and sermons) have revealed, *Boldogasszony* [literally "blessed woman"] has been used as a synonym for the Blessed Virgin Mary since the Middle Ages, cf. Madas 2002. The quest for a lost epic and a missing mythology of the Hungarians, which was inspired by national romanticism, resulted in the term gaining a new, ethnic meaning by the end of the nineteenth century. If *táltos* was considered the high priest in a re-invented Ancient Hungarian religion, than Boldogasszony was the most emblematic figure of its pantheon: the Mother Goddess, cf. Kálmány 1885. Boldogasszony is also interpreted as the Hungarian equivalent of the Goddess by some Neopagan traits, see Bowman 2009.

The hierarchic order of angels above all recalls Christian angelology, but it is easy to recognise the influence of the theosophical-anthroposophical "Zeitgeist" notions:[26] Buddhism ("mentals"); furthermore, the traits of contemporary popular angel cult.[27]

> I would like to hand you a bouquet… about the hierarchy of angels. So that people know that there is more to it than the things they see, what the five sensory organs perceive, there are plenty of invisible creatures around us who help our development, help our work and are looking forward to helping us. We are simply unable to "tune in" to them yet because, as a matter of fact, we are too limited by our senses to be condensed in the material. Three types of spiritual groups are sent down to our physical bodies. One is the previously mentioned group of angels, who are assigned directly to a person; there are archangels, who are assigned to a certain community, to small groups of people, or nations. And there is "arche". Arche is the Zeitgeist. (…) We are currently in the fifth cultural era. The Zeitgeist of this fifth era is Michael arche. Thus, Michael is responsible today for every human being on Earth. (…) Archangels are [assigned to] the astral plane… yes… And then comes the lower "mental"; this spiritual group includes powers, virtues and dominions. And there is the other, the superior mental with thrones, cherubim and seraphim. The spiritual hierarchy consists of twelve groups. The thirteenth group includes the Creator God himself and the Holy Trinity (Kercselics 2006/03).

The image and roles of the guardian angel clearly reflect Christian ideas: he is a spirit guide who is also recording the good and bad deeds of someone. However, it seems that according to the teachings of Psychotronics, each soul has two guardian angels. One of them, whom I would call a "temporary escort", is only present at the person's side during the time of their earthly incarnation. In contrast to the earthly guardian, the other angel is a permanent companion, who follows the soul in each and every new incarnation, and leads the individual book of fate, the *Akasha-chronicle.*[28]

---

[26] Rudolf Steiner had been talking since 1913 about Michael, as a kind of *Zeitgeist* and the "leader of cosmic intelligence" whose mission is to prepare the return of Christ to Earth, see Steiner 1994.

[27] For popular angelic belief in America, see Draper and Barker 2011; in Norway, see Gilhus 2012; in Estonia, see Uibu 2013; in the Republic of Ireland, see Tighe and Butler 2007; in Finland, see Utriainen 2015, 2016 [2013]; in the UK, see Walter 2011; and Engelke 2012, 156–8; in Hungary, see Kis-Halas 2008; 2009a.

[28] In Hinduism, the Sanskrit term *ākāśa* represents one of the five primeval elements: ether. Other connotations are: "sky", "space", "glowing". At the end of

We have no room here to discuss in detail the apocalyptic ideas of spirit surgery. We have to note, however, that Satan, who appears mainly in this context, is far from being equivalent to the creator and an almighty supreme deity. Hell, and Satan in it, have only existed since the birth of Christ, and they exist only on Earth:

> According to the Bible Hell is on Earth. The external crust of the earth is this third dimension, it is in fact the ordinary Hell (Csontos, V. Jr. Interview 2009).
>
> Satan's main adversary is the Archangel Michael, with the help of whom the army of men supporting the evil powers will eventually disappear (because everyone will become good), and Satan will eventually stop existing (Csontos, V. Jr. *SzH* VI/1: 3).
>
> Satan has done and taught so many silly things in the past 2,000 years [sic] on Earth that it is very difficult to turn it into good (Csontos, V. Jr. Interview 2009).

Our texts mention the structure of the universe only sporadically and indirectly. Similar to the cosmogony generally accepted, scientific elements of the cosmology are blended with mythological universals (multi-layered world; Heaven-Earth/earthly Hell-Underworld, duality of this world and the other world, deities living in the sky-people living on Earth) and with elements inspired by science fiction literature and the fantasy subculture (hyperspace, multitude of dimensions).

> There are things regarding the celestial beings, and things that regard the earthlings (Csontos, V. Jr. *SzH* V/4: 3).
>
> From dimension zero to ninety-nine God appears in a human form; in the other nine hundred and ninety-nine he appears as a light creature. […] These are parts of Space where matter is always present in a softer form;

the nineteenth century, Western occultism (primarily Theosophy) took over the term but somewhat reinterpreted the concept: it applied to the "cosmic consciousness" encompassing the past, present and future of the Universe, cf. Minya 2009. Anthroposophy teaches that the individual also has an *akasha*, which flashes before the eye like a movie in the period of three days after death, see Steiner 2010; and Hansson 1991, 37–8. In current esoteric discourse, the Anthroposophical interpretation has become common. For instance, the healer from Győr also used the individual Akashic chronicle to gather information about the patient's former lives; cf. S. Balázs 2004, 216 and 220–1.

> moreover, beyond the ninety-ninth dimension one can only see light creatures (Csontos, V. Jr. *SzH* V/4: 3).

In a short reference, we learn that the Earth itself consists of layers and dimensions (the Earth's crust is the third dimension) with the underworld at its centre.[29]

It seems that the universe of Psychotronics is not associated with the traditional three-dimensional space and time structure in the Euclidean sense, but it is partly a hyperspace. Hyperspace is a multidimensional medium (with four or even more dimensions) in which teleportation and time slips are possible and in which various paranormal phenomena can be experienced. Dimensions with different frequencies, such as the different slices, planes of space and time, are separated by "dimension gates". These portals open up to those who apply various meditation techniques. Narrators describe the experience of passing through a gate as flowing in a whirling bundle of energy (Kis-Halas 2009, 526).

Body and soul

In spirit surgery, the concept of bodily and spiritual alter egos is very characteristic: during the process of creation and over the course of reincarnation rebirths, the physical body is assigned several bodies and souls that are identical in size and appearance, but different in material. It seems as if in the beginning, once the healing method had been established, the trinity of body-soul-spirit was dominant.

This categorisation has been gradually extended to a four-part system by introducing the concept of the etheric body:

> we have four bodies… There is the "physical body", the matter, which is well perceived by the physical eyes. We have an "etheric body" that cannot be seen by the naked eye. It surpasses our physical body by approximately twenty centimetres in a concentric manner. This is called the etheric body, or vital body. Here we find the disembodied projections of our organs. They are present in another material, in a non-physical, intangible matter, in a grand, subtle resonance. Basically, these constitute our physical body, this matter. After that there is an even more subtle body, which is called the soul body or "astral body". The soul is also a body. It contains our organs and systems as well: the lymphatic system, nervous system, circulatory system, digestive system, energy system; it is only with subtler vibration that they appear. And there is a fourth body,

---

[29] "For example, in the centre of the Earth is where Hades reigns": Csontos, V. Jr. Interview 2009.

> the "spiritual body". This is the subtlest. This is our self, our God-equivalence (Kercselics 2009/1).

It is possible that the introduction of new concepts became necessary with the dissemination of healing methods, because Psychotronics was taught in a similar way to the self-improvement and energy healing methods that had already become popular a few years earlier, during weekend courses and group activities. Obviously, there were attempts to make the new method more comprehensible, more acceptable for those who had already acquired knowledge and experience in other fields of energetic medicine (such as Reiki, Prananadi), where the *aura* plays an important role.

> The etheric body was introduced to the healing practice this year. It provides new information from the spirit world and therefore we have immediately incorporated it into our procedures of healing (Kercselics 2009/2).

The denominations of non-material bodies—the astral body and etheric body—might sound familiar from Theosophy, one of the dominant currents of late nineteenth-century Western esotericism and occultism; we will come back to that in a later section. Defining the spiritual body as a "God-equivalence" is also an idea which shows the influence of Theosophy and Anthroposophy.

It is typical that the vocabulary of teachers and followers is not consistent: the notions of body and soul appear as synonyms even in the texts intended as teaching material. This definitely indicates that the lines become blurred and fluid, not only between particular terminologies, but also between body-spirit-soul conceptions.

> It is a new doctrine in healings that our seven souls heal the seven souls of the patients (our seventh soul is our spirit), and that therefore we should always set them outside the aura. (…) The soul has six planes as well (Astral, Mental, Buddhic, Atman, Monadic, Divine). This means that they are on different levels of development in accordance with the place from where God has sent them back (Csontos, V. Jr., *SzH* V/2: 3).

> We are actually down here with seven bodies. The Indians divide each of the seven bodies into a further seven bodies, which gives us a total of forty-nine bodies (Kercselics 2009/1).

The six souls preceding the current incarnation and the seventh soul, the spirit, are located in the respective planes of the *aura* surrounding the physical body:

> The seven souls in the aura are, hence, the seven previous lives; but if we have to accomplish a greater task then they are selected. (…) It is always the soul located at the deepest plane of [the aura]: that first one is "Me" (Csontos, V. Jr., *SzH* V/2: 3–4).

Universal energy, described previously, is an essential component of both the physical and the non-material bodies. The different vibrations of the particles cause the different material quality of the material body and the non-material bodies (soul, spirit), and at the same time, assigns their place in the qualitative hierarchy.

As regards the correspondence between body-universe and microcosm-macrocosm, the different material quality of bodies and souls illustrates the different dimensions of the universe. At the lowest level we have the physical (material) body and the earthly world; while the spirit represents the spiritual world located at the highest level.

Another characteristic motif of the body conceptions of spirit surgery is the mechanical body machine[30] controlled by a computer-like brain.[31] Organs are reparable and replaceable parts: the essence of Psychotronics is a spirit surgery performed in the transcendent sphere, which is also

---

[30] This takes us to the anatomical and organ models of Medicine, to the Mechanical Turk of Kempelen and to robots and various manifestations of the artificial man phenomenon; but we do not have room to follow up on that. Thomas Csordas in his lecture at the *After Post Modernism* conference talked about modern diagnostics in which from the second half of the nineties, they applied computer animated, three-dimensional body models (*kadaver*), which now also serve as models to animate the most various creatures of virtual and fantasy worlds; see Csordas 1997. He referred to the Visible Human Project, which meant a revolutionary change in the field of imaging diagnostics; on the ethical aspects of this, see the study with the identical title by Catherine Waldby 2000. I have discussed body conceptions prevailing in Psychotronics in a brief analysis, see Kis-Halas 2014b.

[31] The Hungarian spiritual teacher, György Sipos proposes an interesting parallel: the matrix of informatics and philosophy, "infosophy". The essence of the doctrine is defined by the author as follows: "…there is an object called Humanity (Steiner calls it etheric body, Jung calls it collective consciousness, Buddhism calls it common mental, and so forth…), which is technically created in the following way: the nine-tenths of certain people's brains that we do not use according to our knowledge is connected to others in the state of sleep and it is part of a shared database network, which aims to live, design and control the future of humanity" (See "Infozófia"). A spirit surgeon from Siklós can also be considered an adherent of these ideas; she believes that János Neumann took an internal journey inside his own brain, and following that model he later created the first computer. (Field notes, Siklós-Máriagyűd, August 18, 2009).

rendered in physical reality. Karma is also defined in a mechanical form: events in life and the actions of a person are stored in the memory on a special "hard drive" updated by the personal guardian angel which goes under the name of the *Akashic chronicle*.[32]

> Because the soul that constitutes the physical body is not material, it is from God. God created it, and He immediately created a guardian angel beside it, which was sent down to it at the moment of birth to look out for us. This guardian angel is assigned to a soul and it observes the development of the soul. And not only in the physical body! When the soul is located on the astral plane, or may be living in another body on another planet, the guardian angel still accompanies it there. And it keeps a record of the development of the soul, of its every movement! This is very interesting because nothing escapes its attention. Ergo, no action can be made by the body, no thought can come out of one's brain, no word can leave one's mouth without the angel (assigned to the soul) taking an unbiased note of it! So there is no selection. Everything that happens in the human mind—actions, words—will be recorded. This is the Akashic record. You surely know this: soul record, Akashic record. This Akashic record contains everything. And as soon as we learn how to read these records we will be able to go back to any hour of any of our past days. And thus… this is an open book, this is our Big Book in which everything is written (Kercselics 2009/2).

Fate: reincarnation and karma

One of the most characteristic elements of New Age religiosity is teaching karmic fate interpretation and reincarnation. Reincarnation regulated by karma plays a fundamental role in the doctrine of spirit surgery as a "central development model" (Szilágyi and Szilárdi 2007, 27–8).

> The soul develops by being born to earth. The "young" soul usually makes a series of mistakes and it needs many, many years to become aware of these mistakes and for the ennoblement of the soul (Margit 2010).

According to the ideas of Psychotronics, in the event of death it is first the material physical body that perishes which is then followed by the etheric body. The spirit returns to the Creator so that it can be reincarnated. The

---

32 The term "Akashic disc" spread in Hungarian esoteric discourse due to the influence of the highly popular works of Bruce Goldberg, published continuously from the early nineties, about life after death and about the spirit world (for instance *Past Lives, Future Lives*, or *Psychic Defense Strategies Against Energy Vampires*); cf. S. Balázs 2004, 221.

souls of previous lives staying in the *aura* remain close to Earth, as do the spirits of dead ancestors who help their descendants:

> …it is always the innermost soul that counts: that first one is Me. If I die that will be the one to return to God, the rest stays here and helps the children and great-grandchildren (Vilmos Csontos Jr., *SzH* V/2: 3).

Karmic fate usually cannot be changed; in certain cases, however, there is a possibility; for instance, by visiting the Heavenly Jerusalem and obtaining absolution:

> …This is important because if your illness is karmic, meaning that it is an illness brought from a past life, and the karma is dissolved—only the Creator is entitled to dissolve someone's karma—, then the karmic illness will be healed (Kercselics 2009/3).

Prophets, teachers, healers

Steven Sutcliffe calls "seekers" and "gurus" the most typical forms of identity in postmodern religiosity. The term "guru", taken from Sanskrit, denotes a spiritual teacher, someone with "the possession of special spiritual insight based on personal revelation" (here he cites the definition of Storr: Sutcliffe 2000, 33). As Sutcliffe explains, a guru starts out as a seeker who seeks to find the mentality and lifestyle that is most in accordance with his own spiritual needs. He becomes a leader or a teacher if his quest is considered exemplary (2000, 25–6).

So far, we have at our disposition only fragmentary information on the person who introduced Psychotronics in Hungary. Vilmos Csontos Junior was born in Zselíz (Želiezovce, Slovakia). His works and teachings are disseminated to his followers in private publications, in the previously mentioned newsletter, and in the notes photocopied by his disciples. Nevertheless, our data, which also mention a few biographical events (accounts by disciples and interviews with him), suggest the character of a self-taught spiritual teacher with undoubtedly Christian features and certain traits that evoke popular religious specialists (pilgrimage leaders, peasant prophets).

It is a common trait in many cultures that the character of a founder of a religion/prophet/religious specialist (also) includes the ability to heal. In the context of our present study, the primary models seem to be Jesus Christ and Ignatius of Loyola, the founder of the Jesuit order (because of their common feature of militant rhetoric).[33] In his words, Vilmos Csontos Jr. interprets his own mission as a healer and teacher of Jesus' mission: humanity is "the army of Jesus", the leaders of which are the healers "trained" by Jesus and by God in Heaven: the psychotronic experts.

> …we were sent to Earth as the army of Jesus in order to heal humanity. This might sound a little weird, mightn't it? It might seem conceited to say that we are the army of Jesus, but (…) the entire humanity can join the army of Jesus if they invite love into their hearts (see Interview 2009).

Besides the accentuated Christian content, as it was in the case of the world view, the signs of religious syncretism can be observed: Egyptian and Sumerian "magician-priests", *táltos*, and shamans appear as historic prefigurations of Psychotronics and healers (Vilmos Csontos Jr., *SzH* VI/1: 4).

> Well, its origins go back to Jesus, even Zarathustra (he lived 1700 years before Jesus [sic]), even to Egypt. To the Egyptian magician-priests and to the Sumerian magician-priests. It can also be shown that the Hungarian magician-priests, the priests of the Sun god also knew these practices; and applied them, too (see Interview 2009).

Previously we have mentioned that certain biographical moments of Vilmos Csontos Jr., such as his vocation and the acquisition of his healing skills, show a stylistic connection to the beliefs related to the figures of popular magical and religious specialists (e.g. healer, seer of the dead, holy person): he lies in a modified state of consciousness (sleeping or unconscious) while he travels to the other world where he is healed and is assigned a mission.[34]

> Spirit surgery or psychotronic surgery as a method of healing arrived on Earth thanks to Vilmos Csontos Junior. He was badly beaten at the age of eighteen, he lost his consciousness, he had a concussion and suffered several bone fractures. His spirit went up before the Almighty, where it

[33] On the Jesuit order, see O'Malley 2014. The papal bull allowing the formation of the Society of Jesus issued by Pope Paul III on 27 September 1570 is the *Regimini militantis Ecclesiae.*

[34] We find an abundance of similar motifs in relation to the vocation of contemporary popular religious specialists showing traditional characteristics, in relation to the case of Ilona Jánó, the holy Moldavian seer, see Kóka 2006; and Pócs 2006. On the folk healers from Töröcske (village in Somogy County, South West Hungary), see Kis-Halas 2005a.

> was revealed to him how he could heal himself. He recovered in twenty-four hours (Zsuzsa9421 2009).

It is noteworthy that Vilmos Csontos Jr. shared this experience only with his disciples; he secluded himself from wider publicity. Seemingly, the story of a heavenly journey and the things he was taught had, by now, become inherent parts of the healing method, and thus an initiation into which only future healers gain an insight. One of his first disciples, Imre Kercselics, briefly refers to this moment:

> When we started to deal with spirit surgery and healing, the founding father of Hungarian spirit surgery was a man from Upper Hungary. His name is Vilmos Csontos. Probably many of you have heard of him, many of you know him. He is the greatest spirit surgeon in Europe today. He is a wonderful man. He was the one to bring this knowledge down here. We learned it from him (Kercselics 2009/02).

As we have previously indicated, the motif of heavenly, otherworldly and—in a wider sense—transcendental initiation and knowledge acquisition plays an important role in New Age ideas. The typical contemporary form of "mediumism", the notion of "channelling", describes accurately the basic "activities" of specialists who are in constant contact with the transcendent sphere, who transmit energy, knowledge and messages. Accordingly, the other half of the narratives relates how Vilmos Csontos Jr. acquired his knowledge. It is extra-terrestrial creatures who treated and taught him and who gave (and still give to this day) tasks to the founder-healer who visited their galaxy/planet. The widespread idea that Psychotronics originates from the planet Sirius clearly reflects the globalisation of esoteric UFO belief.[35]

The motif of the ancient nature and/or special origins of Psychotronics often plays an essential role, and serves as a strategy of legitimisation, in the central narrative of several contemporary esoteric healing systems. The concept of earthly life and civilisation originating from space has also now become commonplace. The relevant works of Erich von Däniken, the best-known author of the topic, were already extremely popular in the eighties in the registers of Hungarian works for public vulgarisation of science and

---

[35] A few texts in the corpus also mention that Hungarians themselves stem from the Sirius star system and they brought this healing practice from there to Earth. There is no room here for discussing the belief in the Sirian origin of the Hungarians, which is one of the most popular alternative ethnic etymologies in contemporary non-academic historical, and Neopagan discourses in Hungary. See Szilágyi and Szilárdi 2007: 68–9; Szilárdi 2013, 236; Kis-Halas 2014.

science fiction literature. Among the recent Hungarian esoteric bestsellers, the same topic appears for instance in the Kryon series.[36] A recurring element in Kryon's messages is that the "enlightened" coming from the Pleiades lifted, with the approval of angels, today's humans from previous human races, by giving them two extra "layers of DNA" ("Magyar Kryon Honlap" 2003). The motif of the Sirian origins of Psychotronics, nonetheless, indicates close connections to the theory by György Kisfaludy, the founder of the Church of the Universe, according to which the Huns (who are generally considered the ancestors of the Hungarians) came to Earth from Sirius to create human civilisation.[37] We find Kisfaludy's ideas partly in the work of the "neo-*táltos*"[38] András Kovács,[39]

---

[36] Kryon is an angel-like entity whose messages have been channelled by several mediums to Earth since the late 1980s. In 1997 American, Lee Carroll, claimed to be the authentic and exclusive channel and he started publishing Kryon's prophecies and messages in the same year. The first Hungarian volume of the Kryon series was published in 2004. For many years it was one of the major sources of knowledge on the angelic realm and the extra-terrestrial worlds among the esoteric healing practitioners in the Siklós region. The charismatic healer from Győr had seemingly heard of Kryon, because she claims that she had gained her knowledge from extra-terrestrials and she had been continuously in contact with them ever since; see S. Balázs 2004, 21).

[37] Excerpt from the credo of the Church: "Don't forget, we came from the ocean of stars to the "Mud", (…) 6045 years ago (March 21, 2004 AD) when a great wave of our ancestors arrived on Earth…" See UC Creed. Attila the Hun is depicted in Anthroposophy as a cultural hero, who is an Atlantean initiate, and who fought the Roman Empire in order to fulfil his Christian mission. See for instance Baji Lázár 2003.

[38] I used the term "neo-*táltos*" in order to clearly distinguish this modern specialist from the *táltos* of Hungarian folk belief. A *táltos* is a type of shamanistic sorcerer in Hungarian folk belief. It is not an exclusively Hungarian phenomenon since it has multiple connections to the sorcerer figure appearing in the beliefs of other European peoples, mostly dealing with agrarian magic. The European relations of the belief figure of the *táltos* were first described by Gábor Klaniczay and Éva Pócs; see Klaniczay 1983; 1984; 2001; and Pócs 1989; 2017. By contrast, for a long time, Hungarian research in linguistics, ethnography and prehistory has interpreted the figure and activities of the *táltos* in the context of Eurasian shamanism; see Diószegi 1958; 1967; 1971. Consequently, the *táltos* has been considered to this day as the *par excellence* Hungarian shaman. In the Hungarian Neopagan discourse, which considers national identity as a central question, this interpretation has become dominant; see Szilárdi 2013, 234–6; Kis-Halas 2014b. Árpád Bajkó (2007) analyses the biography of a neo-*táltos* healer practising in Transylvania. See Bajkó's data collection in Czégényi and Keszeg 2010. I have made a brief overview of the activities of neo-*táltos* healers operating in Hungary, see Kis-Halas 2014b.

a long time collaborator of healers and teachers such as Imre Kercselics and Tibor Tóth who have played a crucial role in spirit surgery.[40]

Treatments: aura cleansing, absolution, spirit surgery

Psychotronics, as we have mentioned on several occasions in this text, is primarily an energetic healing method. Accordingly, the diagnosis is established with the help of the *aura*; the goal of the treatment is to restore and harmonise the energy imbalance of the patient.

> We have our physical body and the body surrounded by an energy field called aura, which has seven colours. It is connected to the seven energy centres. In this aura, if it is injured… An injury might occur from a water vein or earth radiation, magnetic zone radiation or from an inflammation within the organism. Thus, as I have mentioned before, in this subtle body that surrounds our bodies, here and here [he points at them] are our organs, but they are non-material organs, therefore they are not materialised. A dark spot, an alteration appears in the energy field surrounding the body. Those who have the ability to see auras notice at the very beginning that one of the organs, located in the aura, is energetically injured. And our seven energy centres [he points at them on himself]: the hypophysis, the third eye, the throat, the immune system, the pancreas, the spleen and the root. Our organs are connected to these centres in pairs. Each energy centre is linked to two organs. If there is a deficiency in these areas in the aura, in the energy field surrounding the body, then the energy centre cannot accomplish its function properly. The connecting organs will be energetically weakened! There is no pain yet!

---

[39] An excerpt from a poem describing Attila's deeds from András Kovács's website: *"Az V. század első felében a maja királytól, testvérétől, Tantól vezérelve / Jön Dél-Amerikából Európába, / Hogy az eltévelyedett embereket Istenhez vezérelje. / A hun birodalmat világuralommá tette."* [In the first half of the fifth century, guided by Tan, the brother of the Maya king / He comes from South America to Europe / So that he can lead the errant people to God / He made the Hun Empire dominate the world.] (See http://www.szellemvilag.hu/szent-attila/attila-napja-januar-7). According to András Kovács, Hungarians are the founders and the disseminators of earthly civilisation; cf. http://www.szellemvilag.hu/dvd/kovacs-8211-magyar-andras-a-taltosok-kuldetese.

[40] "…a seventeen-year-old boy got encephalitis and was admitted to the László Hospital. At that time, I was still working in the *táltos* consulting room in the *táltos* centre" (Imre Kercselics 2009/3). Allegedly, both healers were initiated as *táltos* by András Kovács personally. Lázár also refers to Kercselics as a *táltos* healer. On the video of the lecture given by Kercselics, he wears a leather sabretache decorated with metal plates, which, according to Lázár, is a typical identity marker of neo-*táltos* healers; cf. Lázár 2006, 40.

> So it does not manifest in the matter, but the injury is already there (Kercselics 2009/4).

Meanwhile, spirit surgery is also a religious medical system: it explains the original cause of illnesses by a deficit in faith, love and virtue, and by the damaging effect of misbeliefs, false beliefs, false convictions and sins. These ideas imply a nosological matrix, in which Christianity's seven cardinal sins are assigned to the concrete "areas" of the human body's microcosm, to its specified organs, to the appropriate layers of the aura and definite illnesses.

> …if someone is unable to love and accept oneself then that person will be unable to love and accept on Earth. (…) That person will start to hate. We know exactly that hate is the cause of cancer. Anger is the cause of diabetes, sclerosis multiplex and these illnesses.

Consequently, Psychotronics is a bipolar belief system based on the archaic dichotomy of "health=physical/spiritual cleanliness"—"illness= physical/spiritual uncleanliness" (Douglas 2001 [1966]). Subsequently, the basic metaphor of the treatments is "cleansing", which only results in successful healing if every plane of existence is cleansed. This is precisely what spirit surgery has to offer in addition, as opposed to any other energy healing method: it also treats the soul, constituting the divine nature of man, because that is where it locates the origin of illnesses.[41] In the karmic development model of spirit surgery, the spirit of a person is a constant entity, which is reincarnated over and over again in order to arrive at a greater perfection in its earthly existence. The spirit creating and constituting the human body,[42] the soul(s) assigned to it, the *aura* and the material body are in perpetual interaction with one another and

[41] Citing the words of a practitioner from Miskolc (North-Eastern Hungary): "While physicians and doctors heal the physical body, we heal the soul or spirit. Psychotronics means spirit healing and our efforts aim to correct problems on a spiritual level, and the solution to the problem is transcribed to a physical level." (Field data collected by Tünde Iván 2007.)

[42] "In the first phase, over the course of nine months the child constructs its physical body from the physical body of the mother. In the first seven years the etheric body is constructed from the mother's etheric body. In the second seven-year cycle—here the child is already fourteen years old—the child builds the astral body from the mother's astral or soul body […] So we've already had the matter, the ether, the soul, now comes the spirit body. This is the third seven-year cycle. This is when a person builds the spirit body from the mother's spirit body." Kercselics 2009/3.

communicate continuously through the vibration/energy generated by the particles they are made of. A psychotronic healer helps to make the communication uninterrupted, to ensure that the bodies and souls are entirely cleansed in every "dimension of existence". After initiation they are able to achieve superior levels of existence and to take the soul of the patient there with them.

> This method has a wonderful basis. We take the patients to the Creator God. They meet Jesus, the Virgin Mary and their own spirit. There the patients put down all their sins committed in previous lives on a spiritual and on a soul level, and the sins committed on a spiritual, soul and physical level in their current lives. They apologise sevenfold for their sins, and tenfold for the sins of their fathers. This is important because if the illness is karmic, that is, brought from a previous life, then the karma has to be dissolved (only the Creator is entitled to do that), and thus they can recover from a karmic illness as well (Kercselics 2009/3).

Cleansing the body and the soul, as I have explained above, is only possible in the corresponding dimension/alternative sphere, which, in the present case, is the "other world" that echoes more or less Christian beliefs. The goal of the patient's and the healer's journey together is—again, in accordance with Christian interpretations, to obtain absolution for both the patient and the healer.[43]

The essence of the method is a form of hypnosis therapy known from psychological practice as "reincarnation hypnosis", which we can achieve through controlled meditation. On the basis of the data at my disposal and my own field experience, I think that the meditation process is schematic and easy to learn for the patient. It is an important criterion for the patient to participate in the therapy relatively actively and deliberately; and this, again, is due to the religious nature of the medical system. The patient's task is not only to attain complete purification, but to believe in his own recovery based on the faith in the creating power of thought: the patients have to create, with the assistance of the healer, their own health. The following two examples reflect the practitioners' view on this topic.

> Now, in order for these healings to occur the patients have to be prepared to participate actively in their own recovery. We teach them to meditate. Meditation is nothing less than taking brain waves into a deep sleep state.

[43] The physical and especially the mental-spiritual immaculacy of the healer are of key importance. So, in order to achieve this, certain healers might take the heavenly journey several times a day to obtain absolution, just like the Siklós spirit surgeon and her partner. (Field notes, June and July 2009).

> So we are not working in hypnosis, but in a state similar to sleep. Brain waves are between zero and four Hertz. This is when a person's spirit eye is activated; it is the third eye [he points between his eyes] with which we see our dreams. They practice this meditative state with the help of a tape recording, and then with this third eye, with brain waves between zero and four Hertz, the patients can see the healing process happening inside their body (see Kercselics 2009/3).[44]

> One of the principles of spirit surgery is that the healer can help if the patient voluntarily asks for it and the Creator allows it. This method is not for everyone, only for those whose hearts are opened towards God (excerpted from a Budapest spirit surgeon's website, see Derzsi, Anna 2010).

Based on my own personal experience, the course of the treatment goes as follows:

1) Achieving a meditative state: the healer counts out loud backwards and leads the patient "downwards" along a staircase.
2) In a meditative state: arriving at the shore of a lake or a sea (meanwhile the healer recounts natural images relaying calm: a clearing in the forest, sunset at the ocean, etc.).
3) Cleansing the *aura*, the soul body and the spirit body, charging them with new energy (the healer describes a specific way of cleansing oneself with water: for instance, rain washes the body, sea water carries the uncleanliness away), removal of contamination (which are taken to the Heavenly Treasury in a bag).
4) Departure to the Heavenly Jerusalem in a whirlwind.
5) Meeting heavenly creatures (the Holy Trinity, God, Jesus Christ, the Virgin Mary, Archangel Michael, angels, saints).
6) Asking for absolution, obtaining it and accepting *heavenly gift*s (usually clothes, weaponry, maybe a crown or a book).
7) If necessary, continuing the journey to the Heavenly Hospital where the surgery of the spiritual body (and further soul bodies) is performed and organs are exchanged with the cooperation of the patient.
8) Releasing the soul of the patient, sending the excised organs to the Heavenly Treasury.
9) Returning to the shore in a whirlwind.

---

[44] A spirit surgeon from Siklós gave almost the same explication to my question concerning the method and aim of meditation. The use of the cassette is described by Lázár 2006.

10) Returning from the meditative state with the help of the healer counting forwards.

In the second part of the treatment, the patient recounts what he/she has seen in response to the questions of the healer, then the healer highlights and analyses certain moments of the events. The gifts given by the heavenly creatures play an important role; they partly serve as symbolic protection against the illness (sword, armour, cloak) and partly initiate the patient into the army fighting against the earthly forces of evil. Let me quote here my field notes taken during a healing session, when I and a healer friend of mine were both purified from our sins:

> Then she [the healer] instructed us to pay attention to the gifts we were going to be given. He talked about receiving a crown each, on which Jesus had exchanged the diamonds for a pink stone. [She later explained that this is the colour of love.] Then she told us that we were also going to get a robe. She asked us to remember its colour. Finally the angels gave us a sword each, which we also had to remember (field notes Siklós-Máriagyűd, 2009).

Similar thoughts are told by one of the Hungarian gurus of spirit surgery (Imre Kercselics).

> When we come back from the level of deep consciousness we always discuss what the patient has seen or experienced because asking and verifying are very important parts of the patient's recovery (Kercselics 2009/3).

The heavenly journey is the most important element of the ritual of psychotronic healing: this is where the actual treatment takes place. The course of the therapy follows, in fact, the structure of the rites of passage: the controlled image-creating meditation corresponds to the separation and reintegration phases, while the events taking place in the dimension of the Heavenly Jerusalem and in the Hospital correspond to liminality. Contrary to rites of passage, the new status gained by the patient is only a temporary state: in order to preserve it, a continuous self-control is needed as well as disciplined and conscious behaviour following the fundamentally Christian moral norms of Psychotronics:

> Everyone should perform self-examination. During self-examination the best is when I look at myself from the outside because then I cannot be biased. These things have to be processed; we have to acknowledge them and work them out from our system, because we can, indeed (Kercselics 2009/4).

The visual world of narratives about the heavenly journey is very heterogeneous: motifs of Judeo-Christian eschatology, medieval literature on visions and popular beliefs of the other world are blended with the galactic townscape of science fiction books and movies, with virtual fantasy worlds and with the "ancient Hungarian" beliefs from alternative history- and mythology-interpretations. An elaborate philological study would be necessary to establish the origin, the potential sources, motivic and genre-related parallels of certain elements. In this present paper, I would like to highlight two motifs from the architecture of heaven in spirit surgery: the heavenly church and the hospital in hyperspace.

The narratives usually describe Heavenly Jerusalem as a shiny edifice (temple, palace). In this case, there is an evident parallel with the Eschatology of the New Testament and with the heavenly city looking inviting with shiny, open gates, appearing in the book of Ezekiel (see Benz 1969, 356).[45] Here I present an excerpt from a student's notes taken during the guided meditation, when the patient is taken to this otherworldly venue. The dialogue form also illustrates the active role the patient plays in the course of this part of the healing session, and which I have already referred to above.

> Healer: Now I will call a whirlwind that will take us to the Heavenly Jerusalem. What is it like?
> Patient: It's shiny, very shiny!
> Healer: Yes it is! [The disciple assisting the healer nods in agreement.] Now the whirlwind puts us down at the gate. What is the gate like? What do you see?
> Patient: It's white, and decorated with gold and silver (Tünde Iván's field notes, Miskolc, 2007).

The dominant element of the building is the large, sometimes shiny, lustrous gate, probably inspired by the gate of the Christian Heaven. However, the design of local buildings may be an important source of inspiration. One of the Siklós healers described it as a glowing church to which countless stairs led the way. "It's like the church in Gyűd, only with wider wooden gates" (field notes, Siklós-Máriagyűd, Aug 18, 2009).[46]

---

[45] Peter Dinzelbacher takes the dream vision of Laisrén to denote the church opening towards heaven where souls are taken by angels: Dinzelbacher 1981, 108.

[46] The eighteenth-century Marian shrine of Máriagyűd (a former village, now a district of Siklós) is a popular pilgrimage destination for both Christian devotees and spiritual seekers from all over Hungary and neighbouring Croatia.

The interior space of the building also reminds us of a Christian temple: aisles with singing figures in shiny clothes (perhaps angels or saints). In place of the altar, God is sitting on a throne, Christ on his right and the Holy Trinity above their heads. Let me quote the minutes of my healing session again:

> After the gates were opened she led us inside the church where many were waiting for us. We passed between the aisles before the Holy Trinity, the Virgin Mary and Our Lady (field notes Siklós-Máriagyűd, Aug 18, 2009).

Obtaining absolution is an indispensable criterion of healing in spirit surgery: purgation every single time is not only necessary for the patient, but for the healer as well, as we discussed earlier.

The hospital in hyperspace, similar to the heavenly church, appears as a lustrous complex. One part of the narratives relates that only initiated healers are allowed in there: angels and hyperspace doctors then take the patient over from him or her. Other beliefs claim that the patients also actively participate in their surgeries: they are the ones who create the appropriate new organs with the guidance of the healer. The following narratives illustrate the first version:

> The initiated spirit surgeon accompanied by his Superior Self takes the spirit body of the patient (who can see and is living a beautiful experience) up to a higher dimension called hyperspace. The spirit surgeon hospital, which was given as a gift by the Creator to the spirit surgeon healers, is located here. Countless healing spirits and healing angels work here with many surgical instruments. (…) The spirit hospital in hyperspace is a building of twice twenty-seven floors with golden crosses, shining in golden light; the structure of which resembles a pyramid. The lower level is nine hundred square metres; it is 30x30 metres. The next floor, and every further floor, overhangs by eight metres. Above the twenty-seventh floor is the two hundred and three thousand, four hundred and forty-four square-metre runway. The entrance is from the East. Flowers are everywhere and everything is bright and clean, in a relaxing light. Four angels take care of administration. Only initiated spirit surgeons are let in. There is a drinking fountain in which the water of life flows; anyone can drink from it. A light elevator takes us to the other floors, but we can also take the stairs up until the seventh floor (see Bubuh, 2009).

The description above mostly uses elements from the genre of science fiction, but we can also easily recognise the desired, idealistic patient care we know from popular medical drama television series.

> They have a much more developed medical instrumentation than the hospitals on Earth; and they are continuously innovating, on a research basis; I, myself, have also been experiencing since 1993 the trial-run of new equipment available in the hyperspace hospital (see Bubuh, 2009).

Summary

The ideological background to the religious healing system of Psychotronics is constituted of extremely heterogeneous and syncretic beliefs. In the search for ideological components, three fields have been outlined thus far: 1) the Anthroposophy by Rudolf Steiner; 2) the Atlantean spirit surgery by Eckard Strohm, who was also the one to introduce the most popular branch of energy medicine: Reiki (for more on this see Kis-Halas 2008, 245–7); 3) the esoteric UFO and ET belief blended with the esoteric trends of contemporary Hungarian Paganism. A subsequent study with detailed analysis would be necessary in order to accurately describe the rather intricate system of sources and origins.

The current state of our research, nonetheless, shows that there are fundamental differences in the attitudes of those who follow and apply the healing method in terms of the preference in trends. Vilmos Csontos Jr., the reformer of the method, besides emphasising international references, expressly propagates a healing method and a philosophy with Christian features. The interventions of Imre Kercselics and the other healers reflect ideas that put national identity more to the centre: for them, spirit surgery is primarily an "ancient Hungarian" method. The following questions can be raised in relation to this: 1) can we interpret the strengthening of nationalistic ideology and rhetoric in spirit surgery as a sign of an ideological paradigm shift, and if yes, how can we explain it? 2) why did *this* healing system lean in a nationalistic direction and not any other, similar method in energy healing? In my opinion, the main direction of further research would be to learn more about these changes.

As we have briefly mentioned earlier, Vilmos Csontos Jr., the reformer and prophet of the healing method in Hungary and Slovakia, appears as a very contemporary type of magical specialist and religious expert: a *guru*. Nevertheless, we can discover several traits in his persona that indicate a strong connection with the traditional characters of peasant prophets, holy men and living saints. The detailed analysis of the self-fashioning and the reception of this charismatic healer on the basis of subsequent sources and interviews could be another direction of research in this topic.

References

Blogs

Zsuzsa9421 2009. "Mi a szellemsebészet vagy pszichotronikai sebészet? [What is spirit or psychotronical surgery?]" Published August 20, 2009. http://onmegvalositas.hu/blog/zsuzsa9421/mi_szellemsebeszet_vagy_pszichotronikai_sebeszet, accessed March 9, 2010.

Websites

Angyalszárny 2009. "Az emberiség története a Föld bolygón [The history of mankind on planet Earth]." Published February 19, 2009. http://www.angyalszarny.eoldal.hu/cikkek/szellemi-uzenetek/az-emberiseg-tortenete-a-fold-bolygon.html, accessed August 23, 2016.

CU Creed. "Az Univerzum Egyháza hitvallása [Creed of the Church of the Universe]." http://www.hunok.hu/egyhaz/index1.html, accessed August 23, 2016.

Derzsi, Anna. 2010. "Derzsi Anna szellemsebész honlapja [Homepage of Anna Derzsi, spirit surgeon and Reiki practitioner]." http://szellemgyogyasz.mindenkilapja.hu/html/22226486/render/kezdolap, accessed August 23, 2016.

"Infozófia [Infosophy]." http://www.sipi46.hu/, accessed August 23, 2016.

"Kafka, B." http://bretislav.kafka.sweb.cz.

Magyar Kryon Honlap 2003. "A földönkívüliekről [On extra-terrestrials]." Published 2003. http://www.kryon.hu/foldonkivuliekrol.php, accessed August 22, 2016.

US Psychotronics. Website of the United States Psychotronics Association. http://www.psychotronics.org, accessed August 22, 2016.

Message boards / Discussion Forums

Aksi and Lalune 2005. Contributions by Aksi and Laune to the topic of Edith Fiore's book entitled "*Megszálló halottak* [The Possessing Dead]." Posted to Agykontroll fórum [Braincontroll forum] 2005, June 9. www.esettanulmanyok.hu/index.php, accessed March 9, 2010.

Bubuh 2009. (2009, Sept 7). Contribution by Bubuh to the topic entitled "*Léleképítés, szellemsebészet* [Spiritual empowerment, spirit surgery]."

Message posted to http://espavo.hu/node/5309, accessed March 13, 2010.

Margit 2009. Contribution by Margit Imre to the topic entitled "*Szellemi gyógyítás (szellemgyógyászat)* [Spiritual healing (spirit healing)]." Posted to the Jézus a fény fórum [Jesus is the light forum] 2009, November 23. http://jezusafeny.hu/index.php?option=com_fireboard&Itemid=58&func=view&id=2080&view=threaded&catid=11, accessed 22.08. 2016.

YouTube videos

Kercselics, Imre. 2006/1. "Video recording of Imre Kercselics's lecture, part 1. Budapest, June 25, 2006." https://www.youtube.com/watch?v=Ha1QntaRkkw, accessed March 12, 2010.

—. 2006/2. "Video recording of Imre Kercselics's lecture, part 2. Budapest, June 25, 2006." https://www.youtube.com/watch?v=Ha1QntaRkkw, accessed March 12, 2010.

—. 2006/3. "Video recording of Imre Kercselics's lecture, part 3. Budapest, June 25, 2006." https://www.youtube.com/watch?v=Fp6SSWmR_t4, accessed March 12, 2010.

—. 2006/4. "Video recording of Imre Kercselics's lecture, part 4. Budapest, June 25, 2006." https://www.youtube.com/watch?v=d5r5DeYii8c, accessed March 12, 2010.

—. 2006/5. "Video recording of Imre Kercselics's lecture, part 5. Budapest, June 25, 2006." https://www.youtube.com/watch?v=H8VBJEj6Zys, accessed March 12, 2010.

—. 2006/6. "Video recording of Imre Kercselics's lecture, part 6. Budapest, June 25, 2006." https://www.youtube.com/watch?v=o_aNWS2ivM0, accessed March 12, 2010.

—. 2006/7. "Video recording of Imre Kercselics's lecture, part 7. Budapest, June 25, 2006." https://www.youtube.com/watch?v=MBdP9ofa4TY, accessed March 12, 2010.

—. 2006/8. "Video recording of Imre Kercselics's lecture, part 8. Budapest, June 25, 2006."

https://www.youtube.com/watch?v=Hg0s0d_wPm0, accessed March 12, 2010.

—. 2006/9. "Video recording of Imre Kercselics's lecture, part 9. Budapest, June 25, 2006." https://www.youtube.com/watch?v=_-aV3HJR2ps, accessed March 12, 2010.

Sources from the author's notes

Csontos, V. Jr. Interview 2009. Interview with Vilmos Csontos Jr. and János Lévai in the programme entitled *Dimenziókapu* [Dimension gate] on Kecskemét's Gong Rádió on July 7, 2009. Author's archive.

Bibliography

Adlam, Robert, and Lorne Holyoak. 2005. "Shamanism in the postmodern world. A review essay." *Studies in Religion/Sciences Religiouses* XXXIV: 517–68.

Aitamurto, Kaarina, and Scott Simpson, eds. 2013a. *Modern Pagan and Native Faith Movements in Central and Eastern Europe.* Durham, UK: Acumen. (Studies in Contemporary and Historical Paganism.)

Aitamurto, Kaarina, and Scott Simpson. 2013b. "Introduction." In *Modern Pagan and Native Faith Movements in Central and Eastern Europe*, edited by Kaarina Aitamurto, and Scott Simpson, 1–9. Durham, UK: Acumen. (Studies in Contemporary and Historical Paganism.)

Albanese, Catherine L. 1991. *Nature Religion in America. From the Algonkian Indians to the New Age.* Chicago: Chicago UP.

—. 1992. "The Magical Staff: Quantum Healing in the New Age." In *Perspectives on the New Age*, edited by James R. Lewis, and Gordon J. Melton, 68–84. Albany: State University of New York Press.

—. 2000. "The Aura of Wellness. Subtle Energy Healing and New Age Religion." *Religion and American Culture. A Journal of Interpretation* XXI (10/1): 201–22.

Baji Lázár, Imre. 2003. "Ikonográf. Történelmi arcképcsarnok rejtett kontúrokkal [Iconograph. Historical portrait gallery with hidden contours]." *Ökotáj* XXXI–XXXII: 23–42.

Bajkó, Árpád. 2007. "Táltos tanítványság—viszonyok és kontextusok. Egy Magyarfenesi gyógyító biográfiája [Being a *táltos* disciple—relations and contexts. Biography of a healer from Magyarfenes (*Vlaha)*]." In *Lenyomatok. Fiatal Kutatók a népi kultúráról* VI. [Imprints. Young researchers on popular culture], edited by Sándor

Ilyés, and Albert Zsolt Jakab, 117–47. Kolozsvár: Kriza János Néprajzi Társaság. (Kriza Könyvek XXVIII.)

Barnes, Linda L., and Susan S. Sered, eds. 2004. *Religion and Healing in America.* Oxford: Oxford UP.

Benz, Ernst. 1969. *Die Vision. Erfahrungsformen und Bilderwelt.* Stuttgart: Ernst Klett.

Bowman, Marion. 2009. "From Glastonbury to Hungary. Contemporary Integrative Spirituality and Vernacular Religion in Context." In *Passageways: From Hungarian Ethnography to European Ethnology and Sociocultural Anthropology*, edited by Gábor Vargyas, 195–221. Budapest, and Pécs: L'Harmattan, and Pécsi Tudományegyetem.

Bowman, Marion, and Steven Sutcliffe, eds. 2000. *Beyond New Age. Exploring Alternative Spirituality.* Edinburgh: Edinburgh UP.

Brennan, Barbara. 1988. *Hands of Light. A Guide to Healing through the Human Energy Field.* New York: Bantham.

Brown, Michael F. 1997. *The Channelling Zone. American Spirituality in an Anxious Age*. Cambridge, Mass.: Harvard UP.

Bruce, Steve. 2000. "The New Age and Secularisation." In *New Age. Exploring Alternative Spirituality Beyond*, edited by Steven Sutcliffe, and Marion Bowman, 220–36. Edinburgh: Edinburgh UP.

Clifton, Chas S. 2006. *Her Hidden Children. The Rise of Wicca and Paganism in America.* Lanham, Md.: AltaMira.

Chryssides, George D. 2007. "Defining the New Age." In *Handbook of New Age* I, edited by Daren Kemp, and James R. Lewis, 5–24. London, and Boston: Brill.

Cowen, Douglas E., and Jeffrey K. Hadden. 2004. "Virtually Religious. New Religious Movements and the World Wide Web." In *The Oxford Handbook of New Religious Movements*, James R. Lewis, 119–40. Oxford: Oxford UP.

Csordas, Thomas J. 1997. *Computerized Cadaveres; Shades of Being and Representation in Virtual Reality.* (Lecture at the conference "After Post Modernism"). http://www.focusing.org/apm_papers/compucad.html, accessed October 25, 2009.

Czégényi, Dóra, and Vilmos Keszeg. 2010. *A beteg ember. Betegségek, betegek és gyógyítók* [The sick man. Illnesses, ill people and healers]. Marosvásárhely: Mentor. (Emberek és kontextusok IV.)

Czeizer, Zoltán. 1998. "A hangos olvasástól a másodlagos szóbeliségig. Bevezetés Balogh József 'Voces paginarum' című írásához [From reading out loud to secondary orality. Introduction to József Balogh's article entitled 'Voces paginarum']." *Replika* XXXI–XXXII: 221–6.

Davie, Grace. 1990. "Believing without Belonging: Is This the Future of Religion in Britain Today?" *Social Compass* 37 (4): 455–69.
DeNio Stephens, Holly. 2004. "Okkultizmus a mai Oroszországban [Occultism in Russia today]." Translated by András Soproni. In *Az okkult az orosz és a szovjet kultúrában*, edited by Bernice G. Rosenthal, 349–383. Budapest: Európa. [*The Occult in Russian and Soviet Culture*. Ithaca: Cornell UP, 1997.]
Dinzelbacher, Peter. 1981. *Vision und Visionsliteratur im Mittelalter*. Stuttgart: Anton Hiersemann.
Diószegi, Vilmos. 1958. *A sámánhit emlékei a magyar népi műveltségben* [Remnants of shamanistic beliefs in Hungarian popular culture]. Budapest: Akadémiai.
—. 1967. *A pogány magyarok hitvilága* [The beliefs of the Pagan Hungarians]. Budapest: Akadémiai. (Kőrösi Csoma kiskönyvtár.)
—. 1971. *Az ősi magyar hitvilág* [Ancient Hungarian beliefs]. Budapest: Gondolat.
Douglas, Mary. 2001 [1966]. *Purity and Danger. An Analysis of the Concepts of Pollution and Taboo*. London, and New York: Routledge.
Draper, Scott, and Joseph Barker. 2011. "Angelic Belief as American Folk Religion." *Sociological Forum* 26 (3): 623–43.
Engelke, Matthew. 2012. "Angels in Swindon. Public Religion and Ambient Faith in England." *American Ethnologist* 39 (1): 155–70.
Faivre, Antoine. 1994. *Access to Western Esotericism*. Albany: Suny.
—. 1998. "Questions of Terminology Proper to the Study of Esoteric Currents in Modern and Contemporary Europe." In *Western Esotericism and the Science of Religion. Selected Papers Presented at the 17th Congress of the International Association for the History of Religion, Mexico City 1995*, edited by Antoine Faivre, and Wouter J. Hanegraaff, 1–11. Leuven: Peeters.
Farias, Miguel. 2006. "A Psychological Study of New Age Practices and Beliefs." *Journal of Alternative Spiritualities and New Age Studies* II: 105–15.
Flaherty, Robert Pearson. 2011. "UFOs, ETs, and the Millennial Imagination." In *The Oxford Handbook of Millennialism*, edited by Catherine Wessinger, 587–610. Oxford: Oxford UP.
Foster, George M. 1976. "Disease Etiologies in Non-Western Medical Systems." *American Anthropologist* LXXVIII: 773–82. http://onlinelibrary.wiley.com/doi/10.1525/aa.1976.78.4.02a00030/epdf, accessed January 20, 2016.
Füvessy, Anikó. 2007. "Egy nagyiváni 'médium' túlvilági utazása és beavatása [The otherworldly journey and initiation of a 'medium' from

Nagyiván]." In *Maszk, átváltozás, beavatás. Vallásetnológiai fogalmak tudományközi megközelítésben* [Mask, transformation, initiation. Interdisciplinary approach to concepts in ethnology of religion], edited by Éva Pócs, 378–99. Budapest: Balassi. (Tanulmányok a transzcendensről V.)

Gaidukov, Alexey. 2013. "The Russian Language Internet and Rodnoverie." In *Modern Pagan and Native Faith Movements in Central and Eastern Europe*, edited by Kaarina Aitamurto, and Scott Simpson, 315–32. Durham, UK: Acumen. (Studies in Contemporary and Historical Paganism.)

Gerber, Richard. 1988. *Vibrational Medicine. New Choices for Healing Ourselves*. Sante Fe: Bear.

Glendinning, Tony, and Steve Bruce. 2006. "New Ways of Believing or Belonging. Is Religion Giving Way to Spirituality?" *The British Journal of Sociology* 57 (3): 399–414.

Goldberg, Bruce. 1991. *Előző életek, jövendő életek. Hipnózis, reinkarnáció, karma*. Translated by Ágnes Hegyi. Budapest: Édesvíz. [*Past Lives, Future Lives*. New York: Ballantine Books, 1982.]

—. 2007. *Energiavámpírok. A lelki önvédelem alapvető technikái*. Translated by Gábor Lovasi. Budapest: Édesvíz. [*Protected by the Light: The Complete Book of Psychic Self-Defense*. St. Paul, Minn.: Llewellyn, 1998.]

Grünschloß, Andreas. 2004. "Waiting for the 'Big Beam'. UFO Religions and 'Ufological' Themes in New Religious Movements." In *The Oxford Handbook of New Religious Movements*, edited by James R. Lewis, 419–44. Oxford: Oxford UP.

Hammer, Olav. 2004. *Claiming Knowledge. Strategies of Epistemology from Theosophy to New Age*. Leiden, and Boston: Brill.

Hanegraaff, Wouter J. 1996. *New Age Religion and Western Culture. Esotericism in the Mirror of Secular Thought*. Leiden, and New York and Köln: Brill.

—. 2007. "The New Age Movement and Western Esotericism." In *Handbook of New Age* I, edited by Daren Kemp, and James R. Lewis, 25–50. London and Boston: Brill.

—. 2012. *Esotericism and the Academy. Rejected Knowledge in Western Culture*. Cambridge, UK: Cambridge UP.

Hansson, Sven Ove. 1991. "Is Anthroposophy Science?" *Conceptus* XXV (64): 37–49.

Harrington, Melissa. 2007. "Paganism and New Age." In *Handbook of New Age* I, edited by Daren Kemp, and James R. Lewis, 435–52. London and Boston: Brill.

Harvey, Graham. 2007. "Inventing Paganism. Making Nature." In *The Invention of Sacred Tradition*, edited by James R. Lewis, and Olav Hammer, 277–90. Cambridge, UK: Cambridge UP.

Hedges, Ellie, and James A. Beckford. 2000. "Holism, Healing and the New Age." In *Beyond New Age. Exploring Alternative Spirituality*, edited by Steven Sutcliffe, and Marion Bowman, 169–87. Edinburgh: Edinburgh UP.

Heelas, Paul. 1996. *The New Age Movement.* Cambridge, Mass.: Blackwell.

Honko, Lauri. 1959. *Krankheitsprojektile. Untersuchung über eine urtümliche Krankheitserklärung.* Helsinki: Academia Scientiarum Fennica. (Folklore Fellows' Communications 178.)

Hubbes, László Attila. 2013. "Romanian Ethno-Paganism. Discourses of Nationalistic Religion in Virtual Space." In *Modern Pagan and Native Faith Movements in Central and Eastern Europe*, edited by Kaarina Aitamurto, and Scott Simpson, 213–29. Durham, UK: Acumen. (Studies in Contemporary and Historical Paganism.)

Jesus Christ, the Bearer of the Water of Life. Christian reflection on the "New Age". Pontifical Council for Culture, Pontifical Council for Interreligious Dialogue.
http://www.vatican.va/roman_curia/pontifical_councils/interelg/documents/rc_pc_interelg_doc_20030203_new-age_en.html,
accessed January 12, 2016.

Jézus Krisztus, az élő víz hordozója. Keresztény reflexió a New Age-ről [Jesus Christ, the bearer of the water of life. Christian reflection on the "New Age". Pontifical Council for Culture, Pontifical Council for Interreligious Dialogue]. Translated to Hungarian by Jakab Várnai OFM. Budapest: A Kultúra Pápai Tanácsa és a Vallásközi Párbeszéd Pápai Tanácsa.
http://www.karizmatikus.hu/images/stories/docs/elo_viz.rtf.pdf,
accessed January 12, 2016.

Jonas, Waynes B., and Cindy C. Crawford. 2009. "Science and Spiritual Healing. A Critical Review of Spiritual Healing, 'Energy' Medicine and Intentionality." *Alternative Therapies in Health and Medicine* IX (2): 56–61.

Kaku, Michio. 1995. *Hyperspace: A Scientific Odyssey Through Parallel Universes, Time Warps, and the 10th Dimension.* Oxford: Oxford UP.

Kálmány, Lajos. 1885. *Boldogasszony, ősvallásunk istenasszonya* [Blessed Woman, the goddess of our ancient religion]. Budapest: Magyar Tudományos Akadémia.

Kamarás, István. 1999. "Új vallási mozgalmak világszerte és Magyarországon [New religious movements around the world and in Hungary]." *Magyar Tudomány* 5: 560–8.
Kemp, Daren, and Lewis, James R. 2007. *Handbook of New Age I–II.* London, and Boston: Brill.
Kercselics, Imre. [n.d.]. "A testi betegségek lelki okai [Spiritual causes of physical illnesses]." Manuscript. http://www.doksi.hu/get.php?lid=12497, accessed August 18, 2009.
Keszeg, Vilmos, Lehel Peti, and Éva Pócs, eds. 2009. *Álmok és látomások a 20–21. századból. Szöveggyűjtemény* 1. [Dreams and visions from the twentieth and twenty-first centuries. Textbook]. Budapest: L'Harmattan, and PTE Néprajz–Kulturális Antropológia Tanszék. (Fontes Ethnologiae Hungaricae VI.)
Ketola, Kimmo. 2007. "Spiritual Revolution in Finland? Evidence from Surveys and the Rates of Emergence of New Religious and Spiritual Organisations." *Nordic Journal of Religion and Society* XIX (1): 29–39.
Kis-Halas, Judit. 2004. "'Amikor gyógyítok, angyalok jelennek meg a szemem előtt'. Egy dél-baranyai szent gyógyító (Esettanulmány) ['When I heal, angels appear before my eyes'. A holy healer from South Baranya (Case study)]." In *Áldás és átok, csoda és boszorkányság. Vallásetnológiai fogalmak tudományközi megközelítésben* [Blessing and Curse, Miracle and Witchcraft. Interdisciplinary approach to concepts in the ethnology of religion], edited by Éva Pócs, 284–319. Budapest: Balassi. (Tanulmányok a transzcendensről IV.)
—. 2005a. "Átformált hagyomány. A töröcskei öntőasszonyok [Re-inventing tradition: a charm and a dynasty of healers and diviners in a Hungarian village]." *Tabula* 7 (2): 191–208.
—. 2005b. "A wiccától a cyberboszorkákig. Újboszorkány kultuszok a 20. században [From Wicca to cyber witches. Contemporary witch cults in the twentieth centuries]." *Rubicon* 7: 56–61.
—. 2007. "'Fejtetőmön arany fénygömb'. Az első lépések reiki ösvényén. Beavatás egy ezoterikus gyógyászati rendszerbe ['Golden light ball on the top of my head'. The First Steps on the Reiki-path. Initiation into an esoteric healing system]." In *Maszk, átváltozás, beavatás. Vallásetnológiai fogalmak tudományközi megközelítésben* [Mask, transformation, initiation. Interdisciplinary approach to concepts in the ethnology of religion], edited by Éva Pócs, 400–20. Budapest: Balassi. (Tanulmányok a transzcendensről V.)
—. 2008. "'Ha eljönnek az angyalok'. Angyallátók, esszénusok, beavatottak a mai magyar New Age mozgalmakban ['When the angels come...'

Angel-seers, Essenes and initiates in Hungarian New Age spirituality].” In *Démonok, látók, szentek. Vallásetnológiai fogalmak tudományközi megközelítésben* [Demons, seers, saints. Interdisciplinary approach to concepts in the ethnology of religion], edited by Éva Pócs, 243–78. Budapest: Balassi. (Tanulmányok a transzcendensről VI.)
—. 2009a. “‘Mihály arkangyal katonái’ Kortárs látók és gyógyítók [‘Archangel Michael’s soldiers’ Contemporary seers and healers].” In *Álmok és látomások a 20–21. századból. Szöveggyűjtemény* 1. [Dreams and visions from the twentieth and twenty-first centuries], edited by Vilmos Keszeg, Lehel Peti, and Éva Pócs, 512–38. Budapest: L’Harmattan and PTE Néprajz–Kulturális Antropológia Tanszék. (Fontes Ethnologiae Hungaricae VI.)
—. 2009b. “New Age hiedelmek cyber köntösben: az energiavámpír [New Age beliefs in cyber disguise: the energy vampire].” *Acta Papensia* VIII: 195–219.
—. 2010. “Jézus katonái a földön és a Mennyei Jeruzsálemben. Szellemsebészet: egy kortárs ezoterikus gyógyászati rendszer [Soldiers of Jesus on Earth and in the Heavenly Jerusalem: Psychotronics, a contemporary esoteric healing system].” In *Mágikus és szakrális medicina. Vallásetnológiai fogalmak tudományközi megközelítésben*, edited by Éva Pócs, 593–622. Budapest, Balassi. (Tanulmányok a transzcendensről VII.)
—. 2012a. “‘I make my saints work…’: A Hungarian Holy Healer’s Identity Reflected in Autobiographical Stories and Folk Narratives.” In *Vernacular Religion in Everyday Life: Expressions of Belief*, edited by Marion Bowman, and Ülo Valk, 63–92. Sheffield: Equinox.
—. 2012b. “Az etnográfus esete az energiavámpírral. Kortárs vallási jelenségek kutatási lehetőségei a világhálón [The case of the anthropologist and the energy vampire: Researching religion on the Internet].” In *Az elkerülhetetlen. Vallásantropológiai tanulmányok Vargyas Gábor tiszteletére*, edited by Zoltán Nagy, and Ildikó Landgraf, 827–48. Budapest: L’Harmattan.
—. 2014a. “A táltos és az emberi lét hét szintje. Ezotericizmus és újpogányság kölcsönhatásainak vizsgálati lehetőségei [Táltos and the seven levels of human existence: on examining the interferences of esotericism and contemporary Paganism].” In *Sámán sámán hátán. A kortárs pogányság multidiszciplináris elemzése*, edited by István Povedák, and Réka Szilárdi, 129–43. Szeged: SZTE BTK Néprajz–Kulturális Antropológia Tanszék. (Szegedi vallási néprajzi könyvtár 38. MTA SZTE vallási kultúrakutató csoport a vallási kultúrakutatás könyvei 6.)

—. 2014b. "Auratisztítás és szellemműtét. Gondolatok egy kortárs alternatív gyógymód, a pszichotronika testképeiről [Aura cleansing and spirit surgery. On the body concepts in an alternative healing system]." *Pannonhalmi Szemle* XXII (4): 25–39.

Klaniczay, Gábor. 1983. "Benandante-kresnik-zduhač-táltos. Samanizmus és boszorkányhit érintkezési pontjai Közép-Európában [Benandante-kresnik-zduhač-táltos. Some points of contact between Shamanism and Witch belief in Central Europe]." *Ethnoghraphia* XCIV (1): 116–134.

—. 1984. "Shamanistic Elements in Central European Witchcraft." In *Shamanism in Eurasia*, edited by Mihály Hoppál, 404–22. Göttingen: Herodot.

—. 2001. "Shamanistic Elements in Central European Witchcraft." In *Witchcraft, Healing, and Popular Diseases*, edited by Brian P. Levack, 267–92. New York, and London: Routledge. (New Perspectives on Witchcraft, Magic and Demonology V.)

Knoblauch, Hubert. 2008. "Spirituality and Popular Religion in Europe." *Social Compass* 55 (2): 140–53.

Kóka, Rozália, ed. 2006. *"Beteljesítem Isten akaratját..." A lészpedi szent leány látomásai.* ["I'm going fulfil God's will." Visions of the holy girl from Lészped]. Budapest: L'Harmattan and PTE Néprajz–Kulturális Antropológia Tanszék. (Fontes Ethnologiae Hungaricae III.)

Kürti, László. 2001. "Psychic Phenomena, Neoshamanism and the Cultic Milieu in Hungary." *Nova Religio* IV: 322–51.

Lázár, Imre. 2006. "Táltos Healers, Neoshamans and Multiple Medical Realities in Post-Socialist Hungary." In *Multiple Medical Realities. Patients and Healers in Biomedical, Alternative and Traditional Medicine*, edited by Helle Johannesen, and Imre Lázár, 35–53. Oxford, and New York: Berghahn Books. (The EASA Series 4.)

Lengyel, Ágnes. 1998. "Halottlátó Lőrinciben [A Seer of the dead in Lőrinci]." In *Szentemberek—a vallási élet szervező egyéniségei* [Holy men—organisers of folk religiosity], edited by Gábor Barna, 188–204. Szeged, and Budapest: Néprajzi Tanszék, and Magyar Néprajzi Társaság.

Lewis, James R. 2004. *The Oxford Handbook of New Religious Movements*. Oxford: Oxford UP.

Lewis, James R., and Murphy Pizza, eds. 2009. *The Handbook of Contemporary Paganism.* Leiden, and Boston: Brill. (Brill Handbooks of Contemporary Religion 2.)

Lewis, James R., and Inga Bårdsen Tøllefsen, eds. 2016. *The Oxford Handbook of New Religious Movements* 2. Oxford: Oxford UP.

Limbacher, Gábor. 1998. "'Magyar országnak egy külön védőszentje'—Szurdokpüspökiből ['Hungary has its own patron saint'—from Szurdokpüspöki]." In *Szentemberek—a vallási élet szervező egyéniségei* [Holy men—organisers of folk religiosity], edited by Gábor Barna, 160–87. Szeged, and Budapest: Néprajzi Tanszék, and Magyar Néprajzi Társaság.

Luhrmann, Tanya M. 1991 [1989]. *Persuasions of the Witches' Craft. Ritual Magic in Contemporary England.* Cambridge, Mass.: Harvard UP.

Lupton, Deborah. 1995. *Medicine as Culture. Illness, Disease and the Body in Western Societies.* London, Thousand Oaks, and New Delhi: Sage.

Madas, Edit. 2002. *Középkori prédikációirodalmunk történetéből. A kezdetektől a XIV. század elejéig* [From the history of our medieval Christian preaching literature. From the beginnings until the fourteenth century]. Debrecen: Kossuth Egyetemi. (Csokonai Könyvtár Bibliotheca Studiolum Litterarium 25.)

Magliocco, Sabina. 2015. "New Age and Neopagan Magic." In *The Cambridge History of Magic and Witchcraft in the West. From Antiquity to the Present*, edited by David J. Collins, 635–63. Cambridge, UK: Cambridge UP.

Minya, Klára. 2009. "A teozófia néhány tanítása szellemi világokról. Az okkultizmus és a tudomány flörtje [Some things Theosophy taught us about spirit worlds. Occultism flirting with science]." Budapest: Private edition.
http://mek.oszk.hu/07400/07456/07456.htm, accessed December 21, 2009.

O'Malley, John W., S. J. 2014. *The Jesuits: A History from Ignatius to the Present*. London: Rowman & Littlefield.

Ong, Walter J. 1971. "The Literate Orality of Popular Culture Today," In idem, *Rhetoric, Romance, and Technology: Studies in the Interaction of Expression and Culture*, 284-303. Ithaca: Cornell University Press.

—. 1982. *Orality and Literacy: The Technologizing of the Word.* London: Methuen.

Östling, Erik A. W. 2016. "What Does God Need with a Starship? UFOs and Extra-terrestrials in the Contemporary Religious Landscape." In *The Oxford Handbook of New Religious Movements* 2, edited by James R. Lewis, and Inga Bårdsen Tøllefsen, 418–27. Oxford: Oxford UP.

Partridge, Christopher. 2002. "The Disenchantment and Re-enchantment of the West. The Religio-Cultural Context of Contemporary Western Christianity." *The Evangelical Quarterly* 74 (3): 235–56.

—. 2004. "Alternative Spiritualities, New Religions, and the Re-enchantment of the West." In *The Oxford Handbook of New Religious Movements*, edited by James R. Lewis, 39–67. Oxford, UK: Oxford UP.

Pócs, Éva. 1989. "Hungarian Táltos and his European Parallels." In *Uralic Mythology and Folklore*, edited by Mihály Hoppál, and Juha Pentikäinen, 251–76. Budapest, and Helsinki: Ethnographic Institute of the Hungarian Academy of Sciences, and Finnish Literature Society.

—. 2006. "Jánó Ilona és az újkori magyar látomások [Ilona Jánó and modern age Hungarian visions]." In "*Bételjesítem Isten akaratját...*" *A lészpedi szent leány látomásai* ["I'm going fulfil God's will." Visions of the holy girl from Lészped], edited by Rozália Kóka, 230–51. Budapest: L'Harmattan, and PTE Néprajz–Kulturális Antrolopógia Tanszék. (Fontes Ethnologiae Hungaricae III.)

—. 2017. "Shamanism or Witchcraft? The *Táltos* Before the Tribunals." In *Witchcraft and Demonology in Hungary and Transylvania*, edited by Gábor Klaniczay and Éva Pócs, 221–289. London, UK: Palgrave Macmillan.

Possamaï, Adam. 2005. *In Search of New Age Spiritualities.* Aldershot: Ashgate.

—. 2007. "Producing and Consuming New Age Spirituality: The Cultic Milieu and the Network Paradigm." In *Handbook of New Age* I, edited by Daren Kemp, and James R. Lewis, 151–66. London, and Boston: Brill.

S. Balázs, Lívia. 2004. "Vallási elemek egy népi gyógyász tevékenységében [Religious elements in a folk healer's practice]." In *Népi vallásosság a Kárpát-medencében* VI. *6. Konferencia Pápán 2002. június,* I–II., edited by Emőke S. Laczkovits, and Veronika Mészáros, II. 213–22. [Folk religiosity in the Carpathian basin VI. Conference in Pápa, June 2002]. Veszprém: Veszprém Megyei Múzeumi Igazgatóság.

Simpson, Scott, and Mariusz Filip. 2013. "Selected Words for Modern Pagan and Native Faith Movements in Central and Eastern Europe." In *Modern Pagan and Native Faith Movements in Central and Eastern Europe*, edited by Kaarina Aitamurto, and Scott Simpson, 27–43. Durham, UK: Acumen. (Studies in Contemporary and Historical Paganism.)

Sontag, Susan. 1983. *A betegség, mint metafora.* Translated by László Lugosi. Budapest: Mérleg. [Illness as Metaphor. New York: Farrar Straus and Giroux, 1978.]

Steiner, Rudolf. 1994. *Die Sendung Michaels. Die Offenbarung der eigentlichen Geheimnisse des Menschen Wesens. Zwölf Vorträge gehalten in Dornach vom 21. November bis 15. Dezember 1919.* Dornach, Schweiz: Rudolf Steiner. http://fvn-archiv.net/PDF/GA/GA194.pdf, accessed: January 15, 2016.

—. 2010. *Aus der Akasha-Chronik. Gesammelte Artikel aus de Zeitshcrift „Luzifer-Gnosis" 1904/05.* http://anthroposophie.byu.edu/schriften/011.pdf, accessed August 22, 2016.

Strmiska, Michael. 2005. *Modern Paganism in World Cultures: Comparative Perspectives*. Santa Barbara, Calif.: ABC-CLIO.

Sutcliffe, Steven J. 2000. "'Wandering Stars': Seekers and Gurus in the Modern World." In *Beyond New Age. Exploring Alternative Spirituality*, edited by Steven Sutcliffe, and Marion Bowman, 17–36. Edinburgh: Edinburgh UP.

—. 2004. "The Dynamics of Alternative Spirituality. Seekers, Networks, and 'New Age'." In *The Oxford Handbook of New Religious Movements*, edited by James R. Lewis, 466–90. Oxford: Oxford UP.

Szilárdi, Réka. 2007. "Posztmodern identitáskultúra a magyarországi neopogány közösségekben [Postmodern Identity-Culture in Hungarian Neopagan Communities]." *Erdélyi Társadalom* V: 103–22.

—. 2013. "Neo-Paganism in Hungary. Under the Spell of Roots." In *Modern Pagan and Native Faith Movements in Central and Eastern Europe*, edited by Kaarina Aitamurto, and Scott Simpson, 230–48. Durham, UK: Acumen. (Studies in Contemporary and Historical Paganism.)

Szilágyi, Tamás, and Szilárdi, Réka. 2007. *Istenek ébredése. Az újpogányság vallástudományi vizsgálata* [The Awakening of Gods. The Religious Study of Neo-Paganism]. Szeged: JATE. (Vallás a társadalomban I.)

Tighe, Maria, and Butler, Jenny. 2007. "Holistic Health and New Age in Britain and in the Republic of Ireland." In *Handbook of New Age* I, edited by Daren Kemp, and James R. Lewis, 415–34. London, and Boston: Brill.

Tomka, Miklós. 1996. "A vallásszociológia új útjai [New ways of sociology of religion]." *Replika* XXI–XXII: 163–71.

Urban, Hugh B. 2005. "Kuṇḍalinī." In *Encyclopedia of Religion* VIII. *Ka'bah–Marx, Karl*, edited by Lindsay Jones, 5266–7. Detroit, Mich.: Thomson Gale.

Utriainen, Terhi. 2015. "Combining Christianity and New Age Spirituality. Angel Relations in Finland." In *Handbook of Nordic New*

Religions, edited by James R. Lewis, and Inga Bårdsen Tøllefsen, 158–72. Leiden, and Boston, Brill.

—. 2016 [2013]. "Doing Things with Angels: Agency, Alterity and Practices of Enchantment." In *Helsinki Study of Religions. A Reader*, edited by Riku Hämaläinen, Heikki Pesonen, and Terhi Utriainen, 138–49. Helsinki: University of Helsinki. (Uskontontiete 17.)

Waldby, Catherine. 2000. *The Visible Human Project. Informatic Bodies and Posthuman Medicine.* London, and New York: Routledge.

Walter, Tony. 2011. "Angels not Souls: Popular Religion in the Online Mourning for British Celebrity Jade Goody." *Religion* 41 (1): 29–51.

Woodroffe, John. 1950. *The Serpent Power. The Secrets of Shaktic and Tantric Yoga.* (4th ed.) Madras: Ganesh and Co. London: Luzac, 1919.

Integrating Ancient and Modern Healing Concepts in Tandem Hypnotherapy

József Pál Vas and Noémi Császár

Introduction

Tandem Hypnotherapy (THT), originating from ancient shamanistic techniques, designates a group of hypnotic methods which can be effectively applied in psychosomatic and mental disorders stemming from intergenerationally mediated, relational traumas. (Vas and Császár 2011a). The word tandem has two meanings: (1) a bicycle with two seats; (2) a mosaic word for **T**ouch of **A**ncient and **N**ew Generations with a **D**ialogue **E**xperiencing Oneness of **M**inds (**TANDEM**). THT involves the participation of more than two persons: the client(s), the co-therapist(s) and the hypnotherapist. It works this way: the co-therapist descends into a trance together with the client in a tandem situation to elicit a positive, corrective experience, with the potential of coping with the client's traumas, while the therapist keeps a distance from those in the tandem trance. Techniques of THT have been elaborated by the authors for the following settings: (1) a joint rebirth trance of two clients by taking the role of mother and daughter or son; (2) a joint twin-type tandem trance in which natural or virtual twins go into a trance to resolve intrauterine traumatic experiences; (3) some forms of intergenerational hypnodrama, for example three persons taking the roles of members of a clan.

All the techniques of THT involve hypnosis with the aim of reliving an imagined communication among ancestors and descendants, including intrauterine experiences and subsequent birth. In the therapeutic setting, touch plays a central role as it helps to resolve the psychopathological outcomes of early relational traumas, because touch is viewed as the first sensory mode of the embryo after conception in the womb. A multi-person trance, when occurring alongside physical proximity, has been found to have the capability of creating an experience of oneness and being conscious of oneness, which can have the power of resolving psychopathological splittings[1]. The healing power of THT is considered to be a type of collective unconscious communication, which is called the "communication of ontological love" among members of generations (Vas and Császár 2011b).

Although THT is treated as an original therapeutic method, it has several theoretical and methodological roots which are the following: ancient shamanistic practice (Jilek 1988, 64–85; Eliade 1993, 15–9),[2] Jungian archetypal therapy,[3] hypnotherapy (Bányai 2008), psychodrama and hypnodrama,[4] contextual family therapy,[5] Hellinger's Systemic Approach,[6] evolutionary psychology (Pléh 2001), ethnopsychology,[7] developmental neuropsychology (Schore 2003, 33–57), prenatal and perinatal medicine and psychology (Blum 1993, 107–31; Janus 1997, 143–58; Chamberlain 1993; Piontelli 1987; Verny 1996), and transpersonal psychology (Grof 2000, 49–107; Wilber 1996, 217–36).

---

[1] Splitting is the name of a primitive defence mechanism of the Ego, which divides psychic contents into two parts—totally good and totally bad—especially those contents relating to the inner images of parents.

[2] Stanley Krippner analyses common and different features of trance methods applied on both natural tribes and western scientific hypnotherapy (Krippner 1993).

[3] It is an application of Jungian archetypes in the framework of psychotherapy (Jung 1978, 83–90).

[4] Jacob Levi Moreno was the first to deal with hypnodrama (Moreno 1987, 341–59).

[5] Iván Böszörményi-Nagy introduced contextual family therapy. According to him, ancestors can pass either constructive or destructive authority to descendants. In a case of constructive authority, the descendant is treated by the message of authority as a person who lives in his or her own right, and she or he is delegated to cope with traumas to reach happiness. Destructive authority is seen as a message to the descendant either not to live in their own right, or where their dignity depends on unrealisable conditions (Böszörményi-Nagy and Krasner 1986, 201–34).

[6] Bert Hellinger's Systemic Approach designates a combination of psychodrama and family therapy, in which the trauma of the protagonist (the person whose problem is acted out by some members of a group), ancestors, and the transmission of this trauma to the descendants are represented (Hellinger 1994, 18–26).

[7] According to ethnopsychology, there are two types of spatial settings in therapies: first, proximate types which are characterised by physical closeness; and the second types, which are distal or distancing therapies, characterised by spatial distance (Vas and Császár 2011c: 460–81).

Some of the forms of Tandem Hypnotherapy illustrated via case vignettes

(1) Mother–Daughter Tandem Hypnotherapy

As an illustration, let us show a THT case: Angie, 18; diagnosis: Anorexia Nervosa; weight: 33 kg; height: 170 cm. Angie was born prematurely, as her mother had an intrauterine infection during pregnancy. It is an interesting parallel that she was approaching her school-leaving exams when the therapy began so she was in a premature (child-like) state; in a sense, both emotionally and in her physical appearance. She had always suspected that she had a twin sibling who was lost prenatally. As a child she was overweight and mocked by her schoolmates. A few years beforehand, she had started a drastic slimming diet after a break-up with a boyfriend. Her grandmother died, and her parents' enterprise went bankrupt. The family atmosphere was very tense. Angie felt she had to starve to spare money for the family. Her weight dropped to 33 kilograms and all she was able to do for a year was lie in bed.

Angie and her mother agreed to take THT. Since Angie had ego-weakness, the therapist (Dr Vas) decided to initiate guided affective imagery with nature symbols of a meadow, a stream, and so on. In tandem trance, her mother's role was to serve as a holding environment because Angie's security had been fragile as a foetus due to the intrauterine infection. Angie enjoyed being in a meadow and watching a stream. Then she was instructed to transform herself into the stream. As a stream she felt she was moving, continually flowing; she could feel her energy ever reviving since spring water would always feed her. This could be regarded both as a symbolic message of purification from prenatal infection and the symbol of gaining ancestral power. The following thoughts are cited from her diary:

> During the previous imagination I had an incredible experience when I transformed into a stream. This little stream is capable of purifying itself because it has immense strength. It is capable of coping with cliffs and other obstacles, and it is capable of attaining its goal. It is beautiful when the sun shines on its surface, it looks like gold and silver. I consider this stream to be my ideal so I am going to attain my goals in every field.

At the next session, Angie and her mother announced that after one year of inactively lying in bed, Angie had suddenly started to study every day, so much so, that she slept only three hours a night. It seemed as if she was identifying herself with a fast stream running down the valley. Then the therapist introduced a change to slow her down. They imagined that as a stream, Angie had reached a little pool in which she slowed and calmed down while deepening, in order to accumulate strength. As a consequence of this suggestion, her sleep gradually became set at between six to eight hours a night. At the following session, she imagined herself transforming into a tree with tropical blossom, which might be seen as a metaphor of her unsatisfied symbiotic foetal needs. By then she had started to acquire feminine features in the eyes of others.

At the next session, they imagined that Angie was a foetus before being born. Angie said she felt joy at being in the uterus. The therapist suggested that she sleep in the womb and have a dream in which she and her twin sibling meet in the realm of unborn babies. She noticed a nice girl, Wendy. It was suggested that Wendy and she say that they love each other so much that they would be born at the same time, but that it would be very hard to make this come true. Wendy stressed that one of them might fail to be born. If this were the case, neither of them would feel sorrow or guilt because the other had failed to be born. Instead, one would have to keep in mind that either Wendy or Angie would love and protect the other twin during her life on Earth. As this suggestion was given, Angie burst into tears.

Four months passed and Angie passed her school-leaving exams with flying colours. Her weight increased to 45 kilograms. This period of therapy, including her mother in a tandem situation, focused on satisfying their symbiotic needs. A year later she had no symptoms.

(2) Matrilineal Tandem Hypnotherapy

In a joint tandem trance undergone in intergenerational matrilineal hypnosis, three women who were not blood relatives were able to experience each other's roles as grandmother, mother and daughter, by being mutually involved in each role. The three women were given names by using the first three letters of the alphabet: Alice, Betty and Charlotte. Alice's great-grandmother had arrived in the south of Hungary, from the Balkans, to improve her fortunes; she had become pregnant and had been rejected by her community when she gave birth to Alice's grandmother out of wedlock. She died at the age of 24 in shame, as the family legend tells. The daughter, Alice's grandmother, was a dependent, helpless person all her life, also giving birth to a child, Alice's mother, out of wedlock. As a child, Alice had to care for her grandmother and mother, who were both suffering from being regularly sick in the street, due to agoraphobia and panic disorder. Alice's mother showed some talent and she found a kind husband, but the matrilineal heritage of "women are always losers" did not allow her talent to become known; she became ill, developed anxiety-depression disorder which was followed by cancer, and died after a long period of suffering. Alice herself developed severe psychosomatic illnesses twice during her adolescence, possibly as a manifestation of the matrilineal "curse", and she was forced to give up her career as an artist. The second participant, Betty, was a lonely, childless woman over 60, whose grandmother had died early, leaving Betty's mother to be brought up without a mother. Having given birth to Betty, she divorced and raised Betty by herself (the intergenerational message of Betty's mother was: "You have to go through everything on your own!"). Regarding the third woman, Charlotte's grandmother married the man she loved, gave birth to Charlotte's mother, and then died of tuberculosis at the age of 24. The mother was brought up in an emotionally cold climate and later gave birth to Charlotte with whom she had a disharmonious relationship.

In hypnosis, Alice was in the role of the "grandmother", Betty of the "mother" and Charlotte of the "daughter". Before the start of the joint hypnosis, the three women lay down on their sides, with Alice, the "grandmother" lying on the outside in the highest position. Betty, the "mother" was lying with her back facing Alice, while Charlotte, the "daughter" was coiled in Betty's lap. During hypnotic induction, attunement of the participants to each other and age-regression were both occurring simultaneously. As a result, each of them could emotionally experience the messages of their fate as women, and the emotional messages of their children and grandchildren, as well as those of their mothers and grandmothers. Here is part of the induction: "As grandmother, mother and daughter, the three of you will experience something that each of you are in need of. You will experience the unity of grandmother, mother and granddaughter, in which the female "fate", overseeing the three generations, appears simultaneously and in a compressed manner. You will see and sense the presence of grandmother, mother and grandchild, their interlocking influences, and their messages transcending the limits of space and time".

First, the behavioural changes that could be observed externally will be described. Following the induction, the therapist told the participants that they could make contact with each other. As a response, Alice, the "grandmother" said: "You are the most important persons for me", while putting her hand on Betty's shoulder, who was in the role of "mother". Betty, in her turn, put her hand on Charlotte, the "daughter's" shoulder. At this point, the "grandmother" Alice and the "daughter" Charlotte began to reach out towards each other with their free hands, without seeing or talking to each other, and with the assistance of the therapist they took each other's hand in such a way that Betty's, the "mother's" hand could touch both. After about ten seconds had passed, a fourth hand, Betty's, joined in by embracing the hands of the others from above. The therapist then said: "Now imagine that a golden light appears in front of you, the light of love which binds you together and shows you the way to follow".

The retrospective accounts of the participants reveal what happened experientially during these moments. To begin with, Betty, as a mother, felt the hands of her trance companions were cold but she felt more and more warmth, support, protection and strength from the "grandmother" Alice, and the "daughter" Charlotte. The following is the experience of Alice, the "grandmother":

> Somehow I was Charlotte's grandmother and Charlotte the "daughter" at the same time, to whom my grandmother was sending a message. As if life was flowing backwards, it was me as a child, who had to support my grandmother. Then I felt that on behalf of my grandmother I had to ask for forgiveness from Charlotte. I wanted to get hold of her hand. I could barely believe that I could actually reach it, and I could hardly believe that she was grasping mine. I felt that I should not burden her hand too much so I kept mine a little away. As if I was protecting her from disasters. As a result my hand got stiff, but then it became very light…

The "daughter" Charlotte's account of her experience:

> I saw my real grandmother whom I had known earlier only from photographs. I saw her from above, as a young, fragile woman, and I could also see my mother as a foetus in her womb, and in my mother's ovary I saw myself as an ovum. My grandmother told me how much she loved my mother, more than her firstborn daughter. I was amazed by the scene. I was standing in the yard of a village hut surrounded by destruction, right after the end of World War II. My grandmother rested her hand on her stomach, indicating to me in a state of radiant happiness, that it was the birth of my mother which really mattered, as if telling me not to pay attention to the outside world but rather to what mattered, the thing that was growing inside. Meanwhile, at the suggestion of the therapist that everyone could make contact with everybody, my mother in the group, Betty slightly moved her hand. I knew she was trying to make contact with me. I took her hand, indicating that I was there for her, she was not alone, and she could lean on me. My real grandmother disappeared and instead of her my grandmother in the group, Alice appeared before me, with Betty in her womb. I felt Alice was almost begging me to take her hand...

Let us remember Alice's account of her experience in those minutes; the grandmother, Alice, felt that she had to ask for forgiveness from Charlotte, whom she was identifying as her childhood self, on behalf of her real grandmother. She wanted to hold Charlotte's hand in a way that would not weigh on her, as if protecting her from disasters. Charlotte's account continues:

> I loosened my hold on Betty's hand and stretched back to include my grandmother, Alice, and with the help of the therapist she took my hand. The therapist also moved Betty's hand over to us. The energy pulsing among the three interlocking hands was immense. In my mind I heard Alice, who begged me, without words, for forgiveness. Then I felt that my arm was getting heavy to the point of almost breaking off. In my mind I answered, saying that I had forgiven her. I felt that Alice was holding my hand more strongly. It suggested that she was helping me hold my arm which immediately became lighter. OK, I told her and the others, without words; I will cope.

Going back to the observable behaviour of the participants in the trance, after about a minute of intimate silence and stillness, the four hands unfolded as if under the will of a single person, without the hypnotherapist giving instruction to this effect. The de-hypnosis, restoration of the temporal and spatial dimensions, occurred as the women checked out of their roles. During this minute of full silence, the participants lived through the following experiences as expressed in their retrospective reports. The "mother" Betty: "Feelings of insight and acceptance followed, I repeatedly say: loving forgiveness!" The "grandmother" Alice: "When our hands grasped each other I suddenly felt immense happiness; I felt numbness from head to toe as if struck by lightning. By then I didn't know who was who; my grandmother, who had never been able to make contact with me before, not even in the cemetery, now did so. Time and space completely ceased to exist. Great strength was streaming from the grasping hands. They were holding me. The female fate can be shared. I don't know how but my social phobia is gone, all my anxieties are gone!" Charlotte's account of this minute: "My arm was no longer heavy. The weight put on it had disappeared, dissolved. I felt that Alice was also relieved. Both of them let my hand loose. My real grandmother told me: Your life is worth living for the people you love…We returned to the present."

The therapist reported that he was in a trance the whole time during hypnosis, attending to the emotional state of the union formed by the three participants, which made him feel that he had to say things that were different from what he had intended. However, he felt that it was the group's unconscious message that emanated from the experience of oneness; from the non-verbal, synchronous emotional experiences of those being in a joint trance. He had a feeling that the hypnosis proceeded along the workings of powers higher than his own will or consciousness, powers which he was merely assisting in.

(3) THT with Therapist-Patient Dyad

Should an individual psychotherapy come to an impasse, THT can be used with a Therapist-Patient Dyad. When peri- or prenatal trauma is suspected behind a patient's resistance, the individual therapist can ask us to mediate by conducting special supervision. Both the patient and their individual therapist come to a supervision session. We are open to communicating in the presence of the patient so he or she is not excluded from supervision. After discussing the problem, the therapist and the patient go into tandem hypnosis with the help of the supervisor hypnotherapist. It is necessary for the therapist to be of the same sex as the patient. The method can be applied during the supervision of difficult or frustrating individual psychotherapies.

What follows is a very interesting double case involving Dr Császár's borderline identical twin patient Samantha, and Kate, the patient of one of our female colleagues. Both of their individual therapies came to a deadlock. Samantha, 42, born prematurely as one of identical twins, suffers from Borderline Personality Disorder. Her psychotherapy, led by Dr Császár for two years, had been unsuccessful. Samantha is extremely fitful, while her twin sister, Myra, is a perfectionist. They have hated each other since their adolescence. Before their birth, their brother became severely sick, which put their mother in constant fear of losing her son. Kate, 39, who is also a twin, had been having panic attacks since her childhood. She always had a feeling that something was missing on her left side. She was told in her early teens that she had had a twin sister who had died a few days after birth. She had serious touch aversion because she could not remember that she had ever been caressed. Kate cancelled several sessions because she could not go out into the street.

One supervision session, the two therapists of these patients decided to take the patients to THT under the leadership of a supervisor psychotherapist, Dr Vas. The plan was for Kate to get the chance to meet and say farewell to her sister in her imagination, while Samantha would experience positive feelings towards her own sister, feelings she once actually felt. At the beginning of the session, the supervisor therapist explained the method and asked for the approval of the patients. It was obvious that the two patients didn't like each other, and so each therapist had to take the role of their patient's mother because it was known that each twin had an exclusive need for one mother. Samantha lay in her therapist's lap while Kate sat on a sofa rigidly with no contact with her therapist "mother". Tale induction was employed, in which a mother and her two daughters left the past together in order to search for the blue bird of happiness. During hypnosis the patients were lying relaxed while the therapists were embracing them just like mothers. After the imagery of conception, the supervisor asked them about their feelings: Samantha felt that she had an affectionate mother while her therapist stated that she had always wanted a daughter and she was eventually getting one. Kate said she felt strong and that she enjoyed being there with her mother. Her therapist responded that she had enjoyed it as well and she was looking forward to giving birth. Both patients stated that they did not want to be born, they were having a good time there as a foetus. Samantha wanted to stay there forever and asked for suggestions to conserve the peaceful feeling of the uterus even after the hypnosis, and so imagery of her birth was postponed for another time. On listening to the suggestion that she let her body move spontaneously in birth, as if it had an unconscious programme for coming into the world, Kate spontaneously turned towards her own therapist as if to her mother and embraced her with open eyes. The atmosphere of the closing discussion was relaxed.

A few days after the THT, Samantha felt she could trust her therapist more than ever before, just as in the case of Kate. Several months later, Samantha's twin sister, Myra divorced her husband who had severe psychological problems, and the twins' relationship improved. A year later, Samantha's symptoms were relieved and her coping mechanisms became more mature. Kate recovered rapidly during her individual therapy, her panic attacks disappeared, and she began to live independently. Now she has a new male partner. Kate wrote in her diary, cited word for word: "I am worthy of love because I was born, just because I AM ALIVE!"[8]

[8] The latter psychotherapeutic frame can be easily questioned because after Ferenczi, therapists hardly ever embraced patients. This feature can be emphasised as resembling shamanistic trancework. Touch is viewed as a normal action among people, expressing friendship, closeness and intimacy. As a matter of fact, the ethics of therapeutic touch is fundamental (Phelan 2009; Young 2007). Experiences during tandem hypnosis are transcendental, conveying not seduction or occupancy but ontological love. For the sake of human dignity this rule must be respected both by therapists and patients. Zur and Nordmarken have recently collected

Discussion

It is known how proximate therapies changed in the history of modern psychotherapies when Freud refused proximate hypnosis for the sake of distancing analysis.[9] According to developmental neuropsychology, touch appears to be the mother of perception and thus the first language. Touch is called skin-ego.[10] The experience of touch is processed in the right hemisphere of the brain, which represents relations and contexts. Thus, touch is responsible for reliving spatial regression that is an attunement with partners, which means to be protected, to feel secure, and to have warmth and love.[11] The neurochemistry of social support emphasises the role of oxytocin which is excreted when people approach each other in

---

developmental, neurophysiological, clinical, ethical and legal data upon therapeutic touch (Zur and Nordmarken 2011).

[9] Freud's follower, a Hungarian analyst, Sándor Ferenczi developed a proximate method and made the patient sit in his lap (Ferenczi 1933). Wilhelm Reich's orgone-therapy was based on bodily massage; later, Frank Lake, Leonard Orr and Stanislav Grof practised psychotherapies called rebirthing therapies to relive the birthing process. Current proximate types comprise somatopsychotherapy, bioenergetic therapy, movement- and dancing therapies, and haptonomy. In the foetal period of our life, touch is absolutely vital to establish the frontier of the body, and to evolve the boundaries of ego and self upon which attachment and relations are built (Grof 2000, 49–107).

[10] Ashley Montagu's famous early work on touch as human significance deals with touch and touching as a key stimulus for evolving ego-functions of the developing personality. The touch of the amniotic fluid on the skin is a stimulus essential for the development of the nervous system and it also provides a continual proof for the foetus of its existence. This foetal heritage represents the basis for any personal attunement, the state of being loved, or the state of sexual or emotional fusion. Skin to skin contact, particularly on the left side of the breast, causes oxitocin release, which is known to be the most important biochemical mediator of caring behaviour, of the sense of being held and loved (Montagu 1986, 19–25). Somatopsychotherapy is based upon the therapeutic effects of touching (Meyer 2010, 43–64). Cells of the neuroimmune system contain inorganic piezoelectric crystals of nanoscale size in their billions, which are capable of photon emission (Bókkon 2005). By creating a hologram these can produce synchronous vibrations in groups of cells in a whole organ, say in the whole body at a quantum wave level. It can be presumed that these synchronous vibrations might be responsible for the energy fields of higher dimensions surrounding the body—see the concepts of oriental healing, like chakras or meridians—which in our hypothesis might constitute the basis for attunement among persons.

[11] Frans Veldman developed haptonomy as a special somatotherapeutic method (Veldman 1994).

order to touch. Touch is said to have the effects of anti-stress, calming and love (Varga 2009).

When a premodern community was involved in the ritual of their origin, members of this community entered temporal regression, that is, a common fate determined by the beginning of time. This may be why participants in inter- or transgenerational THT recognise the life narrative of their tandem partners. In fact, they are able to imagine collective archetypal experiences, which are called "consciousness of oneness".[12]

Contrary to Western medicine, which focuses on the person as an individual, healers of premodern communities (shamans, wizards) represent the faith, morality, traditions and viewpoint of life of the whole community; that is, the community's spiritual power. A transgression of spiritual powers is assumed in the background of illnesses (Krippner 1993). A good example of anomic depression to refer to is of a Salish Indian tribe which lived on the American West Coast by the Pacific Ocean. Symptoms of anomic depression like passivity, aimlessness, drug- and alcohol addiction, and helplessness were observed after the tribe was forced to move onto a reserve.[13] Moving onto the reserve involved leaving behind the original and sacred homeland, tribal unity, way of life, faith, and rites of their own, which was a suspension of tribal identity. This process is shown by the concept of collective oblivion written by Garcia Marquez in his novel, "One Hundred Years of Solitude" (Marquez 1971). The suspension of collective identity was caused by the conquest of Western civilisation, resulting in existential, cultural and spiritual disintegration.

We think that our Hungarian society is subject to such existential, cultural and spiritual disintegration today (Vas and Császár 2011c). Symptoms of anomic depression can be observed, which are the same as

---

[12] In our assumption the oneness-experiences in THT are not the kinds which emanate from the type of consciousness reflecting the dual object-subject relationships, but rather the experiences of an archaic consciousness of oneness which possesses quantum attributes by not being able to be localised within the person and by spreading without the use of conceptual-linguistic symbols. Let us cite from Alice's account on her oneness experience during THT: "When our hands grasped, I suddenly felt immense happiness; I felt numbness from head to toe as if struck by lightning. By then I didn't know who was who. My grandmother, who had never been able to before, not even in the cemetery, got in touch with me. Time and space completely ceased to exist. Great strength was streaming out from the clasped hands. They were holding me. The female fate can be shared. I don't know how, but my social phobia is gone, all of my anxieties are gone!"

[13] Wolfgang G. Jilek describes Spirit Dancing as a healing rite of Salish Indian tribes who inhabited the West Coast at the Pacific Ocean (Jilek 1988, 64–85).

in the case of the Indian tribe mentioned earlier. What kind of essential interests are damaged through cultural and spiritual disintegration? These interests are presumed to be territoriality, race preservation, and self-preservation, which are all viewed as functions of the reptilian brain[14] and mind. If a spiritual disintegration were to take place there would be no effective mental mechanism to control the instincts and drives of the reptilian brain of people. As a result, both aggression and separation anxiety would be released. It is well-documented that the release of aggression and anxiety results in disturbed social adaptation and psychopathology. Therefore, we need the values and tools which ancient shamanistic tribes used to have. We need collective rituals and spirituality. We need a unity of faith, tradition and rituals, which is supposed to form an experience of relatedness, unity and oneness among members of a community. This experience of unity serves as a guarantee against disintegration both among the members of a community and in the history of that community.

Conclusions

What are the advances of Tandem Hypnotherapy?

(1) TH is instrumental in causing people to get close together, resulting in security, warmth and love.

(2) As a new method, its place is among transpersonal therapies, since instead of being symptom-oriented, it is characterised by a holistic, existential-ontological approach which places its focus on the meaning of our lives and its marked events. The physical presence and mutual touches of those in a joint trance can facilitate the resolution of traumatic experiences in the past, not only on an imaginary level but also on the level of reality, with the capability of eliminating pathological splittings, stemming from relational traumas of the prenatal and perinatal period.

(3) In a joint tandem trance, mutual attunement becomes possible on a narrative, experiential, emotional, behavioural, physiological and transferential level, with some of the elements of this state of attunement appearing and becoming conscious in each participant; that is, each member becomes able to experience the inner processes taking place in all of the other members as well. In this way, the members of a small community (for instance, a THT group) can be made conscious of their

---

[14] The reptilian brain is located in the hypothalamus and brain stem, securing the functions of an individual's fundamental biological urges and drives, such as territoriality, self-preservation and sex (Siegel 1999, 175–81).

own clan's spiritual message, that known as the "communication of ontological love".

(4) By being a group therapy, THT effectively goes beyond individual suffering by addressing the collective, archetypal dimension of the individual. It is the holding capacity of a small community which enables all of its members to be immersed in the trance state of rites and myths, which is necessary for the construction of the collective past. A collective trance is essential for the re-writing of burdensome past experiences and for transcending them.

References

Bányai, Éva. 2008. "Hipnózis és hipnoterápia a 21. században: a hipnózis a tudomány főáramában [Hypnozis and hypnotherapy in the 21st century: Hypnosis as mainstrean science]." In *A hipnózis és hipnoterápia alapjai. Szöveggyűjtemény*, edited by Éva Bányai, and L. Benczúr, 15–34. Budapest: ELTE Eötvös Kiadó.

Blum, Thomas, ed. 1993. *Prenatal Perception, Learning, and, Bonding*. Berlin: Leonardo Publishers.

Bókkon, István. 2005. "Dreams and neuroholography." *Sleep and Hypnosis* 7 (2): 61−76.

Böszörményi-Nagy, Iván, and Barbara R. Krasner. 1986. *Between Give and Take: A Clinical Guide to Contextual Therapy*. New York: Brunner/Mazel.

Chamberlain, David B. 1993. "Prenatal Intelligence." In *Prenatal Perception Learning and Bonding*, edited by Thomas Blum, 9–31. Berlin: Leonardo Publishers.

Eliade, Mircea. 1993. *Az örök visszatérés mítosza* [Myth of eternal return]. Translated by Péter Pásztor. Budapest: Európa. [Le mythe de l'éternel retour. Paris: Gallimard. 1949.]

Ferenczi, Sándor. 1933. "Trauma in Psychoanalysis." In *Final Contributions to the Problems and Methods of Psychoanalysis*, 210−33. New York: Brunner/Mazel.

Grof, Stanislav. 2000. *The Psychology of the Future*. New York: State University Press.

Hellinger, Bert. 1994. *Ordnungen der Liebe. Ein Kursbuch*. Heidelberg: Carl-Auer-Systeme Verlag.

Janus, Ludwig. 1997. *The Enduring Effects of Prenatal Experience*. London: Jason Aronson.

Jilek, Wolfgang G. 1988. *Indian Healing*. Surrey: Hancock.

Jung, Carl, G. 1978. *Man and his Symbols*. London: Picador.

Krippner, Stanley. 1993. "Cross-cultural perspectives on hypnotic-like procedures used by native healing practitioners." In *Handbook of clinical hypnosis*, edited by William Rhue, Steven Jay Lynn, and Irwin Kirsch, 691–717. Washington DC: APA.

Marquez, Gabriel G. 1971. *Száz év magány* [One hundred years of solitude]. Translated by Vera Székács. Budapest: Magvető. [Cien años de soledad. Buenos Aires: Sudamericana. 1967].

Meyer, Richard. 2010. *A szomato-pszichoterápia* [La Somato-psychothérapie, dans la mouvance de Ferenczi]. Budapest: Oriold és Társai.

Montagu, Ashley. 1986 [1971]. *Touching. The Human Significance of the Skin*. New York: Harper & Row.

Moreno, Zerka T. 1987. "Psychodrama, Role Theory and the Concept of the Social Atom." In *The Evolution of Psychotherapy*, edited by Jeffrey K. Zeig, 341–66. New York: Brunner/Mazel.

Phelan, John E. 2009. "Exploring the use of touch in the psychotherapeutic setting: A phenomenological review." *Psychotherapy: Theory, Practice, Research, Training* 46 (1): 97–111.

Piontelli, Alessandra. 1987. "Infant observation from before the birth." *International Review of Psycho-Analysis* 16: 413–26.

Pléh, Csaba. 2001. "Az evolúciós szemlélet felmerülése, eltűnése s újra felmerülése a pszichológiában." In *Lélek és evolúció. Az evolúciós szemlélet és a pszichológia* [Soul and evolution. An evolutionary viewpoint and psychology], edited by Csaba Pléh, Vilmos Csányi, and Tamás Bereczkei, 13–59. Budapest: Osiris.

Schore, Allan N. 2003. *Affect Dysregulation and Disorders of the Self.* New York: Norton.

Siegel, Daniel J. 1999. *The Developing Mind. Toward a Neurobiology of Interpersonal Experience*. New York: The Guilford Press.

Varga, Katalin. 2009. "Szexualitás, szülés, kötődés: az oxitocin pszichoemotív hatásai" [Sexuality, delivery, attachment: psychoemotive effects of oxytocin]. In *Polihistória—köszöntők és tanulmányok Buda Béla 70. születésnapja alkalmából* [Polyhistory'—compliments and studies on the occasion of Béla Buda's 70th birthday], edited by Emőke Bagdy, Zoltán Demetrovics, and János Pilling, 449–76. Budapest: Akadémiai.

Vas, P. József, and Noémi Császár. 2011a. "Transnatal Tandem Hypnotherapy (TTH): A New Method for Resolving Prenatal Traumas." *International Journal of Psychotherapy* 15 (1): 55–64.

—. 2011b. "Multipersonal Tandem Hypnotherapy (MTH): A New Method for Resolving Intergenerational Traumas." *International Journal of Psychotherapy* 15 (3): 38–48.

—. 2011c. "Tandem hipnoterápia az elődöktől származó traumák oldására" [Tandem Hypnotherapy for resolving traumas originating from ancestors]. In *Transzperszonális pszichológia és pszichoterápia* [Transpersonal psychology and psychotherapy], edited by Emőke Bagdy, Zsuzsa Mirnics, and Erika Nyitrai, 460–86. Budapest: Kulcslyuk.

Veldman, Frans. 1994. "Confirming Affectivity, the Dawn of Human Life." *The International Journal of Prenatal and Perinatal Psychology and Medicine* 6 (1): 11–26.

Verny, Thomas R. 1996. "Isolation, Rejection and Communication in the Womb." *The International Journal of Pre- and Perinatal Psychology and Medicine* 8 (3): 287–94.

Wilber, Ken. 1996. *A Brief history of Everything*. Boston: Shambala.

Young, Courtenay. 2007. "The Power of Touch in Psychotherapy." *International Journal of Psychotherapy* 11 (3): 15–24.

Zur, Ofer, and Nancy Nordmarken. 2011. *To Touch Or Not To Touch: Exploring the Myth of Prohibition On Touch In Psychotherapy And Counseling. Clinical, Ethical and Legal Considerations.* http://www.zurinstitute.com/touchintherapy.html, accessed September 20, 2011.

CONTRIBUTORS

Albena Georgieva. Professor, IEFSEM BAS Bulgaria. Her books include: *Razkazi i razkazvane v bulgarskiia folklor* [Stories and storytelling in Bulgarian folklore]. Sofia: Figura, 2000; *Obrazi na drugostta v bulgarskiia folklor* [Images of otherness in Bulgarian folklore]. Sofia: PH Gutenberg, 2003; *Folklorni izmereniia na hristiianstvoto. Ustni razkazi i lokalna religioznost v raiona na Bachkovskiia manastir "Uspenie na Presveta Bogoroditsa" i na Hadzhidimovskiia manastir "Sv. Velikomachenik Georgi Pobedonosets".* [Folklore dimensions of Christianity. Oral narratives and local religiosity in the region of Bachkovo Monastery "Dormition of the Virgin Mary" and in Hadzhidimovo Monastery "St. George"]. Sofia: Prosveta, 2012.

Ane Ohrvik. Associate Professor in Cultural History, University of Oslo. Her recent publications include *Magic and Texts from 2014* (co-edited volume) and *Medicine, Magic and Art in Early Modern Norway*, in print 2018 by Palgrave Macmillan.

Anna Judit Tóth. Researcher, HAS Institute of Ethnology, Budapest. Her publications include: "John Lydus as Pagan and Christian." In *Pagans and Christians in the Late Roman Empire: New Evidence, New Approaches (4th–8th centuries)*, edited by M. Sághy, and E. M. Schoolman. Budapest: CEU Press, 2017, 59–68; "Mystical Experience in Theurgical Practice." In *The Immediacy of Mystical Experience in the European Tradition.* (Sophia Studies in Cross-Cultural Philosophy of Traditions and Cultures 18), edited by M. Vassányi, E. Sepsi, and A. Daróczi. Cham: Springer, 2017, 23–30; *Ünnepek a keresztény és a pogány kor határán* [Festivals on the border of Christianity and Paganism]. Budapest: Balassi, 2017.

Ádám Mézes. PhD student, Central European University, Budapest. His publications include: "Visum repertum: Georg Tallar és az 1753-as vámpírvadászat [Visum repertum. Georg Tallar and the vampire hunt of 1753]". In *Boszorkányok, varázslók és démonok Közép-Kelet-Európában*, edited by G. Klaniczay and É. Pócs. Budapest: Balassi, 2014. 109–54.

Dániel Bárth. Associate professor and leader of the Department of Folklore, Eötvös Loránd University, Budapest. Among his books are:

Esküvő, keresztelő, avatás. Egyház és népi kultúra a kora újkori Magyarországon [Marriage, baptism and churching of woman. The church and popular culture in early modern Hungary]. Budapest: Magyar Tudományos Akadémia, 2005; *Benedikció és exorcizmus a kora újkori Magyarországon* [Benediction and exorcism in early modern Hungary]. Budapest, and Pécs: L'Harmattan and PTE Néprajz-Kulturális Antropológia Tanszék, 2010; *A zombori ördögűző. Egy 18. századi ferences mentalitása* [The exorcist of Zombor. The mentality of an 18th century Franciscan friar]. Budapest: Balassi, 2016.

Christa Agnes Tuczay. Associate Professor for Medieval German literature, German Department, University of Vienna. Her monographs include: *Ekstase im Kontext*. Habilitationsschrift. Frankfurt a. Main: Peter Lang, 2009; *Kulturgeschichte der mittelalterlichen Wahrsagerei*. Berlin: De Gruyter, 2012; *Geister, Dämonen—Phantasmen. Eine Kulturgeschichte*. Wiesbaden: Marix, 2015.

Emanuela Timotin. Senior researcher, Institute of Linguistics "Iorgu Iordan—Al. Rosetti" of the Romanian Academy, Bucharest, Department of the Romanian Philology. Her publications include: *Paroles protectrices, paroles guérisseuses. La tradition manuscrite des charmes roumains (XVIIe–XIXe siècle)*. Paris: Presses Universitaires de Paris Sorbonne, 2015; "La tradition roumaine manuscrite de *La Lamentation d'Adam à l'expulsion du paradis*". In *Philologie, herméneutique et histoire des textes entre Orient et Occident. Mélanges en hommage à Sever J. Voicu*, edited by F. Barone, C. Macé, and P. Ubierna. Turnhout: Brepols, 2017, 729–54; "Le roumain ancien". In *Manuel des anthologies, corpus et textes romans*, edited by M. Iliescu and E. Roegiest. Berlin, and Boston: De Gruyter, 2015, 595–611.

Gábor Vargyas. Scientific councillor, HAS Institute of Ethnology, Budapest. His publications include: *A la recherche des Brou perdus, population montagnarde du Centre Indochinois.* (Les Cahiers de PENINSULE 5.) Olizane: Etudes Orientales, 2000; "'Up' and 'Down': 'Zomia' and the Bru of the Central Vietnamese Highlands. Part I: Are the Bru 'Natives' in 'Zomia?'" *Acta Ethnographica Hungarica*, 61/1 (2016): 241–58; and "'Up' and 'Down': 'Zomia' and the Bru of the Central Vietnamese Highlands. Part II: Fleeing the State or Desire for Modernity? Reflections on Scott and Salemink." *Acta Ethnographica* 62/2 (2017): 441–63.

Ildikó Csepregi. Historian of religion, author of several articles on cultic healing, especially incubation, and edited (with Charles Burnett) the volume *Ritual Healing. Magic, Ritual and Medical Therapy from Antiquity until the Early Modern Period,* 2012; co-editor and co-translator of the Latin-English edition *Legenda Vetus, Acta Processus Canonizationis et Miracula Sanctae Margaritae de Hungaria. The Oldest Legend, Acts of the Canonisation Process and Miracles of Saint Margaret of Hungary.* Budapest: CEU Press, 2018.

Janine Rivière. Lead Instructor, New College, University of Toronto. Her publications include: "Demons of Desire, or Symptoms of Disease? Medical Theories and Popular Experiences of the Nightmare in Premodern England." In *Dreams, Dreamers and Visions: The Early Modern Atlantic World*, edited by A. M. Plane, and L. Tuttle, 49–71. Pennsylvania: University of Pennsylvania Press, 2013; *Dreams in early modern England: Visions of the Night*. London: Routledge, 2017.

József Gagyi. Professor, Sapietia University, Kolozsvár/Cluj Napoca. His recent publications include: "Lopás a kollektívből. A falusi társadalom erkölcsi-társadalmi átalakulásáról [Stealing from the cooperative. On the moral and social transformatio of village soceity]." *Erdélyi Múzeum* 2 (2016): 166–73; "Balogh Pál praetextusán: a rituális kommunikáció revíziójáról [On the pretext of Pál Balogh—A revision of ritual communication]." In *Néprajzi intézmények, kutatások, életpályák.* (A Kriza János Néprajzi Társaság évkönyve 22.), edited by V. Keszeg, I. Sz. Szász, and J. Zsigmond. Kolozsvár: Kriza János Néprajzi Társaság, 2014, 509–20; *Hiedelemszövegek Székelyföldről* [Belief narratives from Székler land]. (Edited by Virág Dyekiss, and József Gagyi): Budapest: L'Harmattan, 2015.

József Pál Vas. Reasearcher at the Hungarian Psychiatric Association, Budapest. His publications include: "Diana's Diary: A Case Study of Hypnotherapy." *International Journal of Traditional and Complementary Medicine,* 1/1 (2016): 44–60; "A Theory Upon Origin of Implicit Musical Language." *Health Psychology Research Journal—Music Psychology, Health and Well-being,* 3/3 (2015): 63–9; (with N. Császár, and N. Nagy:) "Multipersonal Tandem Hypnotherapy (MTH): A New Method for Resolving Intergenerational Traumas." *International Journal of Psychotherapy,* 15/3 (2011): 38–48.

Judit Kis-Halas. Researcher, HAS Institute of Ethnology, Budapest. Her publications include: "'I Make my Saints Work...': A Hungarian Holy Healer's Identity Reflected in Autobiographical Stories and Folk Narratives." In *Vernacular Religion in Everyday Life: expressions of belief,* edited by M. Bowman, and Ü. Valk. Sheffield: Equinox, 2012, 63–92; "The Trial of an Honest Citizen in Nagybánya 1705–1705. A Tentative Microanalysis of Witchcraft Accusations." In *Witchcraft Mythologies and Persecutions*, edited by G. Klaniczay and É. Pócs. Budapest: Central European University Press, 2008, 213–35; "Divinatio Diabolica and Superstitious Medicine. Healers, Seers and Diviners in the Changing Discourse of Witchcraft in Early Modern Nagybánya." In *Witchcraft and Demonology in Hungary and Transylvania*, edited by G. Klaniczay and É. Pócs. London: Palgrave 2017, 159–219.

Kateryna Dysa. Associate Professor, History Department of National University of "Kyiv-Mohyla Academy", Kiev. Her publications include: "A Family Matter: The Case of a Witch Family in the Eighteenth-Century Volhynian Town". In *Witchcraft Casebook: Magic in Russia, Poland, and Ukraine, 15th–21st Centuries.* (Special issue of Russian History/Histoire Rus. Vol. 40, nos. 3–4), edited by V. Kivelson. Leiden: Brill, 2013, 352–63; and: "Orthodox Demonology and the Perception of Witchcraft in Early Modern Ukraine." In *Friars, Nobles and Burghers—Sermons, Images and Prints. Studies of Culture and Society in Early Modern Europe. In Memoriam István György Tóth,* edited by J. Miller, and L. Kontler. Budapest: CEU Press, 2009, 341–60; "Ukraine, Witchcraft", and "Ukraine, Witchcraft Trials." In *Encyclopedia of Witchcraft*, edited by R. M. Golden. Texas: ABC-CLIO, 2006, 1139–40, and 1140–2.

Krisztina Kehl-Bodrogi. Independent scholar. Her publications include: *Die Kızılbaş-Aleviten. Untersuchungen über eine esoterische Glaubensgemeinschaft in Anatolien.* (Islamkundlichen Untersuchungen, Band 126.) Berlin, 1988; *Syncretistic Religious Communities in the Near East, edited by* K. Kehl-Bodrogi, B. Kellner-Heinkele, and A. Otter-Beaujean. Leiden: Brill, 1997; "*Religion is not so strong here*". *Muslim Religious Life in Khorezm after Socialism.* Münster: LIT Verlag, 2008.

Laura Iancu. Researcher, HAS Institute of Ethnology, Budapest. Her publications include: *Vallás Magyarfaluban. Néprajzi vizsgálat* [Religion in Magyarfalu. Ethnographic study]. Budapest and Pécs: L'Harmattan, and PTE Néprajz–Kulturális Antropológia Tanszék, 2013; *Peremlétben. Tanulmányok a moldvai katolikusok vallásosságáról* [On the peripheries.

Essays on the religiosity of Moldavian Catholics]. Budapest: Lucidus, 2017; "Isten engedje meg!" Az átok." In *Aranykapu. Tanulmányok Pozsony Ferenc tiszteletére*, edited by A. Zs. Jakab, and I. Kinda. Kolozsvár: Kriza János Néprajzi Társaság, and Szabadtéri Néprajzi Múzeum – Székely Nemzeti Múzeum, 2015, 677–91.

Madis Arukask. Associate Professor and Senior Researcher, University of Tartu. His publications include: "Sorcery, Holiness, the Third Sex—the Role of Herdsman in Finnic and North Russian Folk Culture." In *Storied and Supernatural Places. Studies in Spatial and Social Dimensions of Folklore and Sagas.* (Studia Fennica Folkloristica 23), edited by Ü. Valk, and D. Sävborg. Helsinki: Suomalaisen Kirjallisuuden Seura, 2018, 159–80; "The Personal Rituals of the Finnic Peoples with Forest Trees." *Anthropology & Archaeology of Eurasia*, 56/1–2 (2017): 167–85; "Communication Across the Border: What Burial Laments Can Tell Us About Old Beliefs." "*The Culture of Death". Estonian Journal of Archaeology,* 15/2 (2011): 130–50.

Mirjam Mencej. Professor of Folkloristics, Department of Ethnology and Cultural Anthropology, Faculty of Arts, University of Ljubljana. Her recent publications include: *Styrian Witches in European Perspective. Ethnographic Fieldwork*. London and New York: Palgrave Macmillan and Springer, 2017; "Unwitching. The Social and Magical Practice in Traditional European Communities." *Western Folklore* 74.2 (Spring 2015): 115–59; "Security Guards as Participants in and Mediators of Ghost Tradition." *Fabula* 56.1/2 (2015): 40–66.

Noémi Császár-Nagy. Associate professor, Faculty of Medicine, Semmelweis University, Budapest. Her most important publications from the last five years: N. Császár et al. "Factors affecting quality of life in Hungarian adults with epilepsy: A comparison of four psychiatric instruments." Epilepsy & Behavior 74 (2017): 45–58; N. Császár et al. "The 'Hidden Observer' as the Cognitive Unconscious During Hypnosis." *Activitas Nervosa Superior: Journal of Neuroscience and Cognitive Research* 58 (2016) (3-4): 51–61; N. Császár and J. P. Vas: "Healing Prenatal Traumas with Tandem Hypnotherapy." *Journal of Clinical and Experimental Cardiology* 4 (2016) (7): 256–62.

Nóra Zergi. Independent scholar. Her publications include: "Theophanes Chrysobalantes: Synopsis de remediis. Text edition with translation and commentary." MA thesis, Budapest, University Eötvös Lóránd, 2012; "ΚΥΚΕΩΝ". *Antik Tanulmányok* 54/2 (2010): 265–70.

Svetlana Tsonkova. Independent scholar. Her most important publications: "Megégni tűz nélkül. Betegségdémonok a késő középkori bolgár mágikus szövegekben. [Burned without fire. the illness demons in late medieval Bulgarian magical texts]." In *Mágikus és szakrális medicina,* edited by É. Pócs. Budapest: Ballasi, 2010, 101–18; "The Supernatural Agents in Medieval and Early Modern Bulgarian Charms: Magical Functions and Quotidian Contexts." *Scripta & Scripta* 10–11 (2012): 417–32; "Snake Pernicious and Venomous. The Malicious and Dangerous Other in Medieval Bulgarian and Early Modern Charms." In *Animals and Otherness in the Middle Ages. Perspectives across Disciplines* (BAR International Series 2500), edited by F. de Asís García García, M. A. Walker Vadillo and M. V. Chico Picaza. Oxford: Archaeopress, 2013, 125–32.

Tünde Komáromi. Senior Research Fellow, HAS Institute of Ethnology. Her publications include: *Rontás és társadalom Aranyosszéken* [Witchcraft and society in Ariesului region]. Cluj Napoca: Babes-Bolyai University and Kriza János Ethnographic Society, 2009; "Crossing Boundaries in Times of Personal Crisis: Seeking Help from Orthodox Clergy in Transylvania." In *Religion and Boundaries. Studies from the Balkans, Eastern Europe and Turkey*, edited by G. Valtchinova. Istanbul: The Isis Press, 2010, 155–66; "In Search of Moral balance: Conversion and Church Adherence inside the Russian Orthodox Church during the Post-Soviet Period." *Acta Ethnographica Hungarica* 56/1 (2011): 93–108.

INDEX